# GASTROENTEROLOGY NURSING
## A Core Curriculum

# GASTROENTEROLOGY NURSING
## A Core Curriculum

Coordinated by the
**Society of Gastroenterology
Nurses and Associates**
Core Curriculum Committee

illustrated

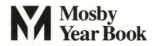 **Mosby
Year Book**

St. Louis  Baltimore  Boston  Chicago  London  Philadelphia  Sydney  Toronto

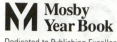

**Publisher:** Alison Miller
**Editor:** Terry Van Schaik
**Developmental Editor:** Jeanne Rowland
**Project Manager:** Mark Stephan Spann
**Production Editor:** Julie Zipfel
**Designer:** David Zielinski

Printed in the United States of America

Mosby–Year Book, Inc.
11830 Westline Industrial Drive
St. Louis, Missouri 63146

**Library of Congress Cataloging-in-Publication Data**

Gastroenterology nursing: a core curriculum / edited by Marjorie Beck
   and Nancy G. Evans for the Society of Gastroenterology Nurses and
   Associates, Core Curriculum Committee. — 1st ed.
      p.   cm.
      Includes bibliographical references and index.
      ISBN 0-8016-6924-3
      1. Gastrointestinal system—Diseases—Nursing.      I. Beck,
Marjorie. II. Evans, Nancy G.   III. Society of Gastroenterology
Nurses and Associates. Core Curriculum Committee.
   [DNLM: 1. Gastrointestinal Diseases—nursing. 2. Nursing Care—
methods.    WY 156.5 G2565]
RC817.G33   1993
610.73′69—dc20
DNLM/DLC                                                                                       92-16189
for Library of Congress                                                                        CIP

93  94  95  96  (GW/MV)  9  8  7  6  5  4  3  2  1

# SGNA CORE CURRICULUM COMMITTEE

**Nancy G. Evans,** RN, BSN, CGRN
Chairperson
Nurse Manager, Gastroenterology Department
Daniel Freeman Memorial and Marina Hospitals
Inglewood, California

**Marjorie Beck,** RN
Nurse Manager, GI Procedure Unit
Abington Memorial Hospital
Abington, Pennsylvania

**Barbara Calvette,** RN, BA, CGRN
Nurse Manager, GI Lab
Swedish American Hospital
Rockford, Illinois

**Gail B. DeCosta,** RN, CGRN
Nurse Manager,
Gastroenterology/Endoscopy
Medical College of Virginia
Richmond, Virginia

**Marcia Gruber,** RN, MSN, CGC
Clinical Nurse Specialist, Gastroenterology
Veterans Affairs Medical Center
Buffalo, New York

**Marcia Hardick,** RN, CGC
Nurse Manager, Section of Gastroenterology
University of Chicago Medical Center
Chicago, Illinois

**Dorothy Sherman,** RN, BS, CGC
Director, Gastroenterology
Hinsdale Hospital
Hinsdale, Illinois

### Editorial Staff

**Julia A. Kneedler,** RN, EdD
Editor
Director, Education Services
Education Design, Inc.
Denver, Colorado

**Linda R. Sexton,** BS
Technical Editor
Education Design, Inc.
Denver, Colorado

# REVIEWERS

The Core Curriculum Committee is especially grateful to the following individuals who reviewed this document for content and accuracy.

**Janice S. Adams,** RN, CGC
Coordinator, Gastroenterology Diagnostic Lab
University of Tennessee Bowld Hospital
Memphis, Tennessee

**Lorna S. Andrews,** RN, CGRN
Manager, Endoscopy Department
Northwest Hospital
Seattle, Washington

**Doris C. Barnie,** RN, MSN, CGRN
Head Nurse, Endoscopy Unit
The Valley Hospital
Ridgewood, New Jersey

**Marjorie Beck,** RN
Nurse Manager, G.I. Procedure Unit
Abington Memorial Hospital
Abington, Pennsylvania

**Wendy L. Biddle,** RNC, PhD
Research Assistant Professor
Department of Medicine
University of Kansas Medical Center
Kansas City, Kansas

**Gretchen N. Bodinsky,** RN, BS, CGC
Director, Endoscopy Services
Rex Hospital
Raleigh, North Carolina

**Fran Briem,** RN
Nurse Manager, G.I. Studies
University Hospital
Albuquerque, New Mexico

**Barbara Calvette,** RN, BA, CGRN
Nurse Manager, G.I. Lab
Swedish American Hospital
Rockford, Illinois

**Norah F. Connelly,** RN, CGRN
Section Director, G.I. Lab
Lutheran General Hospital
Park Ridge, Illinois

**Gail B. DeCosta,** RN, CGRN
Nurse Manager, Gastroenterology/Endoscopy
Medical College of Virginia
Richmond, Virginia

**Carol Durham,** RN, MPPM
Manager, Endoscopy
Harper Hospital, Detroit Medical Center
Detroit, Michigan

**Marsha L. Ellett,** RN, MSN, CGRN
Nurse Clinician, Pediatric Gastroenterology
James Whitcomb Riley Hospital for Children
Indianapolis, Indiana

**Nancy G. Evans,** RN, BSN, CGRN
Nurse Manager, Gastroenterology Department
Daniel Freeman Memorial and Marina Hospitals
Inglewood, California

**Jerelyn S. Fyvolent,** RT, CGT
Office Manager
Joel D. Fyvolent, MD
Tampa, Florida

**Joel D. Fyvolent,** MD, FACG
Clinical Associate Professor of Medicine
University of South Florida College of Medicine
Tampa, Florida

**Agnes Gaber,** RN, BSN, CGRN
Nurse Manager, GI Unit
Veterans Administration
West Side Medical Center
Chicago, Illinois

**Margaret L. Gill,** BSN, CGRN
Nurse Manager, Gastroenterology
  Department
United Health Services
Binghamton, New York

**Marcia Gruber,** RN, MSN, CGC
Clinical Nurse Specialist, Gastroenterology
Veterans Affairs Medical Center
Buffalo, New York

**Marcia Hardick,** RN, CGC
Nurse Manager, Section of Gastroenterology
University of Chicago Medical Center
Chicago, Illinois

**Carolyn A. Harrigan,** RN, BSN, CGRN
Clinical Nurse III, Gastroenterology Lab
Fair Oaks Hospital
Fairfax, Virginia

**Patricia Holland,** RN, BSN, CGRN
Manager, Digestive Disease Center
Saint Joseph Hospital
Denver, Colorado

**Bettie Jean Howard,** RN, CGRN
Full Partner-Charge Nurse
Surgical Endoscopy
University of Maryland Medical Center
Baltimore, Maryland

**Zoraida Hurley,** RN, CGC
Staff Nurse
St. Luke's Hospital
Racine, Wisconsin

**Rebecca Jackson,** RN
Coordinator, Endoscopy Suite
Alexandria Hospital
Alexandria, Virginia

**Michael Kline,** MD
Associate Professor, Gastroenterology
University of California at Los Angeles (UCLA)
Los Angeles, California

**Barbara A. Lencki,** RN, CGRN
Manager, Gastroenterology
Olympia Fields Osteopathic Hospital
  and Medical Center
Olympia Fields, Illinois

**Kathleen A. Maher,** RN, BSN, CGC
Clinical Research Coordinator
Esophageal Studies Section
Division of Gastroenterology
Georgetown University Hospital
Washington, D.C.

**Arlene Margopoulos,** RN, BSN, CGC
Manager, Ambulatory Services
Morton Plant Hospital
Clearwater, Florida

**Janice S. Mathews,** RN
Nurse Specialist, Endoscopy Unit
Georgetown University Hospital
Washington, D.C.

**Patricia Pethigal,** RN, BSN, CGC
Nurse Manager, G.I. Endoscopy/Gastric Lab
Virginia Mason Medical Center
Seattle, Washington

**Donna Reeves,** LPN, CGN
Nurse Manager, Gastroenterology Unit
Victory Memorial Hospital
Waukegan, Illinois

**Dorothy Sherman,** RN, BS, CGC
Director, Gastroenterology
Hinsdale Hospital
Hinsdale, Illinois

**Nancy Shields,** RN, MSN
Nurse Manager, Endoscopy
University of Minnesota Hospital and Clinic
Minneapolis, Minnesota

**Loretta Simonsen,** RN
Clinical Nurse Manager
St. Luke's Hospital
Racine, Wisconsin

**Jim Sutton,** RN, MS, CGRN
Manager, Endoscopy
Osteopathic Medical Center of Texas
Fort Worth, Texas

**Melanie Lynn Swartz,** RN, BSN, CGC
Graduate Student/Clinical Nurse, Endoscopy
SUNY-Binghamton/United Health Services
Binghamton, New York

**Theresa C. Vos,** RN
Staff Nurse
St. Luke's Hospital
Racine, Wisconsin

**Nicolae Weisz,** MD
Clincial Instructor, Gastroenterology
University of California at Los Angeles
  (UCLA) School of Medicine
Los Angeles, California

**Sheridan D. Wiggett,** RN, CGRN
Administrative Nurse, Medical Procedures Unit
University of California at Los Angeles
  (UCLA) Medical Center
Los Angeles, California

**Kathy B. Wright,** RN, MS, CGRN
Nurse Coordinator, G.I. Consultants
University of Texas Southwestern Medical Center
  and Parkland Memorial Hospital
Dallas, Texas

# PREFACE

Since its inception in 1974, the Society of Gastroenterology Nurses and Associates (SGNA) has held the education of its members as its highest priority. This focus on education continued during the ensuing years as publications were developed to supplement the annual educational courses. SGNA's journal *Gastroenterology Nursing,* the *Manual of Gastrointestinal Procedures* (with pediatric and pulmonary supplements), and the SGNA Monograph Series are some of the excellent references published by SGNA for the gastroenterology nurse and associate.

With the establishment in 1986 of a certification examination for gastroenterology clinicians, it became apparent that gastroenterology nurses and associates needed one comprehensive text that consolidated information about gastroenterology/endoscopy and related nursing care considerations. To this end, SGNA began preparation of this core curriculum. The dedicated efforts of the coordinators and reviewers listed at the beginning of this book have resulted in a comprehensive text that reflects current nursing practice.

In preparing this first edition of the core curriculum, the Coordinating Committee identified the body of knowledge that underlies gastroenterology nursing and the information that affects this specialty practice. Prior to publication, the contents of the text were subjected to an intensive review process to ensure the accuracy and currency of the material.

The text is designed to meet the needs of all members of the gastroenterology nursing team. Throughout the book, the word "nurse" is used generically when describing tasks or situations that are shared by all disciplines. The term "RN" is used in instances where tasks or judgments are solely the responsibility of the registered nurse.

Although gastroenterology nurses and associates work in a variety of settings and come from varied educational backgrounds, there is a commonality of knowledge and practice within all disciplines. The RN, LPN, and technician all contribute in different ways to the nursing process. The second section is devoted to the nursing process, in order to assist nurses who are adapting this process to their daily practice. Each practitioner will find in this publication information that is applicable to his or her daily practice and study needs.

This core curriculum is not intended to be all-inclusive. It is designed to serve as a primary source of information for nurses and associates who are preparing for SGNA's certification examination. The material is also applicable for nursing students and nurses in any hospital or office setting. Although all components of the underlying body of knowledge are included, it is not possible to cover each topic in depth. The reader is therefore advised to use this core curriculum as a base for study and to refer to other publications for additional and complementary information. For example, an anatomy/physiology book will enhance the information found in Section 3 and a surgical nursing text will outline surgical implications for gastroenterology patients. SGNA's *Manual of Gastrointestinal Procedures* and its supplements are excellent resources for procedure information and illustrations of equipment. The use of complementary texts will extend the reader's knowledge base and serve as a review where information overlaps.

Most chapters of the core curriculum include a case situation, a list of review terms, and a number of review questions. The review questions are not taken from the certification examinations, but they are similar in format and content to actual test questions. A bibliography at the end of each chapter will enable the reader to obtain additional information on that particular topic. Resources, a glossary, and an appendix at the end of the book provide additional reference material.

*Gastroenterology Nursing: A Core Curriculum* covers the body of knowledge upon which gastroenterology nursing is based. It is a much requested and needed addition to SGNA's list of publications. The information provided will be helpful for all members who are studying for the certification examination. It will also be a welcome addition to every nursing library and GI lab, serving as a daily reference for anyone involved in the specialty practice of gastroenterology nursing.

**Marjorie Beck, RN**
Publications Committee Chairman
Society of Gastroenterology Nurses and Associates

# CONTENTS

# GASTROENTEROLOGY NURSING PRACTICE

# Chapter 1

# THE GASTROENTEROLOGY NURSE AND ASSOCIATE

This chapter reviews the background leading to the development of specialized healthcare workers in the area of gastroenterology. The scope of practice in this setting is outlined, as are the competencies required to provide quality care for patients who are having endoscopic diagnostic and therapeutic treatments. Educational preparation and job qualifications are addressed. Practice settings and the types of positions needed and required responsibilities and functions are emphasized.

**Learning objectives**

After reviewing the content of this chapter, the gastroenterology nurse should be able to:
1. Trace the evolution of gastroenterology nursing as an area of specialization.
2. Discuss the scope of practice in the gastroenterology setting and the educational requirements needed to practice gastroenterology nursing.
3. Describe the general responsibilities and functions of the gastroenterology nurse and associate.
4. Delineate the roles of the gastroenterology nurse and associate, as specified by the Certifying Board of Gastroenterology Nurses and Associates, Inc. (CBGNA).
5. Give examples of the job responsibilities of nurse managers, staff nurses, and associates in a typical gastroenterology unit.

## BACKGROUND AND HISTORICAL PERSPECTIVE

As far back as records show, the care of the sick has constituted a role in everyday life. Witch doctors performed their rituals and departed, leaving someone else to follow through with the care. Nursing care was first differentiated from medicine in the fourth century by Hindu physician B.C. Charaka, who referred to the "aggregate of four," comprised of the physician, the drug, the nurse, and the patient. Hippocrates referred to care givers as assistants to the physician. There are accounts from the pre-Christian era of nurses involved in caring for the sick. Archaeological discoveries describe early nursing procedures as dressing wounds and feeding patients.

The Egyptians had a highly developed medical community wherein the members of the medical profession were organized so they could protect the secrets of their practice. The Egyptians were as progressive as today's physicians in that they had specialists dedicated to one disease, such as treatment of the eyes, head, or stomach. Accounts of the Egyptians, Greeks, and Romans all refer to the existence of midwives, whose art was the care of child-bearing women. When their civilizations declined, medical care of women deteriorated and was not brought back to its former stage of development until the seventeenth century.

During the Middle Ages, nursing was done primarily by women and was the function of many religious orders. Between 500 and 1300 AD, nursing care consisted of only the most menial tasks, such as bathing, feeding, and bed-making. The nuns, who were chiefly responsible for this care, were assisted by women who were being punished for thievery or prostitution. It was not until the nineteenth century that education and dignity were brought to the nursing profession. Florence Nightingale emancipated upper-class women from idleness and encouraged them to serve humanity. As women became educated, the care of the sick began to improve.

Throughout the nineteenth century, prominent women became involved in promoting the cause of nursing. School nursing, industrial nursing, and other nursing specializations began to emerge. As technology increased and physicians needed more time to learn and implement new techniques and practices, the responsibilities of nurses also increased. During the 1940s, Frances Reiter first described the nurse with advanced education and clinical competence as a "nurse clinician." This was the precursor of the nursing specialties that we recognize today.

## Development of gastroenterology

As early as the time of Hippocrates, specific mention was made of the gastrointestinal tract in medicine. Hippocrates recorded use of a candle to inspect the rectum. In 1795, Bozzini documented the use of a rigid sigmoidoscope. Almost 100 years later, Kussmaul made the first attempt to visualize the stomach with a rigid tube. Rigid esophagoscopy developed slowly over the next 50 years, with progress being dependent primarily on the quality of the light source. The rigid instrument was able to survey only a small portion of the stomach and it carried a significant hazard because of the possibility of perforation.

In 1932, a semiflexible instrument was designed by Rudolph Schindler. The Schindler gastroscope remained the model for development of gastroscopes for the next 30 years. The semiflexible gastroscope was based on the principle that a series of convex lenses could transmit light undistorted through a flexible tube if the distal tube was not bent beyond a certain angle. Risk of perforation was reduced by the placement of a rubber obturator at the tip.

In 1958, Hirschowitz, Curtiss, Peters, and Pollard published their report of a new gastroscope, the fiberscope, which revolutionized gastroenterology. The development of fiberoptic scopes was made possible by the earlier work of **Professor Harold Hopkins** of Reading University in the United Kingdom. Hopkins worked with John Logie Baird, the inventor of television, to design fiberoptic bundles that would transmit an image. The optical principles are dependent on the total internal reflection of light in each fiber. The fiber bundles are of two types: noncoherent bundles, which conduct light but not images; and coherent bundles, which produce high-quality images.

Modern, flexible fiberoptic instruments have the same basic features as those developed in the early fifties. The simplicity, ease of use, and safety of the earlier instruments caused the rapid adoption of this new technology.

## Development of gastroenterology nursing

Gastroenterology nursing was first recognized as an area of specialization in 1941, when a group of physicians called the American Gastroscopic Club met at Dr. Rudolph Schindler's home in Chicago. This group was later named the Gastroscopic Society and was the forerunner of the American Society of Gastrointestinal Endoscopy. At that time, Dr. Schindler was the recognized master gastroscopist and his wife, Gabriele, was

the first gastroenterology assistant. **Gabriele Schindler** was always at her husband's side, soothing the patient, helping with positioning, and assisting during the procedure. The memory of Gabriele personifies the spirit of professionalism and caring that has become the mark of excellence for today's gastroenterology nurses and associates. Beginning in 1985, the Society of Gastroenterology Nurses and Associates (SGNA) has annually presented the Gabriele Schindler Award in recognition of high standards and outstanding achievement in gastroenterology nursing.

The next several decades brought about many changes in gastroenterology nursing practice and education. Fiberoptic instrumentation developed rapidly and the demand for skilled personnel to care for patients, instrumentation, and equipment increased, resulting in the need for dedicated personnel to work with patients who were undergoing endoscopic procedures. Physicians demanded a specialized unit within the hospital to perform gastrointestinal procedures. A nurse or assistant was required to attend the patient and assist the physician with the procedure. Initially, the role of the gastroenterology nurse was to support the patient while the physician inserted the scope. It soon became evident that a successful unit called for someone who would not only care for the patient but also set standards and develop some order within the unit. There was a need for procurement and maintenance of instruments, checking patient consent forms, dispensing and documentation of medications, documentation of patient responses to treatment, and recording of information for hospital reports.

As the complexity of procedures increased, government and regulatory agencies added another aspect to the knowledge base required. The Centers for Disease Control (CDC), Joint Commission on Accreditation of Healthcare Organizations (JCAHO), and other organizations all put forth guidelines, which required that gastroenterology personnel be informed of these new regulations and guidelines and integrate them into practice settings. Persons functioning in gastroenterology units felt a need for a support group or network of individuals to unite those associated with the practice of gastroenterology.

## Society of gastroenterology nurses and associates

The new guidelines and the subsequent need for support groups led to the formation of the Society of Gastrointestinal Assistants (SGA) in 1974. The first members of this group sought identification, respect, and national recognition of their activities. Their goals were to collect information, establish guidelines for future professionals, and expand specialized educational opportunities. SGA decided to hold annual meetings in May, concurrently with the annual educational meeting of gastroenterologists.

As the Society grew, the need to communicate information to the membership on an ongoing basis became evident. Therefore, in 1977 the first journal issue of the *SGA Journal* was published. Since 1989, the title of the journal has been *Gastroenterology Nursing*. Also in 1977, nine regional societies were established to give members the opportunity to meet during the year in geographically accessible areas; the number of regional societies has increased gradually to over 60 and continues to increase.

In 1989, SGA changed its name to the **Society of Gastroenterology Nurses and Associates, Inc. (SGNA),** in order to better reflect the composition of its membership. According to a 1992 report, SGNA members include registered nurses (RNs, 85%), licensed practical nurses (LPNs, 11%), and licensed medical technicians or technologists (MLTs or MTs), radiology technologists (RTs), equipment technicians, and assistants (4%). Within the RN group, there are nurses with baccalaureate degrees, diplomas, associate degrees, masters degrees, and doctorates.

Certification for gastroenterology nursing had its beginning in the early 1980s. The American Nurses Association (ANA) and independent specialty groups believed there was merit in establishing a mechanism to measure the competency of nurses in the practice setting. A standing committee on certification was established by SGA to develop a certification program for gastroenterology clinicians. In 1985, the Certification Committee became the independent Certifying Council for Gastroenterology Clinicians, Inc. In 1986, a total of 666 candidates took the first certifying examination. This voluntary certification program is aimed both at assuring the patient that the caregiver has acquired a proficient level of knowledge and at publicly recognizing the individual nurse/associate. The membership of SGNA is continuing to grow as the Society demonstrates its commitment to further education and practice for the member.

In 1990, in order to be consistent with the professional society, the name was changed again to the Certifying Board for Gastroenterology Nurses and Associates (CBGNA). Further refinement of the certifying process began that same year. Task analysis and role delineations serve to differentiate competency areas for the registered nurse and the associate. Two distinctly different examinations are now administered.

## SCOPE OF PRACTICE

Delineating a **scope of practice** is the responsibility of a professional society. The practice of nursing is further defined by state regulatory agencies and institutional policies and procedures.

As the professional society for nursing in the United States, ANA has assumed the responsibility of providing a current definition of nursing that reflects the dynam-

ic, evolving role of professional nurses. In 1978, the Executive Committee of ANA's Division on Medical-Surgical Nursing Practice appointed an ad hoc committee to identify and describe the parameters of medical-surgical nursing. A statement on the scope of medical-surgical nursing practice was published in 1980. This statement defines the practice, delineates its dimensions, and outlines the functions of a professional nurse. This comprehensive definition served as a guide to emerging specialty organizations and societies.

SGNA has developed a scope of practice that is directly related to the development of a task analysis for certification. Gastroenterology nursing practice is defined as the nursing care of patients with known or suspected gastrointestinal problems who are undergoing diagnostic or therapeutic endoscopic procedures. Nursing care includes the care and treatment necessary to provide comfort, assist individuals in the promotion and maintenance of health, provide for the physical and emotional needs of the patient, and provide safe and proficient care during endoscopy and other specialized procedures. It encompasses patient assessment, diagnosis, outcome identification, planning, implementation, and evaluation of patient care. The biologic, psychologic, and social components of the patient's response or adjustment to illness or disability are also taken into account. Gastroenterology nurses and associates use and adapt theories in microbiology, communication, ethics, and the behavioral sciences to form the basis of practice. That practice is continually influenced by the patient's physiologic alteration, the patient's and family's needs for support and assistance, collaboration between medicine and nursing, and the level of professional autonomy in the practice setting.

## EDUCATION AND TRAINING

The Society of Gastroenterology Nurses and Associates continues to broaden its scope of practice and update standards for practice and the certification process. It is also essential to develop requirements for education and training of personnel who will be working in this practice setting because those factors have direct effect on the quality of patient care provided.

Educational requirements for registered nurses include graduation from an accredited school of nursing and a license to practice nursing. SGNA recommends that registered nurses specializing in the field of gastroenterology have at least one year of general medical-surgical experience. This enables the **gastroenterology nurse** to practice acquired skills and be exposed to "first-line" management. In general, individuals should possess the following educational backgrounds:

- Solid education and training in the biologic sciences
- Pertinent experiences in the healthcare field
- Familiarity with hospital and other practice settings

Specific content areas that might be incorporated into a specialty training program include:

- Anatomy and physiology of the GI tract, and relationships to pathophysiology and relevant diagnostic and therapeutic procedures
- Techniques of management and administration of a gastroenterology unit
- Skills in patient care, teaching, and inservice education
- Care and maintenance of clinical instruments
- Pharmacology and IV therapy
- Emergency situations
- Research methods and application of published research to the practice setting
- Ethical, professional, and legal standards inherent in professional conduct

A **gastroenterology associate** is defined as a "health care professional with varied educational background engaged in the field of gastroenterology." This educational background may include licensure, such as LPNs have; certification, such as an RT or operating room technologist (ORT) has; or on-the-job training as a patient care technician receives. In a hospital setting, the associate is legally accountable to an RN (JCAHO 1990).

## JOB RESPONSIBILITIES AND FUNCTIONS

Gastroenterology healthcare workers perform a variety of functions in various practice settings. SGNA members work in hospitals, clinics, free-standing endoscopy units, operating rooms, and physicians' offices. General areas of responsibility include patient care, care of instruments and equipment, management, teaching and research, and documentation. Gastroenterology nurses also perform some gastroenterologic procedures independently, including esophageal and anal manometry, gastric analysis, and rigid and flexible sigmoidoscopy.

### Patient care

Gastroenterology team members are responsible for the care of patients undergoing diagnostic and therapeutic gastroenterologic procedures. Preparation before a procedure includes instruction on physical preparation of the patient, such as food or medication restrictions. It is also important to meet the patient's psychologic needs by reassuring the patient, explaining the procedure, and instilling confidence. A brief history is taken to evaluate and assess any pertinent medical or surgical conditions. Baseline vital signs are recorded and a brief physical assessment is done.

During the procedure, care is directed at ensuring the patient's physical safety and psychologic well-being. Emphasis is placed on monitoring and assessing the patient, because the physician must concentrate his or her attention on the procedure. The nurse or associate must have a thorough understanding of the purpose of the proce-

dure and how the procedure will be performed. He or she assists the physician with various technical aspects of the procedure, such as biopsy, polypectomy, or coagulation. The nurse or associate continues to offer reassurance to the patient throughout the procedure, and the nurse continually assesses the patient's response to sedation and to the procedure, intervening when appropriate.

At the completion of the procedure, the nurse continues to monitor the patient's response to the procedure and to any medication administered. Patients who are sedated during the procedure will require time to recover. Assessment is also directed toward identification of potential and/or actual complications related to the procedure. The nurse must ascertain that the patient has met the institution's discharge criteria before the patient is released. At discharge, the patient receives a written explanation about follow-up care and how to contact health personnel if problems arise. A family member, if available, should be included in any discharge education to ensure a clear understanding of postprocedure instructions.

### Management

The scope of nursing management and the responsibilities of the manager of the gastroenterology department vary depending on the types of procedures performed and the services provided. Management functions include developing the organizational structure of the department (e.g., lines of communication and authority), standards for practice, policies and procedures, position descriptions, and performance appraisals. It also involves developing a budget, determining staffing patterns, coordinating services, and being fiscally accountable to the department.

### Care of instruments and equipment

Gastroenterology nurses and associates must demonstrate technical competency in instrument and equipment care. Knowledge of the decontamination process is essential. Understanding the current facts about disinfection and sterilization ensures safe patient care. Nurses and associates must also know how to maintain the instruments and equipment and arrange for repair when required.

### Teaching and research

Individuals working in the gastroenterology department have a responsibility to share knowledge. This may be done through inservice and orientation programs or through continuing education. Participation in professional organizations also offers an excellent opportunity to exchange information. The manager of the department has the responsibility to assess the level of expertise of the staff and encourage employees to plan for their own personal and professional growth. It remains the responsibility of individual nurses or associates to identify their own learning needs, acquire necessary knowledge, and stay abreast of current technologies.

Participating in and communicating clinical research are also vital parts of the gastroenterology nurse's or associate's role. Research may entail participation in drug trial studies, testing new instruments or procedures, or evaluating the effectiveness of treatment. Whatever the research, the nurse or associate must have some background in data collection, documentation, analysis, and interpretation. Publication of findings is essential for communicating results of research to the healthcare community. In addition, presentation of a paper or poster at professional meetings is an excellent way for the nurse or associate to meet the responsibility of expanding current knowledge. Knowledge of research techniques also allows for critical evaluation of published materials.

## Documentation

Documentation of patient care and maintenance of records and department reports are other responsibilities of the gastroenterology team member. Documentation requirements vary according to institutional policy and the particular endoscopy setting, but JCAHO stipulates the following minimum documentation requirements:

- Documentation of a preprocedural patient assessment, including physical and psychosocial factors, current medications, treatment, and previous medical, anesthesia, and drug history; review of the patient's symptoms and general history of the current gastrointestinal complaint
- Documentation of the procedure performed; equipment used; staff involved; drugs, fluids, and anesthesia administered; unusual events and intervention; patient status at the conclusion of the procedure; type of specimen(s) obtained and disposition; postprocedure diagnosis
- Documentation of the postprocedural physical and mental status of the patient including but not limited to vital signs, level of consciousness, drugs and IV fluids, unusual events and intervention, discharge instructions, disposition of patient

SGNA provides a documentation monograph that details pertinent JCAHO documentation requirements and lists types of information that might be included on preprocedure, procedure, and postprocedure forms, and when providing discharge instructions to outpatients.

## ROLE DELINEATION

The following statements summarize the behaviors that are expected from gastroenterology nurses and associates, respectively, based on the **role delineation** statements issued by the Certifying Board.

**Registered nurse's role (expected behaviors)**

1. Discuss professional and practice issues related to the field of gastroenterology, including:
   a. History of gastroenterology/GI endoscopy
   b. Principles of basic management pertinent to operating the gastroenterology unit, such as scheduling, record keeping
   c. Standards for practice or recommended practices as set forth by SGNA, JCAHO, CDC.
   d. Ethical, professional and legal standards specific to patient care and professional conduct
   e. Quality assurance process
2. Distinguish normal and abnormal GI anatomy, physiology, pathology, histology and microbiology, and alterations that may be imposed by congenital anomaly and/or surgical intervention. This protocol incorporates normal and abnormal structure and function of the following:
   a. Esophagus
   b. Stomach
   c. Small bowel
   d. Large bowel
   e. Gallbladder
   f. Pancreas
   g. Liver
3. Formulate a plan of care that includes assessments, prioritizations, and interventions that are implemented and documented. This includes:
   a. Objective and subjective assessment
   b. Utilizing the nursing process to develop and implement a plan of care
4. Demonstrate knowledge of pharmacology and IV therapy. This includes:
   a. Diagnostic, therapeutic, and emergency medications
   b. IV medications used in the GI lab
   c. Transfusion of blood and blood products
   d. Antibiotic prophylaxis
   e. Electrolyte, colloid, and other IV solutions
   f. Enteral and parenteral nutritional therapy
5. Assist with or perform specific GI diagnostic and therapeutic modalities. This includes:
   a. Assisting with diagnostic and therapeutic endoscopic procedures
   b. Performing or assisting with manometric procedures
   c. Performing or assisting with nonendoscopic specimen collection and administering patient care specific to the procedure
   d. Assisting in the performance of esophageal dilatation
   e. Performing or assisting in the performance of secretory studies and GI tests
   f. Knowledge of related GI diagnostic studies such as contrast radiographs, nuclear scans

6. Identify signs and symptoms of life-threatening situations and respond appropriately. Life-threatening situations include:
   a. Vasovagal reaction
   b. Respiratory depression
   c. Adverse drug reactions, including anaphylaxis
   d. Hemorrhage
   e. Aspiration
   f. Procedural and spontaneous perforations
   g. Shock
   h. Cardiopulmonary arrest
7. Describe the basic research process, including:
   a. Research terminology
   b. Elementary data analysis

### Gastroenterology associate's role (expected behaviors)

1. Discuss professional and practice issues related to the field of gastroenterology, including:
   a. The history of gastroenterology/GI endoscopy
   b. Principles of basic management pertinent to operating a gastroenterology unit, such as scheduling, recordkeeping
   c. Standards for practice and/or recommended practices as set forth by SGNA, CDC, JCAHO
   d. Ethical, professional, and legal standards specific to patient care and professional conduct
   e. The quality assurance process
2. Distinguish normal and abnormal GI anatomy, physiology and pathology, histology and microbiology, as well as those alterations imposed by congenital anomaly and/or surgical intervention. This incorporates normal and abnormal structure and function of the following:
   a. Esophagus
   b. Stomach
   c. Small bowel
   d. Large bowel
   e. Gallbladder
   f. Pancreas
   g. Liver
3. Implement a plan of patient care that includes assessment, observation, intervention, and documentation. This includes:
   a. Performing an objective assessment
   b. Providing pre-, intra-, and postprocedure care
4. Demonstrate basic knowledge of pharmacology and IV therapy. This includes:
   a. Diagnostic, therapeutic and emergency medications
   b. IV medications and solutions used in the GI lab
   c. Signs and symptoms of transfusion reactions and appropriate responses
   d. Indications for antibiotic prophylaxis

5. Have knowledge of GI diagnostic and therapeutic modalities. This includes:
   a. Assisting with diagnostic and therapeutic endoscopic procedures
   b. Performing or assisting with manometric procedures
   c. Performing or assisting with nonendoscopic specimen collection
   d. Assisting with esophageal dilatation
   e. Performing or assisting with secretory studies and GI tests
   f. Knowledge of related GI diagnostic studies such as contrast radiographic studies, nuclear scans
6. Identify signs and symptoms of life-threatening situations and respond appropriately. Life-threatening situations include:
   a. Vasovagal reaction
   b. Respiratory depression
   c. Adverse drug reactions, including anaphylaxis
   d. Hemorrhage
   e. Aspiration
   f. Procedural and spontaneous perforations
   g. Shock
   h. Cardiopulmonary arrest
7. Describe the basic research process, including:
   a. Terminology of research design
   b. Elementary data analysis

Although these role delineation statements are similar, there are several important differences between the roles of the gastroenterology nurse and associate. For example:

- The RN uses the nursing process to formulate and prioritize a plan of care and revise it as needed.
- The RN interprets both objective and subjective assessment data to formulate a nursing diagnosis.
- Based on the patient's individual needs, the RN confers with the patient to establish appropriate outcomes.
- The RN integrates the findings of current nursing research into the practice setting.

In addition to defining the behaviors expected of gastroenterology nurses and associates, these role delineation statements form the basis for the certification examinations. The general areas of knowledge required of the nurse and associate are similar, but the depth of knowledge tested is proportional to the level of expertise required for the performance of each role.

## POSITION DESCRIPTIONS

The categories of individuals who perform functions in the gastroenterology department include:

- Registered nurses, who may have the title of supervisor, manager, head nurse, staff nurse, clinical nurse specialist, nurse clinician, nurse educator, nurse practitioner, or nurse researcher

- Associates, a group that may include LPNs, technicians, technologists, aides, or ancillary personnel

The **position descriptions** for all of these individuals vary according to the practice setting and its organizational structure. The duties also vary depending on the size and number of procedures performed. In a hospital setting the location of the gastroenterology department in the organizational structure also has an effect on the types of responsibilities assigned to different personnel. Another variable is the method used throughout the hospital to formulate position descriptions and the subsequent evaluation mechanisms.

Position descriptions usually include a number of common elements, including the title of the position; the department in which the position belongs; the person to whom the individual is responsible; a job summary; job qualifications, such as level of education, experience required, and personal habits and characteristics; and specific duties or functions.

## Nurse manager

Examples of the duties and responsibilities that may be included for the manager of the gastroenterology department are:

*Planning and organization*
1. Plan, coordinate, and direct the flow of patients through the gastroenterology department.
2. Allocate space and physical resources according to patient and physician need.
3. Develop and review department quality assurance standards.

*Management*
1. Conduct performance reviews for assigned staff.
2. Monitor clinical performance for compliance with established standards and policies.

*Staff allocation*
1. Adjust staffing to meet workload volume.

*Fiscal responsibility*
1. Formulate and implement annual budget.

*Education/orientation*
1. Support staff orientation and cross training through instruction, case selection, assignment of preceptors, and ongoing evaluation.
2. Assist staff in ongoing educational process.

*Professional commitment*
1. Actively participate in meetings or committees as assigned.

Relationships, teamwork, and communication are other areas that might be included in the manager's position description.

## Staff nurse (RN)

Selected examples of some of the duties and responsibilities that may be assigned to an RN staff nurse might be:

*Nursing process*
1. Assessment
   a. Make initial observations of the patient upon arrival at the gastroenterology unit.
   b. Formulate nursing diagnosis based on data collected.
   c. Provide assessment documentation that reflects the full range of patient needs, including physical, psychosocial, spiritual, and safety.
   d. Continue assessment of patient throughout entire stay in gastroenterology unit.
2. Diagnosis
3. Outcome identification
4. Planning
   a. Individualize the plan of care, based on patient assessment.
   b. Prepare rooms, equipment, and supplies to accommodate the patient load.
5. Implementation
   a. Implement the plan of care.
   b. Assist physician with procedures.
   c. Monitor the patient before, during, and after the procedure.
   d. Provide patient education.
6. Evaluation
   a. Evaluate and document the patient's response to the nursing and medical plan of care.

*Patient teaching*
1. Assess patient's needs to include family, or significant other when appropriate.
2. Provide patient with relevant information regarding diagnosis, medications, diet, and other therapy.

The above is only a sampling of the responsibilities that might appear. Other categories may include research and professional development.

## Associates

Examples of duties and responsibilities that might be expected of associates include the following:
1. Assisting the physician with procedures
2. Implementing the plan of care under direction of an RN
3. Assessing the patient under the direction of an RN
4. Decontaminating instruments and equipment
   a. Receive and decontaminate instruments, equipment, and reusable supplies.
5. Sterilization and reprocessing
   a. Prepare items to be sterilized and maintain sterility through proper handling
   b. Operate equipment used for cleaning and disinfecting endoscopic equipment.
6. Handling and storage
   a. Receive and place supplies in assigned storage area.

**gastroenterology associate, gastroenterology nurse, Professor Harold Hopkins, position descriptions, role delineation, Gabriele Schindler, scope of practice, Society of Gastroenterology Nurses and Associates, Inc. (SGNA)**

REVIEW QUESTIONS

1. The first recorded gastrointestinal assistant was:
   a. Florence Nightingale.
   b. Frances Reiter.
   c. Gabriele Schindler.
   d. B.C. Charaka.
2. During what period was medicine so far advanced that they had what is equivalent to today's subspecialties?
   a. Egyptians.
   b. Pre-Christian era.
   c. Middle Ages.
   d. Greeks and Romans.
3. The individual who first developed the fiberoptic telescope used for gastrointestinal procedures was:
   a. Hippocrates.
   b. Hopkins.
   c. Schindler.
   d. Baird.
4. The rationale for the rapid adoption of fiberoptic instruments includes:
   a. Simplicity, ease of use, patient safety.
   b. Complex lens system, noncoherent bundles.
   c. Perfect imaging and ease of use.
   d. Combination of noncoherent bundles and coherent bundles to make a perfect image.
5. The first Society of Gastrointestinal Assistants (SGA) was formed in what year?
   a. 1968.
   b. 1976.
   c. 1972.
   d. 1974.
6. The practice of gastroenterology nursing requires application of the nursing process. The components include:
   a. Communicating, planning, evaluation, follow-up.
   b. Assessing, planning, implementing, evaluating.
   c. Interviewing, observing, communication, listening.
   d. Assessing, planning, evaluating, follow-up.
7. A gastroenterology associate is defined as:
   a. A nurse who is engaged in the field of gastroenterology.
   b. A non-RN healthcare professional with varied educational background engaged in the field of gastroenterology.
   c. An individual with advanced education who is engaged in gastroenterology.
   d. An individual who is responsible for transporting patients and caring for instruments and equipment.
8. Initial assessment of patients upon arrival to the gastroenterology unit is usually the responsibility of the:
   a. Physician.
   b. Nurse manager.
   c. Staff nurse (RN).
   d. Associate.
9. A general requirement for a recently graduated nurse who is interested in practicing gastroenterology nursing is:
   a. To work for one year on a medical-surgical unit to gain experience.
   b. To work for a private gastrointestinal physician to gain knowledge of diagnosis and procedures.
   c. To work in a special procedures unit for one year.
   d. To work in an ambulatory care unit to practice skills for one year.
10. The gastroenterology nurse and associate roles are differentiated in that:
    a. The nurse's role is to formulate a nursing diagnosis and plan care accordingly.
    b. The associate's role is to formulate a nursing diagnosis and plan care accordingly.
    c. The associate is responsible for assisting only with the procedure.
    d. The nurse is primarily responsible for documenting care provided.

**BIBLIOGRAPHY**

Barnie, D. "Evaluation of Nursing Specialties." *SGA Journal* 11(Spring 1989): 214-16.

Bodinsky, G. *Documentation: Charting to Standardize.* SGNA Monograph Series. Rochester, N.Y.: Society of Gastroenterology Nurses and Associates, 1989.

Certifying Board of Gastroenterology Nurses and Associates, Inc. *Role Delineation for Gastroenterology Associates.* March 1990.

Certifying Board of Gastroenterology Nurses and Associates, Inc. *Role Delineation for Gastroenterology RNs.* March 1990.

Connelly, N. "Certification: A Study Primer Covering the Basics." In *Journal Reprints II,* ed. Trivits, S, 5-10. Rochester, N.Y.: Society of Gastroenterology Nurses and Associates, 1990.

Hirschowitz B, Curtiss L, and Pollard A. "Demonstration of a new gastroscope, the 'fiberscope.'" *Gastroenterology* 35(1958):50-53.9.

Joint Commission for Accreditation of Healthcare Organizations. *Accreditation Manual for Hospitals, 1991 Ed.* Volume 1. Standards. Oakbrook Terrace, Ill.: JCAHO, 1990.

Ravenscroft, M, and Swan, C. *Gastrointestinal Endoscopy and Related Procedures: A Handbook for Nurses and Assistants.* Baltimore: Williams & Wilkins, 1984.

Shields, N. "The Role of Professional Organizations in the Practice of GI Nursing." *SGA Journal* 10(Fall 1987): 112-13.

Sugawa, C, and Schuman, B. *Primer of Gastrointestinal Fiberoptic Endoscopy.* Boston: Little, Brown & Co, 1981.

*Chapter 2*

# MANAGING THE GASTROENTEROLOGY DEPARTMENT

This chapter reviews the principles and functions inherent in managing human and material resources in a gastroenterology unit. Five functions of management are addressed, including planning, organizing, directing, controlling, and staffing. Each function is further defined and the process outlined in an effort to provide the manager of the gastroenterology unit with fundamental managerial concepts. "New age" skills the gastroenterology manager should acquire to create excellence within the organization are also reviewed.

**Learning objectives**

After reviewing the content of this chapter, the gastroenterology nurse should be able to:

1. Discuss the five functions of management and provide examples of activities included in each function.
2. Describe the organizational structure of the gastroenterology unit.
3. Outline methods for accomplishing department goals through efficient use of personnel.

## FUNCTIONS OF MANAGEMENT

Management can be defined as a process of getting things completed with the help of others. This means that individuals must be directed toward common goals. There are two criteria used to determine whether or not an individual in an organization is a manager. First, does the individual perform management functions? Second, does he/she have authority? If either of these two components is lacking, the structure of the organization or the individual in the management position should be re-examined. These two criteria are presented here because they are important to the success of any gastroenterology unit and because the manager

must demonstrate competency in the area of management.

The five functions a manager performs are planning, organizing, directing, controlling, and staffing.

- Planning is the first function performed; it determines in advance what should be done.
- Organizing comes after the planning process; it involves dissecting the work into parts so that it can be accomplished.
- Directing is the third management function and includes guidance, coaching, motivating, and supervising subordinates.
- Controlling involves activities that are used to measure attainment of the goals outlined in the planning phase.
- Staffing is not always a separate management function, but when it concerns hospital departments such as the gastroenterology unit, it is important to set staffing apart. It can be a time-consuming process that entails recruiting, training, and promoting of staff.

These five functions are performed by managers at every level of the organization. The amount of time spent on the various functions by the hospital administrator in relation to that of the gastroenterology unit manager will be different. For instance, the administrator probably spends more time planning and organizing, whereas the unit manager spends more time staffing, directing, and controlling.

In addition to performing management functions, the second key criterion that a manager must possess is **authority,** which is the legal or rightful power to command and act. The manager must be given the power to command or enforce order; otherwise, there would be

11

disorganization and chaos. In today's work force the words *responsibility* or *task* are used rather than the word *authority*. Nevertheless, an effective manager must understand his or her authority. Regardless of how an individual manager applies that authority, it is important to have it. This issue will be further explored when the directing function of management is examined.

Coordination should be a byproduct of the performance of the five functions of management described below. It is described as the ability of a manager to direct individuals to perform efficiently.

## Planning

Planning is the first function performed by the gastroenterology unit nurse manager and entails outlining a course of action that is realistic for the unit. Planning involves development of a purpose or mission, philosophy, goals, and objectives for the organization and development of "work maps" showing how these goals and objectives are to be accomplished.

In the planning stage, the gastroenterology manager attempts to forecast how trends in patient treatment modalities and technologies will affect the unit. Gathering data on an ongoing basis from suppliers of equipment, reading current journals, attending professional meetings, and viewing exhibits provide a basis for forecasting.

The manager also has to project the qualifications of future employees based on the level of knowledge and skills needed to perform tasks in the gastroenterology unit. The political climate of the hospital and the timing of any anticipated staffing or management changes are also critical in planning. The manager must choose the best strategy and know when to plan changes that will provide a positive result.

During the planning phase, the manager decides how to best use available resources. This decision requires review of equipment and supplies. Is there a need to purchase or replace medical devices? Are the supplies and materials used in the unit appropriate and the best for the types of procedures being performed? Another important planning task is to look at work methods and processes. Are there ways of being more efficient? Are there activities being done that are not necessary and could be changed? Is there a need to do any space planning? The physical space of the unit and the placement of equipment and furniture should be conducive to a smooth work flow. It is easy to understand the importance of planning and how it affects the ability to perform other management functions.

Budgeting is a managerial task that takes place in both planning and controlling functions. During the planning function, budgeting involves setting goals or policies that guide the unit throughout the year.

A prerequisite to performing the above planning tasks is the manager's ability to make decisions. Identifying problems, exploring alternatives, choosing alternatives, implementing decisions, and evaluating results will help in clarifying the purpose of the unit. The gastroenterology unit nurse manager must be skilled in using decision-making tools to select the best course of action from all of the alternatives presented. Problem solving is a skill that can be learned. Decision-making tools that assist the manager include the probability theory, which operates on the assumption that things occur in a predictable pattern; simulations, models and games that help describe, explain, and predict phenomena; decision trees, which are graphic tools that aid in visualizing alternatives; critical path method, which is useful when looking at costs; and queuing theory, which is used when problems arise around service that is being provided.

## Organizing

Organizing is the second function of management and is the means by which a manager develops order and fosters productivity. Organizing involves the integration of resources in a unit and the assignment of activities within that unit so they can be most effectively executed. This entails establishing lines of authority within activities and between departments and examining the contributions people make to the organization and determining to whom one will report. The organizing process comes from the need for cooperation; the goal is to build, develop, and maintain a structure of working relationships that brings about the objectives of the unit in a positive way.

### Types of organizational structures

The **organizational structure** determines the process by which a specific group of people distribute responsibilities, establish lines of communication, identify relationships, and establish authority.

Organizational structures can be formal or informal. An informal structure develops in all organizations. It is concerned primarily with the personal and social relationships that are not seen on the organizational chart. Formal organizational structures can be designed or rescinded, but informal structures cannot, because they have not been instituted by the manager. The manager needs to know that the informal structure exists, how it operates, and how to use it to advance the objectives of the unit. By knowing how the informal organization works, the manager can avoid activities that will unnecessarily threaten or disrupt it.

Formal organizational structures can be either bureaureaucratic or adaptive. Bureaucratic structures imply subdivision, specialization, technical qualifications, rules, and standards. The newer, adaptive organizational models are more free-form, open systems that are flexible and lend themselves to a more participative atmosphere.

There are no rules regarding which type of organizational structure is best for the gastroenterology unit; whatever works for the unit and institution is acceptable. Different types of formal organizational structures that may be appropriate for the gastroenterology unit include line organization, functional organization, staff organization, matrix organization, and project organization, each of which are described as follows:

- **Line authority** is probably the most traditional and easiest organization structure to use, because each position has authority over a lower one in the organization. It is a chain of command, a leader-follower relationship. This type of structure works well when there are levels of expertise within the unit. For example, the manager would be in charge, with the RN, LPN, or gastroenterology associate reporting to her, and the LPN and associate reporting to the RN. The ideal structure does not always exist and many times associate staff members assist everyone.
- **Functional organization** authorizes a specialist from a given area to enforce recommendations within a clearly defined area. This type of structure might work well in a gastroenterology unit where there is an all-RN staff. One RN would act as the specialist or spokesperson for communication to the institution's administration.
- In a **staff authority** structure, staff members serve in an advisory capacity to the line structure but have no authority. The primary responsibility of the staff is to assist personnel who are in a line authority or chain of command. Unfortunately, this structure does not allow personnel to take the initiative to implement change. Staff personnel function primarily through influence and by offering suggestions to assist line personnel to be more effective.
- A **matrix organization** looks at individual subsystems within a complex structure. Depending upon the complex structure, these subsystems can be totally dependent or have total autonomy. This is demonstrated in many decentralized systems in whichsubsystems are given the authority to work independently of other groups but toward a common goal.
- **Project organization** is usually used to accomplish a specific task; when the task is completed, the group is disbanded. This type of structure is beneficial when a specific task must be accomplished, such as evaluating a new product and recommending whether or not to purchase it.

Regardless of the type of organizational structure used, it must be clearly defined for the unit to deliver quality care. Each team member must know the process for distributing responsibilities and how to communicate through appropriate channels. The organizational structure should facilitate the communication of staff ideas and concerns and the integration of **quality.** If it does not accomplish this, it should be reevaluated and a different type of structure should be tried. However, individual departments such as the gastroenterology unit may not be able to exert much influence and many times structure is imposed without input from all involved departments. The emphasis should be on a team approach to delivery of quality care.

**Organizational principles**

Certain principles help maximize the efficiency of the organizational structure and help the manager and employees function more effectively within that structure. These principles include unity of command, requisite authority, and continuing responsibility.

- Unity of command implies clear lines of authority. The employee knows who to report to and who is the final authority. This means that each member of the organization has a single immediate supervisor.
- Requisite authority implies that when a subordinate has been delegated a task, he or she is given the final authority to accomplish the task.
- Continuing responsibility refers to the fact that when a manager delegates responsibility for a function to a subordinate, the manager is still responsible for that function.

Recognition of these few basic principles assists the manager by enhancing the efficiency of the organizational structure.

**Organizational tools**

Organizational tools that are helpful for the gastroenterology manager include organization charts and job descriptions.

The organization chart is a graphic representation of how the unit is organized. It depicts formal organizational relationships, areas of responsibility, persons to whom one is accountable, and channels of communication. It is used for planning, administrative control, and policy making.

Job descriptions are important because they assist the manager with organizing the administration of the various functions. Descriptions specify the title of the position, the qualifications necessary to complete the duties listed, and the person to whom the employee is responsible.

**Span of control**

The span of control is often referred to as the span of management; it is used to identify the scope of managerial responsibility. Most managers know there is a limit to the number of employees they can effectively supervise. Therefore, while the manager remains the final authority, he or she delegates authority to subordinates, who in turn supervise a group of employees.

Factors that influence the manager's capability to supervise include:

- The amount of experience and management training he or she has acquired. An experienced and well-trained manager is able to supervise more employees.

- The amount and the nature of work a manager has to do.
- The characteristics of the employees themselves. If they are self-directed and possess a high degree of knowledge and skill they may not need as much direction.
- The design and complexity of procedures and activities that take place in the unit.

One caution regarding the span of control for a small unit is that overly prudent supervision discourages problem solving and independent thinking, and may give subordinates the feeling of being smothered. Today we see the influence of the concept of continuous quality improvement permeating the hospital structure. This type of management philosophy will prevail through the 1990s and we will soon begin to see benefits, such as reduced waste, improved services, increased success, and decreased cost of healthcare services.

### Directing

After organizing, the next step in the process of management entails directing personnel and activities in such a way that goals of the unit are met. Managers must demonstrate the ability to lead and motivate employees through the issuance of directives, instructions, assignments, and orders. The two main objectives are to complete work and to teach employees. The gastroenterology unit manager should build an effective work force and motivate each member of the team. Regardless of the level of management, directing is always an important function. It requires that a manager possess leadership skills and the ability to integrate a participative management style into the daily coordination of the gastroenterology unit. Every manager should become familiar with his or her own leadership style, managerial philosophy, and sources of power and authority.

#### Leadership

The emphasis in management today is on human skills. Leadership is defined as the process of influencing the activities of an individual or group in efforts directed at goal achievement. In other words, leadership involves accomplishing goals with and by means of people. People have not always been the focus of leadership theory. Some of the more popular schools of thought in organizational theory have been:

- The theory of scientific management (Taylor, 1947), in which the function of the manager is to set up and enforce performance criteria to meet organizational goals. The focus is on the organization and not the needs of the people within the organization.
- The human relations theory, which stresses concern for the needs of the people versus the task. Some have felt that a predominant concern for the task represents authoritarian leadership behavior, while

concern for relationships represents democratic leadership. The human relations theory is based on the idea that the real power of the organization is the interpersonal relations that develop within the working unit. Mayo illustrated this concept in the famous Hawthorne experiment done with the Western Electric Company (Mayo, 1949).

- The managerial grid, which includes both task and relationship concepts. This model tends to be an attitudinal model because it measures the values and feelings of the manager. This theory considers five different types of leadership, based on the manager's concern for tasks versus people within the organization (Blake and Mouton, 1964).
- The contingency model of leadership, which holds that a manager's leadership style can be effective or ineffective, depending upon the situation. This model defines three aspects of a situation that structure the leader's role: leader-employee relations, task structure, and position power. Like the managerial grid model, this model is two-dimensional, in that it reverts back to the basic leader behavior styles: task-oriented and relationship-oriented (Fiedler, 1922).
- The authoritarian–democratic leader behavior model is another theory of leadership style. In this theory, the authoritarian leader places more emphasis on tasks. On the other end of the continuum, the democratic leader is more concerned about relationships. This popular theory is still used today. Basically it coincides with McGregor's X and Y theory. There are two basic leadership styles on a continuum: on one end, the leader directs employees by telling them what to do and how to do it; on the other, the leader influences employees by sharing responsibilities with them and involving them in decision making. In some cases the continuum is extended beyond democratic behavior into a permissive style of leadership known as laissez-faire. In this style, employees do as they please. There are no policies and procedures, and there is no sign of any formal leadership.

Regardless of which model is used, the manager must develop and implement the leadership style that works best in accomplishing the goals of the unit.

#### Motivating

To be successful at directing employees, the manager must understand human behavior and what motivates employee performance. Much has been written on the topic of motivation, and there are classic theories with which all managers should be familiar. In the 1950s, however, advocates of the behavioral sciences became concerned about the lack of scientific validation behind the management theories that had been applied in the past. The management theories in use today developed from this concern.

Maslow was one of the first to initiate the human behavior school with his hierarchy-of-needs theory. He classified human needs into five categories: physiologic, safety, love, esteem, and self-actualization. Maslow's theory has been and still is very influential in management and continues to stimulate much research.

Another popular theory today is Herzberg's motivation-hygiene theory, wherein job factors are classified as either dissatisfiers or satisfiers. Satisfiers, or motivators, are achievement, recognition, work, responsibility, advancement, and growth. The idea is that as an employee receives positive feedback, his level of performance increases. The job dissatisfiers, or hygiene factors, are supervision, company policy, working conditions, interpersonal relations, job security, and salary. These are not motivators because for the most part, they do not cause any improvement in performance. They only prevent poor morale. Herzberg believes that if a person finds the job interesting, he or she can tolerate the dissatisfiers.

In management theory the manager's style affects the degree to which he or she can stimulate employee performance. McGregor's X and Y theory is a good example. Theory X assumes that most people prefer to be directed, are not interested in assuming responsibility, and have to be constantly supervised. Theory Y assumes that the employee is mature, independent, and self-motivated. Managers who believe that people are inherently lazy tend to use fear and threats to motivate personnel, delegate little responsibility, and do not include personnel in planning. Managers who philosophically believe that people are self-motivated and enjoy work use praise and recognition and provide opportunities for growth. Theory Y complements Herzberg's theory in that positive incentives are used to stimulate personnel.

Personal management styles reflect managers' beliefs about motivation. Webster's dictionary defines motive as "that within the individual, rather than without, which incites him to action; any idea, need, emotion, or organic state that prompts to an action." If managers want to motivate employees, they have to provide the motive — in other words, incite action from the employee. If this is true, one of the roles of the manager is to understand what really motivates employees and what stimulates certain behaviors. This can be determined by identifying what employees want from their jobs. Different people have different needs. Today, the trend seems to be toward recognition, flexibility in the work setting, and a sense of responsibility. Employees want to participate in decision making, particularly as it relates to them and their own jobs.

### Participative management

Current management philosophy holds that the better a manager treats an employee, the better the employee will perform. The trend in nursing is toward participative management. This philosophy is based on the belief that employees are self-directed and self-motivated and can be self-managed. Group problem solving and decision making give employees a sense of ownership. They are motivated to implement the decisions they have helped develop. Professional employees have a need for autonomy and for some control over their own behavior. The challenge presented to managers is to integrate the needs of the organization with those of the employees. It is essential to have a balance.

Gastroenterology managers must possess well-developed human interaction skills. Instead of being autocratic, they need to be encouraging when interacting with employees. To be most effective, managers must relinquish control in the traditional, autocratic sense in order to maintain management control.

One skill the manager must use to the best of his or her ability is that of listening. The manager should spend some time each day interacting with the staff, in order to develop a personal relationship with each of the employees within the department. The effective manager tries to be available to discuss issues, problems, and concerns that come up during the usual workday. He or she listens to employees' ideas and assists with problem-solving. Communication is one of the biggest challenges for managers. It is important to share information, to keep employees informed of happenings, and to gain their cooperation.

Managers who deliver positive rewards in some form for productive behavior find that the behavior is repeated. Employees need to be told when they do something right. Acknowledgement of good work performance is a strong motivating force. It lets employees know they are doing what is expected of them. The better employees feel about themselves, the more eager they are to work hard and be productive.

### Controlling

Controlling is the fourth step in the management process. It entails setting standards, measuring performance, reporting results, and taking corrective action. In controlling, the manager is concerned with making certain that the solution to a problem is properly implemented. This involves feedback of results and follow-up to determine the extent to which the predetermined goals have been accomplished. The success of the gastroenterology department depends on the degree of difference between what should be done and what is done. Having set the standards, the manager has a responsibility to stay informed of the actual performance. This can be achieved through observation, reports, and verbal feedback.

The controlling function of management should not be separated from the other management functions. In the managerial process of planning, the manager sets goals that become standards against which performance is continually checked and appraised. There is a direct connection between planning and controlling. Control is directly interwoven with other managerial functions, in that a manager cannot expect to have good control over the department without following sound managerial principles in pursuing his or her duties. Well-made plans, workable policies and procedures, continual training of employees, and appropriate supervision all play a significant role in control.

A gastroenterology department is part of a total system. In order for the system to be under control there are certain essential requirements:

- Procedures through which control is maintained must be understandable.
- Deviations from the controls or procedures must be identified quickly.
- Controls or procedures must be appropriate and economical.
- There must be flexibility in the system.
- Corrective action must be taken when required.

Controlling entails three basic steps: setting standards or objectives, checking and appraising performance, and taking corrective action.

### Setting standards

The overall objectives of the hospital are broken down into relative objectives for each department. These objectives are established by the department manager and include parameters such as quality, time standards, quotas, schedules, budgets, and patient procedures. Both internal and external types of standards affect the department and both must be taken into consideration by the manager.

The manager should keep in mind that standards must be realistic. They must be achievable and must be considered fair by the employees as well as the manager. It is essential that the employees be involved in identifying realistic and attainable standards.

Not all standards are tangible. Some types of intangible standards are important, particularly in the hospital setting. These might be the reputation of the hospital and even the individual department, high morale among employees in the department, and effective patient care, so recovery is quick and the patient's stay is pleasant.

Setting standards may seem overwhelming when considering the many types of activities in the department. Therefore, the manager might break down the task to a more manageable task by focusing on selecting strategic standards and looking for critical performance indicators.

### Checking performance

The second step in the process of control is to check on the performance. Once the standards have been set, it is the manager's responsibility to compare actual performance with these standards. This is done by observing the work, by personally checking on employees, and by studying various reports.

### Taking corrective action

The third part of controlling is taking corrective action. The manager is not really controlling if he or she does not take corrective action when indicated. Ideally, there are no deviations from expected performance. Realistically, however, there will be discrepancies or variations that will need attention. When deviations do occur, the manager must analyze the situation and look at the total picture. He or she must then decide what remedial action is necessary and what modifications will secure improved results in the future.

### Managing the budget

One of the most important control devices available to the manager is the budget. The budget is prepared during the planning process and provides direction for the manager. The budget is simply a statement of estimated expenses and revenues for a predetermined time period. The two types of budgets are the operating budget and the capital budget.

#### Operating budget

The operating budget consists of consumable items and resources used to provide direct patient care. Operating expenses vary depending on the volume of patients and the procedures performed in the gastroenterology unit. In most cases, the operating budget is further divided into direct or indirect expenses. Direct costs include items such as salaries, medical and surgical supplies, repairs and charges from other departments. Indirect costs are expenses assigned for overhead and facility use. Table 2-1 provides examples of items that are considered direct and indirect expenses.

An important part of the operating budget is determination of staffing requirements. The goal is to secure enough budgeted positions to provide the quality of care projected. Some hospitals use a patient classification system or acuity to determine appropriate numbers. Others look at the total number of shifts per week required by category of staff. The staffing budget must take into account the number of patients that will be seen in the unit each day and the hours the unit will be staffed.

The supply part of the operating budget is usually based on the previous year's expenses and projection of costs for the next fiscal year. Other factors to consider include inflation rates, changes in work load by procedures or patients, and any new or different supplies.

#### Capital budget

The second type of budget is the capital budget. This budget includes large purchases, such as equipment, furniture, or construction projects that amount to more than $500 and are usually depreciated. Most hospitals expect the department manager to make a formal request in a proposal format that incorporates data specific to the item requested; alternative solutions, such as purchase, rent, or lease; priorities and recommendations;

**Table 2-1.** Examples of direct and indirect expenses

| Direct expenses | Indirect expenses |
| --- | --- |
| Salaries and wages | Equipment depreciation |
| Per diem staff | Building depreciation |
| Overtime | Malpractice insurance |
| On-call personnel | Employee health benefits |
| Disposable items | Accounting |
| Instruments | Purchasing |
| Medical and surgical supplies | Utilities |
| Repairs | Housekeeping |
| Pharmacy | |

cost and benefits analysis; and an implementation plan.

Whatever budgetary goals are in place, the manager who is administering the budget should have a part in preparing it. The gastroenterology manager should remember that budgets are merely a tool for management and not a substitute for good judgment.

### Staffing

Staffing is the final managerial function. Once planning and organizing have been accomplished, the manager of the gastroenterology unit must assign staff to carry out the unit's goals. Staffing involves employee selection, placement, training, and compensation. The manager's function is to hire, place, develop, and train the employees for the unit. In addition, the manager evaluates and appraises the performance of employees and either rewards their efforts and abilities, or disciplines and at times even discharges employees who are not performing at acceptable levels.

#### Staffing functions

The staffing function is not done only at the time the department or unit is established; it is ongoing. The manager has a responsibility to make certain that employees possess the necessary capabilities and are competent to perform the tasks required in the gastroenterology unit. To ensure that the right employees are hired for the necessary positions, the manager has to "determine the need." This step entails deciding on the number and type of employees needed. In a small unit, several functions may be combined. Staffing needs can be determined only after careful study of the entire unit. The manager must match jobs with people. Using job descriptions that fully delineate the requirements of the job facilitates this process.

The manager will determine the number of employees and the staffing budget requirements based on the volume of procedures. He or she generally hires individuals to replace those who voluntarily resign, are dismissed, or transfer. When an additional employee must be hired, the goal is to recruit and select a person who is qualified to perform the duties outlined in the job description.

#### Selection of employees

The human resources department may initially interview and screen job applicants; however, qualified individuals will ultimately be presented to the manager before being hired. A copy of the applicant's curriculum vitae or resume should always be obtained to review the applicant's experience and qualifications. An interview provides additional information about the applicant's job knowledge and personality. At this point, the interview should focus on the individual's competencies and qualifications to perform the required duties in the gastroenterology department. Questions asked in the interview must follow guidelines established by the Equal Employment Opportunity Commission (EEOC). The manager compares prospective employees' strengths and weaknesses to choose the one who best fits the needs of the department. It is also a good practice to follow up on references provided by prospective employees. Sometimes these can be invaluable. Following up may entail making telephone calls or requesting letters of recommendation. A record should be kept of all prospective employees and should include the position applied for and the decision to hire or not to hire.

#### Orientation and staff development

Once the manager has hired the desired employee, it is the manager's responsibility to orient the new person to the hospital and the unit. Orientation should include introduction to policies and procedures, rules and regulations specific to the hospital, and a thorough review of the tasks, duties, and responsibilities outlined in the employee's job description.

The purpose of staff development is to provide opportunities for the individual employee's professional growth and development; as such, it goes beyond orientation and should be available for all employees on an ongoing basis. Staff development opportunities might include hospital or department inservices, courses, seminars, and independent study or projects.

#### Staffing assignments

Providing for patient care on a daily basis is also a function of staffing. Schedules should provide staff with information as to where and when they should be on duty. There are a variety of staffing patterns that can be used; however, the hospital nursing service or human resources department usually provides the guidelines and determines the type of delivery that will be used. The delivery system may be managed care, functional nursing, team nursing, or primary nursing. Any of these delivery systems will accommodate the various theoretical models of nursing.

Another consideration for the gastroenterology unit manager is whether centralized or decentralized staffing is in place. Today, computers are used for centralized staffing by many nursing service departments. This type of scheduling is cost-effective and reduces the hours allocated to developing and implementing staffing needs. Decentralized staffing is accomplished by a manager at the unit level. The advantage of decentralized staffing is that employees get more personalized attention.

## BEYOND FUNDAMENTAL MANAGERIAL SKILLS

The managerial thoughts and ideas presented are merely overviews and therefore are not discussed in depth. The gastroenterology nurse manager should be able to assess his/her level of competency and seek out resources that will enhance his or her motivation skills. In addition to the fundamental managerial skills required for success, it is critical to stay abreast of new ideas and approaches to accomplishing the task.

Managing in today's environment is not an easy task. Emphasis is being placed on increasing productivity and quality through team development. The role of the manager is to coach, facilitate, and develop the staff. Essential skills include the abilities to delegate power, encourage staff to expand their talents, and encourage risk taking.

Some people believe that the individual leaders, rather than the organization, create excellence. In other words, it does not just happen; an individual makes it happen. The challenge for managers is to integrate a set of skills that Hickman and Silva (1984) believe are essential for the "new age" executive. The following leadership skills enable the gastroenterology unit manager to engage in laying a strong foundation of excellence.

- *Creative Insight: Asking the Right Question.* Insight means being able to get to the root of the problem. The manager is able to readily see opportunities, advantages, and strengths that result in new strategies for success.
- *Sensitivity: Doing Unto Others.* Because people are the organization's greatest asset, the manager must find a way to bind them together so they will achieve high goals. The manager may choose to unify employees through one-on-one communication, ongoing education programs, creative incentive programs, and job security.
- *Vision: Creating the Future.* This skill enables the manager to have a clear vision of changes that may occur.
- *Versatility: Anticipating Change.* The versatile manager is prepared and readily adapts to the ever-changing world. A manager must be able to anticipate and accept change and use it to predict the future.
- *Focus: Implementing Change.* A successful manager gives undivided attention to the task at hand. By focusing on priorities, the manager increasingly controls the situation.

- *Patience: Living in the Long Term.* Patience is a virtue. The manager who is able to integrate and orchestrate the other five skills will, through patience, know how and when to use them. If every manager would commit to acquiring the above skills, organizations would evolve into a high level of excellence.

Managers in hospitals are being pressured to develop new skills and abilities which will improve the productivity, and quality of services provided in every department. These skills cannot be mastered overnight, but hard work and commitment will result in success.

---

CASE SITUATION

---

Patsy Bartlett is the gastroenterology unit nurse manager at Piedmont Hospital. Her daily activities include managing the unit as well as being clinically competent to assist with scheduled procedures. This combination produces frustration because she must also develop a marketing plan to keep her hospital competitive in the healthcare market place.

*Points to think about*

1. Patsy realizes that it is essential that she devise a plan for the new laparoscopic procedures that will be implemented in her unit. What kind of information must she put together?
2. Sometimes Patsy wonders if she is capable of managing the gastroenterology unit, because it gets rather hectic and time is precious. What types of activities would demonstrate management ability?
3. Patsy believes that a participative management style works best for her gastroenterology department. What are some examples of behaviors that would reinforce this management style?
4. Patsy had a situation where an employee would call in at 5 AM and request the day off. What type of plan might Patty use to alter this employee's behavior?
5. Patsy has been asked to develop a marketing plan to increase the volume of procedures performed in the gastroenterology unit. How might she approach this challenge?

*Suggested responses*

1. In order to prepare for the introduction of new laparoscopic procedures, Patsy should:
   - Perform a financial forecast based on the projected number of laparoscopic procedures.
   - Determine capital equipment needs relative to this new procedure.
   - Design an orientation/training program for personnel.

- Revise the existing budget to include income and expenses associated with this procedure.
2. Examples of management activities might include:
   - Making changes in staffing schedules based on requests of personnel.
   - Reviewing monthly financial statements and justifying variances.
   - Meeting with staff to discuss problems encountered with cleaning the new laparoscopes.
   - Conducting a performance appraisal of an associate.
3. Examples of behaviors that would reinforce the participative management style include:
   - Staff involvement in the decision of who would cover weekend call.
   - Staff meeting regarding general low morale throughout the institution.
   - Staff meeting to obtain input regarding the replacement of obsolescent equipment.
   - Staff involvement in developing a policy for monitoring sedated pediatric patients.
4. In order to improve this employee's behavior, Patsy might:
   - Set up a meeting with the employee and attempt to gather objective data about the reasons for her behavior.
   - Explain to the employee that the schedule has already been completed and only needed personnel are assigned.
   - Explain that her request should be made in advance, in accordance with written leave policies.
   - Provide positive feedback on behaviors which should be recognized.
   - Set mutual goals relative to requesting time off.
   - Schedule a follow-up meeting to review progress.
   - Document the counseling session plus anecdotal notes.
5. To develop a marketing plan, Patsy might:
   - Use creative insight to begin looking at what problems currently exist and possible solutions that would result in identification of opportunities.
   - Use these opportunities to create a vision of what she would like the department to do and to outline a plan for accomplishing the goals set forth.
   - Be open to accepting the changes that have taken place and use them to advance toward the anticipated goals.

---

**REVIEW TERMS**

**authority, functional organization, line authority, matrix organization, organizational structure, project organization, quality, staff authority**

---

**REVIEW QUESTIONS**

1. Management of the gastroenterology department entails:
   a. Coordination of the five functions of management.
   b. Getting things done through others.
   c. Doing tasks yourself to ensure they are done correctly.
   d. Ensuring that the employee knows who to report to.
2. The management function that entails establishing authority relationships between activities and departments is:
   a. Staffing.
   b. Controlling.
   c. Organizing.
   d. Directing.
3. Managerial components of planning include:
   a. Developing goals and objectives.
   b. Maintaining a structure of working relationships.
   c. Assigning work activities.
   d. Hiring new personnel.
4. Activities that the gastroenterology nurse manager performs in the directing function of management include:
   a. Counseling employees.
   b. Leading and guiding employees.
   c. Developing position descriptions.
   d. Performance appraisal.
5. The emphasis in management today should be on:
   a. Motivation.
   b. Pay increases.
   c. Flexible staffing.
   d. Human skills.
6. For the manager to determine the staffing budget, it will be necessary to calculate:
   a. Full-time equivalents and flexible staff.
   b. Volume of procedures and required staff.
   c. Qualifications of the required staff.
   d. Volume and cost of procedures.
7. A person who delegates authority to others is accountable for:
   a. The tasks allocated to other workers.
   b. The tasks unassigned to staff.
   c. The tasks delegated to staff.
   d. The tasks of other managers.
8. The process of measuring the degree to which predetermined goals of the gastroenterology unit are achieved is called:
   a. Planning.
   b. Controlling.
   c. Staffing.
   d. Directing.

9. In an operating budget, salaries, overtime, benefits, and medical-surgical supplies are usually considered:
   a. Indirect expenses.
   b. Fixed assets.
   c. Direct expenses.
   d. Capital budget items.
10. The management skill that focuses primarily on the assets of people in the organization would be:
    a. Focusing on being a change agent.
    b. Constructing the operating budget.
    c. Performing a financial forecast.
    d. Developing sensitivity.

## BIBLIOGRAPHY

Blake, R, and Mouton, J. *The Managerial Grid.* Houston: Gulf Publishing, 1964.

Caruthers, C. "Strategic Management: The Human Element." *Gastroenterology Nursing* 11(Winter 1989): 164-66.

Fielder, F. *A Theory of Leadership Effectiveness.* New York: McGraw-Hill, 1967.

Garfield, C. *Peak Performers.* New York: Avon Books, 1986.

Gruber, M. "Practical Time Management for GI Nursing Staff." *SGA Journal* 10(Winter 1988): 150-52.

Gruber, M, and Gruber, M. "Communication: A Pound of Prevention." *Gastroenterology Nursing* 12(Winter 1990): 183-86.

Hersey, P, and Blanchard, K. *Management of Organizational Behavior: Utilizing Human Resources.* Englewood Cliffs, N.J.: Prentice-Hall, 1982.

Hickman, C, and Silva, M. *Creating Excellence.* New York: New American Library, 1984.

Marriner, A. *Guide to Nursing Management.* St. Louis: Mosby–Year Book, 1980.

Mayo, E. "Hawthorne and the Western Electric Company." In *The Social Problems of an Industrial Civilization,* 60-76. Boston: Routledge, 1949.

Pethigal, P. "Positive Effective Communication: A Key to Success at Work." *SGA Journal* 10(Spring 1988): 205-07.

Salmore, R. "Praise as a Means to Increase Job Satisfaction." *Gastroenterology Nursing* 13(Fall 1990): 98-100.

Schaffner, M. "Interviewing, Orientation and Evaluation." *Gastroenterology Nursing* 13(Winter 1990): 172-78.

Shields, N. "Budgeting Responsibilities of the GI Laboratory Manager." *Gastroenterology Nursing* 12(Summer 1989): 55-58.

Shields, N. "Participative Management." *Gastroenterology Nursing* 12(Winter 1990): 196-99.

Shields, N. "Management of the GI Laboratory. Part 1: Planning and Organizing." *SGA Journal* 10(Summer 1987): 9-11.

Taylor, F. *Scientific Management.* New York: Harper & Row, 1947.

# Chapter 3

# INFECTION CONTROL

This chapter describes the precautions that must be taken in the gastroenterology unit to control the risk of infection for patients and healthcare personnel. Guidelines are provided for the decontamination and disinfection of instruments and patient care items present in endoscopy settings. **Sanitation** and waste management considerations are outlined and precautions for the protection of healthcare workers are discussed.

**Learning objectives**

After reviewing the content of this chapter, the gastroenterology nurse should be able to:
1. Discuss general principles of infection control.
2. Explain appropriate measures for the decontamination and disinfection of instruments and patient care items, and the cleaning of environmental surfaces in the endoscopy setting.
3. Describe how to deal with infectious waste in the endoscopy setting.
4. Discuss the application of universal precautions for the protection of patients and personnel in the gastroenterology unit.

## INFECTION CONTROL PRINCIPLES

It is imperative that all healthcare personnel be educated regarding appropriate infection control measures. An infection results when **microorganisms** enter the human body, multiply, and produce a reaction. For an infection to develop, all three of the following interlinking components in the chain of infection must be present: an infectious organism, a means of transmission, and a susceptible host.
- The infectious organisms may be in the form of bacteria, viruses, fungi, protozoa, or helminths (worms). Bacteria are the most common infectious agents in hospital settings. The source of infection may be within the patient's own body (endogenous) or outside the patient's body (exogenous).
- Direct and indirect contact are the most common

methods of transmission in hospital settings. Other methods include airborne transmission, a concern in operating rooms; vehicle transmission, such as liquid antiseptics; and vector transmission via an animal or insect.
- A susceptible host can be anyone who has a lowered resistance. Factors that contribute to host susceptibility are age, immune status, or underlying disease. Because of their inefficient immune systems, patients infected with the AIDS virus are highly susceptible to infection.

An infection can occur only if all three components of the chain of infection are present under the right conditions. If any one of these components can be eliminated, the chain is broken and infection cannot occur.

To break the chain of infection the gastroenterology nurse must recognize the need for appropriate decontamination, disinfection, and, in some cases, sterilization of instruments and patient care items. Hospital policies must identify whether decontamination, disinfection, or sterilization is indicated based on the item's intended use. Classifications for levels of disinfection and categorization of equipment and patient care items were devised in the 1960s by Earl H. Spaulding. Spaulding classified equipment and patient care items as critical, semicritical, and noncritical, based on the risk of infection involved in their use.
- **Critical items** are those that present a high risk of infection if they are contaminated. These are objects or instruments that come in contact with body tissue below the skin surface or mucous membranes, the vascular system, or other normally sterile areas of the body. Examples of critical items used in the gastroenterology unit would be biopsy forceps and intravenous catheters. Sterilization is recommended for critical items.
- **Semicritical items** come in contact with intact skin and mucous membranes but usually do not penetrate body surfaces. Sterilization of semicritical

items may be preferable, but high-level disinfection is usually sufficient because intact skin and mucous membranes are generally resistant to bacterial spores. Endoscopes are considered semicritical items.

• **Noncritical items** come in contact with intact skin but not mucous membranes. There is relatively little risk of transmitting infection with these items. Some examples of noncritical items used in the gastroenterology unit are bedpans, blood pressure cuffs, pulse oximeters, and stethoscopes.

## DECONTAMINATION

In the endoscopy unit the primary objective of **decontamination** is to prevent drying of secretions on instruments, supplies, and surfaces immediately following a procedure. According to guidelines issued by SGNA, the endoscope insertion tube and all channels must undergo scrupulous mechanical cleaning with a detergent (e.g., an enzymatic detergent). A thorough cleaning is always necessary before disinfection or sterilization because any remaining soil may inactivate germicidal solutions and thus protect microbes.

One important consideration in cleaning is the type and amount of bioburden on an item. Bioburden refers to the microbial population with which a specific object is contaminated, also known as bioload or microbial load. Unfortunately, no quantitative standard exists for decontamination processes; therefore, it is very difficult to assess their efficacy.

The following lists the steps required for decontaminating flexible endoscopes:

• Immediately after use, perform leak test (see leak tester endoscope instruction manual) and inspect all scopes for damage. If damage is detected, do not soak equipment; instead, consult the manufacturer.
• Disassemble the endoscope according to the instruction manual.
• Scrupulously clean all channels and immersible parts of the endoscope with detergent and a channel brush, following the manufacturer's instructions.
• For nonimmersible portions of endoscopes, meticulously clean and wipe with alcohol-moistened pads.
• Following the cleaning process, rinse the endoscope and all channels thoroughly with water.

After thorough decontamination, the next step is sterilization or disinfection.

## STERILIZATION OR DISINFECTION

**Sterilization** is defined as the destruction of all forms of microbial life, including spores. In the hospital, it is commonly carried out by using steam under pressure, **ethylene oxide** (EtO), or prolonged soaking with EPA-approved sterilant/disinfectants. Sterilization of endoscopic equipment is not usually practical: EtO sterilization is time-consuming, conventional heat sterilizing methods will destroy flexible endoscopes, and prolonged immersion in sterilant/disinfectants may result in endoscope damage. Nevertheless, endoscopes are sometimes sent for EtO sterilization or for prolonged immersion in an EPA-registered sterilant/disinfectant. There is also a peracetic acid-based automated system on the market that allows endoscopes to be sterilized after each procedure.

If sterilization is not practical, **disinfection** is the alternative. The Centers for Disease Control (CDC) classify disinfectants according to the system originally proposed by Spaulding, which defines high, intermediate, and low levels of disinfection:

• High-level disinfectants are effective against vegetative bacteria, the tubercle bacillus, some bacterial spores, fungi, and viruses.
• Intermediate-level disinfectants are effective against vegetative bacteria and the tubercle bacillus, but not bacterial spores; they are effective against most fungi and against lipid and medium-size viruses. They may have limited activity against nonlipid and small viruses.
• Low-level disinfectants are effective against vegetative bacteria, but not the tubercle bacillus or bacterial spores; they are effective against fungi and lipid and medium-size viruses.

The CDC recommends that any semicritical medical equipment that touches mucous membranes, including endoscopes and accessories, receive high-level disinfection. According to SGNA's *Recommended Guidelines for Infection Control in Gastrointestinal Endoscopy Settings,* disinfectants such as certain **glutaraldehyde** or hydrogen peroxide–based chemical germicides may be used. Those germicides registered with the Environmental Protection Agency (EPA) as sterilant/disinfectant agents are appropriate. Following are the SGNA guidelines:

• Follow the chemical manufacturer's instructions for immersion time and other special considerations.
• Make sure all surfaces, lumens, and channels come in contact with the chemical agent.
• Routinely test the potency of the disinfectant solution, following the instructions provided with the test kit.
• Avoid entrapment of air. Use syringes to fill channels.
• Cover containers during immersion period.
• Remove equipment after the allotted time.

If an automated washer/disinfector is used, prior cleaning is required to remove gross contaminants. All nonimmersible parts of the endoscope should be cleaned with 70% alcohol-moistened pads. The washer/disinfector should circulate the detergent and/or disinfectant through all channels at equal pressure without trapping air. The disinfectant should not be diluted with wash or rinse water. Washing and disinfection cycles should be followed by thorough rinse cycles and forced-air drying. No residual water should remain in the water hoses or reservoirs. All mechanical washer/disinfectors must be routinely disinfected according to the manufacturer's instructions and institutional policy.

To remove toxic chemicals, adequate rinsing must follow any type of disinfection. Sterile water is ideal for rinsing, but may be impractical or impossible in most gastroenterology settings. Rinsing must be followed by thorough drying. Seventy percent alcohol can be flushed through the channels to facilitate drying, followed by air to remove any residual alcohol. The scopes should then be hung vertically in a well-ventilated closet to prevent recontamination or damage between uses.

Because of the increase in the number of patients seen with hepatitis B (HBV) or HIV, there has been some controversy regarding the care of endoscopes used on these patients. Because scopes may be used on patients with both recognized and unrecognized infections, it is important that they be cleaned and disinfected thoroughly after *each* use, regardless of the patient's status.

### Accessory equipment

The use of disposable accessories is optimal because it eliminates the need for reprocessing. It is imperative that the gastroenterology nurse categorize reusable accessories to determine how to disinfect or sterilize them. For example, biopsy forceps break the mucosal barrier, a fact that places them in Spaulding's critical category and requires that they be sterilized after each use. Only steam under pressure will penetrate the metal coils of this springlike structure and any residual debris on these forceps. It is important to note, however, that the sterile forceps will be handled and passed through a nonsterile scope when in use and therefore the forceps will not be sterile during the procedure.

Another accessory used in the gastroenterology unit is the water bottle and its connecting tube which, according to SGNA guidelines, should be sterilized daily. Sterile water should be used to fill the bottle for endoscopic irrigation. A fresh, sterile bottle and sterile water should be used for each endoscopic retrograde cholangiopancreatography (ERCP) examination.

Every unit must have policies and procedures that govern the way patient care items are managed. The personnel involved with decontamination/disinfection/ sterilization processes must be well qualified and educated regarding proper cleaning methods and hazards associated with the work environment. Personnel must receive instruction on the basic principles of microbiology, infection-control practices, decontamination/ disinfection/sterilization processes, and employee safety

procedures. Ongoing education must be provided and documented.

### SANITATION

Safe and effective sanitation methods are an essential component of infection control practices within any gastroenterology unit. Such methods are necessary to remove sources of contamination, thereby minimizing the hazards of cross-contamination and lessening the risk of nosocomial infections.

SGNA guidelines recommend the use of an EPA-registered tuberculocidal "hospital disinfectant" for general wipe-down of noncritical items, such as procedure carts and stretchers. Environmental surfaces such as walls and floors should also be wiped down on a routine basis. Policies and procedures must be developed and adhered to for routine housekeeping.

Visible spills of blood or blood-contaminated body fluid should be blotted up *immediately* with disposable towels. The spill area should then be wiped with clean, disposable towels soaked in freshly prepared household bleach or an EPA-registered tuberculocidal hospital disinfectant, and allowed to dry.

Endoscopy schedules should be planned so there is sufficient time for adequate processing of instruments and for the cleaning and set-up of the unit for the next patient.

### WASTE MANAGEMENT

Confinement and removal of potentially **infectious waste** is another important aspect of infection control. Healthcare facilities must have written policies and procedures for handling waste from the point of generation to the point of disposal. Clear guidelines that spell out minimization and segregation standards of infectious versus noninfectious waste are essential. Having standardized policies and procedures for the disposal of non-infectious and infectious waste helps to eliminate accidental exposure of personnel, cross-contamination of patients, and fines for improper disposal.

There is a plethora of waste management guidelines and regulations that must be taken into account when devising a waste management plan, including information provided by JCAHO and by various federal, state, and local agencies. For example, EPA guidelines specifically state that isolation wastes, cultures, stocks of infectious agents and associated biologic materials, human blood, blood products, pathologic wastes, and contaminated "sharps" (needles, lancets, and so on) are infectious waste and must be handled according to specific rules. The institution has the option of designating other materials as infectious waste. When the gastroenterology unit manager develops waste disposal guidelines, he or she must consider protection of staff and patients, regulatory compliance; risk management;

the cost of disposal, including personnel, special containers, and fees for transport and disposal; and environmental effect. Guidelines must address the following issues:

- Use of personal protective equipment
- Handwashing
- Suctioning patients and changing suction tubing
- Handling of specimens
- Handling of contaminated instruments
- Segregation and disposition of trash
- Handling and disposition of linen, suction or body fluid contents, and sharps

Needles and sharps must be discarded in designated disposal containers. They must not be bent, cut, or broken by hand before disposal. Use of needle cutters is not recommended. Used needles must not be recapped by hand. Many gastroenterology nurses use recapping devices.

To carry out an effective waste management plan, all personnel must be educated about proper methods of handling and disposing of waste, penalties for noncompliance, and their respective responsibilities.

## HEALTHCARE WORKER SAFETY

Protection of healthcare personnel from exposure to infectious agents is another aspect of a comprehensive infection control program. It is important that gastroenterology nurses be aware of common viruses and bacteria and their methods of transmission. The CDC defines **Universal Precautions** that should be followed in all endoscopic procedures, including the following:

- Gloves must be worn when touching blood or contaminated body fluids, mucous membranes, or nonintact skin of all patients; for handling items or surfaces soiled with blood or body fluids; for all cleanup procedures; and for vascular access procedures.
- Masks and eye protection and protective clothing must be worn when performing tasks where blood or blood-contaminated body fluids are encountered and where splashing is likely to occur.
- Personnel with open skin lesions should not perform or assist with any endoscopic procedures or handle equipment used for procedures.
- Jewelry, watches, glue-on nails, and fingernail polish can harbor microorganisms and hinder effective handwashing; they should not be worn by gastroenterology personnel. To avoid puncturing gloves, fingernails must be kept short.
- Hands must be washed when entering or leaving the endoscopy unit, when removing gloves, and between contact with patients and/or their secretions.
- All gastroenterology personnel, if not seropositive for anti-HBs, should be immunized with the hepatitis B vaccine.

In addition to the recommendations outlined in this chapter, it is essential that gastroenterology personnel know and abide by institutional policies and procedures pertaining to infection control, and that manufacturers' guidelines for the decontamination and disinfection of patient care items be strictly followed.

---

**CASE SITUATION**

---

Peter Kraus is a 25-year-old male who has recently been diagnosed as HIV positive. He has a history of migraine headaches and has suffered from constipation for a long time. His migraines have been brought under control; however, the constipation is getting progressively worse. At this time he is having a bowel movement once every 5 days and then only when taking a laxative. Other diagnostic tests have been performed and the physician is planning to do a colonoscopy.

*Points to think about*

1. Keeping in mind that Mr. Kraus is HIV positive, what protection should be considered for personnel during the colonoscopy?
2. Upon completion of the procedure, how should the accessories be cleaned?
3. How would the environment be cleaned at the conclusion of the procedure?
4. At the completion of the procedure, what steps must the gastroenterology nurse take to properly decontaminate and disinfect the flexible colonoscope before use on subsequent patients?

*Suggested responses*

1. Regardless of the patient's immune status, personnel should apply consistent infection-control practices, including:
   - Wearing gloves when touching blood or blood-contaminated body fluids or instruments
   - Wearing masks and eye protection
   - Wearing moisture-resistant gowns or aprons when soiling of clothing with blood or body fluids is anticipated
   - Not performing or assisting in procedures if they have open lesions or dermatitis
   - Not wearing jewelry, watches, glue-on nails, or fingernail polish, because these items harbor microorganisms and make effective handwashing difficult
   - Washing hands thoroughly between endoscopy procedures and patient contacts
2. Disposable accessories may be used. If nondisposable accessories are used, they must be meticulously cleaned, and disinfected or sterilized according to manufacturers' instructions.

3. At the conclusion of the colonoscopy, the environment should be cleaned by:
   • Confining and removing organic material
   • Using moisture-proof disposable drapes as protective coverings for procedure carts and equipment
   • Using an EPA-registered "tuberculocidal" hospital disinfectant for general wipe-down of all noncritical equipment
   • Using a 1:100 dilution of household bleach or an EPA registered tuberculosidal hospital disenfectant for visible spills of blood or blood-contaminated body fluids
   • Discarding moist, grossly contaminated waste in a disposable, leak-proof container
   • Transporting grossly soiled linen with minimal handling in labeled, leak-proof bags
4. In order to properly decontaminate and disinfect the flexible colonoscope, the gastroenterology nurse should:
   • Consider the flexible colonoscope as a semicritical item that has been in contact with mucous membranes
   • Wash hands, don rubber gloves and goggles, and protect skin and clothing by wearing a protective cover gown
   • Thoroughly inspect the colonoscope for damage
   • Clean, decontaminate, and dry the scope in accordance with SGNA infection-control guidelines and the manufacturer's instructions
   • Provide high-level disinfection for the colonoscope and its accessories by using an appropriate "sterilant/disinfectant"
   • Know the required precautionary measures and potential adverse reactions to the agent used for high-level disinfection
   • Following the appropriate disinfection process, thoroughly rinse and dry all colonoscope components to remove any residual toxic chemicals
   • Store the colonoscope by hanging vertically in a well-ventilated closet to prevent recontamination and damage between uses
   • Dispose of gloves and protective coverings according to hospital policy and wash hands thoroughly

**REVIEW TERMS**

**critical items, decontamination, disinfection, ethylene oxide, glutaraldehyde, infectious waste, microorganisms, noncritical items, sanitation, semicritical items, sterilization, Universal Precautions**

**REVIEW QUESTIONS**

1. Which of the following is *not* one of the links in the chain of infection?
   a. Susceptible host.
   b. Contamination.
   c. Means of transmission.
   d. Infectious organism.
2. An example of a noncritical item that has little risk of transmitting an infection might be a(n):
   a. Intravenous catheter.
   b. Pulse oximeter.
   c. Biopsy forceps.
   d. Flexible endoscope.
3. According to SGNA guidelines, the first step in processing an endoscope following a procedure is to:
   a. Clean it with a detergent.
   b. Inspect it for damage.
   c. Rinse it with water.
   d. Hang it vertically in a well-ventilated cabinet.
4. As part of the decontamination process, the nonimmersible portions of an endoscope should be:
   a. Wiped with alcohol-moistened pads.
   b. Rinsed with water.
   c. Sterilized with ethylene oxide (EtO).
   d. Cleaned with a detergent.
5. Ethylene oxide sterilization of endoscopes is not always practical because:
   a. It does not destroy all microorganisms.
   b. Ethylene oxide is toxic.
   c. It can damage the scope.
   d. It takes too long.
6. An example of a conventional heat sterilization method that will destroy a flexible endoscope is:
   a. Steam sterilization.
   b. Ethylene oxide.
   c. Peracetic acid-based systems.
   d. EPA-registered sterilants/disinfectants.
7. High-level disinfectants destroy all of the following microorganisms *except:*
   a. Fungi.
   b. Bacteria.
   c. Spores.
   d. Viruses.
8. For patients with AIDS or hepatitis B:
   a. Endoscopes should be sterilized overnight with glutaraldehyde.
   b. Endoscopes should be processed as usual.
   c. Endoscopes should be kept in a separate cabinet and used only for those patients.
   d. Endoscopic procedures are contraindicated.
9. After use, biopsy forceps should be:
   a. Sterilized with ethylene oxide.
   b. Steam sterilized.
   c. Disinfected with glutaraldehyde.
   d. Disinfected with hydrogen peroxide.
10. After use, needles and sharps should be:
    a. Bent or cut before disposal.
    b. Recapped by hand.

c. Discarded in designated containers.
d. Discarded as noninfectious waste.

## BIBLIOGRAPHY

Beck, M, ed. *Recommended Guidelines for Infection Control in Gastrointestinal Endoscopy Settings.* 2nd ed. SGNA Monograph Series. Rochester, N.Y.: Society of Gastroenterology Nurses and Associates, 1990.

Environmental Protection Agency. *EPA Guide for Infectious Waste Management.* EPA/530-SW-86-014, NTIS No. PB86-199130. Washington, D.C.: EPA Office of Solid Waste, 1986.

Garner, J, and Favero, M. *Guideline for Handwashing and Hospital Environmental Control.* Atlanta: Centers for Disease Control, 1985.

Graham, G. "Decontamination: A Microbiologist's Perspective." *Journal of Healthcare Material Management* 5(January-February 1988): 36-41.

Rutala, W. "APIC Guidelines for Selection and Use of Disinfectants." *American Journal of Infection Control* 18(April 1990): 99-117.

# Chapter 4

# ENVIRONMENTAL SAFETY

This chapter identifies the different types of environmental hazards that are present in gastroenterology settings and the precautions the gastroenterology nurse can take to protect both patients and healthcare personnel. The hazards associated with electrical equipment, ionizing radiation, chemical agents, and accidents are explored and the importance of disaster planning is stressed.

**Learning objectives**

After reviewing the content of this chapter, the gastroenterology nurse should be able to:
1. Identify hazards in the endoscopy unit that have a potential to cause harm to patients or personnel, including electrical equipment, radiographic equipment, chemical agents, and accidents.
2. Describe steps that may be taken to minimize the dangers associated with these hazards, including disaster planning.
3. Explain the responsibilities of gastroenterology personnel for assuring a safe environment.

Basic safety regulations that govern hospitals are found in the standards, guidelines, and codes of local, state, and federal agencies, such as the Occupational Safety and Health Administration (OSHA), and voluntary standard-setting groups, such as the Joint Commission on Accreditation of Healthcare Organizations (JCAHO) and the National Fire Protection Association (NFPA). It is the legal, ethical, and moral responsibility of all gastroenterology personnel to be aware of these safety standards and how they affect patient care in the gastroenterology suite. This chapter highlights only the most important safety precautions.

## ELECTRICITY

Electrical equipment is everywhere in the endoscopy suite. Light sources, cautery devices, lasers, and video equipment are all powered by electrical energy, as are lights, many operating tables, and radiographic equipment. The three most common hazards relative to electricity are fire, burns, and shock, or electrocution.

- Fires can be started by faulty wiring, extension cords, poorly maintained equipment, and unsafe practices.
- Burns can occur from direct contact with overheated electrical wires or by contact with other items that have been heated by contact with faulty wires. In the GI lab, the primary danger of electrical burns occurs with the use of electrocautery devices and lasers.
- Any direct contact with 110- or 220-volt wiring has the potential for **electrocution.** If the voltage is high enough, it can damage the brain and respiratory center, resulting in apnea. Low-voltage currents frequently affect the heart, causing ventricular fibrillation. Complications of electrical **shock** may include vascular injury, loss of consciousness, damage to the respiratory center, infection, cardiac arrhythmias, and eye damage.

To prevent fires associated with electrically powered ignition sources, gastroenterology personnel can take the following measures:
- Use appropriate precautions with flammable gases or liquids.
- Before use, check the integrity of all electrical equipment, including cords, switches, plugs, and wall receptacles.
- Be sure that all electrical equipment is properly grounded.
- Do not use multiple-outlet adapters or two-wire extension cords. Do not remove ground pins from three-pin plugs.
- Avoid routing power lines through heavy traffic areas and avoid rolling equipment over electrical cords.
- Follow manufacturers' recommendations and standards for all electrical equipment.

- Enforce and document maintenance routines for electrical devices.
- Remove and report any questionable electrical equipment.
- Never place containers of liquid on electrical equipment.

Even when staff take all reasonable precautions, it is still possible for a fire to occur in the endoscopy suite. To handle a fire quickly and effectively, gastroenterology personnel must participate in periodic fire drills in which they practice using firefighting equipment. In addition, there should always be written procedures for handling a fire emergency. Fire policies and procedures should be reviewed regularly and whenever a new type of equipment is installed.

If a fire occurs, it is important to proceed with the following steps:

- Sound the alarm.
- Smother or extinguish the flames, if possible, using a **Halon** extinguisher for an electrical fire. Never use water to extinguish an electrical fire.
- Disconnect electrical equipment from its power source and throw the appropriate circuit breaker.
- Close all gas supply valves.
- If the fire involves an endotracheal tube, disconnect the tube and remove it.
- Treat materials that are melting, dripping, or smoking as if they are actually burning, in order to eliminate the possibility of their igniting or re-igniting.
- Remove patients and staff from the immediate danger zone, if feasible.
- Close all doors to confine smoke and flames.
- Direct firefighters to the location of the fire.

When a fire involves a patient directly, personnel should remove burning articles or smother the flame with a blanket. Smoldering, charred debris should be extinguished and removed from the patient immediately. Personnel should never use fire extinguishers directly on a patient because of the danger of cryogenic tissue damage or deposition of dangerous residues. After the fire has been extinguished, all burned material and equipment should be saved so the cause of the fire can be determined.

Additional details on the safe operation of specific electrical devices used in the endoscopy unit are provided below.

### Endoscopes

Like any other electrical device, endoscopes must be checked for proper functioning before each use. Gastroenterology personnel should adhere to the following procedures:

- Check the integrity of all electrical cables before use.
- Follow institutional policies and procedures regarding testing electrical equipment; for example, never use an electrical device that has not been given a stamp of approval from the biomedical department.
- Do not handle equipment when hands, feet, body, or floor is wet.
- Never use the light source as a supply table.
- Turn on the light source and suction to make sure both are functioning properly.
- Turn the light source off when not in use.
- Look through the scope for broken fiber bundles, presence of fluid, or poor visualization. (Never tightly coil the endoscope because this causes the fiber bundles to break.)
- Check for bite marks or any indications of damage on the scope.
- Manipulate all controls.
- If there is a malfunction, do not use. Send equipment out for repair.

### Electrosurgical devices

Electrosurgical units (ESUs) are among the most hazardous electrical devices used in the GI lab. Burns can result from poorly applied **grounding pads** or when electrical current seeks alternative pathways out of the body, such as through ECG electrodes or metal objects like IV poles and stirrups. Bipolar electrosurgery may be safer than the monopolar modality because the current returns through the electrode itself.

To avoid problems with electrocautery devices, it is important to follow the manufacturer's instructions for testing the equipment before the procedure. It is also important to properly ground the patient and equipment. In monopolar electrocautery, the grounding pad should be attached securely to a muscular site, well vascularized, and away from bony prominences or places where circulation is likely to be impaired.

Electrosurgery probes, when out of use, should be placed in a safe location. The handpiece should always be in direct view when activated and the ESU should be used on the lowest possible power setting. The unit should have an audio tone so everyone knows when it is activated. The unit should be turned off or placed in a standby mode following each use.

If power settings above normal are required to cut or coagulate, the electrical return pathway could be faulty and the machine should be removed from service until the problem is corrected.

### Lasers

The most dangerous aspects of lasers are misdirection, scattering of the laser beam, and smoke inhalation. Whenever lasers are in use there is a potential for damage to the skin or eyes of patients and personnel. To prevent such injuries, personnel should follow the guidelines below:

- Place a warning sign on the door leading into the room where the laser is in use.
- Provide protective eyewear for all patients and personnel. The optical density of the eyewear should be equivalent to the wavelength of the laser used.
- Use instruments that are anodized or covered with a nonreflective coating to prevent inadvertent beam reflection.
- Place the laser in the standby mode when it is not in use and allow the physician access to only one foot pedal when it is in use.
- Use lasers with a tamperproof audio tone that sounds when the beam is being activated.
- Use smoke evacuators to minimize the inhalation of the smoke produced in laser procedures.

## Maintenance

Every piece of electrical equipment must have an operation manual, and routine preventive maintenance checks should be performed by the biomedical engineering department. "Inservice" seminars should be held on a regular basis to update staff members on new equipment or changes in old equipment.

All malfunctioning electrical equipment must be reported immediately, and appropriate action taken. Policies and procedures must specify what to do about equipment problems.

## RADIATION

Waves of electromagnetic energy can penetrate almost anything by disrupting bonds between atoms and creating electrically charged ions, hence the term **"ionizing radiation."** Radiation is a hazard because of its ability to modify molecules within body cells, thus causing cell dysfunction, alteration or halt in cell replication, or cell destruction. The effects of radiation may be somatic or genetic.

The primary source of ionizing radiation in the endoscopy suite is fluoroscopy. Fluoroscopy allows the physician and nurse to quickly view and monitor the placement of catheters, stents, dilators, or colonoscopes. In addition, portable x-ray machines may be used for diagnostic purposes. Government regulations limit permissible levels of exposure to radiation to 5 rem per year for workers over the age of 18 years.

There is no level of ionizing radiation that is not potentially harmful. Unnecessary exposure can be minimized in the following three ways:
- Decreasing the time of exposure
- Increasing the distance from the source
- Placing a shield between the radiation source and the body

All female patients of childbearing age should be questioned about the possibility of pregnancy before radiographic procedures. Pregnant employees should not be permitted to assist with such procedures.

The following protective guidelines may help minimize the exposure of gastroenterology patients and personnel to ionizing radiation:
- Wear lead-lined aprons, collars, gloves, and protective eyewear in accordance with institutional guidelines. Use gonadal shielding as appropriate.
- Wear film badges during procedures in which radiation exposure is encountered.
- Analyze exposure levels monthly.
- Alternate personnel for procedures that require radiation and limit exposure time for personnel holding patients and/or films.
- When the fluoroscope is in use, instruct personnel not to turn their unshielded backs to the radiographic equipment and to maintain as great a distance from the x-ray beam as possible.
- Allow only trained personnel to operate and maintain all radiographic equipment.
- Be certain that the contrast medium selected is effective for the type of study being done.
- To help reduce unnecessary repeat procedures, be sure the patient is properly prepared and positioned. Expose only the area of study to the film or fluoroscopy.
- Consult with a radiation safety officer regarding equipment inspection, analysis of radiation exposure badges, and educational inservices.

When handled properly and efficiently, ionizing radiation can be an effective diagnostic and therapeutic tool in the endoscopy suite, but it is important to treat such tools with respect.

## CHEMICALS

Gastroenterology personnel come into daily contact with a large number of chemicals, some of which carry high exposure risks. There are certain common-sense rules for handling chemicals.
- Always read and follow label directions. Obtain medical safety data sheets on all hazardous chemicals.
- Mix chemicals only in accordance with directions.
- Use the rules of Universal Precautions as if the chemicals were body fluids: if it will come in contact with the hands, wear gloves; if it might splash, use protective eyewear and clothing, if necessary; wash hands after using any chemicals.
- After the use of disinfectants, rinse instruments or surfaces thoroughly to remove any harmful residue.

One of the most frequently encountered hazardous chemicals in the endoscopy suite is glutaraldehyde. Because glutaraldehyde is water-soluble, its main effects are on the mucous membranes and the eyes. Short-term exposure can cause nose and throat irritation, burning of the eyes, and headaches.

When handling glutaraldehyde, gastroenterology personnel should wear rubber gloves, goggles, a mask, and an apron. Glutaraldehyde should be stored in a covered container in a cool, dry place. Sinks, showers, and eyewash stations should be available. If glutaraldehyde comes in contact with the eyes, the eyes should be flushed with water for a full 15 minutes. Skin should be washed thoroughly; clothing should be removed and washed before reuse. In case of excessive inhalation, the individual should be moved to fresh air and treated medically as symptoms warrant.

Another hazardous chemical that gastroenterology personnel are exposed to is formaldehyde, which is used primarily as a tissue fixative. Like glutaraldehyde, formaldehyde is highly soluble in water and therefore mainly affects the mucous membranes and the eyes. To minimize exposure, personnel should wear gloves, goggles, aprons, and masks. Formaldehyde should be stored in an airtight container. Personnel should be informed about possible adverse reactions. First-aid measures are the same as for glutaraldehyde.

Isopropyl (rubbing) alcohol is also found in endoscopy suites. Gloves should be worn when using this chemical and care should be taken to avoid splashing, because it may cause corneal burns and eye damage. Isopropyl alcohol is highly flammable and therefore should be stored in tightly closed containers, away from heat, flames, or sparks. In case of excessive inhalation, the individual should be moved to fresh air and possibly given medical support. In case of ingestion, the individual must receive immediate medical treatment.

To avoid leakage, mercury-filled dilators should be inspected on a set schedule to ensure that they are intact and that their expiration dates have not passed.

## ACCIDENTAL INJURY

A few simple preventive measures go a long way toward helping gastroenterology personnel reduce the risk of accidental injury to themselves and/or their patients.

Human errors related to the operation of medical devices in the endoscopy suite can be minimized by utilizing built-in safety features such as the audible activation indicator on an ESU; providing adequate operator training; and servicing equipment regularly.

With the enactment of the new Safe Medical Devices Act, healthcare facilities are now required to report device-related injuries and illnesses to the Food and Drug Administration (FDA) and to the manufacturer. If problems develop, the FDA has the authority to recall certain devices.

Accidental falls are another potential source of injury. To avoid accidental falls in the endoscopy suite, the following steps should be taken:

- Hallways and doorways should be free of equipment and carts.

- Rooms should be kept neat and orderly.
- Electrical cords, cable, and tubing should be placed so personnel do not trip and fall.

Mental or physical exhaustion can also contribute to the risk of accidents. Proper lifting techniques must be practiced. Comfortable temperatures, noise control, ventilation, and adequate lighting are essential.

OSHA is the federal agency responsible for regulating workplace environments to ensure safety. It is important that the endoscopy unit comply with all applicable OSHA standards.

## DISASTER PLANNING

Hospital staff must be prepared to respond quickly and effectively to internal or external disasters. Although rare, the occurrence of such events is a real possibility and must be anticipated. Personnel must be familiar with institutional policies for fire, severe weather, and other disasters.

An internal disaster plan that includes procedures for moving patients out of the unit or evacuating them from the building should be devised and posted. Simulated disaster drills help personnel evaluate how they would function in a crisis.

---

**CASE SITUATION**

Mr. Marks is a 63-year-old male who has been admitted to the endoscopy unit for laser vaporization of multiple sessile polyps of the colon. The treatment room has been set up for a flexible video colonoscopic procedure using the contact Nd:YAG laser system.

*Points to think about*

1. In setting up the treatment room, what precautions must the gastroenterology nurse take to minimize the potential dangers associated with electrical equipment?
2. During set-up, how might the gastroenterology nurse minimize any hazards associated with the use of the Nd:YAG laser system?
3. Mr. Marks is admitted to the treatment room, properly sedated, and positioned on his side. The physician begins the colonoscopy, identifies the sessile polyps to be treated, and requests the laser fiber. During the procedure, what measures must the gastroenterology nurse take to protect the patient and personnel from accidental exposure to laser energy?

*Suggested responses*

1. To avoid problems with electrical equipment, it is important that the gastroenterology nurse accomplish the following precautionary steps:

- Check the integrity of all electrical cords.
- Position equipment and power lines away from heavy traffic areas and out of the paths of rolling equipment.
- Verify proper operation of all equipment and remove and report any questionable equipment.
- Keep liquids away from electrical equipment.
- Know the location of the nearest Halon fire extinguisher.

2. To avoid accidental injury associated with the use of the Nd:YAG laser system, setup procedures should include the following:
- Post the appropriate laser warning sign on all doors leading into the treatment room.
- Ensure that appropriate eyewear for the Nd:YAG laser is readily available outside each entrance to the treatment room.
- Because the Nd:YAG, KTP, and argon laser beams can transmit through glass, cover all windows in the treatment room to prevent accidental exposure.
- Remove all volatile liquids, such as alcohol or benzoin, from the treatment room when the laser is to be used.
- Use a smoke evacuator to remove potentially harmful smoke.

3. To avoid accidental exposure of the patient and personnel to laser energy during the procedure, it is important that the gastroenterology nurse take the following precautions:
- Ensure that Mr. Marks and all personnel are wearing the appropriate protective eyewear.
- Use the appropriate scope filters, shutter, or protective eyepiece to avoid video interference and to protect the physician's eyes from scattering of laser energy.
- Instruct Mr. Marks on the importance of wearing protective eyewear and caution him to avoid unnecessary movement while the laser is being used.
- Limit entrance to and exit from the treatment room while the laser is activated.
- To prevent accidental damage to the internal components of the scope, ensure that the tip of the laser fiber is completely clear of the flexible endoscope channel before activating the laser.
- Prevent traffic between the physician and the laser machine to avoid accidental extraction and/or fracture of the laser fiber.
- Verify fiber integrity by visualizing a clear, concentric timing beam only at the distal tip of the fiber, and by confirming that there is no escape of light along the axis of the fiber.
- Ensure that all laser settings are clearly understood by the person operating the laser and the physician.
- Do not allow the physician access to more than one foot pedal.

- When suction is used in conjunction with laser vaporization, ensure that a disposable laser plume filter is placed between the collection bottle and the suction source.

**REVIEW TERMS**

**electrocution, grounding pads, Halon, ionizing radiation, shock**

**REVIEW QUESTIONS**

1. An electrical fire that does not involve the patient directly should be handled by:
   a. Using a Halon extinguisher.
   b. Throwing water on it.
   c. Immediately removing the patient from the room.
   d. Suffocation with a fire blanket.
2. When out of use, an ESU probe should:
   a. Be set down on a drape.
   b. Be placed in a safe location.
   c. Remain in the endoscopist's hand.
   d. Be handed to an assistant.
3. To avoid accidental injuries to patients and personnel when a laser is in use, it is important to:
   a. Use protective eyewear.
   b. Post "laser in use" signs.
   c. Use nonreflective instruments.
   d. All of the above.
4. For laser procedures, the optical density of the protective eyewear used is determined by:
   a. The physician's preference.
   b. The procedure that will be performed.
   c. Institutional policies and procedures.
   d. The wavelength of the laser being used.
5. If a piece of electrical equipment malfunctions, it should be:
   a. Fixed by gastroenterology personnel.
   b. Removed from service and reported according to institutional policy.
   c. Used again to see if the problem recurs.
   d. Reported to the FDA.
6. When ionizing radiation is in use, pregnant healthcare workers should:
   a. Wear a lead-lined apron.
   b. Limit exposure to 5 rem per year.
   c. Not assist at all.
   d. Wear a film badge.
7. The primary source of ionizing radiation in the endoscopy suite is:
   a. Portable radiographic equipment.
   b. Fluoroscopy.
   c. Radionuclides.
   d. CT scans.

8. If glutaraldehyde accidentally comes in contact with a healthcare worker's skin, he or she should:
   a. Wash the area thoroughly.
   b. Rinse the area with water only.
   c. Apply burn ointment.
   d. Cover the area with a bandage.
9. Under the new Safe Medical Devices Act, healthcare facilities are required to report device-related illnesses and accidents to:
   a. The manufacturer.
   b. OSHA.
   c. The FDA.
   d. The FDA and the manufacturer.
10. Plans for evacuating patients in the event of an internal disaster should be:
   a. Posted in an obvious location.
   b. Recorded in institutional policies and procedures manuals.
   c. Practiced in simulated disaster drills.
   d. All of the above.

## BIBLIOGRAPHY

Association of Operating Room Nurses. *AORN Standards and Recommended Practices for Perioperative Nursing.* Denver: Association of Operating Room Nurses, 1991.

Cwalina, W, Gust, C, Lorenzo, C, Monica, M, Nelson, A, and Stone, K. "Occupational Hazards in the Endoscopy Suite." *SGA Journal* 11(Fall 1988): 100-05.

Joint Commission on Accreditation of Healthcare Organizations. *Accreditation Manual for Hospitals, 1991 Ed.* Oakbrook Terrace, Ill.: JCAHO, 1990.

Kneedler, J, and Dodge, G. *Perioperative Patient Care.* 2nd ed. Boston: Blackwell Scientific Publications, Inc., 1987.

Marousky, R. "The Material Safety Data Sheet: A Guide to Chemical Safety in the OR." *Today's O.R. Nurse* 13(June 1991): 6-11.

Patterson, Pat. "Advice for Users on Compliance with Devices Act." *OR Manager* 7(May 1991): 1, 14-15.

# Chapter 5

# STANDARDS FOR PRACTICE

This chapter acquaints the gastroenterology nurse with the standards for practice that guide gastroenterology nursing. Standards for practice in the context of this chapter are viewed as any standards used by gastroenterology nurses and associates to define the scope of their professional practice. These include the Society of Gastroenterology Nurses and Associates (SGNA) *Standards for Practice,* the **American Nurses' Association (ANA)** *Standards of Clinical Nursing Practice,* and the Joint Commission on Accreditation of Healthcare Organizations (JCAHO) hospital standards. The JCAHO statement of patients' rights and responsibilities and SGNA's infection control guidelines are summarized. Pertinent standards, regulations, and guidelines issued by governmental agencies are also reviewed.

## Learning objectives

After reviewing the content of this chapter, the gastroenterology nurse should be able to:
1. Outline the expected behavior of the gastroenterology nurse as set forth in the SGNA *Standards for Practice.*
2. Discuss the JCAHO standards that influence gastroenterology practice in the hospital setting, and the JCAHO statement of patients' rights and responsibilities.
3. Explain how regulations and guidelines developed by specific government agencies guide practice in the endoscopy unit.

## STANDARDS DEFINED

Standards provide guidelines for professional behavior. They are the yardstick by which professionals are measured in job evaluations, and by which they may be judged in malpractice actions.

**Standards for practice** are qualitative, conceptual statements that describe practice outcomes. They are not intended to specify how an outcome is to be achieved, but rather what is to be achieved. **Standards of care,** on the other hand, are measurable statements that define the means to accomplish practice outcomes. They define criteria against which the nurse's level of performance may be measured.

Standards of care cannot be static. As technology and knowledge advance, so must the approach to care. Standards must be continually validated in the practice setting. Their relevance must be evaluated critically as technology and scientific knowledge develop.

## SOURCES OF STANDARDS AND GUIDELINES IN GASTROENTEROLOGY NURSING

Standards and guidelines that provide directions for gastroenterology nurses include standards of nursing practice, accreditation standards, community standards, standards of technical practice, and the regulations and guidelines issued by various government agencies.
- Standards of nursing practice have been developed by SGNA, ANA, and other specialty nursing organizations.
- Accreditation standards include those developed by the JCAHO.
- Community standards based on legal and ethical principles also affect practice in the endoscopy unit, as exemplified by statements of patients' rights and responsibilities.
- Standards of technical practice may be developed in individual endoscopy units, with reference to guidelines issued by professional associations, such as SGNA's *Recommended Guidelines for Infection Control.* Technical standards must be congruent with other standards that apply to the gastroenterology nurse and associate.
- A number of federal regulations and guidelines also affect the practice of gastroenterology nursing.

## SGNA STANDARDS FOR PRACTICE

In 1986, when it became apparent that the organization had outgrown the standards written in 1979, the SGNA Standards of Practice Committee began working toward the development of an innovative set of practice standards. The final standards were developed with the assistance of a facilitator and presented at the 1990 fall course.

These unique standards for practice are qualitative, conceptual outcome statements that are intended to specify the expected result of the care provided. They describe what is to be accomplished, not how those outcomes are to be achieved. The criteria necessary to meet these standards should be individualized for each work setting, based on the policies, procedures, and practices of the employing institution and the education and professional licensure of its staff.

The SGNA *Standards for Practice* reflect the organization's values of collegiality, continuity of care, collaboration, commitment, and patient advocacy. They are broad enough to encompass the practice of all gastroenterology staff members (RNs, LPNs, NAs, or technicians) within their job descriptions, professional licensure, and institutional constraints.

The standards are designed to be applicable across a continuum that covers independent, collaborative, and dependent aspects of practice. SGNA members perform some tasks independently, some in collaboration with others, and some dependent on the performance or judgment of another individual. Whether or not an action can be performed independently depends on state Nurse Practice Acts, educational background, and institutional policy. For example, an RN might conduct a patient assessment independently, collaborate with a physician when assisting with an endoscopic biopsy, and be dependent on the physician for ordering diagnostic tests or transfusions. Similar examples may be devised for independent, collaborative, and dependent activities of an LPN or technician.

The SGNA *Standards for Practice* are listed below and accompanied by examples of measurable criteria or standards of care that might be created to specify how each standard should be adapted to an individual practice setting.

The gastroenterology nurse or associate:

I. Performs the technical procedures required by the patient need/assignment without causing harm and consistent with one's own scope of practice and the practice setting's legal constraints.

*Example:* Cleans and disinfects all endoscopes according to institutional policy and procedure.

II. Initiates actions to insure continuity of effective care before, during, and/or after the patient's contact with the practice setting.

*Example:* Provides a written set of preparatory instructions, including a phone number, to each outpatient scheduled for an endoscopy.

III. Documents actions and interventions, outcomes and responses, and/or assessment data consistent with the policy and procedures of the practice setting.

*Example:* Documents pre-, intra-, and post-endoscopy vital signs, level of consciousness, and nursing assessment on the periprocedure nursing care overprint.

IV. Participates in activities to maintain and/or enhance the competent practice of self and others as defined by the nursing profession/SGNA and consistent with the practice setting's legal constraints.

*Example:* All RNs obtain 20 continuing education credits per annum.

V. Acts on behalf of patients before, during, and/or after contact with the practice setting to ensure that their rights and/or values are not compromised.

*Example:* Assures the patient's right to privacy and confidentiality in the GI endoscopy unit.

VI. Initiates actions to prevent, correct, and/or reduce identified risks to individuals' health.

*Example:* Carries out Universal Precautions.

VII. Uses internal and/or external resources to prevent, resolve, and/or minimize patient/family health problems.

*Example:* Refers patient newly diagnosed with inflammatory bowel disease to the Ileitis and Colitis Foundation, or refers new ileostomy patients to community nursing care agency for follow-up after discharge.

VIII. Provides evaluative evidence of effective, efficient, and/or satisfying care in the practice setting.

*Example:* Conducts or participates in a research or quality assurance (QA) review to examine gastroenterology/endoscopy nursing or patient care-related questions.

IX. Changes, continues or discontinues practice on the basis of evaluative evidence.

*Example:* Shows evidence of a written plan to correct deficiencies identified during quarterly QA reviews.

X. Uses communication or interpersonal skills with individuals and/or groups to achieve desired/intended outcomes and/or feelings of satisfaction/acceptance.

*Example:* Conducts annual colorectal cancer screening program for the community.

XI. Supports actions/inactions/decisions with logical, ethical, legal rationale and/or proven experience.

*Example:* When referring a patient care problem to the ethics committee or ombudsman, provides evidence of the violation in question and reason for referral.

In addition to the *Standards for Practice* listed above, JCAHO accreditation standards demand that all gastroenterology nurses and associates adhere to JCAHO requirements in the hospital setting.

## JCAHO STANDARDS

The **Joint Commission on Accreditation of Healthcare Organizations (JCAHO)** is a voluntary accrediting agency that was established for the purpose of encouraging high standards of institutional health care. Standards developed by JCAHO reflect optimal achievable healthcare practices. They are reviewed and revised continually as warranted by technological developments, new knowledge, changes in government regulations, and consumer demands for accountability. Experts in applicable areas, government agencies, and responses to hospital surveys all provide input for new standards.

During a JCAHO accreditation survey, four sources are used to assess the healthcare organization's compliance with JCAHO standards, including:

- Documentation of compliance provided by the hospital
- Verbal answers to questions concerning the implementation of a standard, or examples of its implementation, that will enable a judgment of compliance to be made
- Interviews with patients and staff members
- On-site observations by JCAHO surveyors

To be accredited, a hospital must demonstrate that it is in substantial compliance with the standards in general. If a hospital is in substantial compliance with JCAHO standards, it is awarded accreditation for 3 years.

To meet JCAHO standards, in-hospital endoscopy/gastroenterology units must have certain specific characteristics. The *Accreditation Manual for Hospitals, 1991* has 24 separate sections covering different aspects of hospital management and patient care. Of these, the section most pertinent to gastroenterology nurses and associates is that of surgical and anesthesia services. (Gastroenterology departments are specifically assigned to this category.) Other relevant requirements deal with hospital-sponsored ambulatory care; infection control; nursing care; and plant, technology, and safety management.

- *Surgical and Anesthesia Services.* JCAHO requires that surgical and anesthesia services are available to meet patients' needs; that patients with the same health status and condition receive comparable surgical and anesthesia care throughout the hospital; that there is effective collaboration among departments/services providing and supporting surgical and anesthesia services; and that surgical and

anesthesia services participate in the hospital's quality assurance program.
- *Hospital-Sponsored Ambulatory Care Services.* JCAHO requires that ambulatory care services are safe and effective, and are integrated with other departments/services of the hospital; that staff participate in relevant educational programs or activities; that written policies and procedures address specific issues; that structures, systems, policies, and procedures are in place for safety management, life safety, equipment management, and utilities management; that comprehensive medical records are kept; that structures are in place that are designed to improve the quality of patient care; and that the ambulatory care unit participates in the hospital's quality-assurance program.
- *Infection Control.* JCAHO requires that there is an effective hospital-wide program for infection surveillance, prevention, and control; that a multidisciplinary committee is responsible for monitoring and correcting infection control practices; that a qualified individual(s) has responsibility for infection control activities; that there is written infection control policies and procedures; and that the infection control program is coordinated with support services, such as central services, housekeeping, and linen and laundry.
- *Nursing Care.* JCAHO requires that patients receive nursing care (based on a documented assessment of their needs) conducted by a registered nurse; that all members of the nursing staff are competent to fulfill assigned responsibilities; that patient care programs, policies, and procedures *based on nursing standards of patient care and standards of nursing practice\** are developed; that the hospital's plan for providing nursing care is designed to support improvement and innovation in nursing practice and is based on patient needs and the hospital's mission; that nursing leaders participate in the hospital's decision-making structures and processes; and that nursing care is monitored and evaluated as part of the hospital's quality assurance program.
- *Plant, Technology, and Safety Management.* JCAHO requires the existence of a safety management program concerned with the physical environment and staff activities; a life safety management program covering fire safety and the safe use of buildings and grounds; an equipment management program; and a utilities management program.

Relevant standards may also be found in the sections of the JCAHO manual on diagnostic radiology, medical records, pathology and medical laboratory services, quality assurance, and utilization review.

*Emphasis added.

## PATIENTS' RIGHTS AND RESPONSIBILITIES

When sickness occurs, it is difficult for patients to exert their rights; therefore, the gastroenterology nurse has the responsibility to assure that these rights are preserved for the patient. Patients also have responsibilities that they and their significant others should consider.

The JCAHO *Accreditation Manual for Hospitals* lists a number of basic patient rights and responsibilities that emphasize independence of expression, decision, and action and concern for personal dignity and human relationships.

According to JCAHO the patient has the following rights:

- Access to care. All patients have a right to access to treatment or accommodations that are available or medically indicated.
- Respect and dignity. Patients have the right to considerate, respectful care at all times and under all circumstances, with recognition of their personal dignity.
- Privacy and confidentiality. Patients have the right to expect that any interviews, examinations, or consultations will be conducted with consideration for their privacy and that their hospital records will remain confidential.
- Personal safety. Patients have the right to expect reasonable safety insofar as hospital practices and environment are concerned.
- Identity. Patients have the right to know the identity and professional status of individuals providing service to them, to know which practitioners are primarily responsible for their care, and to know of any professional relationships among individuals or institutions involved in their care.
- Information. Patients or their legally authorized representatives have the right to obtain complete, current, and understandable information concerning their diagnosis, treatment, and any known prognosis.
- Communication. Patients have the right of access to people outside the hospital by means of visitors and by verbal and written communication; interpreters should be provided where language barriers are a problem.
- Consent. Patients have the right to reasonable informed participation in decisions involving their care and the right to refuse participation in any research involving human experimentation.
- Consultation. Patients have the right to consult with specialists at their own request and expense.
- Refusal of treatment. Patients have the right to refuse treatment to the extent permitted by law.
- Transfer and continuity of care. Patients have the right to receive a complete explanation of the need for and alternatives to any transfer to another facility or organization and the right to be informed of any continuing healthcare needs following discharge from the hospital.
- Hospital charges. Patients have the right to an itemized and detailed explanation of the total bill for services rendered in the hospital.
- Hospital rules and regulations. Patients should be informed of hospital rules and regulations applicable to their conduct and about the hospital's mechanisms for handling patient complaints.

Furthermore, JCAHO states that hospitals have the right to expect behavior on the part of patients and their significant others that is reasonable and responsible, in view of the nature of their illness. Each patient's responsibilities include the following:

- Provision of information. Patients have the responsibility to provide an accurate and complete medical history, to report unexpected changes in their condition, and to communicate their understanding of the contemplated treatment regimen.
- Compliance with instructions. Patients are responsible for following the treatment plans recommended for their care and for keeping appointments or notifying the appropriate person if they are unable to do so.
- Refusal of treatment. Patients are responsible for their actions if they refuse treatment or do not follow the practitioner's instructions.
- Hospital charges. Patients are responsible for assuring that the financial obligations to the hospital are fulfilled as promptly as possible.
- Hospital rules and regulations. Patients are responsible for following hospital rules and regulations affecting patient care and conduct.
- Respect and consideration. Patients are responsible for being considerate of the rights of other patients and hospital personnel and respectful of the property or other persons and of the hospital.

Gastroenterology nurses and associates should respect the rights of all patients and their families, regardless of race, religion, sex, disease status, national origin, or sources of payment for care. At the same time, gastroenterology patients and their families must be made aware of their responsibilities to care givers, healthcare institutions, and other patients.

## SGNA RECOMMENDED GUIDELINES FOR INFECTION CONTROL

In addition to its general standards for practice, SGNA has published technical guidelines specific to infection control (Beck, 1990). These guidelines are intended to communicate the most current infection-control trends and techniques to practitioners in the endoscopy setting.

These guidelines include not only actions that minimize the potential of transmitting infectious agents from patient to patient but also actions that address the safety and health concerns of the gastroenterology nurse. They include recommendations for decontamination, disinfection, and sterilization of endoscopes and accessories; methods and practices to assure a safe environment; and guidelines for the protection of personnel.

These infection control guidelines should be reviewed in depth by each gastroenterology nurse, but may be adapted as appropriate for use in individual hospital-based and private practice settings. The guidelines are discussed in greater detail in Chapter 3.

## FEDERAL REGULATIONS AND GUIDELINES

In addition to the infection control guidelines developed by SGNA, several government agencies, including the **Centers for Disease Control (CDC),** the **Environmental Protection Agency (EPA),** the **Food and Drug Administration (FDA),** and the **Occupational Safety and Health Administration (OSHA),** have promulgated guidelines and regulations that have an impact on disinfection and sterilization practices in the endoscopy suite.

### Centers for Disease Control

The CDC has formulated a set of general guidelines for the prevention and control of nosocomial (hospital-acquired) infections. Most applicable to patient care in the endoscopy unit is the *Guideline for Handwashing and Hospital Environmental Control,* which covers hand washing; cleaning, disinfecting, and sterilizing patient care equipment; microbiologic sampling; management of infective waste; housekeeping; and laundry.

Although the CDC guidelines have no force of regulation or law and may be modified as appropriate in individual healthcare settings, they represent the best available compilation of practical, well-founded infection control practices. Some of the recommendations are based on well-documented epidemiologic studies; in areas where little scientific evidence is available, the guidelines are based on reasonable theoretic rationales.

### Environmental Protection Agency

The EPA is the federal agency that approves products for disinfectant registration after review of labeling and supporting data submitted by manufacturers. The EPA classifies chemical germicides as sporicides, general disinfectants, hospital disinfectants, sanitizers, and "others."

The role of the EPA is to carry out certain laws enacted by Congress. One of its functions is to regulate solid waste, which includes hazardous waste, such as toxic, ignitable, corrosive, and reactive waste. In November, 1988, this agency was commissioned to establish a demonstration program for tracking medical waste when federal regulations were signed into law.

The EPA developed specific guidelines for handling infectious waste from "the cradle to the grave." The guidelines cover designation of waste; handling, storage, packaging and transporting waste; selection of appropriate treatment and disposal methods; monitoring of treatment methods; and compliance with state and local requirements. The demonstration project was established for a 2-year period and the comprehensive goals were to collect information on the scope of the problem, the usefulness of the tracking system, and other alternatives to managing infectious medical waste.

### Food and Drug Administration

The FDA is the federal regulatory agency responsible for controlling the safety and effectiveness of drugs, devices, and instrumentation.

The complexity of medical devices and the increased number of new products resulted in Congress developing the comprehensive Medical Device Amendments of 1976 to the Federal Food, Drug, and Cosmetic Act. The primary reason for the amendments was to ensure that any new device was safe and effective before it was put on the market. Congress divided medical devices into two groups; according to three classes based on the potential hazards of the device, and according to a set of seven basic categories: preamendment, postamendment, substantially equivalent, implant, custom, investigational, and transitional.

There are essentially two ways that a new device gets on the market. If the manufacturer can establish substantial equivalence, premarket notification is all that is required. However, if the new device is not similar to a preamendment device, a Premarket Approval Application (PMA) must be filed.

Therefore, most manufacturers file a "Premarket Notification," which is referred to as a 510(K), before introducing a new product. This is a request by the manufacturer to the FDA to market a device. If the FDA does not approve, the only alternative is the lengthy process of submitting a PMA.

In some situations, the manufacturer may need to conduct clinical studies to support a PMA or 510(K) submission. If this is the case, the device may need to be distributed and used for investigational purposes. An Investigational Device Exemption (IDE) is obtained to ensure that the preclinical testing makes use of a predetermined protocol.

The FDA has also established a reporting system whereby the healthcare practitioner must report problems with medical devices. The new Safe Medical Device Act of 1990 requires healthcare facilities to submit a report twice a year regarding device-related injuries and serious illnesses. Based on the user reports, the FDA has the authority to recall devices.

### Occupational Safety and Health Administration

OSHA is the federal regulatory agency responsible for enforcing safety and health regulations in the workplace. The primary function of OSHA is to protect the healthcare worker by making sure that employers comply with health and safety provisions of the federal laws. OSHA can inspect the workplace at any time on request of the employees. OSHA issued a compliance directive, Instruction CPL 2-2.44A, "Enforcement Procedures for Occupational Exposure to Hepatitis B Virus (HBV) and Human Immunodeficiency Virus (HIV)." These are guidelines used by enforcement officers who conduct inspections of practices required to implement CDC Universal Precautions. Other proposed rules for protecting employees in the work setting were published in OSHA 29 CFR Part 1910 "Occupational Exposure to Bloodborne Pathogens."

## CASE SITUATION

Jeannie Allan, a 56-year-old woman, has just been admitted to the gastroenterology unit for a colonoscopy. She has had rectal bleeding for the past 2 months and is concerned about what the doctor will find when he performs the colonoscopy. She has a history of ulcerative colitis and has had problems with her bowels for the past 25 years. She is concerned that she may have cancer and does not want her husband to know until a diagnosis is defined. The nurse preparing Mrs. Allan for her procedure, follows a set of predetermined standards for practice. These standards are put forth by the SGNA and serve as a guide to gastroenterology staff members.

### Points to think about

1. What activities might a gastroenterology nurse perform on behalf of Mrs. Allan to ensure her right to privacy and confidentiality in the gastroenterology unit?
2. In preparing for Mrs. Allan's colonoscopy, what types of activities might be conducted to meet the standard of "preventing harm to the patient?"
3. What type of information about Jeannie Allan should the nurse document that would demonstrate nursing actions and the patient's responses to those actions?

### Suggested responses

1. To ensure Mrs. Allan's right to privacy and confidentiality, the gastroenterology nurse might:
   - Establish mutually with the patient what information she would like discussed in front of her family
   - Make sure that any information discussed with other staff and the patient's physician is communicated discreetly and in a professional manner, so it is not overheard by the patient's family or by other patients and their families

- When preparing for the colonoscopy, take care to keep the patient covered with an appropriate drape
2. The types of activities that might be performed to protect the patient from harm would include:
   - Decontaminating and disinfecting endoscopic instruments
   - Ensuring that informed consent has been obtained before the procedure
   - Performing safety checks of electrical equipment that has the potential to burn the patient or cause fires
3. Examples of a nursing action and patient response the nurse would document are:
   - Nursing action: administration of midazolam (Versed)
   - Response: patient is calm

## REVIEW TERMS

**American Nurses' Association (ANA), Centers for Disease Control (CDC), Environmental Protection Agency (EPA), Food and Drug Administration (FDA), Joint Commission on Accreditation of Healthcare Organizations (JCAHO), Occupational Safety and Health Administration (OSHA), standards for practice, standards of care**

## REVIEW QUESTIONS

1. Which of the following is *not* a source of standards of nursing practice?
   a. Professional consensus.
   b. Expert opinions and theories.
   c. Scientific research.
   d. State licensing authorities.
2. The federal agency responsible for monitoring the safety of medical devices is:
   a. OSHA.
   b. EPA.
   c. FDA.
   d. CDC.
3. Accreditation standards are developed by:
   a. SGNA.
   b. CDC.
   c. JCAHO.
   d. ANA.
4. SGNA standards for practice specify the types of behavior expected of all:
   a. Hospital staff.
   b. Gastroenterologists.
   c. Registered nurses.
   d. SGNA members.
5. Qualitative, conceptual statements that define practice outcomes are called:

a. Standards of care.
b. Guidelines.
c. Standards for practice.
d. Criteria.

6. JCAHO standards apply to:
a. In-hospital endoscopy/GI units.
b. Independent endoscopy labs.
c. Physician's offices.
d. All of the above.

7. JCAHO considers endoscopy units to be in what category of services:
a. Ambulatory care.
b. Surgical and anesthesia services.
c. Nursing care.
d. Outpatient services.

8. According to the JCAHO *Accreditation Manual for Hospitals,* patients are responsible for:
a. Ensuring their own safety.
b. Providing an accurate medical history.
c. Providing an interpreter if they do not speak English.
d. Participating in medical research.

9. Which of the following is *not* covered in the SGNA infection control guidelines?
a. Decontamination, disinfection, and sterilization of endoscopes and accessories.
b. Recommendations for a safe environment.
c. Protection of personnel.
d. Isolation practices.

10. The Centers for Disease Control guidelines for the prevention and control of nosocomial infections:
a. Have the force of law.
b. Are an accepted compilation of practical recommendations.
c. Are applicable only to hospital settings.
d. Are all based on conclusive scientific research.

**BIBLIOGRAPHY**

Patterson, P., ed. "Advice for Users on Compliance with Devices Act." *OR Manager* 7(May 1991): 1, 14-15.

American Nurses' Association. *Quality Assurance Workbook.* Kansas City, Mo.: American Nurses' Association, 1976.

American Nurses' Association. *Standards of Clinical Nursing Practice.* Kansas City, Mo.: American Nurses' Association, 1991.

Barnie, D. "Professionalization of the GI Unit: Standards and the GI Assistant." In *SGA Journal Reprints,* ed. Trivits, S, 271-74. Rochester, N.Y.: Society of Gastrointestinal Assistants, 1988.

Beck, M., ed. *Recommended Guidelines for Infection Control in Gastrointestinal Endoscopy Settings.* 2nd ed. SGNA Monograph Series. Rochester, N.Y.: Society of Gastroenterology Nurses and Associates, 1990.

Garner, J, and Favero, M. *Guideline for Handwashing and Hospital Environmental Control.* Atlanta: Centers for Disease Control, 1985.

Joint Commission on Accreditation of Healthcare Organizations. *Accreditation Manual for Hospitals, 1991.* Volume I. Standards. Oakbrook Terrace, Ill.: JCAHO, 1990.

Kessler, D, Pape, S, and Sundwall, D. "The Federal Regulation of Medical Devices." *New England Journal of Medicine* 366(August 6, 1987): 317-57.

Kneedler, J. "A Standard: What Is It and How to Use It." *AORN Journal* 23(March 1976): 551-54.

McAloose, B, and Gruber, M. "SGNA Standards for Practice for Gastroenterology Nurses and Associates." *Gastroenterology Nursing* 12(Spring 1990): 229-31.

Society of Gastroenterology Nurses and Associates. *Standards for Practice.* SGNA Monograph Series. Rochester, N.Y.: SGNA, 1991.

Thomson, E. "The Surgical Patient's Rights." In *A Commitment to Caring,* 139-45. Papers Presented at the Second World Conference of Operating Room Nurses, Lausanne, Switzerland, August 12-15, 1980. Denver: Association of Operating Room Nurses, 1980.

# Chapter 6

# QUALITY IMPROVEMENT

One of the challenges to healthcare professionals is to transform the commitment to quality care from an idea into a reality. The emphasis on quality is being driven by customer demand for better products and services. This chapter provides guidelines for integrating a quality improvement (assurance) process in the gastroenterology unit.

## Learning objectives

After reviewing the content of this chapter, the gastroenterology nurse should be able to:
1. Define the term "quality" as it pertains to patients undergoing gastroenterology procedures.
2. Outline the steps that must be taken to develop a quality improvement program.
3. Identify indicators for measuring quality of care for gastroenterology patients.
4. Formulate ideas for improving quality within the gastroenterology unit.

## RATIONALE FOR A QUALITY PROGRAM

The demand for **quality** in products and services in the United States and the rest of the world has forced healthcare workers to examine ways of improving quality in the healthcare setting. Many individuals believe quality is undefinable and therefore not measurable. In the book *Quality Is Free,* Crosby defines quality as "conformance to requirements," and argues that it is precisely measurable. Some say that quality constitutes a value or standard. Webster's dictionary defines quality as "a degree of excellence or a distinguishable attribute." The American Society for Quality Control defines quality as the "totality of features and characteristics of a given product or service that bears on its ability to satisfy a given need."

Leaders in health care have defined quality as the "degree to which actions taken or not taken maximize the probability of beneficial outcomes." Quality care is appropriate, is delivered efficiently, and conforms to the patient's expectations.

In **quality assurance** terminology, *quality* is the degree of adherence to generally recognized and accepted standards of practice. Quality assurance entails establishment of a plan that ensures optimal patient care and clinical performance within the constraints of available resources. Standards are developed and measured using appropriate indicators. The main goal is to provide patients and their families with care that helps to resolve their problems and result in satisfaction.

## INTEGRATING QUALITY INTO THE GASTROENTEROLOGY DEPARTMENT

To implement any type of quality assurance program, the management team must have a commitment to quality. The manager must evaluate his or her own beliefs regarding quality because they are directly and indirectly communicated to the staff. Quality problems are not limited to certain employees or managers; they involve all members of the healthcare team.

A solid foundation for a comprehensive quality assurance program includes clear definitions of the unit's mission, its scope of services, and specific goals and objectives. In addition, standards of performance must be developed and reviewed on a regular basis.

### Mission statement/philosophy

A **mission statement** should be established or reevaluated for the gastroenterology department. The statement should reflect the overall **philosophy** of the unit, based on the beliefs of the team members. A commitment to quality is one belief that makes up the philosophy of a unit.

If the unit is hospital-based, it is important that the philosophy and mission statement reflect the global mission statement and philosophy of the institution. The JCAHO is shifting its emphasis toward developing uniform standards that provide quality care throughout the entire facility. A patient should be able to receive the same quality of care in all units within the institution.

There are a number of ways to express a unit's mission and philosophy. The following is one idea that may be used in the gastroenterology unit:

*The gastroenterology unit services are organized to deliver personalized, state-of-the-art, quality care to every individual who uses the service.*

It is important that all members of the team be aware that a mission statement exists and that their *own* beliefs match the unit's philosophy. When interviewing prospective candidates for hire, managers have a responsibility to communicate the unit's mission statement and philosophy and to determine whether the candidate's beliefs match that philosophy.

## Scope of services

For the unit to function efficiently, it is important to identify the scope of services that the gastroenterology unit provides. The scope of service encompasses the physical areas and the nursing activities or services provided in those areas. The elements of the service can vary in different gastroenterology units. The scope of service for a hospital-based gastroenterology unit should address the following:

- Departments where gastroenterology services are delivered (e.g., gastroenterology unit, emergency room, intensive care units)
- Diagnostic or therapeutic interventions performed in those areas
- Types of anesthesia provided in the areas of service
- Types of patients served in the different areas
- Types of healthcare providers and their clinical responsibilities
- Other ancillary duties performed, such as care and handling of equipment, specimen transportation

Each member of the team must be aware of the areas of service, what type of anesthesia can be given in each specific area, and the clinical responsibilities of different team members with regard to the various procedures and areas. It is imperative that the gastroenterology unit list its scope of services and the team members' clinical responsibilities so a uniform standard of care is delivered by all parties.

JCAHO (SA.2) requires that patients with the same health status and condition receive a comparable level of quality care throughout the hospital. This standard implies that if an endoscopic procedure is performed in the gastroenterology unit with IV sedation and the patient is monitored via a cardiac monitor and pulse oximeter, the same type of monitoring must also be provided for the same procedure with IV sedation at the patient's bedside. The bottom line is that the quality of care delivered should be uniform, regardless of where it is delivered.

## Goals and objectives

The mission statement and scope of services act as the base or foundation of the unit. The challenge is to translate those broad statements into measurable objectives and goals.

A **goal** is a desired outcome and should reflect the mission statement. There are specific elements that must be included in a goal, such as a measurable target, a time frame, and some type of activity which, when implemented, will deliver a result that reflects the mission statement.

An **objective,** on the other hand, is an observable activity developed to help achieve the established goals. Objectives are much more specific than goals. The following is an example of a goal and an objective that may be implemented in the gastroenterology unit to fulfill the unit's mission of delivering personalized quality care:

*Goal:* To improve the patient education program

*Objective:* To develop postprocedure instruction sheets with procedure-specific care instructions

Achievement of the goal and objective could be measured by placing postprocedure telephone calls to determine each patient's status and to inquire about his or her care and level of satisfaction with the service provided. A specific start date and time frame for completion of the goal would also have to be established.

It is important that the manager evaluate goals and objectives carefully to determine if they are realistic. Asking personnel to achieve unattainable goals and objectives will only set them up for failure and create negative attitudes.

## Performance standards

Performance standards provide a framework against which to measure the success of the organization in meeting the goals and objectives put forth in the mission statement. As detailed in Chapter 5, standards are derived from many sources. They may be defined in terms of structure, process, or outcome.

The continual development of medical care and technology requires ongoing evaluation of current standards. It is advisable to make a list of the standards that are currently in place within the gastroenterology unit and to update them regularly. This endeavor will help to ensure that the standards reflect the expected outcomes and quality of care.

In review, the steps to assuring quality are as follows:

1. Establishing a commitment to quality by all team members

2. Establishing a mission statement and philosophy that reflect quality as an end result
3. Clearly defining the scope of services to be delivered, including where and by whom they will be delivered
4. Establishing attainable goals and objectives that reflect the mission statement
5. Developing and regularly reevaluating performance standards that address structure and process for achieving favorable outcomes

## MEASURING QUALITY

Once all of the components of a quality assurance program have been defined and put in place, a system must be developed to measure the extent to which the organization delivers the quality of care to which it aspires.

### Quality indicators and thresholds

A clinical **indicator** is a measurable variable used to assess the degree to which outcomes or expectations are being met. The identification of indicators for the gastroenterology unit is a complex process that requires a high level of clinical expertise. Those responsible must develop suitable indicators so the important aspects of care may be measured or evaluated effectively.

There are certain criteria for developing effective indicators. They should include the following qualities:
- Objectivity
- Specificity
- Measurability
- Comprehensiveness
- Clinical validity
- Relevancy
- Efficiency

Because indicators are used to measure standards, and there are three types of standards (structure, process, and outcome), there must also be three types of indicators. Following are some examples of structure, process, and outcome indicators that might be appropriate for the gastroenterology unit:
- Proper disposal of contaminated needles after each procedure (structure)
- Emergency equipment available and functional for all procedures (structure)
- Number of incomplete procedures because of poor bowel prep (process)
- Number of patients who do not have necessary lab work preprocedure (process)
- Patient/family who rate satisfaction with nursing care as 80% or above (outcome)
- Patients having sclerotherapy who have blood pressure and pulse within ±5% of their baseline value (if available) before discharge (outcome)

To facilitate the data collection, indicators must be stated in a concise manner. For example, it would be easy to check the chart for preprocedural and postprocedural vital signs to see if the last outcome standard was met properly. Keep in mind that indicators must be easy to use or they will probably not be used at all.

Once indicators are developed, it is important to establish thresholds or acceptable rates of activity that determine when to evaluate care. Indicators can be designated as either rate-based or sentinel events.

- Rate-based indicators are established on the premise that there are usually exceptions to standards of care. When establishing a threshold, acceptable rates for clinical events are established based on the literature, on expert opinion, or on hospital experience. A good approach for the gastroenterology unit manager or nurse is to use the expertise and judgment of his or her staff and briefly justify a selection of 85%, versus 90% or 95%.
- Sentinel event indicators represent standards of care that, if not followed, may result in serious outcomes. A sentinel event is a negative outcome that is so serious, every case is investigated. An example might be a transfusion reaction or a perforation of the bowel during a procedure. Nurses in the gastroenterology department probably will not establish sentinel event indicators because these are usually monitored by the medical staff quality committee.

### Monitoring quality

The JCAHO *Accreditation Manual for Hospitals* requires that, "There is an ongoing quality assurance program designed to objectively and systematically monitor and evaluate the quality and appropriateness of patient care, pursue opportunities to improve patient care, and resolve identified problems." The manual also requires that, "There is a written plan for the quality assurance program that describes the program's objectives, organization, scope, and mechanisms for overseeing the effectiveness of monitoring, evaluation, and problem-solving activities."

In determining quality, the gastroenterology nurse must rely on facts rather than opinions. It is not enough to have all the goals, objectives, standards, and indicators written. There must be a formal process for monitoring the quality of care. It is helpful to involve the entire staff in this process, because it gives each person an inside look at measuring quality. If the gastroenterology unit is hospital-based, there is usually a quality assurance program in place and a coordinator to help facilitate this process. It is imperative that someone assume the responsibility for monitoring and evaluating the quality of care delivered in the freestanding gastroenterology unit.

Monitoring the quality of care involves data collection, tabulation, evaluation, and reporting. It begins with the task of data collection. Data collection specifications must detail exactly what indicators to use, how much data to collect, and how often. It may not be necessary to create new forms for data collection. Existing forms, such as the patient's record, incident reports, patient satisfaction questionnaires, infection rates, and the observations of the staff providing care, may be appropriate.

The frequency with which information is collected should be based on the volume of patients and recurrence of problems. It is recommended that data be gathered, reviewed, and reported regularly, based on a calendar developed for that purpose. Any indicators exceeding the established threshold require investigation of the quality and appropriateness of care.

Once the information has been collected, it must be tabulated so it can be evaluated and compared to acceptable variance levels. It is important to determine in advance what percentage of variance will be acceptable for a specific standard. If one of the indicators in the gastroenterology unit states that *all* patients' allergies are verified before the delivery of any medication, there would be no variance. The expectation is that this standard is met 100% of the time.

Evaluation involves determining the degree to which the key quality elements were met, and taking a look at whether or not the care delivered is still considered state-of-the-art.

The next step is to report the findings. This may require developing a form to serve as a tracking mechanism. It may be helpful to use control charts that depict trends or patterns of performance.

In conclusion, to measure the quality of care provided, it is necessary to establish the following components:

- Written indicators and thresholds
- Tools for data collection and tabulation
- Predetermined acceptable levels of variance for evaluating each indicator
- A means for reporting the findings

Taking the above steps will provide a means of measuring and documenting the quality assurance program that is recommended by JCAHO.

## IMPROVING QUALITY

Once the data have been collected and evaluated, the next step is to identify the areas that need corrective action or improvement. There are always opportunities for improving performance within the gastroenterology unit. It is critical that the staff be involved with the results of the evaluation so they can also receive praise for the indicators that were met. If corrective action is needed, it is prudent to focus on the origin of the problem, not just on the result. The emphasis should then be placed on developing strat-

egies that will correct the problem, thus improving patient care.

Effective methods for improving quality start with a commitment to making changes. The following is a brief list of ideas or strategies for implementing change and improvement.

- Education and training. Education is essential when implementing any new change. Without adequate knowledge, people cannot be expected to understand the need for change.
- Team approach. Involve the entire unit. A team approach gives the employee an opportunity to participate and promotes a more positive attitude.
- Recognition and reward system. Rewards are essential strategies for motivating people and thus can be very effective.

Once the strategies for **quality improvement** have been established, they must be written, communicated, and monitored. Program effectiveness relies on a clearly written plan of action. The written plan is so important that JCAHO has made it a required part of the quality assurance program. If the gastroenterology unit is hospital-based, the written plan should include the overall hospital-wide quality program and the unit's program.

Once the written plan is developed, it must be reviewed on a regular basis to ensure the changing needs, expectations, and outcomes of clients are being met in a timely, effective manner.

---

**CASE SITUATION**

Mrs. Ethel Jones is a 68-year-old female who has been admitted to the gastroenterology unit because she reported blood in her stools and vague abdominal discomfort. She has been scheduled for a colonoscopy.

Mrs. Jones lives alone and has expressed concern about returning home after the procedure. She has also indicated that her husband recently died of esophageal cancer.

*Points to think about*

1. What type of goals would be set for this patient?
2. What types of standards would already be in place within the gastroenterology unit that would pertain to Mrs. Jones?
3. What indicators would be used to measure the effectiveness of the care provided?
4. What methods would be used to collect data for the identified criteria or indicators?
5. Note some outcome standards that would be appropriate for Mrs. Jones.

*Suggested responses*

1. Some goals for Mrs. Jones might include the following:
   • Mrs. Jones will verbalize an understanding of postprocedure instructions.
   • Mrs. Jones will be escorted home by an individual(s) who will assume responsibility for her care, such as a family member.
   • Mrs. Jones will be cooperative and respond appropriately to directions given during the procedure.
2. Some standards that are applicable to Mrs. Jones might include:
   • Verification of allergies before delivery of medications.
   • Assessment of cardiac and respiratory status before, during, and after the procedure.
   • Universal Precautions.
   • Safety straps and side rails in use at all times on procedure cart during transportation.
3. Indicators to measure the effectiveness of the care given might include:
   • Mrs. Jones' vital signs return to her admission baseline vitals before discharge.
   • Mrs. Jones is free from injury related to positioning and/or electrical hazards.
   • Mrs. Jones follows postprocedure instructions.
4. The methods that may be used to collect data are:
   • The chart for documentation of vital signs and patient's skin integrity.
   • Postoperative telephone call to patient and/or family regarding patient's satisfaction and ability to follow instructions.
5. Outcome standards that may apply to Mrs. Jones are:
   • Mrs. Jones is free from injury related to the use of electrical devices.
   • Mrs. Jones is able to return to her normal activities of daily living.

**REVIEW TERMS**

**goal, indicator, mission statement, objective, philosophy, quality, quality assurance, quality improvement**

**REVIEW QUESTIONS**

1. Leaders in health care have defined quality as:
   a. Undefinable and not measurable.
   b. Conformance to requirements.
   c. The degree to which actions taken or not taken maximize the probability of beneficial outcomes.
   d. A distinguishable attribute.
2. The mission statement of the gastroenterology department should include:
   a. Goals and objectives.
   b. Clinical indicators.
   c. Quality improvement program.
   d. Philosophy of care to be provided.
3. An objective:
   a. Is an observable activity.
   b. Is more specific than a goal.
   c. Should be realistic.
   d. All of the above.
4. The extent to which the organization delivers the quality of care to which it aspires is measured by using a series of:
   a. Indicators.
   b. Standards.
   c. Goals.
   d. Objectives.
5. For indicators to be effective, they must:
   a. Be subjective.
   b. Evaluate outcomes.
   c. Be complex.
   d. Be measurable.
6. "Number of incomplete procedures due to poor bowel prep" is an example of a(n):
   a. Structure indicator.
   b. Process indicator.
   c. Outcome indicator.
   d. Outcome standard.
7. The purpose of a threshold is to:
   a. Determine when to evaluate care.
   b. Avoid serious outcomes.
   c. Facilitate data collection.
   d. Monitor vital signs.
8. "Eighty percent of patients are satisfied with nursing care" is an example of a(n):
   a. Sentinel event.
   b. Rate-based indicator.
   c. Process indicator.
   d. Structure standard.
9. Which of the following steps is *not* part of the process of measuring the quality of care?
   a. Data collection.
   b. Establishing standards.
   c. Evaluation.
   d. Reporting.
10. One effective strategy for improving the quality of care is to:
    a. Provide education and training.
    b. Assign the manager total responsibility for making changes.
    c. Discipline those who are responsible for failure to meet objectives.
    d. Change the goals and objectives.

**BIBLIOGRAPHY**

Cline, J. "Quality Assurance." In *SGA Journal Reprints,* ed. Trivits, S, 277-88. Rochester, N.Y.: Society of Gastrointestinal Assistants, 1988.
Crocker, O, Charney, S, Chiu, L, and Sik, J. *Quality Circles: A Guide*

*to Participation and Productivity.* New York: New American Library, 1984.

Crosby, P. *Quality is Free: The Art of Making Certain.* New York: New American Library, 1979.

Dayton, G. "Development, Distribution and Interpretation of a Patient Survey." *SGA Journal* 8(Summer 1985): 47-49.

Joint Commission on Accreditation of Healthcare Organizations. *Accreditation Manual for Hospitals, 1991 edition.* Oak Brook Terrace, Ill.: JCAHO, 1990.

Joint Commission on Accreditation of Healthcare Organizations. *Primer on Indicator Development and Application.* Oak Brook Terrace, Ill.: JCAHO, 1990.

Maradieque, A. "Quality Assurance as Reflected in Documentation." *SGNA Journal* 12(Fall 1989): 135-37.

Society of Gastrointestinal Assistants, Education Committee. *Quality Assurance for the Endoscopy Department.* Rochester, N.Y.: Society of Gastrointestinal Assistants, 1988.

# Chapter 7

# THE RESEARCH PROCESS

This chapter provides an overview of the steps involved in the nursing research process and reviews some of the statistical methods used to analyze data derived from descriptive research. In addition, the measures of central tendency and ethical considerations in nursing research are reviewed. The chapter ends with a case situation in which nursing research is conducted in a clinical setting and applied to clinical practice.

## Learning objectives

After reviewing the content of this chapter, the gastroenterology nurse should be able to:
1. Define basic terms used in research design.
2. Outline the seven steps performed in a research study.
3. Identify indexes of central tendency used to describe typicality and variability in study samples.

Research in nursing has occurred only over the past 15 to 20 years. During this time, whole texts have been written on the nursing research process. Many nurses are intimidated by the word *research* because they may associate it with unfamiliar terms and concepts. Yet nurses are well prepared for research; like the nursing process, research is a form of rigorous problem solving. Hence, the requisite skills for competent practice are also essential in research; that is, careful observation, strict documentation, and systematic assessment. Clinical nurses stand to contribute greatly to nursing science by identifying researchable problems and by applying research findings to clinical practice.

Regardless of whether a research study is straightforward or complex, no investigation is productive without thoughtful planning. Careful contemplation and planning culminate in valuable research.

## THE GOALS OF RESEARCH

Four aims predominate in research: description, exploration, explanation, and prediction and control.

### Description

Description is the primary aim in many nursing studies. When controlled, systematic, empirical observations are made, descriptive accounts of the phenomenon under study may become significant contributions. In nursing, descriptive studies have focused on nutritional habits, pain management, and rehabilitation success.

### Exploration

Unlike descriptive research, the aim of exploratory studies is to expose factors that influence, relate to, cause, or affect a phenomenon. Coexisting variables are observed and the frequency with which they coexist is analyzed in this type of research. For instance, in gastroenterology nursing, the incidence of gastric ulcers in rural, urban, and suburban populations might be explored as part of a larger effort to link stress factors to gastric ulcer formation.

### Explanation

Research aimed at explanation is related to theory-building. Theories represent a method of deriving, organizing, and integrating ideas about the manner in which phenomena are related. A study based on the effects of preprocedural teaching on the level of anxiety experienced by patients who have undergone a colonoscopy might use the information theory to explain the role of nursing in stress reduction. In nursing, there has been particular emphasis on the need for developing theories of nursing.

### Prediction and control

A **variable** is defined as a characteristic or attribute that takes on different values within a given population. Many research studies attempt to demonstrate a relationship between variables by manipulating one, the **independent variable,** and observing for a predicted change in another, the **dependent variable.** In such studies, a researcher must be able to predict the influence of the independent variable and control the influence of extraneous variables. For example, a researcher may study the relation between midazolam (Versed) dosage (the independent variable) and the loss of memory subsequent to endoscopy (the dependent variable). While the objective may be to determine an optimal dose of midazolam that will minimize amnesia, the researcher may have to control other confounding variables, such as sex or age. Note that predictive studies of a phenomenon need not take into account the reason for the phenomenon.

Nursing research may also be classified as either basic or applied research.

- Basic research is concerned with adding to the body of knowledge. It links the study in question to accepted models or theories.
- Applied research focuses on an immediate solution to a practical problem. Most nursing research has been applied research.

The next section describes the seven steps performed in the research process.

## STEPS IN THE RESEARCH PROCESS

The scientific research process is reiterative. Investigation at one stage of the study often casts light on an earlier stage, causing the researcher to return to the earlier step to refine a research problem or to revise study methods. Rarely does discovery proceed in a linear, sequential manner. Seldom does a researcher start at the first step in the process and proceed in orderly fashion through the remaining sequence of steps. Nonetheless, all research includes the following seven steps:

- Identify the problem
- Review the literature
- State the aims of the study and formulate a hypothesis
- Design the study
- Carry out the study plan
- Analyze the data
- Share the results

### Step 1. Identify the problem

Good research begins with appropriate questions. The act of stating a research question or problem initially gives the project direction. In the beginning, problem statements are often too broad and vague. Frequently, they must be refined and limited to make the project manageable.

By examining the level of interest in the topic and exploring the feasibility of the investigation, the researcher may be able to narrow the focus of the study and arrive at a research problem or question that is practical. In fact, the feasibility of a study is sometimes

a study in itself. When a study does not appear feasible, it is important to consider the level of outside interest and the researcher's own motivation before pursuing a research idea. Is there interest among the professional community in the findings to come out of the proposed research? Is the researcher sufficiently interested in the topic to sustain motivation to study the problem until the work is completed?

Interest level and motivation are only two of the factors that influence the feasibility of a project. Following are several others:

- Time. Is the scope of the problem such that it can be studied within the time allotted for the study?
- Availability of subjects. Can the researcher obtain a sufficient number of subjects to investigate the problem?
- Cooperation of others. It is rare that a researcher is able to conduct an investigation independently. Are the necessary resources available? Will it be a problem to get the necessary permissions from subjects, guardians, institutional administrators, and so on?
- Facilities and equipment. What facilities and equipment will be needed, and will they be available to complete the study?
- Money. Will funding be needed? If so, how much? Does the anticipated cost outweigh the value of the expected findings?
- Experience of the researcher. Is the problem from a field in which the researcher has some experience? If not, is there another, more experienced investigator who has substantive knowledge of existing concepts, findings, and theories who can guide the researcher in developing methods of study, and who can help avoid research problems requiring sophisticated measuring instruments and/or complex statistical analyses?
- Ethical considerations. Could the study impose unfair or unethical demands on the participants? (See the section on Moral and Ethical Issues in Nursing Research.)

### Step 2. Review the literature

Before beginning research it is wise to review existing literature related to the topic, including previous research on the same or a similar topic. Several objectives are met in doing so. The researcher may learn:

- That the proposed problem has already been solved
- That it is necessary to investigate a different question en route to the problem
- That the problem has been studied, but not sufficiently to rule out further investigation, in which case it may be feasible to replicate the study according to methods outlined in the literature
- That certain research designs are appropriate for

the proposed topic, while others are not
- That certain important variables must be examined
- That other researchers have made mistakes that must be avoided

In short, searching existing literature will help to clarify and refine the focus of the research, thus enabling the researcher to define the scope of the study so it becomes more feasible.

### Research reports: what to look for

When reviewing previous research, various types of information may be uncovered:

- Facts, statistics, or findings. This is probably the most important category of information because it represents the results of other research efforts. It includes progress other investigators have made in examining the topic.
- Theory or interpretation. This type of information is also significant because it concerns the relation between the idea or topic of interest and an existing body of knowledge surrounding that topic.
- Methods and procedures. Literature focused on research instruments and procedures is useful because it saves the researcher from redeveloping and revalidating measurement tools that already exist.
- Opinions, speculation, anecdotes, clinical impressions, or narrations of incidents and situations. These categories of information are value-laden and subjective. They serve to broaden the researcher's understanding of the problem and help deal with snags that may occur. Because it is important to remain as objective as possible, the researcher should avoid the temptation to rely heavily on such sources.

### Research reports: where to find them

Individual books, journals, and other periodicals are permeated with information. However, browsing through these sources to access pertinent information may be a bit overwhelming. Fortunately, there are tools that allow for more efficient retrieval of relevant data, including abstracts, indexes, computerized databases, bibliographies, and personal contact:

- Abstracts. Abstracts contain summaries of journal articles. While not detailed, they are useful in determining whether or not an article will be relevant to the topic at hand.
- Indexes. Printed indexes, such as *Index Medicus,* can unlock vast stores of literature on every subject imaginable. If the topic requires information from disciplines other than nursing (e.g., chemistry, genetics, or psychology), a librarian can identify relevant indexes on these subjects.
- Computer databases. Relevant information can be identified quickly by searching computerized databases such as *Medline.* The cost of a computer database search varies, depending on the database used and the extensiveness of the search. However,

the expense may be worthwhile if the time saved can be spent more productively. Limiting the scope of the search minimizes expense. A librarian can help develop an efficient search strategy.
- Bibliographies. Bibliographies provide compilations of references to books, periodicals, and reports on a particular topic. Annotated bibliographies provide additional comments about the purposes or findings of studies and sometimes include information about the quality of the work. Bibliographies can also identify other investigators with experience in the area of interest.
- Personal contact. Contacting other investigators can help clarify information they have published and help the researcher refine his or her own purpose and methods.

Any or all of these tools may be a fruitful means of retrieving pertinent literature on the topic of interest.

### Research reports: how to evaluate and screen them

The researcher should critically consider all sources of information. When written by the person or persons who performed the study, a research report is considered a primary source of information. A secondary source describes research performed by other investigators. Reviews of the literature, for example, are secondary sources. Primary information sources should be used as much as possible. In addition, when reviewing a study, the researcher should examine its relevance, the validity and reliability of the instruments used (as discussed in the section on study design), control of extraneous variables, the sample size, and the statistical and clinical significance of the results. Finally, negative findings should not be disregarded. It is not uncommon to encounter conflicting reports; this is generally an indication that more research is necessary.

## Step 3. State the aims of the study and formulate a hypothesis

Stating the purpose of the proposed research helps focus it and clarify its significance with respect to nursing practice. At the same time, it may be useful to predict the outcome of the study; for example, what outcomes are expected as the result of this work? This statement is the research **hypothesis.** A hypothesis defines the researcher's expectations about the relationship between variables in the study. A hypothesis differs from a problem statement, which identifies the phenomena under investigation, while the former predicts how those phenomena are related. A problem statement is really a question, while a hypothesis is a declaration.

## Step 4. Design the study

Steps in actual study design are as follows:
- Determine how to sample the study population (e.g., a random sample, a convenience sample)

- Decide on a setting in which to carry out the study (e.g., a hospital, an office endoscopy setting, a specific geographic location)
- Select measures for collecting data (e.g., develop a new survey instrument, use a previously validated instrument)
- Specify procedures to collect the data (e.g., being certain to protect the rights of human subjects and to isolate the variables under examination)
- Decide which statistical procedures should be used, if any (e.g., mean, median, standard deviation)

In nursing research, three study designs are predominantly used. They are the survey, the experiment, and the case study. While all surveys are partially descriptive in nature, the primary intent of the experiment and the case study is explanation.

- To conduct a survey, interviews or self-completion questionnaires are used.
- An experiment generally involves **quantitative** measurement before and after some treatment or intervention is rendered.
- A case study is almost exclusively **qualitative.** When using this design, data are collected through observation.

Although each step in the study design process deserves elaboration, this section details two: sampling methods and measures for collecting data.

### Sampling the population

**Sampling** refers to the process of selecting a study group to represent the entire population. The overriding concern in assessing a sample is its representativeness. Sampling plans are essentially one of two types: probability sampling and nonprobability sampling.

**Random sampling** is the simplest of the probability sampling designs. It involves selection from the **population** (or a subpopulation) at large, and is performed in such a way that each member of the population has equal probability of being included in the sample. Probability sampling is the more respected of the two types because greater confidence can be placed in the representativeness of the sample.

The nonprobability approach to sampling generates the majority of samples in most disciplines, including nursing research. Accidental sampling is a nonprobability sampling technique that entails using the most readily available persons or objects as subjects in the study. Because it is difficult to argue for the representativeness of an accidental sample, researchers must be careful about generalizing results to the population at large when sampling by this nonprobability technique.

In many experimental designs, an **experimental group** and either a control group or a comparison group are selected. The experimental group is comprised of subjects who receive an experimental treatment or intervention. The **control group** is comprised of subjects who do not receive an experimental treatment or intervention. Their performance provides a baseline against which the effects of the treatment can be measured. A **comparison group** is a sort of alternative control group. A comparison group is a selection of subjects whose scores on a dependent variable are used as the basis for evaluating the scores of an experimental group or the group of primary interest. The phrase *comparison group* is used rather than the phrase *control group* when the investigation does not use a true experimental design.

The terms **"double-blind"** and **"placebo effect"** refer to design features of research studies that recur in investigative literature. A double-blind experiment is one in which neither subjects nor investigators are aware of which subjects are in the experimental group and which subjects are in the control group. In an investigation of the effects of a drug, for example, neither the drug administrator nor the subjects are aware of whether the drug administered is the experimental drug. Double-blind drug investigations frequently involve the administration of a placebo to the control group. A placebo is a material whose appearance is identical to the drug under investigation. Using a placebo sometimes helps researchers to separate psychological effects induced by drug administration (the placebo effect) from the real effects of the drug.

### Measures for collecting data

Measurement, which enables researchers to specify and agree on standardized procedures of observation and description, has been defined as the assignment of numbers to objects (or events or situations) in accord with some rule. This definition suggests that whenever a phenomenon is described—be it a person, place, event, or thing, a rule or set of rules must be followed that prescribe how descriptive numbers will be assigned. It is the measurement *procedures* that are important because they determine the legitimacy of the measure.

The type of data collected determines and sometimes constrains the statistical procedure used to analyze the data. For this reason, it is important to think about the optimal level of measurement while planning the study. In quantitative studies, four types of data are collected: nominal data, ordinal data, interval data, and ratio data.

- To derive nominal data, individuals or objects are simply placed in categories (e.g., sex, occupation).
- Ordinal data are ranked or ordered hierarchically. Disease states, for example, are sometimes roughly characterized as Grade 1, Grade 2, Grade 3, and so on, based upon the severity of symptoms.
- Interval data carry not simply rank order information but rank order at specific *intervals*. These intervals allow for comparison of differences.
- Ratio data combine the properties of rank order, equal intervals, and a genuine zero point.

The handling of the different types of data is controversial. Nominal and ordinal data are more appropriately tested with nonparametric statistics such as chi-square, a test of frequency distributions. Interval and ratio data can be tested with any statistical test; for example, parametric tests such as t-test or nonparametric tests. There is controversy over the importance of these classifications and how particular types of data, such as psychological measures, should be classified. It is important to remember that the research question and/or hypothesis of the study should be the prime determining factor in deciding how to analyze data. The conclusions drawn from the analyses are made not only from the statistical results but also from the clinical significance of the results.

Like the procedures for measurement, the instrument used to perform measurement must fulfill two requirements: it must be valid and it must be reliable. A valid instrument is one that measures what it is supposed to measure. Reliability, on the other hand, refers to the reproducibility or consistency of the measurement. If a researcher must design a data collection instrument, its validity and reliability must be tested via a pilot study before it can be used with confidence. Because instrument testing can be a complicated process, nurses who are new to research should seek, whenever possible, to use an instrument that has been previously developed and tested.

### Step 5. Carry out the study plan

There is little to be said about this step in the research process, except to emphasize that this phase requires careful observation, strict documentation, and systematic assessment. This phase of research is labor-intensive, and is the most important in terms of the outcome and reliability of the results.

### Step 6. Analyze the data

The act of analyzing research data has been revolutionized by the advent of computers, thus leading to a kind of democratization of knowledge. Researchers today have ready access to computers that can store, search, compare, and produce information with a speed that was unheard of in the pretechnological age. In research, computers are useful not only in searching the literature but also in streamlining the once-tedious task of data analysis. Many statistical programs are available to help analyze research data. It is important, however, to apply statistical methods that are appropriate to the type of data generated by a given measurement instrument.

Once the data analysis is complete, but before conclusions can be drawn, it is wise to pause and consider the nature of the scientific approach as it pertains to nursing research. Respect for the powers of the scientific approach must be tempered by a familiarity with its limitations and flaws. Because many of the persistent and intriguing questions in nursing concern morality and ethics, and because no scientific method can be used to answer these questions, it is inevitable that the nursing process will never rely solely upon scientific information. Moreover, the problem of measurement is a substantial one in nursing. While there are reasonably accurate measures of physiological phenomena, comparable measures for psychological phenomena, such as pain and anxiety, have not been developed.

Finally, every study, no matter how sophisticated, has some flaws. Investigators are inevitably faced with compromises and constraints that must be acknowledged when conclusions are drawn. Consumers of research need to understand these limitations to evaluate the usefulness of the information provided.

### Step 7. Share the results

The information derived as the product of a research study is valuable, even if it concludes with a null hypothesis. A **null hypothesis** states that there is no relationship between the variables under study. While it may seem that the study's efforts were wasted, a null hypothesis rules out one conclusion, a step that can be as valuable as confirming one. Other times, when the purpose of a research study was to replicate a previous study, conflicting results may signify the need to continue investigation of the topic. Thus it is always important to communicate research findings.

The results of a research study may be disseminated in the following ways:

- Writing and publishing an article that describes the study and the results obtained
- Giving an oral presentation of the study findings at a local or national meeting
- Presenting the findings with a poster at a local or national meeting
- Presenting the findings within the local area at informal group meetings, at inservices, at work, or at local research conferences

### ELEMENTARY DESCRIPTIVE STATISTICS: A REVIEW OF CENTRAL TENDENCY

When conducting a study, nurse researchers are frequently interested in the typical member of a group. They may care to know, for example, how much information typical colostomy patients have about diet or how much postprocedure pain the typical endoscopy patient experiences.

The lay person tends to think of typicality in terms of a group *average*. However, this term is ambiguous because there are three commonly used kinds of averages, or measures of **central tendency:** the mode, the median, and the mean. Furthermore, an average alone sometimes gives inadequate information about the typicality of a characteristic, as is true when there is considerable variability in the group. Variability refers to the spread or dispersion of data values around the mean, and may be quite different between two groups, while the mean value in either group is the same. Consequently, it becomes necessary to talk about typicality not only in terms of averages (the mode, the median, or the mean), but also in terms of variability.

In this section, measures of central tendency are reviewed. In addition, two indexes of variability are described: the range and the standard deviation.

## Mode

The **mode** is the numerical value that occurs most frequently in a set of values. It is not necessary to calculate to derive the mode; rather, the researcher simply inspects the set of values. For example, in the following set of values it is easy to see that the mode is 14:

14 10 12 14 14 14 22 16 14 8 12 12 14

## Median

The **median** is an index of average *position* in a set of values. It does not take into account the quantitative values of individual scores. Specifically, the median is that point in a set of values above which and below which 50% of the values lie. Notice that to find the median, it is necessary first to order the values. In this first set of values, there are five elements:

2 8 6 0 5

Once they are ordered, it is easy to see that 5 is the median value:

0 2 5 6 8

Also notice that in a set of values containing an even number of elements, finding the median requires computing a midpoint between two values. Examine the set of values below. The median of this set of values is 6:

0 2 5 7 8 9

Because the median is insensitive to extreme values, it is often preferred as the index of central tendency when the distribution of values is skewed, as in this example:

0 2 5 7 8 99

Despite the extreme value of one element in the set (e.g., 99), the median remains 6. In this instance, the median gives a truer picture of what is *typical* of the set.

## Mean

The **mean** is the index of central tendency that is usually referred to as the average. The mean is simply the sum of the values in a set, divided by the number of elements in a set. So, for the following set of values:

4 2 6 15 8

The mean is calculated in this way:

$$\frac{4 + 2 + 6 + 15 + 8}{5} = \frac{35}{5} = 7$$

Of the three indexes of central tendency, the mean is the most stable. If repeated samples are drawn from a population and some characteristic is measured, the means for these samples would fluctuate less than the modes or the medians. When researchers work with interval- or ratio-level measurement, the mean, rather than the mode or median, is almost always the statistic reported. However, as in the instance above in which 99 was an extreme value, there are some circumstances in which the mean would give a distorted picture of what is typical for a group.

The concept of **variability** is concerned with the degree to which subjects in a sample vary from one another with respect to some critical attribute. Sampling strategies can have a dramatic effect on variability. If, for instance, the aim of a study is to determine the variability of systolic pressure in any given sample of the population, and the sample studied is an accidental sample of patients seen in one emergency room, the variability of systolic pressures is likely to be greater than if the sample were selected from the junior class of a local high school. Because emergency room patients are more likely to present with extremes of pressure, the range of pressures may be greater than those among a young, healthy population. Consequently, it is necessary to describe variability in ways that account for situations like this one. Indexes like the range and standard deviation are used to give meaning to the concept.

## Range

The **range** is simply the highest score (or value) minus the lowest score in a given set of values. Examine the range of systolic pressures in an accidental sample of emergency room patients:

110 138 88 246 122 116

The range of systolic pressures in this sample is 246 minus 88, or 158. Now examine the range of systolic pressures in a random sample of high school juniors:

110 118 122 116 112 118

The range in this sample is 118 minus 110, or 8. The systolic pressures among the first group sampled are widely dispersed, while pressures in the second group are more narrowly dispersed.

## Standard deviation

A more complicated measure of variability is the standard deviation. The **standard deviation** measures the spread among values in a set around the average value in the set, or simply how far away the numbers in a list are from their average. The standard deviation is considered more reliable than the range as a measure of variability because, like the mean, it takes into account every value in the set of values. To calculate the standard deviation, examine systolic pressures from the high school juniors sample:

$$110 \quad 118 \quad 122 \quad 116 \quad 112 \quad 118$$

The formula for finding the standard deviation is as follows:

$$SD = \sqrt{\frac{\Sigma \ (\text{deviation scores}^2)}{n}}$$

where $\Sigma$ indicates "the sum of," and n = the number of subjects in the sample.

The first step in finding the standard deviation is to compute the mean pressure. After adding the six pressures and dividing by 6, it can be seen that the mean pressure is 116. The next step is to find the spread or *deviation score* for each pressure in this group. A deviation score is equal to the sample score minus the mean score. For this group, the deviation scores are, respectively:

$$-6 \quad 2 \quad 6 \quad 0 \quad -4 \quad 2$$

Because the standard deviation is a type of average deviation, it might seem logical to find the standard deviation by totalling the deviation scores and then dividing by the number of subjects. The difficulty in this approach is that the sum of a set of deviation scores is always 0. The standard deviation overcomes this problem by squaring each deviation score before summing them. So the third step in computing the standard deviation is to square the deviation scores:

$$36 \quad 4 \quad 36 \quad 0 \quad 16 \quad 4$$

Where n = 6 subjects in the sample, the equation looks like this:

$$SD = \sqrt{\frac{(36 + 4 + 36 + 0 + 16 + 4)}{(6 - 1)}}$$

Finishing the computation, the standard deviation is calculated as follows:

$$SD = \sqrt{\frac{96}{6}} = \sqrt{16} = 4$$

What does the standard deviation indicate about variability? In general, the greater the standard deviation, the more variable the data. Conversely, the smaller the standard deviation, the less variable the data. If the mean blood pressure of two populations is equal, yet the standard deviation in one sample is 17, while the standard deviation in the second sample is 3, it is obvious that the blood pressures of the first sample are more variable than the blood pressures of the second sample. The standard deviation provides a picture of the distribution of the data base. In a normal distribution, 67% of the sample will be within one standard deviation of the mean, 95% within two standard deviations of the mean, and 99% within three standard deviations of the mean.

The standard deviation can also illustrate the relative value of using the mean to describe typicality of an entire data set. The larger the standard deviation, the less reliable the mean is as an indicator of typicality. Conversely, the smaller the standard deviation, the more reliable the mean is as an indicator of typicality.

## MORAL AND ETHICAL ISSUES IN NURSING RESEARCH

The fundamental principles that are discussed in this chapter should guide nurse researchers when they study human problems. First, subjects should be protected from harm and discomfort. The phrase "Harm and discomfort" is not limited to physical injury. Nurse researchers also need to be wary of intruding upon their subjects' psyches.

The second principle is that participation in research must always be voluntary. Sometimes this seemingly obvious principle conflicts with practical considerations or the concerns of research. Occasionally, when the aim is to improve human welfare, but the requirement of voluntary participation threatens the value of a research study, the consequences of involuntary participation must be weighed against the potential contribution of the study.

The participant in a research study also has the following rights:
- Self-determination
- Privacy
- Confidentiality
- The right to maintain self-respect
- The right to withdraw without penalty
- The right to services

The right to self-determination requires further explanation. To voluntarily participate in a research study the participant needs to give informed consent. The subject should have access to the following information:
- The purpose of the project and its general value
- All procedures used in the study and why
- The subject's part in the study and how much time and energy will be required

- Any possible pain, discomfort, stress, or loss of autonomy or dignity
- How privacy, confidentiality, and anonymity will be guarded and the process whereby data will be used.

---

Denise Heckel is a gastroenterology nurse in a metropolitan hospital. For over a month the staff will cooperate with Denise by helping her study the effects of preprocedural visits on the anxiety level of endoscopy patients. The subjects Denise selects for the study must be adults (18 years or older) who are scheduled for upper and lower endoscopies, and who are English-speaking, oriented to their surroundings, and able to hear and give accurate information. Denise is also measuring the amount of diazepam used for patient sedation before and during the endoscopic procedure.

### Points to think about

1. What steps should Denise follow to study her target population?
2. What purpose or purposes (e.g., description, exploration, explanation, or prediction and control) might Denise fulfill in performing her study?
3. What factors should Denise have explored to determine whether or not her study will be feasible?
4. What hypothesis might Denise test in a study of this nature?
5. What variables might influence her results? Which variables has she controlled? Which variables may she yet need to control?

### Suggested responses

1. Denise should take seven steps when conducting her study:
   - Identify the research problem
   - Review the literature
   - State the aims and expected outcome of research
   - Design the study
     a. Sample the population to be studied
     b. Decide on a setting in which to do the study
     c. Select measures for collecting data
     d. Specify data collection procedures
     e. Decide how the data will be analyzed
   - Collect the data
   - Analyze data and draw conclusions
   - Share research results
2. Denise might fulfill any of the predominant aims of research, depending on the nature of her study:
   - Description. Describe the clinical manifestations of stress before endoscopy by using Selye's model of stress.
   - Exploration. Explore factors that influence anxiety, such as content of preprocedural information (sensory versus procedural information); age; sex; contact with nurse versus admission clerk; and patient's past experiences.
   - Explanation. Explain the nursing role in preprocedure visits as reduction of uncertainty, using information theory.
   - Prediction. Predict that some action will reduce patient anxiety before endoscopy.
3. To determine whether or not her study will be feasible, Denise should explore the following factors:
   - The time allotted
   - Availability of a sufficient number of subjects
   - Cooperation of others and availability of the necessary permissions
   - Availability of facilities and equipment
   - The amount of funding needed, if any, to perform the study and whether the anticipated cost outweighs the value of the expected findings
   - The availability of an experienced investigator who can provide guidance in developing methods of study and can help avoid research problems requiring sophisticated measuring instruments and/or complex statistical analyses
   - Whether the study could impose unfair or unethical demands on the participants; whether she can obtain informed consent and, if not, whether she can justify not obtaining informed consent in terms of the benefits to patients versus the harm done
4. Some hypotheses that Denise might test in a study of this nature include:
   - That sensory information and procedural information, rather than procedural information alone, reduces patient anxiety.
   - That patients who receive information the evening before their procedure experience less anxiety than patients who receive information immediately before endoscopy.
   - That preprocedure information is more effective in reducing both anxiety and the need for sedation during endoscopy when patients have had positive experiences or no experience with outpatient surgery than when patients have had negative experiences; that is, negative prior experience influences preprocedural anxiety.
   - That diazepam premedication offers no benefit over no premedication in reducing anxiety when preprocedure visits have been performed.
5. Variables that might influence Denise's results include patient age and sex; timing of preprocedure visits; content of information provided; predisposition toward anxiety; length of visit; format of visit; past experiences; present emotional circumstances; reason for procedure; and many others.

Variables that Denise has controlled are age, type of procedure, and ability to communicate with an English-speaking investigator. She has yet to control all other variables.

---

### REVIEW TERMS

**central tendency, comparison group, control group, dependent variable, double-blind, experimental group, hypothesis, independent variable, mean, median, mode, null hypothesis, placebo effect, population, qualitative, quantitative, random sampling, range, sampling, standard deviation, variability, variable**

---

### REVIEW QUESTIONS

1. If a research study examines the effects of preprocedural visits on the anxiety level of patients undergoing upper and lower endoscopies, and controls the amount of sedative used, what is the dependent variable?
   a. Anxiety level.
   b. Preprocedure visits by an endoscopy nurse.
   c. The amount of sedation required.
   d. Type of endoscopic procedure scheduled.

2. In the case situation described in this chapter, "adults (18 years or older) who are scheduled for upper and lower endoscopies, and who are English-speaking, oriented, and able to hear and give accurate information" describes:
   a. All patients seen in the endoscopy clinic.
   b. The population selected for the study.
   c. A random sample from the population at large.
   d. All of the variables in Denise's study.

3. Patients who are participating in a study of the effects of preprocedure visits (by an endoscopy nurse) on patient anxiety are assigned to one of two groups by a coin toss. Group 1 receives routine preprocedure care, including an instructional pamphlet. Group 2 receives the same care and pamphlet, but also receives a visit from an endoscopy nurse. Which statement best describes Groups 1 and 2?
   a. Group 1 is a random sample, while Group 2 is not.
   b. Group 2 is the experimental group, while Group 1 is the control group.
   c. Group 2 is the comparison group, while Group 1 is the control group.
   d. Group 1 is the experimental group, while Group 2 is the control group.

4. If, in doing a preliminary literature review on the topic of interest, a researcher reads a review article that mentions another study that contradicts her hypothesis, how should the researcher evaluate this information?
   a. She should consider it irrelevant information.
   b. She should consider it a primary source of information and rely on it heavily.
   c. She should disregard it, as other information she has found conflicts with this.
   d. She should view this conclusion skeptically until she has had a chance to read the contradictory study herself.

5. To calculate how long it will take her to complete her study, a researcher must compute the *average* number of patients treated each day in her clinic. How might she find this average?
   a. She could read it in a review of the literature.
   b. She could scan clinic records and see that, on most days, there are 20 patients treated.
   c. She could sum the total number of patients treated last year and divide it by the number of days the clinic operated.
   d. She could compute the difference between the highest number of patients treated and the lowest number of patients treated per day over the last year.

6. If the most sedation required by a member of a study group was 1.7 mg/kg, while the least amount required was 0.8 mg/kg, the range of sedation required for this group would be:
   a. The least and the greatest amount required to produce sedation.
   b. The average of the greatest and least amounts required to produce sedation.
   c. 1.7 mg/kg minus 0.8 mg/kg.
   d. 2.5 mg/kg.

7. The participants in one research study did not sign an informed consent before submitting to the experiment. Because this violates basic moral and ethical principles of research on human subjects, which explanation seems most valid?
   a. The study parameter and goals take precedence over the rights of experimental subjects.
   b. It was a double-blind study and knowing that the experiment was taking place would alter the validity of the study results.
   c. The potential benefits to the subjects far outweigh the need for informed consent.
   d. B and C.

8. Which statement best describes a null hypothesis?
   a. A conclusion statement saying that the study results are inconclusive.
   b. A hypothesis which states that there is no relationship between the variables under study.
   c. A hypothesis to be ignored.
   d. A hypothesis that was never pursued because the idea is too preposterous.

9. A placebo is:
  a. A treatment.
  b. A measure of central tendency.
  c. A theory.
  d. A sample.

10. $\sqrt{\dfrac{\Sigma\ (\text{deviation scores}^2)}{n-1}}$

  is the formula for:
  a. The mean of a sample.
  b. The mode of a sample.
  c. The standard deviation.
  d. The deviation scores.

## BIBLIOGRAPHY

Aker, J. "Review of Current Research on Midazolam and Diazepam for Endoscopic Premedication." *Gastroenterology Nursing* 13(Fall Supplement 1990): 24S-28S.

Biddle, W. "Survey Results: Identification of Research Interests and Needs in SGNA." *Gastroenterology Nursing* 13(Fall Supplement 1990): 12S-16S.

Biddle, W, Mikels, C, Buzby, M, Gallagher, J, Frederick, S, and Cornelius, M. "A Beginner's Guide to Research." *Gastroenterology Nursing* 13(Fall Supplement 1990): 2S-11S.

Ellett, M. "Clinical Nursing Research: Recipe for Success." *Gastroenterology Nursing* 13(Summer 1990): 18-23.

Emmert, P, and Barker, L. "Philosophy of Measurement." In *Measurement of Communication Behavior,* 97-101. New York: Longman Publishing, 1989.

Harrigan, C. "Smart Chart: Research Terminology." *Gastroenterology Nursing* 13(Spring 1991): 241.

Holland, P. "A Model Research Grant Proposal." *Gastroenterology Nursing* 13(Fall Supplement 1990): 17S-22S.

Polit, B, and Hunger, B. "Essentials of Nursing Research." In *Methods and Applications.* Philadelphia: Lippincott, 1985.

Seaman, C, and Verhoniak, P. *Research Methods for Undergraduate Students in Nursing.* Norwalk, Conn.: Appleton-Century-Crofts, 1982.

Waltz, CF, and Bausell, R. *Nursing Research: Design, Statistics and Computer Analysis.* Philadelphia: F. A. Davis, 1981.

# NURSING PROCESS

# Chapter 8

# ASSESSMENT

This is the first of a series of chapters that address the components of the nursing process. The nursing process is composed of six steps: assessment, diagnosis, outcome identification (setting patient goals), planning, implementation, and evaluation. Assessment, which is the primary focus of this chapter, is considered the most crucial step.

This chapter discusses the process of assessment as it applies to gastroenterology nursing. Assessment is defined and the scope of assessment is addressed. Data collection methods are described and in-depth examples of the assessment of gastroenterology patients are provided.

**Learning objectives**

After reviewing the content of this chapter, the gastroenterology nurse should be able to:

1. Delineate the essential elements that constitute the basis of the nursing process used by the gastroenterology nurse.
2. Describe the nursing activities used by the gastroenterology nurse in performing a comprehensive patient assessment.
3. Identify the sources and types of data collected that are specific to gastroenterology patients.
4. Discuss data collection methods that are effective in assessing patients with gastrointestinal disorders.

As a basis for discussing each component of the nursing process, it is appropriate to provide an introduction to the framework of nursing practice in the gastroenterology unit. The **nursing process** is defined as a systematic approach to nursing care using problem-solving techniques. This term is used to describe the intellectual and physical activities a nurse performs in giving care. The word *process* indicates movement in a forward direction. Viewing process as an action implies deliberate efforts to progress toward an identified outcome. The nurse's experience and educational background provide the basic knowledge and skills needed to assist patients in meeting identified outcomes systematically and progressively. The nurse continuously and systematically collects information, formulates nursing diagnoses, identifies outcomes, plans nursing actions, implements those actions, and evaluates the results.

## ASSESSMENT PROCESS

The first step in the nursing process is **assessment,** a continuous activity performed by the gastroenterology nurse throughout contact with a patient. It entails gathering data about the patient that are then analyzed to form a nursing diagnosis. To obtain valid data, the gastroenterology nurse must be able to use well-developed communication, interviewing, and physical assessment techniques.

The assessment process entails collection, validation, and communication of data in relation to the health status of a patient. It has been described as an ongoing process of cue and pattern recognition, in which the cues trigger pattern recognition and/or validate an already recognized pattern.

Assessment precedes other phases in the nursing process so a nurse may make judgments about the patient's health status, the patient's ability to manage his or her own health care, and the patient's need for nursing. An initial assessment provides a means of developing a plan of care, which outlines how specific patient outcomes are to be achieved. But assessment at the time of initial patient contact is in itself insufficient. To continually evaluate the appropriateness and effectiveness of therapy, and to refine the plan of care, assessment must be ongoing.

In nursing practice, it is always desirable and helpful to draw data for care planning from a *comprehensive assessment* of health. Ideally, a comprehensive assessment is performed during initial contact with a patient. As its name suggests, this baseline assessment involves collecting data on *all* aspects of the patient's health.

In particularly acute contexts, in which the expected duration of nurse–patient contact is brief, a *focused assessment* may be more practical and effective in terms of care planning. A focused assessment may be performed during any nurse–patient interaction to gather data about a specific problem. An example of a focused assessment is one performed before a diagnostic or therapeutic procedure such as endoscopy.

As trends in specialization and cost containment mold the nature of acute nursing care, similar trends in focused assessment and collaborative practice have followed. This is not to say that nurses within any specialty attend narrowly to health problems within the special scope of their practice while remaining oblivious to others. Rather, the trend suggests an evolution toward cooperation and collaboration with other nurses and healthcare professionals whose collective goal is to assist the injured or ill patient toward renewed health or toward optimal adaptation to an altered state of health.

A nursing assessment differs in purpose from a medical assessment. The aim of a medical assessment is to define the existence of medical problems and identify underlying pathology. The purpose of a nursing assessment, on the other hand, is to identify adverse patient *responses* to health problems. A *health problem* is any condition related to health that requires intervention if disease or illness is to be prevented or resolved and if coping and wellness are to be promoted.

Assessment involves gathering physical and psychosocial information. In the following sections, the process of collecting data is reviewed in general and as it pertains to assessment of the gastroenterology patient.

## DATA COLLECTION: GENERAL

The quality of the **data** collected to plan the care of gastroenterology patients is a result of the completeness, accuracy (i.e., unbiased nature), and relevance of the data to the health problems. The quality of the data also depends on the nurse's knowledge, experience, and communication and observation skills. Nurses' knowledge and experience enable them to plan data collection, while communication and observation skills enable them to collect data effectively.

Following are the six steps involved in collecting data for a nursing assessment:
1. Identify assessment priorities
2. Prioritize types of data to be collected
3. Establish the data base
4. Continuously update the data base
5. Validate data
6. Communicate data

### Step 1. Identify assessment priorities

Assessment priorities and the type of data collected depend on the purpose of the assessment. If the purpose is to assess a patient's preparation for a laparoscopic cholecystectomy, the first priority may be to assess the patient's understanding of the upcoming procedure rather than to assess compliance with a prescribed low-fat diet. Similarly, the patient's condition should be considered when identifying assessment priorities. Clearly, there is little point in assessing the gait of a patient who presents in shock with a bleeding peptic ulcer. Other factors that may determine assessment priorities include the health orientation of the patient, his or her need for nursing, and the developmental stage of the patient. Nursing standards also play a role in determining assessment priorities.

### Step 2. Prioritize the types of data to be collected

Systematic guidelines for collecting data ensure that comprehensive, holistic data will be collected. If data collection is well planned, nursing diagnoses follow easily. Problems in data collection arise when the data are inappropriately organized, when pertinent data are omitted, when irrelevant or duplicate data are collected, when erroneous or misinterpreted data are collected, when too little information is acquired, when interpretation of data (rather than observed behavior) is recorded, and/or when failure to update the data base occurs.

### Step 3. Establish the data base

The next step in assessment requires the establishment of a foundation of patient information on which to base the design and implementation of a comprehensive and effective plan of care. When an assessment is performed on initial contact with the patient, the data collected are referred to as baseline (i.e., starting point) data, hence the term **data base.** Patient data are derived from many sources, including the nursing history, the nursing examination, a review of the patient's record, and/or consultation with the patient's support persons or healthcare professionals. Data are also available from other sources, including the medical history, physical exam, progress notes, and reports of diagnostic studies or other therapies by other healthcare professionals.

### Step 4. Continuously update the data base

The data base must be continually revised as the patient's therapy and condition change. Updating the data base not only ensures that it remains accurate and current but it also becomes a means of identifying patterns or trends. How often the data base must be updated depends on the data type, the patient's condition, the cost to acquire the data in terms of expense and patient comfort in relation to the benefit in obtaining the data, and many other factors.

Sweeney (1990) has suggested that assessment should occur periodically throughout a patient's stay in the gastroenterology department. According to Sweeney, initial assessment should take place on a patient's admission to the preprocedural area. Second and third assessment reviews should be done on admission and discharge from the procedure room. A fourth assessment should be done on return to the postprocedural area, and a final assessment should be done when the patient is discharged from that area. During each assessment, patient problems and needs should be clearly stated to assure pertinent ongoing assessment and care.

### Step 5. Validate data

To keep the data free from error, bias, and misinterpretation, it must be confirmed or verified periodically. The act of verifying or confirming data is also known as **validation.** Validation becomes particularly necessary when data discrepancies exist. For example, a nurse who receives verbal communication of an allergy to streptomycin, yet notes a recorded allergy to penicillin, should validate a patient's drug allergies.

### Step 6. Communicate data

Data are of no benefit unless they are effectively communicated in a timely and accurate manner. Timeliness of the communication is particularly important if the data are critical to a patient's condition. Data collected in an assessment should be documented in the medical record and/or verbally reported to other members of the healthcare team. In addition, comprehensive, concise, and easily retrievable summaries of these data should be written to convey a unique sense of the patient.

Documentation of patient data fulfills the standard of care that requires a patient's health status be communicated. Data should be recorded legibly, good grammar should be used, and only standard medical abbreviations should be included. Moreover, to speed data retrieval, the data should be formatted under headings and organized categorically whenever possible. Some information is more appropriately recorded in narrative form, while other information should be charted on a flow sheet.

Documentation of patient data must comply with certain legal requirements. (Written records are the most readily acceptable as evidence in a trial.) Specifically, the nurse must chart everything observed, carried out, changed, taught, evaluated, or initiated. The data base should contain descriptive, objective, and subjective information supported by documented facts.

To avoid ambiguity when documenting data derived from conversation or interview, the patient should be quoted verbatim or the entry should be otherwise noted as a paraphrase. Similarly, clarifying errors avoids miscommunication of data. A nurse can fix an error, by striking the notation with a single line, enclosing it in parentheses, writing "error" above it, and initialing it.

### DATA COLLECTION METHODS

During the assessment phase of the nursing process, a nurse relies on the following three techniques to gather data: observation, the nursing interview, and the nursing examination.

### Observation

Observation during the assessment process entails conscious, deliberate use of the five senses. It is employed during both the nursing history and the physical examination. By learning to sense and interpret meaningful stimuli, both subjective and objective data can be collected.

**Subjective data** are those that can only be perceived by the affected person and cannot be perceived or verified experimentally. **Objective data** are perceptible to the senses and verifiable by another person observing the same data. Both data types are important cues in pattern recognition.

### Nursing interview

The intent of the **nursing interview** is to record a patient's unique qualities. When this goal is met, the planning of individualized care becomes possible. Sensitivity to the patient's vulnerability and to the timing of the interview, the environment in which it takes place, and the patient's comfort ensures productive, nonthreatening nurse patient contact.

In addition, well-developed interpersonal communication skills promote a climate of cooperation and involvement. Direct questioning, for instance, may be a useful means of validating or clarifying information, or of placing events in a meaningful sequence. Open-ended, reflective questions encourage respondents to freely vocalize their thoughts and feelings. Both types of questions have a place in the nursing interview. On the contrary, other techniques, including use of cliches, questions requiring the answers "yes" or "no" only, probing or loaded "why" or "how" questions, judgmental comments, false assurance, and advice can impede communication and intimidate respondents.

### Nursing examination

The **nursing examination** is a third means of collecting information with which to establish the patient data base. The nursing examination verifies information uncovered in the nursing history interview and also contributes new objective data. While the physician's physical assessment focuses on pathology and etiology, the nursing examination focuses primarily on the patient's functional abilities, which might affect his or her ability to comprehend or communicate information, the nature of therapeutic intervention, or compliance with a therapeutic regimen. Some nurses in expanded roles perform comprehensive physical examinations. All nurses conduct selected aspects of physical assessment for nursing purposes.

## DATA COLLECTION: THE GASTROENTEROLOGY ASSESSMENT

Because of the vague nature of symptoms of gastrointestinal disorders, digestive diseases are among the most difficult to assess. Systemic diseases, including Graves' disease, diabetes, congestive heart failure, emphysema, neoplasms, rheumatoid arthritis, myxedema, drug reactions, and renal disorders may elicit gastrointestinal manifestations such as nausea, vomiting, abdominal pain, altered appetite, and/or bowel changes. On the other hand, certain gastrointestinal disorders produce systemic manifestations. For example, ulcerative colitis is associated with dermatitis eczema, and dependent edema secondary to protein loss or electrolyte imbalance is common to malabsorptive disease, hepatic disease, and neoplasia. To complicate matters further, some digestive disorders may not be disease-related at all but may be a side effect of medication. For this reason, *all* complaints are potentially meaningful and therefore merit attention.

A gastrointestinal assessment generally follows the same format and guidelines as a general assessment. Data are derived from:

- The nursing history
- The nursing examination
- Other sources, including the results of laboratory tests, radiographic examinations, and special diagnostic procedures

Obviously, however, certain areas of assessment take on greater significance with specific gastrointestinal disorders. In addition, as the nurse begins to recognize patterns in the cues derived, areas on which it is appropriate to focus become more apparent. The following discussion concerns the types of information that should be sought during an initial interview of a gastroenterology patient.

### The nursing history

When taking a **nursing history,** there are five aspects of a patient's profile on which a gastroenterology nurse should focus:

- The nature of the health problem
- History of gastrointestinal symptoms
- A medication profile
- Nutritional status
- Psychosocial factors

### The nature of the health problem

The first objective is to arrive at a clear statement of the patient's health problem or chief complaint. The nurse must be alert to manifestations of pain, noting the location, intensity, and whether or not the pain radiates. Associated symptoms may also be significant. For example, testicular atrophy, gynecomastia, and alopecia may be associated with hepatic cirrhosis. Commonly experienced symptoms that should cue an interviewer to the presence of gastrointestinal disease are nausea and vomiting, changes in bowel habits, dysphagia, weight loss or gain, and changes in appetite.

### History of gastrointestinal symptoms

Equally important is the pattern with which symptoms occur. The nurse should record any relevant history of gastrointestinal symptoms, including the duration of the diagnosed gastrointestinal problem, (if it has been diagnosed), and any evidence of complications stemming from gastrointestinal disease. The nurse should also record any possible familial tendency toward the problem as manifest in parents, brothers, or sisters, and the presence of risk factors for gastrointestinal disease. Examples of familial problems and risk factors might include familial polyposis, a family history of colon cancer, excessive alcohol intake, and smoking.

### Medication profile

Because medications are frequently the cause of gastrointestinal disease and because these disorders can disrupt the normal uptake of certain medications, a medication profile should be obtained. The patient's profile should include medication or food allergies. The patient's past and present use of medications taken for gastrointestinal problems should be explored. If the patient has experienced or is presently experiencing side effects from these medications, this fact should also be recorded. Likewise, it is important to evaluate whether or not the patient is experiencing or has experienced the desired effects of the medication. Finally, current use of other prescription and nonprescription medications should be described.

### Nutritional status

Considering that 40 to 60% of patients admitted to U.S. hospitals exhibit varying levels of malnutrition and that nutritional status directly affects immunity and wound healing, nutritional assessment takes on great importance. The nurse should note patterns of consumption and elimination and relationships between diet and symptoms, diet and medications, diet and lifestyle, and diet and emotional states.

Nutritional problems can be the result of poor intake caused by an impaired appetite or by diseases such as intestinal obstruction or diarrhea. Poor digestion or absorption of nutrients may result from intestinal hypermotility, impaired intrinsic mechanisms of absorption, decreased bile salts, the absence of normal digestive secretions (e.g., secondary to pancreatic deficiency), or from drugs. These effects may also result from decreased utilization of nutrients, as might be seen in liver dysfunction or neoplasms of the GI tract. Increased excretion or protein loss characterizes many gastrointestinal disorders, including abscesses, fistulas, and ulcerative colitis. They also may present as sequelae of gastric surgery.

Nutritional problems also arise when body nutrient requirements increase, as during bouts of fever or during periods of rapid growth and development. In addition, they frequently accompany conditions marked by increased tissue destruction, including cancer, ulceration, and necrosis. (Nutritional assessment is discussed in greater detail in Chapter 23.) Serum albumin level, total lymphocyte count, and unintentional weight loss are three criteria useful as instant assessment parameters of nutritional status. These criteria are especially useful when screening patients at risk for complications related to malnutrition when minimal time is available for nutritional assessment.

**Psychosocial factors**

*Control* and *compliance* are terms that recur in the literature describing gastrointestinal disorders. *Control* refers to a patient's state of health, while *compliance* refers to patient behavior. An implicit relationship exists between compliance and control; the patient in good control is presumed to be compliant, and the patient in poor control is presumed to be noncompliant. Gardner (1987) explains this relationship with the health belief model, which holds that when an individual recognizes personal susceptibility and believes that becoming ill will bring serious organic and/or social repercussions, action will be taken. An individual must believe that the benefits from treatment outweigh the costs of compliance, including drug costs, side effects, lifestyle changes, inconvenient regimens, and so on.

An assessment based on this model focuses on a patient's perceptions surrounding health and illness, which might influence treatment outcome. It also explores a patient's perceptions of the impact of the health problem on his or her life and the cost and benefit of the prescribed treatment regimen. Deficits in knowledge or comprehension, psychological disturbances, social disruption, and/or the nature of the therapeutic regimen may cause an interruption in therapy and consequently, patient noncompliance.

It may be possible to assess the likelihood of compliance. A patient with previously documented low compliance is at high risk for repeating low-compliance behavior; a patient who admits to low compliance shows the most favorable response to compliance improvement strategies. Gardner also believes that an important component of the psychosocial assessment of a gastroenterology patient is the evaluation of the need for education, as well as the need for social, emotional, and financial support.

Others explain compliance or noncompliance in terms of self-concept, suggesting that the psychosocial assessment of a gastroenterology patient should center on factors that affect self-concept. Similarly, nursing diagnoses should reflect disturbances of one or more factors affecting self-concept. According to this model, the role of a nurse assessing the psychological status of patients exceeds evaluation of barriers to compliance to include promotion of healthy psychosocial responses.

Still others define the psychosocial assessment as an assessment of mental status. The major focus of a mental status assessment is the determination of an individual's strengths, capabilities, and resources for environmental, social, and intrapsychic adjustment. The goal of this assessment is to identify cognitive processes, emotions, and behaviors that interfere with a patient's ability to achieve an optimal level of function. Numerous aspects of a patient's psychological functioning are assessed, as manifest in the patient's appearance, behavior, and conversation. In the course of a psychosocial assessment, the nurse first collects and analyzes the data, then makes inferences about the patient's psychological state. Such inferences allow the nurse to plan, implement, and evaluate nursing care during the patient's entire procedural experience.

**Physical examination**

Physical measurements of any patient in a gastroenterology unit must include vital signs. Height and weight may also be included. In addition, the patient's heart, lungs, and abdomen should be assessed. Assessment of other systems may be appropriate, depending on the patient's condition and health problem(s). This section describes techniques used in inspection, auscultation, palpation, and percussion of the abdomen. Physical assessment of the rectum, skin, extremities, chest, reproductive organs, and renal system may be important where a cause and effect relationship exists. The nurse should consult a textbook on physical assessment for comprehensive information.

Physical assessment of the abdomen is performed in four phases: inspection, auscultation, percussion, and palpation. Inspection and auscultation should always precede percussion and palpation. This order is particularly important when assessing the abdomen because stimulation of the abdomen caused by percussion and palpation increases bowel sounds. Therefore, it is important to complete one technique before starting the next.

**Inspection**

The examiner should note the patient's breathing pattern (chest versus abdominal breathing) and be alert for scars, distended veins, and signs of abdominal trauma that may be relevant to the present illness. In addition, striae, which may evidence significant weight loss, should be noted. Upon inspection of the contour, the examiner should observe symmetry of the abdomen (above and below the umbilicus). Distention will present as a rounded contour. The umbilicus is useful as an aid when distinguishing causes of distention. It may be everted in ascites, whereas it remains unchanged in gaseous distention. Peristaltic waves can sometimes be observed, particularly if the patient is thin. This sign becomes even more significant when an obstruction is present.

**Auscultation**

The nurse should observe the frequency and rhythm of bowel sounds by listening with the diaphragm of a stethoscope. Bowel sounds vary considerably in normal individuals, and may be present or absent. Normal bowel sounds do not rule out bleeding or other pathology. Normal bowel sounds are soft, high-pitched sounds. Before declaring that no bowel sounds are present, it is important to listen in each quadrant for a total of 4 to 5 minutes. Findings significant on auscultation include the following:

- Bruits, which may indicate cardiovascular abnormality rather than gastrointestinal pathology
- High-pitched tinkles and peristaltic rushes, which are audible when intestinal obstruction occurs
- Decreased or absent bowel sounds, which are evidence of paralytic ileus, gangrene, peritonitis, or inflammation

**Percussion**

Based on much the same concept as ultrasound, percussion is performed with two hands. Sound waves produced by striking one object against another allow an examiner to note the presence of air, fluid, and solid matter in the abdomen.

To perform percussion, the examiner should place the distal phalanx of the middle finger of the nondominant hand flat against the area to be percussed. This finger is the only part of the examiner's hand that should be in contact with the abdomen. With the tip of the flexed middle finger of the dominant hand, the examiner should sharply strike the distal joint of the phalanx on the abdomen. Notes generated by this action reflect the size, density, and characteristics of the underlying abdominal structures and can be described as flat, dull, resonant, hyperresonant, and tympanic. Tympany generally denotes large amounts of gas in the stomach and intestines, while dullness is normally noted over a full bladder, mass, or organs such as the liver or spleen. The presence of fluid is not always easy to differentiate from other conditions but is suspected when there is abdominal distension with bulging flanks, a fluid wave, and shifting dullness when the patient is turned on one side.

**Palpation**

Touch is most useful in identifying tenderness, temperature changes, and masses. Both shallow and deep palpation should be performed during assessment. Findings significant to digestive diseases include fluid waves, abnormal organ size, rebound tenderness, masses, and hernias. Examination of the size, shape, position, consistency, mobility, and tension of the major organs concludes physical assessment of the abdomen.

It is important for the examiner to refrain from palpating a large pulsating mass in the abdominal midline because the mass might be an aortic aneurysm. In addition, an enlarged spleen should not be overpal-

---

| Potential diagnostic data in gastroenterology | |
|---|---|
| *Laboratory* | *Radiology* |
| CBC: Hb, HCt, lymphocytes | Chest radiograph |
| Electrolytes | Flat plate of abdomen |
| Ketones and protein | Upper GI series |
| Amylase | Lower GI series |
| Lipase | Contrast radiographs |
| Creatinine | |
| Serum cholesterol | *Special diagnostic procedures* |
| LDH, AST, ALT | |
| Glucose | CT scans |
| Bilirubin | Nuclear imaging |
| Serum albumin | Ultrasound |
| | Rectal examination |

---

pated and the kidneys should not be palpated in patients who have had transplants.

**Diagnostic tests**

Diagnostic studies provide another major source of information when collecting patient data. In conjunction with each study, gastroenterology nurses should be aware of why the study is done, the significance of abnormal findings, and the implications for nursing care and patient teaching with each finding. The box above lists laboratory, radiologic, and special diagnostic procedures that may be prescribed in the course of a medical assessment, the results of which should inform a nursing data base.

**Preprocedural assessment**

As described early in the chapter, nursing assessment may be comprehensive or focused. In gastroenterology departments, a preprocedural assessment is typically a focused assessment. Preprocedural assessment of the gastroenterology patient should follow this or a similar format:

- Verify informed consent
- Verify length of NPO status
- Obtain or verify the patient's history, including past surgery, allergies, current medications and information pertinent to current complaint
- Obtain laboratory results per institutional policy
- Verify that preparation for procedure was accomplished (e.g., bowel prep)
- Obtain baseline vital signs
- Be aware of any significant concomitant disease involving the heart, lungs, kidneys, or liver

**Intraprocedural assessment**

In the gastroenterology unit, the primary objectives of an intraprocedural assessment are to help the patient tolerate the procedure with minimal anxiety, fear, and discomfort; to prevent untoward reactions where possible; and to provide a safe, efficient procedure in a therapeutic milieu. As part of the intraprocedural assessment of the gastroenterology patient, the nurse should evaluate and be prepared to deal with:

- The patient's emotional response to the procedure (e.g., fear, anxiety, hostility, or anger)
- Potential procedural complications (e.g., hypovolemia, gastrointestinal bleeding, untoward drug reactions, perforation, or aspiration)
- Any concurrent medical problems (e.g., history of coronary disease, pulmonary disease, allergies, seizure disorders, diabetes mellitus, or chemical dependency)

**Postprocedural assessment**

The primary objectives of postprocedural care in the gastroenterology unit are to help the patient recover in comfort without any untoward event and to provide postprocedural education with regard to diet, medication, activity restrictions, and disease state. Potential problems that the gastroenterology nurse should be aware of in the postprocedural period are as follows:

- Decreased sensory response caused by sedation
- Alteration in comfort: abdominal pain
- Untoward response to medication (e.g., nausea and vomiting)
- Knowledge deficit with respect to postprocedure instructions, disease, and treatment

Thorough preprocedural, intraprocedural, and postprocedural assessments lay the foundation for the rest of the nursing process; identifying appropriate nursing diagnoses, setting patient goals and outcomes, planning patient care, intervention, and evaluation.

---

CASE SITUATION

Eleanor Russell, age 73, arrives in the gastroenterology department holding area. She originally went to the Emergency Room (ER) complaining of nausea and vomiting, severe right upper quadrant abdominal pain, and sternal pain with pressure radiating to her back. The ER nurse did not have time to take a comprehensive history, but he communicates to you that Mrs. Russell described a family history of gallbladder disease and was diagnosed with cholecystitis several months ago. In addition, he reports that Mrs. Russell's symptoms became worse after eating a peanut butter and Swiss cheese sandwich and a milk shake yesterday for lunch. Her ECG is normal, and she is currently on coumarin for thrombophlebitis in her right leg.

The ER nurse tells you that Mrs. Russell's stool is negative for occult blood but that her prothrombin time (PT) partial thromboplastin time (PTT) is abnormal.

Her physician has diagnosed Mrs. Russell with cholecystitis and cholelithiasis. He now awaits the results of further lab studies and an abdominal ultrasound examination to confirm or rule out gallstone obstruction of the common bile duct. The physician asks you to prepare for diagnostic laparoscopy.

As you greet Mrs. Russell, you notice that her face is rigid and pale. She is scanning her environment nervously and her eyes are open wide. Her hands are cool, moist, and trembling; you observe a large bruise near her left wrist. Her respirations are rapid and shallow as she tells you, "I've never had *anything* like this before. My daughter was supposed to have talked to my doctor about my diet...."

*Points to think about*

1. What steps should a nurse carry out in assessing Mrs. Russell before diagnostic laparoscopy?
2. What subjective data is evident thus far? What objective data?
3. Which data might need validation?
4. Which data would require documentation in Mrs. Russell's records?
5. What additional preprocedure assessment should the nurse undertake before preparing for the laparoscopic procedure?

*Suggested responses*

1. In assessing Mrs. Russell before diagnostic laparoscopy the nurse should take the following steps:
   - Identify assessment priorities
   - Prioritize types of data to be collected
   - Establish the data base
   - Continuously update the data base
   - Validate data
   - Communicate data
2. Thus far the following subjective and objective data are evident
   *Subjective data:* Nausea, sternal pain with pressure radiating to her back, symptoms became worse after eating a peanut butter and Swiss cheese sandwich and a milk shake
   *Objective data:* Mrs. Russell's ECG is normal; her face is rigid and pale; she is scanning her environment nervously with eyes open wide; her hands are cool, moist, and trembling; she has a large bruise near her

left wrist; respirations are rapid and shallow; reported history of gallbladder disease in the family; she admits, "I've never had *anything* like this before. My daughter was supposed to have talked to my doctor about my diet. . . ."

3. Because the ER nurse did not take a comprehensive history, but communicates that Mrs. Russell was diagnosed with cholecystitis several months ago, that her symptoms became worse after lunch yesterday, that her stool is negative for occult blood, and that her PT/PTT is abnormal, the nurse might need to validate these data in the record and/or with the patient.

4. The nurse must document everything observed, carried out, changed, taught, evaluated, or initiated.

5. During a preprocedure assessment the nurse should:
   - Verify informed consent
   - Perform nursing physical examination
   - Verify length of NPO status
   - Obtain or verify the patient's history
   - Obtain necessary preprocedural diagnostic tests
   - Obtain baseline vital signs
   - Obtain medication profile
   - Verify allergies

### REVIEW TERMS

**assessment, data, data base, nursing interview, nursing examination, nursing history, nursing process, objective data, observation, subjective data, validation**

### REVIEW QUESTIONS

1. A nursing assessment:
   a. Is an ongoing process of cue and pattern recognition.
   b. Is always comprehensive and systematic.
   c. Is a process of identifying a patient problem.
   d. Should precede a nursing history.

2. Which statement is true of physical assessment of the abdomen?
   a. The order in which inspection, palpation, percussion, and auscultation are performed is only important if the patient is in pain.
   b. Percussion and palpation should be performed before auscultation and inspection.
   c. Bowel sounds are normal if none are heard in four abdominal quadrants over a period of 4 to 5 minutes.
   d. Bowel sounds characterized by high-pitched tinkles and peristaltic rushes are abnormal.

3. A preprocedural assessment includes:
   a. Determination of baseline vital signs.
   b. Verification of current medications in use.
   c. Verification of NPO status.
   d. All of the above.

4. Validation is the act of:
   a. Clarification.
   b. Verification.
   c. Repeating a patient's responses twice.
   d. Checking to be sure a nursing history was taken.

5. Which of the following might the gastroenterology nurse record as objective nursing assessment data concerning a patient who presents in the ER with apparent biliary colic?
   a. A medical diagnosis of choledocholithiasis.
   b. "Patient is anxious."
   c. "Patient ate a peanut butter cheese sandwich yesterday at lunch."
   d. "Patient is scanning her surroundings with wide open eyes."

6. By which method(s) could a patient's medication history be validated?
   a. By asking the patient what medications he or she takes.
   b. By reading the prescription labels on the bottles of medicines the patient provides.
   c. Both a and b.
   d. Neither a nor b.

7. A medication history, a nutritional history, and a psychosocial history are:
   a. Three components of a nursing history.
   b. Only performed during a comprehensive assessment.
   c. Three phases of a nursing assessment.
   d. Barriers to compliance.

8. The purpose of nursing assessment is to:
   a. Identify underlying pathology.
   b. Identify teaching needs.
   c. Identify adverse responses to health problems.
   d. Collect pertinent patient data.

9. The focus by the nurse on the functional abilities of the patient takes place during the:
   a. Interview.
   b. Observation.
   c. Nursing examination.
   d. Physician's assessment.

10. Which of the following statements would indicate that a psychosocial assessment was performed?
    a. Patient is complaining of nausea.
    b. Patient states she is having sternal pain.
    c. Patient admits she has not adhered to prescribed diet.
    d. Patient's hands are cold and moist.

### BIBLIOGRAPHY

Barnie, D. "Care Planning in the Endoscopy Unit: Master Care Plan for the Intraprocedure Patient." *SGA Journal* 11(Winter 1989): 153-55.

Barnie, D. "Care Planning in the GI Endoscopy Unit: Master Care Plan for the Postprocedure Patient." *Gastroenterology Nursing* 11(Spring 1989): 266-67.

Bodinsky, G. *Documentation: Charting to Standardize.* SGNA Monograph Series. Rochester, N.Y.: Society of Gastroenterology Nurses and Associates, 1989.

Gardner, S. "Assessment of Barriers to Compliance or Why Did Eve Go Wrong?" *SGA Journal* 10(Fall 1987): 105-10.

Given, B, and Simmons, S. *Gastroenterology in Clinical Nursing.* 4th ed. St. Louis: Mosby–Year Book, 1984.

Gruber, M, and Gruber, M. "Nursing Malpractice: The Importance of Documentation, or Saved by the Pen!" *Gastroenterology Nursing* 12(Spring 1990): 255-59.

Hardick, M, and Beck, M, eds. *Manual of Gastrointestinal Procedures.* 2nd ed. Rochester, N.Y.: Society of Gastroenterology Nurses and Associates, 1989.

Kneedler, J, and Dodge, G, eds. *Perioperative Patient Care.* 2nd ed. Palo Alto: Blackwell Scientific Publications, Inc. 1989.

Rowland, G, Marks, D, and Torres, W. "The New Gallstone Destroyers and Dissolvers." *American Journal of Nursing* 89(1989): 1473-76.

Stephens, N, and Messner, R. "Nutritional Assessment: Implications for Infection Prevention and Control." In *SGA Journal Reprints,* ed. Trivits, S, 163-66. Rochester, N.Y.: Society of Gastrointestinal Assistants, 1988.

Sweeney, J. "Endoscopy Assessment Tool—A New Approach." *Gastroenterology Nursing* 13(Fall 1990): 71-76.

Taylor, C, Lillis, C, and LeMone, P. "The Nursing Process." In *Fundamentals of Nursing, The Art and Science of Nursing Care,* 241-325. Philadelphia: J.B. Lippincott, 1989.

# Chapter 9

# NURSING DIAGNOSIS

This chapter discusses the nurse's role in diagnosing actual or potential health problems specific to patients with gastrointestinal disorders. Nursing diagnosis is defined and differentiated from medical diagnosis. Examples of functional health patterns and the subsequent nursing diagnoses for gastroenterology patients are presented.

## Learning objectives

After reviewing the content of this chapter, the gastroenterology nurse should be able to:

1. Define nursing diagnosis.
2. Differentiate between nursing diagnosis, medical diagnosis, and collaborative diagnosis.
3. Formulate a nursing diagnosis using an approved classification system.
4. Discuss actual, potential, and possible nursing diagnoses applicable to gastroenterology patients.

During the 1950s the term *nursing diagnosis* first appeared in the literature. Because of the implications associated with diagnosis and the idea that only physicians made diagnoses, nurses were reluctant to use the term. They were more comfortable using the word *"problems"* to refer to a patient's need requiring nursing intervention. Periodically through the '60s and '70s the literature proposed descriptions of nursing diagnoses. Finally, an article by Lester King, M.D., in the *Journal of the American Medical Association* refuted the idea that only physicians could diagnose, thereby clearing the way for more exploration of the concept of nursing diagnosis (McFarland and McFarlane, 1989). King outlined three criteria that must be present to make a diagnosis:

1. A preexisting series of categories or classes that provide a reference for the diagnosis.
2. An entity to be diagnosed.
3. A judgment that the assessed response or phenomenon belongs to a particular class or category.

At that point, nurses began to develop a classification system for nursing diagnosis. This work was started through conferences on classification of nursing diagnoses and is still in progress today through the North American Nursing Diagnosis Association (NANDA). Other individuals and groups have played a role in identifying and testing human response patterns that result in a diagnostic label. The nursing field is now attempting to use the concept of nursing diagnosis as the linchpin in establishing autonomy and bringing unity to the profession. Only the future holds the results of these efforts.

## NURSING DIAGNOSIS DEFINED

Nursing diagnoses are based on the data obtained from the patient in the course of the nursing assessment. A nursing diagnosis provides a concise statement of the interpretation of data collected. This concise statement describes the nature, source, and manifestations of health changes that the nurse is licensed to identify and treat through independent and interdependent nursing intervention.

Nursing diagnosis has become a critical link in the application of the nursing process. The same problem-solving skills are required to analyze the data obtained during an assessment and to make judgments and decisions about the problems that prevent patients and families from responding in a normal, healthy fashion. The process of determining a nursing diagnosis entails the use of clinical reasoning and judgment, which result in labeling the patient's health problem. This labeling is the product of collecting data, interpreting the information collected, grouping and clustering related facts, and assigning a name to the groupings.

Carpenito (1987) has defined nursing diagnosis as a statement of an individual or group that describes a human response (health state or actual/potential altered interaction pattern) that the nurse can legally identify and for which the nurse can order definitive interventions to maintain the health state or to reduce, eliminate, or prevent alterations.

Alternatively, Shoemaker (1984) defines nursing diagnosis as a clinical judgment about an individual, family, or community derived through a deliberate, systematic process of data collection and analysis. It provides the basis for prescriptions for definitive therapy for which the nurse is accountable. It is concisely expressed and includes the etiology of the condition when known.

A **nursing diagnosis** is simply a statement of the results of analyzing and interpreting assessment data. The value of the nursing diagnosis is that it provides a scientific basis for nursing practice so that desired patient outcomes and planned interventions are consistent with the patient's health problems.

### Nursing diagnosis versus medical diagnosis

The process used to identify a diagnosis or a patient problem is the same for nursing and medicine. Both nursing and medical diagnoses are concerned with gathering, sorting, interpreting, and analyzing data. However, **medical diagnosis** focuses on identification of a disease based on pathology and etiology, whereas nursing diagnosis focuses on the patient's present **health problems,** strengths and limitations, and methods of adapting to health problems. Table 9-1 provides examples of how nursing diagnoses and medical diagnoses differ.

### COLLABORATIVE DIAGNOSIS

Recently a distinction has also been drawn between nursing diagnosis and collaborative diagnosis. Taylor, Lillis, and LeMone (1989) have defined **collaborative**

**Table 9-1.** Nursing diagnosis versus medical diagnosis

| Nursing diagnosis | Medical diagnosis |
| --- | --- |
| Directs nursing acts to be performed | Diagnoses medical condition |
| Identifies patient problems that the nurse is licensed to treat | Indicates a course of treatment |
| Made with the intention that nurses will perform interventions to alleviate, diminish, modify, or prevent a state of unwellness and maintain an optimum health state | Made with the intention of prescribing specific treatments to cure the disease or reduce injury |
| May change from day to day as the patient's response to therapy, health, and illness change | Remains the same as long as the disease persists |

**diagnoses** as statements of actual or potential health problems that occur from complications of disease, diagnostic studies, or therapeutic procedures or other treatment regimens. These are problems for which the nurse identifies a need to work with other members of the healthcare team toward resolution. Collaborative diagnoses require both nursing and medical intervention to diagnose, prevent, or treat. Carpenito (1987) defines collaborative problems as "the physiological complications that have resulted or may result from pathophysiological and treatment-related situations." Nurses monitor patients to detect their onset/status and collaborate with physicians for definitive treatment.

It is important to remember that medical diagnoses, medical pathologies, diagnostic tests, treatments, and/or equipment names are not nursing diagnoses. And while the following data are considered when identifying health problems, they are not nursing diagnoses: therapeutic patient needs, therapeutic patient goals, a single sign or symptom, or invalidated nursing inferences.

### FORMULATING A NURSING DIAGNOSIS

The chapter on assessment discusses collection of data. It is essential that nurses understand what data are significant and how to obtain that important information. Knowledge of nursing science and other related biopsychosocial sciences is important to interpret the data and to accurately formulate the nursing diagnosis. Interpretation means sorting information and making a hypothesis for the occurrence of related events, conditions, or behavior. Nurses use clinical inferences in inductive reasoning when looking at functional patterns and observing patient responses. They then ask the questions, "What does this mean? Why is he saying this?" Gordon (1987) notes that interpretation involves the ability to (1) pay attention to and recognize diagnostic cues, (2) clarify or search for clearer understanding of cues, (3) verify or double-check the cues, (4) recognize the direct or concealed meaning of cues, and (5) evaluate the cues.

Cues are explored, data are collected, and the cues are *clustered.* Clustering involves making a judgment as to whether cues are consistent or inconsistent. The conclusion might be that the evidence does not support the existence of an actual problem, but that the patient is at risk for the problem to occur (a potential problem). Inconsistencies might be caused by conflicting reports from other members of the healthcare team, the patient, or the family or by unrealistic expectations on the part of the nurse because of inexperience or lack of knowledge.

The diagnosis made may be an actual problem, a potential problem, or a possible problem, each of which is described as follows:

- **Actual problems** are conditions that presently produce a difficulty. They are identified by observation or statement of fact about the patient and his or her behavior. They may also vary from day to day depending on the circumstances. Example: Non-compliance with prescribed regimen.

- **Potential problems** are problems that do not currently exist; however, the patterns indicate that certain risk factors are in place and nursing actions to prevent these problems are in order. Example: Potential burn resulting from electrical device.
- **Possible problems** are conditions that have a high probability of developing because of an existing condition or disease. Example: Bowel elimination, altered: constipation.

Developing a nursing diagnosis is a three-step process, which is described by Gordon (1976) as the PES format, as follows:

P = Health problem
E = Etiology
S = Signs and symptoms

The diagnosis statement states the health problem as related to the etiology and manifested by the signs and symptoms. To identify these three factors, the nurse performs the following activities:

1. Clusters groups of patient data to point to the existence of a health problem.
2. Compares the collection of cues against established standards to identify any of the following:
   a. Changes in a patient's usual health pattern that are unexplained by expected norms for growth and development
   b. Deviation from an appropriate population norm (e.g., lab values)
   c. Behavior that is nonproductive in the whole-person context
   d. Behavior indicating a developmental lag or evolving dysfunctional pattern
3. Identifies the patient's strengths and the patient's problem areas, and anticipates problems the patient is likely to experience

Several conclusions are possible:

- There is no problem and intervention is unnecessary
- There is an actual or potential problem
- There is a possible problem, which suggests the need to collect more data
- There is a clinical problem other than a nursing problem (a collaborative problem) that requires the nurse to consult with and sometimes cooperate with appropriate healthcare professionals

Identifying specific nursing problems and prioritizing them helps to focus gastroenterology nursing practice and improve the quality of nursing care. Table 9-2 contains a partial list of approved nursing diagnoses classified by functional health problems. The classification system reflects areas in which assessment takes place.

## COMMON NURSING DIAGNOSES FOR THE GASTROENTEROLOGY PATIENT

Nurses caring for patients in the gastroenterology unit have reported a need for the use of standards of care when performing an assessment and identifying patient problems. In many situations it is not evident that the plan of care reflects activities specifically related to an individual nursing diagnosis. Sweeney has suggested a new approach, based on a gastrointestinal assessment form completed by the nurse. Once completed, this assessment form serves as a preprocedural and postprocedural care plan. The nursing assessment and subsequent care plan include data regarding the patient's complaint, nursing diagnosis, plan of care, documentation, and discharge information.

Assessment is the initial component of the nursing process; it should always be done when the patient is admitted to the preprocedural area. The plan of care is initiated when the nurse interprets assessment findings and determines pertinent nursing diagnoses.

Sweeney (1990) identifies selected nursing diagnoses that are common to many gastroenterology patients:

- Anxiety
- Knowledge deficit
- Alteration in sensory perception
- Ineffective airway clearance
- Alteration in comfort
- Alteration in bowel elimination
- Potential for injury
- Potential for infection

---

**CASE SITUATION**

In Chapter 8, Mrs. Russell, who has been medically diagnosed as having cholecystitis and cholelithiasis, was scheduled for a diagnostic laparoscopy. During the preprocedural assessment, certain subjective data were identified, including:

- Nausea
- Sternal pain with pressure radiating to her back
- Symptoms becoming worse after eating peanut butter, swiss cheese, and a milk shake

Objective data were also gathered, including:

- Normal ECG
- Face rigid and pale
- Scanning environment nervously with eyes open wide
- Hands cool, moist, and trembling
- Large bruise near left wrist
- Respirations rapid and shallow

*Points to think about*

1. Based on observations thus far, what are at least three functional health problems for Mrs. Russell?

**Table 9-2.** Potential nursing diagnoses for gastroenterology patients

| Functional health problem | Nursing diagnoses |
|---|---|
| Nutritional metabolic pattern | Fluid volume deficit, actual |
| | Fluid volume deficit, potential |
| | Nutrition, altered: less than body requirements |
| | Nutrition, altered: more than body requirements |
| | Nutrition, altered: potential for more than body requirement |
| | Injury, potential for: (specify) |
| | Skin integrity, impairment of: actual |
| | Skin integrity, impairment of: potential |
| | Oral mucous membrane, altered |
| | Body temperature, altered, potential |
| | Breathing pattern, ineffective |
| Elimination pattern | Bowel elimination, altered: constipation |
| | Bowel elimination, alteration in: diarrhea |
| Activity-exercise pattern | Activity tolerance, decreased |
| | Mobility, impaired physical |
| | Rest-activity pattern, ineffective |
| Cognitive-perceptual pattern | Knowledge deficit related to disease and therapy |
| | Comfort, altered: pain |
| | Comfort, altered: chronic pain |
| | Communication, impaired verbal |
| | Thought processes, altered |
| Sleep-rest pattern | Sleep pattern disturbance |
| | Rest-activity pattern, ineffective |
| Self-perception/self-concept pattern | Body image disturbance |
| | Self concept, disturbance in sensory perceptual alterations |
| Role relationship pattern | Family process, altered, |
| | Social isolation |
| | Social interaction, impaired |
| Sexuality pattern | Sexual dysfunction |
| | Sexual patterns, altered |
| Coping-stress tolerance pattern | Coping, ineffective |
| | Anxiety |
| | Fear |
| | Depression |
| | Hopelessness |
| Value-belief pattern | Health-seeking behaviors (specify) |
| | Unilateral neglect |
| Health perception-management pattern | Noncompliance with prescribed regimen |
| | Home maintenance management, impaired |

2. According to Table 9-2, what are specific nursing diagnoses for Mrs. Russell's health problems?
3. Into which of the following would these nursing diagnoses be categorized: actual problems, potential problems, and possible problems?
4. Using the PES format, how would a nurse diagram two of the nursing diagnoses identified for Mrs. Russell?
5. Is there a collaborative diagnosis for Mrs. Russell? If interdependent nursing and medical interventions are necessary, what would the difference be in the nursing focus versus medical focus?

*Suggested responses*

1. Functional health problems the gastroenterology nurse might identify are:
   • Health perception—health management pattern
   • Coping—stress tolerance pattern
   • Nutritional metabolic pattern
   • Cognitive-perceptual pattern approved

2. Specific nursing diagnoses that correspond to these health problems might be:

| Functional health problem | Nursing diagnosis |
|---|---|
| Health perception—health management pattern | Noncompliant with prescribed regimen |
| Coping—stress tolerance pattern | Anxiety |
| Nutritional metabolic pattern | Injury, potential for bruising, hemorrhage |
| Cognitive-perceptual pattern | Knowledge deficit related to disease and therapy |

3. Nursing diagnoses might include the following actual, potential, and possible problems:
   • Actual problems: noncompliance with prescribed regimen, anxiety, and knowledge deficit

- Potential problem: injury, potential for bruising, hemorrhage
- Possible problem: nutrition, altered: possible less than body requirement because of pain when eating

4. Two nursing diagnoses might be diagrammed in the following manner:

| P: Health problem | Anxiety |
| E: Etiology | Related to procedure |
| S: Signs/symptoms | Scanning environment nervously with eyes wide open |
| | Hands cool, moist and trembling |
| P: Health problem | Nutrition altered: less than body requirements |
| E: Etiology | Loss of necessary nutrients |
| S: Signs/symptoms | Nausea, sternal pain with pressure radiating to back |

5. In Mrs. Russell's case the diagnosis of cholecystitis with cholelithiasis is a medical diagnosis. The nursing focus is on collecting data related to functional needs, with the outcome being care of the patient. The medical focus is on the medical history and a physical examination, with the desired outcome being care of the disease.

---

### REVIEW TERMS

**collaborative diagnosis, health problems, nursing diagnosis, medical diagnosis, potential health problems, actual health problems, possible health problems**

---

### REVIEW QUESTIONS

1. Which of the following was *not* one of King's criteria for making a diagnosis?
   a. A preexisting series of categories to provide a reference.
   b. An entity to be diagnosed.
   c. The existence of a medical pathology.
   d. A judgment that the assessed phenomenon belongs to a particular category.
2. The organization responsible for classification of nursing diagnoses is the:
   a. American Nurses' Association.
   b. North American Nursing Diagnosis Association.
   c. Society of Gastroenterology Nurses and Associates.
   d. American Medical Association.
3. "Cholecystitis with cholelithiasis" is an example of a:
   a. Collaborative diagnosis.
   b. Nursing diagnosis.
   c. Medical diagnosis.
   d. Medical history.
4. A health problem is a:
   a. Problem all healthcare professionals attend to.
   b. Deficit in knowledge about nutrition, exercise, and rest.
   c. Behavior.
   d. Condition related to health.
5. A collaborative diagnosis:
   a. Calls for both medical and nursing intervention.
   b. Requires cooperation between nurses responsible for pre-, intra-, and postprocedure patient care.
   c. Involves the nurse in identification, but not treatment.
   d. Is identified by more than one member of the healthcare team.
6. A model of the three essential components of a nursing diagnosis proposed by Gordon is the:
   a. PSE Format.
   b. SPC Format.
   c. PES Format.
   d. PCE Format.
7. Formulating a nursing diagnosis provides:
   a. Important assessment data.
   b. An interpretation of the data collected.
   c. Interdependent nursing interventions.
   d. Outcome criteria for evaluation.
8. Nursing diagnosis focuses on the patient's:
   a. Pathology and etiology.
   b. Pathophysiology.
   c. Present health state.
   d. Health perceptions.
9. An example of an actual problem would be:
   a. Potential burn resulting from ESU.
   b. Knowledge deficit related to disease and therapy.
   c. Fluid volume deficit, possible, due to nausea and pain.
   d. Skin integrity, potential for impairment.
10. A nursing diagnosis for a patient admitted to the endoscopy unit for a diagnostic esophagogastroduodenoscopy who is not responding to treatment for a gastric ulcer might be:
    a. Knowledge deficit related to new experience.
    b. Sensory perception, altered.
    c. Bowel elimination, altered.
    d. Airway clearance, ineffective.

### BIBLIOGRAPHY

Beare, P and Myers, J. *Principles and Practice of Adult Health Nursing.* St. Louis: Mosby–Year Book, 1990.

Carpenito, L. *Handbook of Nursing Diagnosis.* 2nd ed. Philadelphia: J. B. Lippincott, 1987.

Gordon, M. "Nursing Diagnosis and the Diagnostic Process." *American Journal of Nursing,* 76(1976): 1296.

Gordon, M. *Nursing Diagnosis: Process and Application.* New York: McGraw-Hill, 1987. p. 212.

McFarland, G and McFarlane, E. *Nursing Diagnosis and Intervention.* St. Louis: Mosby–Year Book, 1989.

North American Nursing Diagnosis Association. *Taxonomy 1 with Official Diagnostic Categories.* St. Louis: NANDA, 1989.

Shoemaker, J. "Essential Features of a Nursing Diagnosis." In *Classification of Nursing Diagnosis: Proceedings of the Fifth National Conference,* eds. Kim, M, McFarland, G, and McLane, A, 109. St. Louis: Mosby–Year Book, 1984.

Sweeney, Jeanne. "Endoscopy Assessment Tool: A New Approach." *Gastroenterology Nursing* 13(Fall 1990): 75-6.

Taylor, C, Lillis, C, and LeMone, P. "The Nursing Process." In *Fundamentals of Nursing, the Act and Science of Nursing Care,* eds. Cleary, P, Faven, E, and Intenzo, D, 241-325. Philadelphia: J. B. Lippincott, 1989.

# Chapter 10

# OUTCOME IDENTIFICATION

This chapter addresses outcome identification, another important component of the nursing process. Determining expected outcomes is a nursing activity that occurs as soon as the nursing diagnosis is formulated. In this chapter, the process of setting goals or outcomes is explained and examples specific to gastroenterology patients are provided. Ways in which outcomes are congruent with patient problems are explored and methods for measuring goal attainment are examined. The importance of documenting outcomes to provide direction to other members of the healthcare team and to provide continuity of care is emphasized.

## Learning Objectives

After reviewing the content of this chapter, the gastroenterology nurse should be able to:
1. Set realistic patient outcomes for gastroenterology patients.
2. Develop outcomes that are congruent with the existing or potential health problems of the patient.
3. Outline methods used to measure the result of nursing interventions.
4. Document expected outcomes to provide continuity of care.

## DEFINING OUTCOMES

The term *outcome* is not new; however, its use as a standard has evolved from what recently was referred to as the *patient goal*. The terms *goal* and *expected outcome* have been used interchangeably, although a goal generally describes what is wanted, while an outcome is thought of as the results achieved.

Today, **outcome identification** is the appropriate terminology to use when referring to the third component of the nursing process and also when referring to standards of practice. **Outcome** is the appropriate term to use to describe the end result of nursing actions. When referring to goals, it is best to speak of them in relation to specific amounts of intervention. They may be

short-term or long-term and can be used to measure the level of goal achievement. For example, a patient undergoing a gastrointestinal procedure may have a nursing diagnosis of "alteration in comfort, abdominal pain" with a desired result being "no perforation." Goals associated with this outcome might be "patient evacuating flatus." This indicates that there may not be a perforation; however, it does not ensure the result of "no perforation." In summary, all patient outcomes articulate in behavioral terms the prevention, reduction, or resolution of a health problem.

## IDENTIFYING EXPECTED OUTCOMES

Once the priorities of the nursing diagnosis have been determined the gastroenterology nurse participates in determining outcomes that can realistically be achieved by the patient. It is anticipated that the result of providing nursing care will be a change, resolution, or improvement in the patient's problem because the nursing actions taken will modify the problem. For example, a patient who is scheduled to have a gastroscopy may have a concomitant hematologic disorder. The nurse determines that the patient has a potential for bleeding during the procedure. The expected outcome is "no uncontrolled bleeding as a result of the procedure." To achieve this outcome, the nurse plans interventions that will result in a positive outcome for this patient.

The identification of outcomes requires that the gastroenterology nurse possess communication skills and make good nursing judgments based on decision-making skills. Communication skills are needed when interacting with the patient, the family, and other members of the healthcare team. Determining desired outcomes for patients is not solely a nursing responsibility. If there is any hope of a positive outcome, outcome identification must be a mutual activity that involves both the patient and the nurse. Nurses can make excellent plans for their patients; however, unless patients provide input about what is realistic for them, what has worked in the past, and how they individually respond to situations, the desired results may never be achieved. The outcomes devised will be more realistic when there is an effective nurse-patient relationship. Input from other members of the team is also needed to validate the appropriateness of care.

Nursing judgment is used when the gastroenterology nurse makes decisions related to patients' needs and the care required to meet those needs. Nurses use judgment to challenge, question, examine, and validate principles and procedures. For instance, if the patient has a hematologic disorder, preventing excessive bleeding during the procedure must be a conscious nursing intervention when the plan for care is being implemented. The nurse makes a conscious decision to become involved with the patient and begins to focus on the individual patient, anticipating the potential bleeding problem based on what was heard or observed in the patient.

The nurse may also seek additional data from the patient or from other resources. In the case described above, the patient's current hematology report may provide information on hematocrit, hemoglobin, and platelet count. There may or may not be information on clotting time. If the patient describes a past history of bleeding problems, the nurse may order previous medical records that will confirm this. The gastroenterology nurse must integrate this additional information with current nursing practice to determine the expected outcome for this patient.

Decision-making skills are used in the processes of identifying problems and devising achievable plans to alleviate or solve those problems, thereby assisting the patient to return to normal activities of daily living.

One important step of decision-making is to identify and clarify the personal values of the nurse and the patient. The patient's personal values play an important role in the identification of realistic expected outcomes. The patient's values also affect his or her level of compliance and the ability to respond to various therapeutic regimens. Every nurse and every patient has a slightly different value system based on individual experiences and interactions with people throughout life. Some common values held by nurses include the worth of life and preservation of health. Not all patients hold these same values, a fact that can easily present a conflict for nurses. Therefore, in making decisions specific to patient care, the gastroenterology nurse must clarify the effect of the values held by the patient, the family, the institution, and all members of the healthcare team.

## BASING OUTCOMES ON NURSING DIAGNOSES

Outcomes that gastroenterology nurses establish with their patients should be based on nursing diagnoses that apply to patients undergoing gastrointestinal procedures. Because it is difficult to identify meaningful outcomes without clearly understanding the patient's health problems, gastroenterology nurses should refer to the North American Nursing Diagnosis Association (NANDA) taxonomy for approved nursing diagnoses. Use of this taxonomy facilitates reliable communication between nurses concerning health problems and expected outcomes. This reference not only defines health problems associated with each nursing diagnosis but also provides defining characteristics of health problems to differentiate them from other problems (e.g., perceived constipation from colonic constipation). These definitions and characteristics may help clarify patient outcomes during planning. Examples of accepted nursing diagnoses and corresponding expected outcomes are presented in Table 10-1.

## CHARACTERISTICS OF PATIENT OUTCOMES

When identifying patient outcomes, it is well to remember that the focus is the patient. Many times, when outcomes are being considered, nurses tend to develop *nursing* goals, which indicate what the nurse will do for the patient, rather than *patient* goals, which indicate what the patient will be expected to achieve.

Gastroenterology nurses should keep in mind desirable characteristics of patient outcomes. Outcomes should be stated concisely and should be congruent with the assessment, the nursing diagnosis, and current knowledge and practice. Patient outcomes should also be realistic, usable, observable, and specific:

- Outcomes must be realistic. They must be practical

**Table 10-1.** Nursing diagnoses and corresponding expected outcomes

| Nursing diagnosis | Expected patient outcome |
|---|---|
| Constipation | The patient will identify his or her normal pattern of bowel elimination. |
| | The patient will spend 10 minutes after one meal each day seated on the toilet. |
| | The patient will alter his or her diet to include adequate amounts of fiber and fluids. |
| | The patient will avoid straining to defecate. |
| | The patient will engage in physical exercise for at least 15 to 20 minutes daily. |
| Anxiety | The patient will experience 0 to 1+ anxiety evidenced by relaxed state, behavior appropriate to stimuli, physiological arousal within expected parameters (heart rate, blood pressure, and respiratory rate), and ability to attend to and learn salient details. |

Modified from McFarland, G and McFarlane, E. *Nursing Diagnoses and Intervention: Planning for Patient Care.* St. Louis: Mosby–Year Book, 1989.

and attainable, with consideration of the nature of the health problem and the therapy, and the patient's values. "Mrs. Hunter will demonstrate no disorientation about people, time, or place" may not be a realistic outcome statement if Mrs. Hunter is experiencing advanced stages of Alzheimer's disease. On the other hand, an outcome defined for a patient undergoing endoscopy that states, "Mr. Blumsted's temperature will remain between 97.7 and 99.5 degrees F," is attainable under normal circumstances.

- Outcomes must be usable. They should be consistent with the patient's health problem, based on the nursing diagnosis, and achievable within the scope of independent nursing practice. They must provide direction for nursing intervention. The diagnosis "nasogastric tube," for example, does not suggest an achievable goal or even a problem that nursing intervention might prevent, reduce, or resolve. On the other hand, the diagnosis "skin breakdown, potential for, related to nasogastric tube" and the subsequent goal "skin intact around nostrils" do provide direction for nursing intervention. Similarly, goals based on medical diagnoses are not practical because a nurse has no authority to treat medical problems.
- Outcomes must be observable. An outcome must be stated so it is perceptible. Whether or not an outcome is observable has much to do with the way it is stated. Verbs used in defining outcomes distinguish observable from imperceptible outcomes.
- Outcomes must specify behavior or measurable criteria. Furthermore, a time frame should be assigned to the outcome. For example, the outcomes "applies dressing independently by 8/24," "pupils are equal and reacting to light q 2 hrs × 24 hrs," and "denies nausea 12 hrs postprocedure" are all specific outcomes.

Goals may be written in a long-term or short-term context. They are used to monitor progress toward achieving the end result. In general, short-term goals can be satisfied within 1 week, while long-term goals may require a significantly longer period to be fulfilled. Long-term goals may, in some cases, be written as discharge outcomes, in which case they are more broadly written and communicate to an entire nursing team the desired end result of nursing care (e.g., "By 8/25, patient can describe the importance of natural aids to bowel elimination, including high-fiber foods, daily fluid intake of 40 oz, regular time for elimination, and daily walking"). Short-term goals may apply over a period as brief as a few hours (e.g., "Patient exhibits no break in skin integrity or neurovascular impairment related to positioning intraprocedure").

Goals (outcomes) may also be classified as cognitive, psychomotor, or affective:

- Cognitive outcomes describe increases in patient knowledge or intellectual behaviors (e.g., "Patient lists two benefits of dietary management of upper gastric distress").
- Psychomotor outcomes describe achievement of new skills (e.g., "Patient performs safe, effective esophageal self-dilatation").
- Affective outcomes describe changes in patient values, beliefs, and attitudes (e.g., "Patient accepts need for supervised practice sessions in colostomy care in the home").

## DETERMINING THE END RESULT

Methods used to measure the effectiveness of nursing care are outlined in detail in Chapter 13. However, it is essential that the nurse ask questions about outcomes before outlining nursing interventions. Standards of practice and standard nursing care plans serve as valuable tools when thinking through criteria that will be used in measuring end results. Criteria included in the outcome statement should correspond with the desired end result of nursing care provided in the gastroenterology unit. Evaluation criteria for an outcome such as "the patient will not exhibit signs of shock" might include the following:

- No evidence of skin mottling
- Pulse regular
- Skin warm to touch
- Blood pressure within normal range

Questions that the nurse should have about the outcome identified and appropriate answers include the following:

- Is the outcome derived from a nursing diagnosis? If the diagnosis is that the patient was having considerable pain, the nurse would expect the goal to be directly related to pain.
- Will the nurse be able to observe the patient's response to nursing intervention and determine if the desired outcome is met? If the outcome is "the patient will have minimal pain 12 hours postprocedure," the gastroenterology nurse should be alert for signs and symptoms of pain.
- Has the outcome been identified with input from the patient, family, significant other, and other healthcare personnel? Without input from all persons, there is no assurance that the outcome will be attained. The amount of the patient's involvement depends on the patient's medical diagnosis and the type of procedure being performed. When planning patient care, the nurse has the responsibility to involve the patient and family in identifying and defining important information and then orga-

nizing, analyzing, and interpreting that information.

- Is the outcome congruent with the patient's present and potential physical capabilities and behavior patterns? This question is answered by reviewing the assessment data. Baseline observations made on admission as well as the nursing diagnosis provide this information. The nurse also learns about the patient's potential through the nursing assessment, the family's input, and the opinions of other health professionals who have worked with that patient.
- Is the outcome attainable through available human and material resources? In most cases the services provided by the institution dictate the types of personnel and equipment available. Policies of the gastroenterology unit also enter into the picture.
- Can the outcome be achieved within an identified period of time? To measure outcomes the nurse must establish a deadline or time frame when identifying the expected outcome.
- Are the outcomes assigned a priority? Once outcomes have been identified, they are ranked in order of importance. The patient, family, nurse, and other members of the healthcare team all participate in assigning priorities. The nurse must determine what care is required immediately, what care can wait for a time, and which actions may be long-term. Like the nursing diagnosis and patient problems, goals are defined as immediate, intermediate, or long-term.

The patient outcomes for gastroenterology nursing provide definitive goals for measuring patients' responses to endoscopic treatment. It must be noted that even those published as guides for the practicing nurse must be individualized to the patient depending on the nursing diagnosis. For example, not all patients will have adverse reactions to procedural drugs; however, all may have the potential. The gastroenterology nurse once again must have a thorough knowledge of the patient and know what is realistic in terms of expected outcomes.

## DOCUMENTING EXPECTED OUTCOMES

When documenting expected patient outcomes, it is essential that they be included on some record that is retrievable. This practice will provide accrediting and credentialing organizations with information that not only validates the use of the nursing process but also meets the requirements for accreditation. SGNA's documentation monograph provides examples of charting formats that can be used. One of these formats begins with documenting the assessment information and then provides space for preendoscopic and postendoscopic diagnosis. The nurse should be sure that the nursing diagnosis, the medical diagnosis, and the expected outcomes are all included in this section. It is critical that gastroenterology nurses document the nursing process and those aspects of care that are traditionally part of the medical regimen.

Guidelines that may be helpful when documenting the expected outcomes for patients having gastroenterology procedures might include the following:

- Write one clearly stated outcome and, if necessary, add immediate, intermediate, and long-term goals. Remember that outcome is the end result of care. It may be that along the way there are appropriate goals for the patient to attain, but nonetheless the end result or outcome is the most important.
- The documented outcomes should reflect the patient's values. It should be reemphasized that the patient, the family, and everyone else involved should be considered when identifying patient outcomes. The patient plays a primary role in achievement of the outcomes.
- The outcomes must support the total medical treatment plan. The nurse must have knowledge regarding the medical treatment regimen and the process whereby outcomes based on the nursing diagnoses interface with the overall treatment plan.

Common errors that can be made when documenting patient outcomes include the following:

- Using verbs that do not describe observable or measurable behavior
- Writing vague or ambiguous outcome statements
- Expressing patient outcomes as nursing goals
- Including more than one behavior

The box below provides a list of verbs that the gastroenterology nurse can use when documenting the expected outcomes for patients having gastrointestinal procedures.

## EXAMPLE OUTCOMES FOR GASTROENTEROLOGY PATIENTS

The following examples list potential nursing diagnoses and appropriate outcome statements for patients with malabsorption syndromes and intestinal infections (Beare and Myers, 1990).

---

**Useful verbs to use when writing outcomes**

| | | | |
|---|---|---|---|
| Choose | Define | Cooperate | Dilate |
| Explain | Describe | Agree | Irrigate |
| Verbalize | Perform | Demonstrate | Apply |
| List | Identify | Ask | Ambulate |

### Malabsorption syndromes

Potential nursing diagnoses for patients with malabsorption syndromes are as follows:

- Diarrhea related to increased stool volume or dietary fat
- Altered nutrition: less than body requirements, related to malabsorption
- Fluid volume deficit related to increased fluid loss
- Sensory/perceptual alterations related to neuromuscular irritability from decreased calcium
- Potential for injury related to decreased bone density

Appropriate patient outcomes for patients with malabsorption syndromes are listed as follows:

- Patient will have soft, formed stool of normal color and frequency
- Patient will return to and maintain a desired weight
- Patient and family will prepare meals that are free of gluten or lactose and that provide sufficient nutrients
- Patient will be able to accomplish desired activities of daily living without fatigue or injury

### Intestinal infections

Potential nursing diagnoses for patients with intestinal infections are as follows:

- Fluid volume deficit related to excessive losses from diarrhea and vomiting
- Diarrhea related to intestinal inflammation
- Abdominal pain
- Altered nutrition: less than body requirements related to decreased intake and decreased absorption
- Impaired anal skin integrity related to irritation from diarrhea

Appropriate patient outcomes for patients with intestinal infections are listed as follows:

- Decrease in the frequency and volume of bowel movements
- Fluids and electrolytes balanced
- Adequate nutritional intake
- Relief of abdominal pain
- Perianal skin intact

---

**CASE SITUATION**

Mrs. Kearney has had portal hypertension for some years and is now experiencing upper GI bleeding. Her physician has scheduled an esophageal endoscopic variceal ligation (EVL) for tomorrow. The nurse in the gastroenterology unit performed an assessment on the patient and found that Mrs. Kearney had previously been treated with endoscopic sclerotherapy for hemorrhage from esophageal varices. Mrs. Kearney also has a previous history of cirrhosis and has a problem with alcohol. In addition to her medical history, the nurse checks the laboratory results, paying particular attention to the hematology reports. It may be necessary to have the patient's blood typed and screened for two units of packed red cells in case of emergency.

In developing a plan of care for this patient, the nurse formulated four nursing diagnoses. For each diagnosis, what might be identified as appropriate outcomes for this patient?

*Points to think about*

1. The first nursing diagnosis is "actual or potential injury related to EVL procedure." What are the desired outcomes?
2. The second nursing diagnosis is "actual or potential knowledge deficit related to EVL procedure." What are the desired outcomes?
3. The third nursing diagnosis is "actual or potential knowledge deficit related to disease process." What are the desired outcomes?
4. The final nursing diagnosis is "actual or potential knowledge deficit related to postprocedure routine." What are the desired outcomes?

*Suggested responses*

1. For the nursing diagnosis "actual or potential injury related to EVL procedure," measurable patient outcomes might be:
   - Patient will have minimal or no side effects during the procedure.
   - Patient's condition will be stable before discharge from endoscopy unit.
2. For the nursing diagnosis "knowledge deficit specific to the procedure," one measurable patient outcome might be:
   - Patient and significant other will verbalize basic understanding of purpose, expectations, and potential side effects of the procedure.
3. Appropriate outcomes for the nursing diagnosis "knowledge deficit related to disease process" might be:
   - Patient and significant other will be able to verbalize possible causes and results of esophageal varices.
   - Patient and significant other will be aware of lifestyle modifications needed because of the disease process.
4. An outcome specific to "knowledge deficit related to the postprocedure routine" might be:

• Patient will verbalize expected or associated side effects related to EVL procedure.

REVIEW TERMS

**outcome, outcome identification**

REVIEW QUESTIONS

1. What is the *most important* reason for the nurse to possess good communication skills for the process of outcome identification?
   a. To tell the patient what outcomes the nurse has identified.
   b. To document outcomes clearly.
   c. To communicate outcomes to other healthcare professionals.
   d. To establish realistic outcomes through mutual agreement with the patient.
2. In an initial plan of care, the patient outcome "to provide for patient comfort" is listed. Which statement best describes the problem with this outcome statement?
   a. The goal does not indicate whose comfort is to be provided for.
   b. The goal is a nursing goal, not a patient goal.
   c. The goal does take into consideration the patient's values.
   d. The goal is based on a medical diagnosis.
3. Compared with the concept of patient goals, patient outcomes:
   a. Are more likely to refer to short-term achievements.
   b. Refer to a specific end result of nursing actions.
   c. Are the same thing.
   d. Represent less current terminology.
4. The primary advantage of basing patient outcomes on nursing diagnoses that are defined in the NANDA taxonomy is that:
   a. It facilitates reliable communication among nurses.
   b. The nurse does not have to make up new diagnoses.
   c. The taxonomy also lists appropriate patient outcomes.
   d. The NANDA nursing diagnoses correspond to patients' medical diagnoses.
5. Once patient outcomes have been identified, the next step is to:
   a. Identify nursing diagnoses.
   b. Evaluate the patient's achievement of those outcomes.
   c. Prioritize the outcomes identified.
   d. Develop a plan of care.
6. While updating the plan of care to accommodate for the known presence of *Giardia lamblia* in the stool of a pediatric patient, the nurse documents this outcome: "Parents will demonstrate proper hand-washing technique by 3:00 PM of 2/14." Why is this outcome achievable?
   a. Because it is short-term.
   b. Because it indicates an observable, measurable behavior.
   c. Because it is realistic to teach families during the day shift.
   d. Because teaching need not be documented.
7. When developing a strategy for evaluating whether patient outcomes have been met, it is important to:
   a. Indicate who is to evaluate them, when they are to be evaluated, and how they are to be evaluated.
   b. Always require the nurse who admitted the patient and performed initial planning to evaluate expected outcomes.
   c. Suggest that an evaluation should occur before discharge planning begins.
   d. Consider leaving the task for the subsequent shift.
8. All of the following verbs describe observable behaviors except one:
   a. Cooperates.
   b. Agrees.
   c. Is knowledgeable of.
   d. Asks.
9. Outcomes (goals) describing increases in patient knowledge or intellectual behaviors are classified as:
   a. Affective.
   b. Long-term.
   c. Psychomotor.
   d. Cognitive.
10. Short-term goals are those that depict:
    a. Progress towards the identified outcome.
    b. Expectations that will occur in 10 days.
    c. Nursing diagnoses.
    d. None of the above.

**BIBLIOGRAPHY**

Barnie, D. "Care Planning in the Endoscopy Unit: Master Care Plan for the Intraprocedure Patient." In *Journal Reprints II,* ed. Trivits, S, 322-24. Rochester, N.Y.: Society of Gastroenterology Nurses and Associates, 1990.

Barnie, D. "Care Planning in the Endoscopy Unit: Master Care Plan for the Postprocedure Patient." In *Journal Reprints II,* ed. Trivits, S, 325-26. Rochester, N.Y.: Society of Gastroenterology Nurses and Associates, 1990.

Barnie, D. "Care Planning in the Endoscopy Unit: Master Care Plan for the Pre-Endoscopy Patient." In *Journal Reprints II,* ed. Trivits, S, 319-21. Rochester, N.Y.: Society of Gastroenterology Nurses and Associates, 1990.

Beare, P, and Myers, J. *Principles and Practice of Adult Health Nursing.* St. Louis: Mosby–Year Book, 1990.

Bodinsky, G. *Documentation: Charting to Standardize.* SGNA Monograph Series. Rochester, N.Y.: Society of Gastroenterology Nurses and Associates, 1989.

Carpenito, L. *Nursing Diagnosis: Application to Clinical Practice.* 2nd ed. Philadelphia: J.B. Lippincott, 1987.

Edel, E, Johnson, P, and Tiller, S. "Perioperative Documentation: Incorporating Nursing Diagnoses into the Intraoperative Record." *AORN Journal* 50(1989): 596-600.

Flaherty, G, and Fitzpatrick, J. "Relaxation Techniques to Increase Comfort of Postoperative Patients." *Nursing Research* 27(1978): 352-55.

Griffith, H, Thomas, N, and Griffith, L. "MDs Bill for These Routine Nursing Tasks." *American Journal of Nursing* 91(1991): 22-27.

Hardick, M, and Beck, M, eds. *Manual of Gastrointestinal Procedures.* 2nd ed. Rochester, N.Y.: Society of Gastroenterology Nurses and Associates, 1989.

Kim, M, McFarland, G, and McLane, A, eds. *Classification of Nursing Diagnosis: Proceedings from the Fifth National Conference.* St. Louis: Mosby–Year Book, 1984.

Kleinbeck, S. "Developing Nursing Diagnoses for a Perioperative Care Plan: A Classroom Research Project." *AORN Journal* 49(1989): 1613-25.

Kneedler, J, and Dodge, G, eds. *Perioperative Patient Care.* 2nd ed. Palo Alto, Calif.: Blackwell Scientific Publications, Inc., 1989.

Labar, C. "Filling in the Blanks on Prescription Writing." *American Journal of Nursing* 86(1986):31-33.

MacKenzie Page, S, and Beresford, L. "Planning and Documentation: Addressing Patient Needs in a Day Surgery Setting." *AORN Journal* 47(1988): 526-37.

Malen, A. "Perioperative Nursing Diagnoses: What, Why, and How." *AORN Journal* 44(1986): 829-39.

McFarland, G, and McFarlane, E. *Nursing Diagnoses and Intervention: Planning for Patient Care.* St. Louis: Mosby–Year Book, 1989.

North American Nursing Diagnosis Association. *Taxonomy I with Official Diagnostic Categories.* St. Louis: NANDA, 1989.

Shaffer, F. "Nursing Care Plan for Fiberoptic Procedures." *SGA Journal* 11(Fall 1988): 124-25.

Taylor, C, Lillis, C, and LeMone, P. "The Nursing Process." In *Fundamentals of Nursing: The Art and Science of Nursing Care.* eds. Cleary, P, Faven, E, and Intenzo, D, 241-325. Philadelphia: J.B. Lippincott, 1989.

# Chapter 11

# PLANNING

This chapter will acquaint learners with the planning component of the nursing process. **Planning** entails determining what nursing activities will help the patient achieve the goals set forth in the outcome identification process. Trends in care planning are discussed, followed by an elaboration of the purposes of planning, responsibility for planning, and the activities involved in initial, ongoing, and discharge planning. The identification of treatment options, documentation of nursing orders, and outlining of care plans are also covered. Finally, considerations in planning care for gastroenterology patients are summarized.

## Learning objectives

After reviewing the content of this chapter, the gastroenterology nurse should be able to:
1. List the advantages of planning patient care based on accepted nursing diagnoses.
2. Compare nursing and medical plans of patient care.
3. Describe three basic types of planning, including who performs each type.
4. Describe four means by which nurses can expand their existing repertoire of treatment options.

## TRENDS IN PATIENT CARE PLANNING

Whenever nurses respond to an actual or potential health problem by determining expected patient outcomes and by identifying nursing activities for preventing, reducing, or resolving health problems, they are planning patient care. A plan of care may be a formal, documented plan or it may be implied by a documented set of nursing interventions. At this writing, the Joint Commission for Accreditation of Healthcare Organizations (JCAHO) no longer requires that a formal nursing care plan be documented in a patient's hospital records. Nonetheless, planning and documentation of care based on accepted nursing diagnoses, etiology, and scientifically sound intervention remain the hallmark of professional nursing practice.

## Rationale for care planning

Although formal written care plans are no longer required, the planning of patient care is essential. Once assessment data are obtained and a nursing diagnosis is made and desired outcomes are identified, a plan of action must be developed. Planning is the process of identifying nursing actions that are directed toward achieving desirable outcomes and resolving patient problems. This process involves **setting priorities** for care, determining expected outcomes, deciding on appropriate nursing actions, and documenting the plan of care. For example, if a patient is anxious about an impending procedure, the gastroenterology nurse assesses the patient's fear and considers the types of interventions that will alleviate the patient's anxiety. The patient will no doubt have less anxiety if the nurse explains the procedure in detail. The desired outcome in this situation is decreased anxiety. The planned intervention is to explain the procedure to the patient.

There are a number of important reasons listed for developing a plan of care:
- A plan of care can identify patient problems that may be resolved by nursing interventions. Once again, it must be recognized that the nurse cannot solve all patient problems. The patient may have problems that the family or significant other should assist in solving. There may be problems that should be referred to other members of the healthcare team.
- A plan of action helps the gastroenterology nurse assign priorities for care and select interventions that meet the unique needs of the individual patient.

- A documented plan provides a means of communicating information that will help other members of the healthcare team provide continuity of care.
- The planning of care based on nursing diagnoses uses a universal language with which nurses can communicate about health problems, thus helping to build on the existing knowledge base of nursing science.
- The planning of care based on nursing diagnoses gives a professional quality and character, rather than merely vocational assistance, to the act of nursing. It serves to separate nursing and medicine, bringing the two professions into a collegial relationship in which nurses can acknowledge and demonstrate their own unique knowledge base and contributions to their patients' health.

The planning of patient care has also taken on economic importance. Since the inception in 1983 of Medicare's system of prospective payment based on diagnosis-related groups, providers have been under increasing pressure to render quality care while accepting decreasing compensation for increasing costs. More than ever, it has become important for the nursing profession to delineate its product and to demonstrate that this product is cost-effective.

### Nursing and medical plans of care

In some ways, nursing and medical plans of care are similar. Nursing and medical diagnoses share certain characteristics; both are abstractions derived from assessment and inferences based on scientific knowledge that summarize a cluster of signs and symptoms. Therefore, both nursing and medical plans of care prescribe monitoring of signs and symptoms, both are instituted and refined following initial and ongoing assessments, and both prescribe measures based on bodies of scientific knowledge. But because nursing and medical diagnoses differ (see Chapter 9), there are differences between nursing and medical plans of care. For example, because nursing and medical diagnoses differ in causality,* nursing plans of care address psychologic, environmental, and sociologic factors contributing to disturbances in health, as well as biologic factors. Moreover, because the act of diagnosis carries legal implications regarding the right to initiate treatment, nursing care plans based on nursing diagnoses focus on patient *responses* to medical treatment or on

---

* The concept of causality concerns how a profession views cause-and-effect relationships between health problems and the factors that produce them. Medicine recognizes and seeks to treat biological causes of health problems. Nursing recognizes multiple causes or contributors to a problem, including psychologic, environmental, sociologic factors, as well as biologic causes.

health problems nurses can independently treat.† It follows that interventions prescribed in nursing care plans include only those actions that nurses can lawfully perform.

## COMPREHENSIVE PLANNING

The three basic types of planning that take place in the course of comprehensive care planning are listed as follows:

- Initial planning
- Ongoing, problem-oriented planning
- Discharge planning

### Initial planning

Initial planning is usually performed by the nurse who admits the patient and performs a nursing history and physical examination. Providing they are tailored to the needs of individual patients, standardized care plans, including computerized care plans, agency-developed plans, and textbook plans, may be initiated at this time.

To illustrate initial planning, it may help to look at the nurse's role with a patient having an endoscopic variceal ligation (EVL). When the nurse is notified that a patient is going to undergo EVL, he or she completes initial planning, which includes assessment of the supplies and equipment needed to perform the procedure. Items to consider might include the following checklist:

- Flexible gastroscope
- Overtube with bite block
- Suction apparatus including suction tip
- Ligation kit
- Topical anesthetic
- Sedative, depending on patient's hemodynamic stability
- Devices for intraprocedure monitoring of vital signs

The policies and procedures of the institution also guide the initial planning phase. Such things as ensuring the accessibility of an emergency cart, typing and crossmatching blood for patients with potential bleeding problems, and providing the staff with protective attire are all integral components of comprehensive planning.

As previously stated, the gastroenterology nurse uses assessment data obtained at admission when outlining the plan of care, including any current medications, allergies that might cause complications, history of bleeding problems, and any procedures the patient has already undergone that are related to the problem at hand. In addition, laboratory reports are reviewed to identify any abnormal values that should be communicated to other members of the healthcare team.

---

† The modes of therapy physicians and nurses may undertake independent of one another are defined by medical and nurse practice acts. Thus, because the nursing profession has defined its role as having independent, interdependent, and dependent aspects, nursing diagnosis focuses on the independent aspects of nursing practice.

To ensure that the patient will understand the purpose and expected outcomes of an endoscopic procedure, planned nursing interventions might include the following:

- Allow the patient to ask questions and verbalize any concerns
- Support the patient by listening, showing concern, and encouraging questions
- Be prompt when performing procedures to avoid delays or postponement of procedures
- Involve family and significant others in discussions and questions about the procedure and care needed

### Ongoing planning

Ongoing problem-oriented planning is carried out by any nurse who has contact with the patient. This type of planning involves updating and individualizing nursing interventions. Typically, ongoing planning encompasses the following activities:

- Clarifying nursing diagnoses
- Revising expected outcomes to make them more realistic
- Developing new outcome statements and/or new diagnoses, as indicated by analyses of new data
- Identifying nursing actions that promote achievement of identified outcomes
- Documenting patient responses to nursing interventions

Any changes in the patient's health status, either actual or potential, that might occur before, during, or after the procedure should be documented. During the procedure, monitoring of physiologic and hemodynamic parameters should continue. Changes may affect the nursing diagnosis, identified outcomes, and/or the original plan of care. If changes occur, modification would be essential to better accomplish the desired end results of care. Again, documentation is needed to ensure continuity of care and to facilitate measurement of the effectiveness of care provided.

### Discharge planning

Discharge planning should be performed by the nurse who has had the most consistent contact with a patient and family, with or without assistance from a nurse who has broad knowledge of existing community resources. Ideally, discharge planning begins at admission.

When a patient is admitted for an endoscopic procedure, an informed consent is usually signed. Thus, the patient is agreeing to prescribed care. However, informed consent does not affect the patient's right to participate in or refuse treatment. Patient participation in the plan of care should begin when the patient is first seen by the gastroenterology nurse and should continue to discharge. Patients and their families may or may not take an active role in the therapeutic management of the patient's illness. When taking the nursing history, the nurse should assess the role the patient wants to assume.

The establishment of a nurse-patient relationship with a participative patient will result in the patient actively assuming a role as a member of the healthcare team. This means that before, during, and after endoscopic diagnosis and treatment, the participative patient will want to stay informed about his or her health status, methods available to alter it, and ways to assist health professionals. If desired, the patient can be involved in all decisions, beginning at admission and ending at discharge. The patient should also be involved in establishing the outcomes expected from prescribed treatment.

In discharge planning, the nurse working with the patient assists in identifying appropriate community resources or options, such as home health care, respiratory therapy, or other appropriate agencies. In some institutions, a discharge planner may be available to assist the gastroenterology nurse in planning for care after discharge from the hospital or for care following procedures or treatments performed in a physician's office or outpatient setting.

There are certain factors the gastroenterology nurse must be aware of that influence patients' ability to participate in planning their own care. First are the basic beliefs about health to which the patient subscribes. A patient who does not believe in his or her susceptibility to illness may not want to take preventive measures. A typical example is the patient who consumes large amounts of alcohol and has cirrhosis of the liver. In many cases, family superstitions or folklore affect behavior toward health care. Other barriers to patient participation include distrust, lack of knowledge, pride, modesty, fear, impatience, religious beliefs, and cultural diversity.

It is important to remember that a patient's level of involvement in his or her care can vary depending on the ability to overcome many of the above-mentioned barriers. However, nurses can influence their patients by providing them with support and encouraging them to be self-directed consumers of health care.

### DETERMINING NURSING ACTIVITIES

Care planning involves determining what nursing activities will help the patient achieve predetermined health outcomes. While patient outcomes are related to nursing diagnoses, nursing interventions stem from the etiology of the health problem. Consequently, whenever they are known, measures that address the etiology of the problem must be prescribed. Thus, for example, if the problem identified is "ineffective individual coping related to fear of hospitalization," then a nurse might prescribe information on coping strategies. Similarly, the nurse might write the orders "apply warming blanket to procedure table" and "increase room temperature to 75 degrees F" in response to the diagnosis "body temperature, altered; potential" for an infant who is scheduled to undergo an endoscopic procedure.

### Identifying treatment options

There are no substitutes for knowledge, experience, and resourcefulness when it comes to prescribing care. Furthermore, the nurse who responds to every patient problem with a procedure limits the effectiveness of the patient. The array of treatment options documented in research and in the empirical literature ranges from skilled nursing procedures to teaching and counseling, and simple acts of humanity, such as silence, humor, and touch. Strategies that may help nurses broaden their repertoire of nursing actions include the following:

- Consult with successful colleagues, observe them and talk with them about what they do.
- Research the nursing literature for suggestions to improve care.
- Talk with patients and family members about measures they have found most helpful in addressing their problems.
- Consult standards of care, including those of ANA and SGNA, institutional standards, standards of accrediting agencies such as JCAHO, and so on.

Selected treatment strategies should be tailored to the patient and compatible with the total plan of care. They must be consistent with the patient's values, beliefs, culture, and psychosocial background and must be realistic in terms of the abilities, time, and resources available.

### Writing nursing orders

The following requirements pertain when writing **nursing orders:**

- Describe clearly and concisely the action to be taken (i.e., what, where, who, when, and how).
- Date and sign the order, and note when the care plan is reviewed.
- Use only accepted abbreviations.
- For lengthy procedures, refer to policy manuals or other agency guidelines for steps in the routine.

Below are examples of nursing orders written in regard to endoscopy care:

- "Assess patient's breath sounds immediately after the procedure and with each set of postprocedural vital signs."
- "Instruct parent not to lift the child up by the arms or sides for a period of 24 hours after the procedure."
- "Explain to caregiver signs and symptoms of bleeding or hematoma and what to do if bleeding occurs."

### Documenting the plan of care

The final phase of care planning is to document the plan. These written guidelines comprise nursing diagnoses, desired outcomes, and nursing orders. A well-documented plan directs nursing efforts and advances the four goals of nursing: to promote wellness, to prevent disease/illness, to promote coping, and to prevent injury. It is tailored to the individual patient and is based on scientific principles and incorporates findings of nursing research. A plan of care also addresses dependent and interdependent nursing functions and thus is compatible with the medical plan of care and other interdisciplinary efforts. It includes nursing responsibilities for fulfilling the medical plan of care, yet it guides nursing assessment priorities, teaching and counseling activities, and advocacy behaviors. It is designed to meet the patient's psychologic, environmental, sociologic, and physiologic needs.

### PLANNING CARE IN GASTROENTEROLOGY

Resources have been identified in this chapter to aid in gastroenterology care planning. In addition, Table 11-1 contains nursing care plans based on nursing diagnoses relevant to patients who undergo endoscopic procedures. Diagnoses in the first column represent health problems that gastroenterology nurses frequently treat. The patient outcomes listed are realistic and achievable within the short duration of the patient's stay in the endoscopy suite. Notice that all patient outcomes are behaviors or states that nurses can readily and objectively observe. The far right column lists the actions that nurses caring for these patients would take to treat each problem. These actions are based on scientific principles and incorporate the most recent findings of nursing research. Finally, notice that each intervention has a time frame. Time frames become important in evaluating patient care. When caring for patients in the endoscopy unit, these time frames may be short or long, which suggests that followup is required beyond the expected length of stay.

Barnie (1990) has identified short-term goals applicable before, during, and after endoscopic procedures , and plans of care for the gastroenterology patient undergoing endoscopy. Although these plans incorporate medical diagnoses, they are based in part on nursing diagnosis and suggest useful interventions. Additional worthwhile guides to care planning are offered in the reference list.

---

**CASE SITUATION**

Two-year-old Nathan Mitchell has experienced persistent diarrhea for more than 10 days before

**Table 11-1.** Sample endoscopy care plan

| Nursing diagnosis | Patient outcome | Nursing activity |
|---|---|---|
| Anxiety/fear | Patient demonstrates effective coping mechanisms. | Instruct in relaxation techniques, for example, deep breathing and imagery preprocedure. |
| | Patient exhibits reduced physiologic manifestations of anxiety/fear. | Refer patient concerns to MD when appropriate, all phases of endoscopy experience. |
| | | Allow time for questions preprocedure. |
| | | Involve family/significant other for support preprocedure and postprocedure. |
| | | Minimize noxious stimuli; keep environment calm and unhurried, all phases. |
| | | Use therapeutic communication and touch, all phases. |
| | | Monitor patient for subjective and objective signs of anxiety, (i.e., shakiness, perspiration, increased heart rate, extraneous movement, hesitation, poor eye contact), all phases. |
| Alteration in comfort, actual or potential | Patient tolerates procedure, asking for medication as needed. | Teach patient system of ranking pain preprocedure. |
| | | Support patient through discomfort by coaching patient in deep breathing, visualization, etc. intraprocedure. |
| | | Assess positioning for maximum comfort preprocedure and intraprocedure. |
| Knowledge deficit related to unfamiliar environment and procedure | Patient describes expected physiologic and psychologic responses to endoscopy. | Provide information about impending procedure using visual aids or appropriate literature preprocedure. |
| | | Provide sensory information about procedure and sedation preprocedure. |
| Injury related to change in vital signs related to sedation; potential | Patient remains stable while sedated. | Obtain baseline vital signs on admission. |
| | | Monitor BP, temperature, respirations and pulse intraprocedure and post-procedure. |
| Injury related to instrumentation trauma (perforation and/or hemorrhage); potential | Patient experiences minimal trauma from endoscope. | Check lab work (CBC, PT/PTT, platelets) preprocedure. |
| | | Insert bite block to protect teeth and pharynx intraprocedure. |
| | | Verify emergency equipment in working order preprocedure. |
| | | Monitor intake and output intraprocedure. |
| Aspiration, potential for | Patient's airway remains clear and unobstructed. | Position patient on left side preprocedure. |
| | | Suction secretions prn preprocedure and intraprocedure. |

admission and is severely dehydrated. The gastroenterology unit nurse reviews Nathan's nursing history and visits Nathan, who is combative and uncooperative despite the fact that his parents are doing all they can to comfort him. The nurse who admitted Nathan initiated a standard care plan used in the department for pediatric patients. He diagnosed Nathan by selecting the following from a list of health problems:

- Impaired verbal communication
- Potential for injury, secondary to development (and combativeness)
- Defensive coping
- Noncompliance, secondary to development

- Powerlessness
- Anxiety, secondary to hospitalization

He also added the following health problems:
- Actual fluid volume deficit
- Impaired skin integrity (rectal excoriation)
- Altered health maintenance
- Ineffective family coping, disabling

On examination, the gastroenterology nurse notices that the IV in Nathan's forearm has infiltrated, leaving it quite swollen and sore. The nurse discontinues the boy's IV, wraps his forearm in a warm compress, and elevates it on his teddy bear.

Nathan's parents accuse the doctors of giving Nathan medicine that he does not need, saying that rice cereal and milk have always been good for diarrhea. They believe the medicine is responsible for their child's poor appetite and vomiting. They also are grumbling about the day care center where they take Nathan, reporting that Nathan is the eighth child from the center to come down with severe diarrhea. While listening to their account of the day care center, another nurse takes the gastroenterology nurse aside to show the result of Nathan's stool culture: Nathan is infected with *Giardia lamblia*.

### Points to think about

1. Which basic types of planning have occurred in this scenario? Which type of planning might be initiated at this time?
2. In choosing three priority health problems, what factors would be taken into consideration?
3. The nursing diagnosis "altered health maintenance," which was selected by the admitting nurse, is unfamiliar to the gastroenterology nurse. How would its meaning be determined?
4. In what ways will the nursing plan of care differ from the medical plan of care?
5. The gastroenterology nurse in this case usually cares for adults, and therefore feels somewhat limited in her existing repertoire of pediatric treatment options. How might she expand her repertoire?

### Suggested responses

1. The basic types of planning that have occurred in this scenario include:
   - Initial planning, which was instituted by the admitting nurse
   - Ongoing, problem-oriented planning, which occurred when the gastroenterology nurse responded to a health problem (i.e., impaired skin integrity, secondary to IV infiltration) by setting a patient-centered outcome (to reduce pain and swelling due to fluid extravasation) and identifying means of reducing or resolving the problem (i.e., discontinuing the IV, applying the warm compress, elevating the arm)

   At this time, the gastroenterology nurse might initiate discharge planning with the parents. This planning may include contacting the public health department to investigate the day care center for the presence of *Giardia lamblia*.
2. Factors the nurse may take into consideration in choosing three priority health problems include:
   - The actual or potential threat of each problem to Nathan's well-being
   - The parents' preferences and values, which will determine their participation in Nathan's therapy
   - Potential problems; that is, risks peculiar to Nathan's age, health status, medical management, and so on

3. To determine the meaning of the nursing diagnosis "altered health maintenance" the gastroenterology nurse should refer to the NANDA taxonomy of nursing diagnosis. This reference not only defines health problems associated with each nursing diagnosis but also provides defining characteristics of health problems that differentiate them from other problems.
4. The nursing plan of care would differ from the medical plan of care in the following ways:
   - It addresses psychologic, environmental, and sociologic factors contributing to disturbances in health, as well as biologic causes.
   - It focuses on patient *responses* to medical treatment or health problems that nurses can independently treat. Interventions prescribed in it include only those actions that nurses can lawfully perform.

5. The gastroenterology nurse might expand her repertoire of treatment options by:
   - Consulting with successful colleagues, observing them, and talking with them about what they do
   - Researching the nursing literature for suggestions to improve care
   - Talking with patients and family about measures they have found most helpful in addressing their problem
   - Consulting standards of care, including ANA and SGNA standards, institutional standards, standards of accrediting agencies, and so on

---

**REVIEW TERMS**

---

**nursing orders, planning, setting priorities**

---

**REVIEW QUESTIONS**

---

1. Which of the following is *not* a valid reason for planning patient care based on nursing diagnoses?
   a. It is required by JCAHO.
   b. It enhances continuity of patient care.
   c. It improves the clarity of communication among nurses.
   d. It emphasizes the collegial relationship between nursing and medicine.
2. The nursing care plan:
   a. Is based on scientific principles and incorporates findings of nursing research.
   b. Advances nursing's four aims and is tailored to the individual patient.
   c. Is designed to meet developmental, psychologic,

and sociologic needs of patients, as well as their physiologic needs.

   d. All of the above.

3. A nursing plan of care addresses:
   a. Only the biologic causes of the patient's health problems.
   b. Only those health problems that nurses can treat independently.
   c. Only nursing diagnoses.
   d. Independent, dependent, and interdependent aspects of nursing practice.

4. Assessment of the supplies and equipment needed to perform an endoscopic procedure is an example of:
   a. Initial planning.
   b. Admission planning.
   c. Ongoing planning.
   d. Discharge planning.

5. Intraprocedural changes in the patient's health status may affect:
   a. The nursing diagnosis.
   b. The expected outcomes.
   c. The plan of care.
   d. All of the above.

6. Discharge planning should be the responsibility of:
   a. The physician.
   b. The admitting nurse.
   c. The nurse who has had the most consistent contact with the patient.
   d. Family members and significant others.

7. To help broaden the array of treatment options available to them, nurses should consult successful colleagues, the literature, standards of care, and:
   a. The taxonomy of nursing diagnoses.
   b. The plan of care.
   c. Patients and their families.
   d. Physicians.

8. In response to a patient's fluid deficit secondary to persistent diarrhea, which of the following nursing orders would be appropriate for the gastroenterology nurse to write?
   a. "Increase the IV rate following bouts of diarrhea."
   b. "Prepare patient for electrosurgery."
   c. "Monitor vital signs every 2 hours until diarrhea stops. Observe for signs of hypotension with widening pulse pressure."
   d. "Stools for culture in AM and PM."

9. The final product of the planning phase of the nursing process is:
   a. A well-documented plan of care.
   b. Resolution of the patient's health problems.
   c. A series of outcome statements.
   d. Nursing intervention.

10. The activity concerned with ranking nursing diagnoses in order of actual or potential threat to the patient's well-being is known as:
   a. Planning.
   b. Outcome identification.
   c. Establishing problem priorities.
   d. Cost containment.

## BIBLIOGRAPHY

Barnie, D. "Care Planning in the Endoscopy Unit: Master Care Plan for the Intraprocedure Patient." In *Journal Reprints II,* ed. Trivits, S, 322-24. Rochester, N.Y.: Society of Gastroenterology Nurses and Associates, 1990.

Barnie, D. "Care Planning in the Endoscopy Unit: Master Care Plan for the Postprocedure Patient." In *Journal Reprints II,* ed. Trivits, S, 325-26. Rochester, N.Y.: Society of Gastroenterology Nurses and Associates, 1990.

Barnie, D. "Care Planning in the Endoscopy Unit: Master Care Plan for the Pre-Endoscopy Patient." In *Journal Reprints II,* ed. Trivits, S, 319-21. Rochester, N.Y.: Society of Gastroenterology Nurses and Associates, 1990.

Beare, P, and Myers, J. *Principles and Practice of Adult Health Nursing.* St. Louis: Mosby–Year Book, 1990.

Carpenito, L. *Nursing Diagnosis: Application to Clinical Practice.* 2nd ed. Philadelphia: J.B. Lippincott, 1987.

Edel, E, Johnson, P, and Tiller, S. "Perioperative Documentation: Incorporating Nursing Diagnoses into the Intraoperative Record." *AORN Journal* 50(1989): 596-600.

Flaherty, G, and Fitzpatrick, J. "Relaxation Techniques to Increase Comfort of Postoperative Patients." *Nursing Research* 27(1978): 352-55.

Gordon, M. *Manual of Nursing Diagnosis* 1984-1985. New York: McGraw-Hill, 1984.

Griffith, H, Thomas, N, and Griffith, L. "MDs Bill for These Routine Nursing Tasks." *American Journal of Nursing* 91(1991): 22-27.

Hardick, M, and Beck, M, eds. *Manual of Gastrointestinal Procedures.* 2nd ed. Rochester, N.Y.: Society of Gastroenterology Nurses and Associates, 1989.

Kim, M, McFarland, G, and McLane, A, eds. *Classification of Nursing Diagnosis: Proceedings from the Fifth National Conference.* St. Louis: Mosby–Year Book, 1984.

Kleinbeck, S. "Developing Nursing Diagnoses for a Perioperative Care Plan: A Classroom Research Project." *AORN Journal* 49(1989): 1613-25.

Kneedler, J, and Dodge, G, eds. *Perioperative Patient Care.* 2nd ed. Palo Alto, Calif.: Blackwell Scientific Publications, Inc., 1989.

Labar, C. "Filling in the Blanks on Prescription Writing." *American Journal of Nursing* 86(1986): 31-33.

MacKenzie Page, S, and Beresford, L. "Planning and Documentation: Addressing Patient Needs in a Day Surgery Setting." *AORN Journal* 47(1988): 526-37.

Malen, A. "Perioperative Nursing Diagnoses: What, Why, and How." *AORN Journal* 44(1986): 829-39.

North American Nursing Diagnosis Association. *Taxonomy I with Official Diagnostic Categories.* St. Louis: NANDA, 1989.

Shaffer, F. "Nursing Care Plan for Fiberoptic Procedures." *SGA Journal* 11(Fall 1988): 124-25.

Taylor, C, Lillis, C, and LeMone, P. "The Nursing Process." In *Fundamentals of Nursing, The Art and Science of Nursing Care,* eds. Cleary, P, Faven, E, and Intenzo, D, 241-325. Philadelphia: J.B. Lippincott, 1989.

Winchester, C. "A New Approach to Esophageal Varices: Endoscopic Variceal Ligation." *Gastroenterology Nursing* 14(August 1991): 5-8.

# Chapter 12

# IMPLEMENTATION

This chapter will familiarize gastroenterology nurses with the implementation phase of the nursing process. General information about a variety of issues that arise during implementation of planned care is provided, followed by a discussion of variables that influence the way care is implemented and a list of specific guidelines for nursing intervention. The role of the gastroenterology nurse in communicating about the care provided in the gastroenterology unit is explored. The last part of the chapter examines nursing activities that surround teaching, counseling, and advocacy of patient rights in gastroenterology nursing.

**Learning objectives**

After reviewing the content of this chapter, the gastroenterology nurse should be able to:
1. Describe the three broad areas of nursing activity that occur in the implementation phase of the nursing process.
2. Distinguish between independent, interdependent, and dependent nursing functions when implementing a plan of care.
3. Discuss six variables that influence the way a plan of care is implemented.
4. Define general guidelines for implementing care of the gastroenterology patient.
5. Describe four means of communicating nursing actions performed during the implementation phase of the nursing process.
6. List documentation requirements when implementing care of the gastroenterology patient undergoing endoscopy.
7. Discuss the nurse's role as teacher/counselor when implementing care of the gastroenterology patient.
8. Discuss the nurse's advocacy role as it applies to informed consent and ethical decision-making.

## FROM PLANNING TO IMPLEMENTATION

During the planning phase a patient's health problems are identified. Risks peculiar to the patient's age, health status, and medical management are considered to anticipate and prevent potential problems. During the planning phase these health problems are ranked or prioritized in order of actual or potential threat to the patient's well-being. Nursing actions that will assist the patient toward achievement of identified outcomes are identified and prioritized.

Once documented, the plan outlines a set of nursing actions in a logical sequence that is designed to promote wellness, prevent disease and illness, promote recovery, and facilitate coping with altered functioning. It specifies *what* will be done, and *how, when, where,* and *by whom* (i.e., nurse, patient, or significant other). Each plan of care is tailored to the patient's individual needs, and each incorporates criteria for evaluating the effectiveness of nursing actions in assisting the patient toward achievement of desired outcomes.

In the implementation phase the plan becomes a blueprint that guides nursing care. Each nursing action performed is based on scientific principles and reflects the rights and desires of the individual and significant others. All actions are carried out safely, skillfully, and efficiently in a manner that provides continuity of care during each phase of recovery.

During the implementation phase, the following three broad areas of nursing activity occur:
- The plan is put in motion
- The data base is updated as data collection continues
- Nursing care and patient progress are documented and communicated

This chapter examines these three activities and the role of the gastroenterology nurse as teacher, counselor, and patient advocate.

## PUTTING THE PLAN IN MOTION

During implementation, all of the steps outlined in the plan of care should be carried out efficiently and effectively. Whether or not all steps are executed by a nurse depends on the particular practice setting. The amount of time an institution and its nursing professionals allocate for teaching, counseling, and advocacy depends on the value and benefits they associate with each activity.

Carrying out the plan of care requires cognitive ability, interpersonal skill, and technical skill, each of which is discussed as follows:

- Cognitive ability is necessary not only to think critically about a patient's health problem but also to apply nursing theories to solve problems.
- Interpersonal skill is a component of overall professional skills. Possession of such skills, including the ability to communicate clearly, competently, and with caring, helps elicit patients' trust and cooperation. A nurse's well-developed intellectual and interpersonal skills not only maximize the chance that healthy outcomes will be achieved but also ensure efficient implementation of care.
- Technical skill is often necessary when implementing care. Required technical ability ranges from minimal to extensive, depending on the nature of equipment used to execute procedures and whether they are simple or complex. Examples of implementation measures that require technical skill are noninvasive measurement of arterial hemoglobin oxygen saturation during gastrointestinal procedures using a pulse oximeter, insertion of a duodenal or nasogastric tube, performance of esophageal manometry studies, and monitoring of cardiac status using a cardioscope.

Independent, dependent, and interdependent nursing functions are addressed in the plan of care and carried out during the implementation phase. These functions are explained as follows:

- **Independent intervention** is action initiated without direction or supervision of other healthcare professionals, and is instituted as the result of a nursing assessment. Actions taken in the course of independent intervention are those for which a nurse is legally accountable. Teaching, counseling, and advocacy of patient rights are examples of activities nurses can initiate freely.
- **Interdependent intervention** is action performed in concert with the efforts of other healthcare professionals. For example, case study conferences organized by nurses and attended by related health professionals for the purpose of discussing patient care frequently result in action requiring cooperation and coordination between nurses and other professionals. These cooperative activities reflect nurses' interdependent function in providing care.
- **Dependent intervention** is action performed under the supervision or direction of a physician. It constitutes the bulk of nursing activity in traditional practice settings.

Nurse practice acts in all states clearly indicate that nurses are to fulfill orders written or otherwise given by physicians. Yet it is important for nurses to understand their responsibility in dependent intervention; that is, although physicians are ultimately responsible for actions performed at their direction or under their supervision, nurses are required to clarify any doubts concerning the activities prescribed. The nurse who fails to do so risks a liability suit for the action.

Safety is the focus of many nursing activities carried out during implementation. Adhering to disinfection guidelines during processing of contaminated equipment, monitoring the environment for safety, and positioning according to physiologic principles during or after operative procedures to avoid neurovascular damage and skin breakdown are typical nursing activities performed to safeguard patient safety. Verification of identification and informed consent, validation of reports of essential laboratory findings and diagnostic procedures, and routine inspection of hospital equipment to ensure proper function are other safety measures a nurse may carry out.

### Managing time constraints

Huey (1988) has suggested three ways to free available time for implementing comprehensive nursing care:

- Delegating technical and nonnursing tasks
- Revising policies to prune obsolete practices
- Preventing complications

### Delegating tasks

Making high-quality nursing care possible is a matter of understanding nursing objectives and sticking to them. This frequently requires delegation of nonnursing tasks. Many practice settings have instituted professional practice models to allow nurses to use their time more efficiently and effectively. For example, Jakobsen (1990) suggests the following practical alternatives that reserve professional nurses for independent nursing functions:

- The Professionally Advanced Care Team (Pro-ACT) model instituted at the Robert Wood Johnson Hospital in New Brunswick, New Jersey, has restructured nursing services based on two nursing roles—the primary nurse, whose role is to remain with the patient throughout his or her hospital stay; and a clinical care manager, an RN whose role is to manage that stay. Added support is provided by pharmaceutical services, who manage everything related to medication and IV therapy (except administration), and "support service hosts," who provide housekeeping, dietary trays, and supplies.
- In Miami, the Partners in Practice (PIP) model allows a nurse to team with a "practice partner." The nurse acts as mentor to a partner (usually an LPN or technician) who has been screened for interest in a nursing career. Once teamed, the RN's

practice partner attends to tasks that do not have to be performed by an RN, and any other tasks the RN chooses to teach the partner (e.g., urine testing). Nurses acting as mentors find that they have more time to teach and counsel patients and to consult with other members of the care team.

Another trend in nursing practice has the dual effect of allowing nurses to carry out planned care more efficiently and involving patients in self-care. Many professionals believe that alert, oriented, and reasonably intelligent hospitalized patients are quite capable of taking their own medications. Successful medication self-administration programs have been implemented with physician permission in clinical areas, including postpartum, cardiac, geriatrics, and oncology units.

### Revising practice policies

To make high-quality nursing care possible through increased efficiency, nurses must cast off unnecessary rituals and adapt old techniques to accommodate new information. Protective isolation, for example, is a time-consuming ritual that has been found ineffective in preventing infection. In 1983 the Centers for Disease Control (CDC) deleted protective isolation from their isolation guidelines because it was shown that individuals at risk of infection are infected with their own organisms. Other related studies demonstrated that outcomes of patients treated in isolation versus in rooms with other patients do not differ significantly. Clearly, discarding policies surrounding protective isolation augments nursing care by increasing efficiency without diminishing the overall effectiveness of nursing intervention.

### Preventing complications

Adapting procedures to incorporate new research findings can also free available time by minimizing the risk of complications. For example, recent nursing research suggests that using shorter, smaller catheters minimizes irritation to local veins while still allowing blood transfusion. If the catheter must be retained and thrombophlebitis occurs, a short catheter minimizes the extent of involvement. Thus, taking this measure minimizes the risk and severity of a complication of IV therapy, potentially increasing time available for important nursing functions.

### Variables that affect the way care is implemented

Variables that influence how a plan of care is implemented fall into the following six categories:
- Patient variables
- Nurse variables
- Standards of care
- Research findings
- Resources
- Ethical and legal guides to practice

### Patient variables

Every plan of care must be tailored to individual needs, a requirement that frequently calls for creative solutions to health problems. For example, a patient's previous response to nursing measures may affect his or her receptiveness to further intervention. Obviously, the patient whose past experiences with nursing care were unpleasant or unrewarding is less likely to be receptive. Diminished ability to participate in self-care also influences the way a plan of care is implemented. For example, a quadriplegic may require an assistant for bowel care, whereas a patient with normal neuromuscular function will not. Sometimes a patient's willingness to participate in care becomes a factor when the nurse implements planned care. Psychologic perceptions, religious beliefs, or socioeconomic factors may prompt a patient to reject all or some nursing intervention. For instance, an otherwise receptive patient who lacks the means to purchase meat may not comply with a high-protein diet regimen for weight loss that includes meat. In this case, interim measures to attain the outcome "Patient will select three servings of protein daily from a menu" may include teaching the patient how to identify complete proteins in combinations of vegetable proteins (e.g., grains, legumes) and dairy products.

Developmental differences can substantially influence planned care, especially among pediatric patients. Not only do actual and potential health problems (and therefore desired outcomes) differ within developmental age groups (see Table 12-1), but means of achieving outcomes vary according to the child's unique developmental task for his or her age group. Thus, when taking action (e.g., to reduce the fear and anxiety every child or adolescent experiences during endoscopy), it is necessary to identify the developmental task for the child's age group and select treatment options that meet the child's developmental needs. Similarly, it is necessary to consider whether outcomes and treatment options are realistic, given the patient's developmental circumstances.

### Nursing variables

A nurse's cultivated level of expertise determines the number and kind of treatment options implemented. Moreover, nurses vary in the degree to which they like patient contact. The nurse who enjoys patient contact clearly has greater willingness and motivation to provide comprehensive care during implementation. How well or poorly a nurse manages time affects his or her efficiency and therefore the available time for carrying out all measures planned. On the other hand, many nurses continually struggle to provide time to implement total patient care yet remain frustrated by unpredictable and uncontrollable events.

### Standards of care

Current standards of care determine nursing responsibilities and suggest liability limits. (**Liability** refers to the legal responsibility for nursing acts or failure to act, including the responsibility for financial restitution in

**Table 12-1.** Health Problems Specific to Four Pediatric Age Groups

| Age | Developmental stage | Actual or potential health problems |
|---|---|---|
| **Birth to 1 year** | Trust versus mistrust | Sleep pattern disturbance<br>Swallowing, impaired<br>Hypothermia/hyperthermia, potential<br>Fluid volume, altered: deficit or increase<br>Impaired skin integrity<br>Aspiration potential: related to existing or coexisting conditions<br>Infection, potential: related to existing or coexisting conditions<br>Impaired gas exchange<br>Ineffective thermoregulation<br>Ineffective airway clearance<br>Self-concept disturbance: maturational, related to deprivation<br>Health maintenance, altered: maturational, related to inadequate health practice<br>Self-care deficit, inability to feed, toilet, or dress self |
| **1 to 3 years** | Autonomy versus shame and doubt | Impaired verbal communication<br>Sleep pattern disturbance<br>Impaired skin integrity<br>Infection, potential: related to existing or coexisting conditions<br>Self-concept disturbance: maturational, related to deprivation<br>Health maintenance, altered: maturational, related to inadequate health practice<br>Injury potential for: related to development (e.g., poisoning, falls)<br>Impaired social interaction<br>Powerlessness, maturational or situational<br>Coping, ineffective: situational or maturational<br>Anxiety, situational<br>Fear, situational<br>Self-care deficit, inability to feed or toilet self |
| **3 to 6 years** | Initiative versus guilt | Coping, ineffective: situational or maturational<br>Powerlessness, maturational or situational<br>Anxiety, situational<br>Fear, situational<br>Sleep pattern disturbance, related to nightmares or fears<br>Injury potential for: related to development (e.g. poisoning, falls)<br>Infection, potential: related to existing or coexisting conditions<br>Self-care deficit, inability to dress self<br>Self-concept disturbance: maturational, related to deprivation |
| **7 to 11 years** | Industry versus inferiority | Self-concept disturbance: maturational, related to peer pressure<br>Noncompliance, situational<br>Anxiety, situational<br>Fear, situational<br>Self-care deficit, inability to bathe self completely<br>Impaired social interaction<br>Violence, potential for: situational, related to inability to control behavior<br>Health maintenance, altered: maturational, related to inadequate health practice |

Modified from Carpenito, L, 1983 and North American Nursing Diagnosis Association, Taxonomy I with Official Diagnostic Categories, St Louis, NANDA, 1989; developed with assistance form Zelasny, B, BSN, CCRN, Denver Children's Hospital, Denver.

the event of demonstrable damages resulting from negligent acts.) For example, among SGNA standards, Standard II requires that nurses "initiate actions to ensure the continuity of effective nursing care before, during and/or after endoscopic procedures in the GI unit." Associated with this standard are seven criteria, including "instructs patient(s)/family(ies) in the proper preparation for diagnostic studies" and "provides writ-

ten postendoscopy instructions to outpatients undergoing endoscopy and reviews those directions with the family/significant other, as appropriate." Gastroenterology nurses must therefore involve family and significant others in preendoscopy teaching.

**Research findings**

New information emerges continually, thereby giving rise to new treatment strategies. The nurse who is aware of research findings implements a more creative, varied, and comprehensive set of actions when solving health problems.

### Resources

The best-laid plans are doomed to fail without adequate resources to enable implementation of the plan. Inadequate staffing, equipment, supplies, and other resources may reduce or alter the type of care rendered.

### Ethical and legal guides to practice

Within the past decade, laws governing delivery and ethical dimensions of health care have become more complex. In many settings, hospital risk managers and ethical committees counsel hospital policy makers whose policies, in turn, influence modern nursing practice.

## Guidelines for nursing intervention

The following guidelines for implementation of nursing care have been offered:

- Before instituting any measure to treat a health problem, the patient must be assessed to be sure action is still necessary.
- The nurse should be fully prepared to perform the planned action when he or she approaches the patient. All equipment should be ready and the nurse should either know how to perform the nursing action or come with a nurse associate who does. The nurse should tell the patient why the action is being taken. Also patients should be informed of any potential adverse responses to the procedure.
- The nurse should approach the patient with a caring attitude, using language the patient understands. By communicating genuine concern for what the patient is experiencing, the nurse conveys regard for the patient's well-being.
- The nurse should develop a large repertoire of skilled nursing interventions. The larger an array of options he or she has to choose from when treating health problems, the greater the likelihood of success.
- The nursing actions chosen must comply with standards of care and be within ethical and legal institutional guidelines to practice.
- The nurse should think critically about the plan of care, always questioning whether routines are really the best method of treatment. He or she should consult immediate colleagues and colleagues in related nursing fields and relevant literature to discover more effective ways of managing health problems. The effectiveness of each action in terms of its positive and negative effects on the outcome should be evaluated.
- The nurse should modify the prescribed interventions to accommodate patients' developmental and psychosocial circumstances, ability and willingness

to participate in achieving desired outcomes, previous responses to nursing measures, and progress toward expected outcomes.

## CONTINUED DATA COLLECTION AND DATA BASE UPDATING

Data collection continues throughout the implementation phase, and the data base is continually updated. These activities serve three important functions during implementation in the following ways:

- Comparing new data against the baseline data base enables nurses to identify patterns and trends
- Collecting data following nursing intervention allows nurses to evaluate the effectiveness of nursing actions according to evaluation criteria listed in the care plan
- As the data base is updated, nurses can revise their plans of care

Just as during the assessment phase, nurses collect both subjective and objective data. During implementation, however, subjective data are derived from confirmation or validation of responses to therapy, and perceived progress as noted by the patient or significant others. Objective data are obtained by monitoring both the patient's response to nursing activity and the medical plan of care.

## COMMUNICATING ABOUT CARE

Communicating about care with patient and family, colleagues, and other health professionals is vitally important for several reasons. It not only sparks involvement of patients and significant others but also ensures continuity of care as the responsibility for the patient's care shifts from one provider to the next. Communication is essential to the coordination and continuity of care, and it also promotes efficiency among members of a nursing team. Informing colleagues of action enables nurses to supplement and complement each other's efforts, thus avoiding duplication and omission of effort. Communication about care should focus not only on nursing care provided and patient progress toward specified outcomes but also on the total plan of care rendered by physicians and all health professionals. Communication takes many forms, including documentation, discussion and verbal reports, conferences or consultation, and referrals.

### Documentation

Documentation of care in written records is the most visible and permanent medium of communication with regard to implementation of nursing care. Documentation can refer either to an action or to a written record. As a process, documentation refers to the act of collecting, abstracting, and coding of client data and therapeutic processes for the purposes of communicating about patient care, supplying a supporting reference concerning the status or progress of a patient, and archiving evidence of care rendered.

**Documentation,** the most formal of all methods of communication, constitutes written, legal evidence of all pertinent intervention involving a patient. Since 1982, it has been subject to specific requirements by the Joint Commission for Accreditation of Healthcare Organizations (JCAHO), which requires that "the nursing process shall be documented for each hospitalized patient from admission through discharge."

Documentation of care that has been rendered serves purposes beyond communication between colleagues, including the following:

- Planning. Because patient records document not only baseline and ongoing data but also how a patient is responding to therapies, they are useful as resources for planning and modification of planned care.
- Quality assurance audit. Records provide a medium for studying the quality of care provided and the competence of nurses rendering care. Charts selected at random are audited against standards of care to determine if standards are being met. If discrepancies between practice and standards are found, action involving inservices, policy changes, counseling, and so on may be initiated to remedy substandard practices.
- Research. The nursing record serves as a valuable source of data in nursing research. Each record represents a unique case study from which researchers hope to learn how to improve recognition and treatment of patient health problems.
- Education. By reading a patient's chart, one can learn a great deal about clinical manifestations of disease, effective or less-effective treatment modalities, and factors that affect patients' abilities to achieve health outcomes.
- Legal evidence. The nursing record serves an important function in implicating or absolving nurses when entered into court proceedings as evidence.
- Historical document. Finally, because records are dated and retained for many years, they are sometimes useful as an indicator of a patient's past health.

**Documentation requirements in the endoscopy unit**

The following are examples of the types of documentation required for endoscopic procedures:

- Procedure performed
- Date and time of the procedure
- Equipment used
- Staff present
- Anesthesia/sedation administered and patient's response
- Medications and response

- Vital signs and monitoring methods
- Oxygen therapy
- Use of cautery, electrocoagulation, or laser
- Dilators used
- Solution injected
- Specimens taken
- Photographs and/or x-rays taken
- Postprocedural diagnosis
- Nursing notes and procedure nurse signature

In addition to these procedural notes, SGNA's documentation monograph also lists the information required for preprocedural, postprocedural, and discharge documentation.

**Discussion and verbal reporting**

Communication of care takes several forms. Discussion between two or more individuals to identify problems and work toward their solution constitutes informal communication of care. More formal communication of care is accomplished by oral or written reporting. Formal reports convey new patient data and information about the patient's status and progress toward desired outcomes.

**Conferences or consultation**

Two types of conferences, which are listed as follows, are held in many practice settings for the purpose of communicating about care:

- **Nursing care conferences,** during which a specific case situation or situations are reviewed. Impressions are shared, treatment options are explored, and care is planned.
- **Nursing rounds,** which are on-site conferences from which patient and family input is sometimes elicited and from which direct observation can be made. At the same time, nursing care and patient progress can be evaluated.

**Consultations** with other healthcare professionals to seek advice, instruction, or information, or to exchange ideas concerning patient care may be considered another form of conference communication. For example, gastroenterology nurses consult with clinical nurse specialists in their area concerning mutual patients.

**Referrals**

More and more, nursing has been recognized for its role in screening and referring patients who require or would benefit from adjunct services or existing community resources. The process of sending a patient to another source for aid or to another professional for appropriate action is known as **referral.** Both internal referrals to departments elsewhere within a facility and external referrals to other hospital facilities or outside agencies are useful in providing comprehensive holistic care. Most agencies have policies governing referrals that require submitting special forms. In addition, these policies specify who can make the referral, how it is to be done, and so on. When it is appropriate to make a referral, the nurse must give information to the receiving agency or department that will ensure continuity of patient care. Answering the question, "What would I need to know if I were to continue care of this patient?" will help to accomplish this end.

## INDEPENDENT INTERVENTION: TEACHING, COUNSELING, AND ADVOCACY

During implementation, nurses actively determine their patients' needs for assistance and ability to meet basic human needs. The promotion of self-care through teaching, counseling, and advocacy frequently becomes important when assisting patients to meet desired outcomes.

### Patient teaching

Whether teaching patients about an upcoming endoscopic examination or about self-care during or after their hospital stay, a nurse's role in teaching remains the same. Nurses implement patient education through the following four broad areas of activity:
- Diagnosing a patient's knowledge deficit
- Planning learning activity
- Providing learning opportunities
- Evaluating learning

### Diagnosing knowledge deficits

When identifying a knowledge deficit as a health problem, nurses base this diagnosis on an assessment of the patient's learning needs. This assessment must include not only evidence that the patient is unaware of information that might improve health behaviors but also that the patient is ready to learn. Before nurses can effectively implement a teaching plan, they must also assess their own knowledge on the subject and become informed. It is oftentimes necessary to contact appropriate resource persons or obtain additional information to provide accurate, up-to-date facts to substantiate the lessons.

### Planning the learning activity

Setting goals for the learning activity is an action very similar to that of identifying health outcomes. (See Chapter 11.) Learning goals must be realistic; they may be short-term or long-term. McGregor (1988) advises that gastroenterology nurses and their patients agree in writing or via verbal contract concerning respective roles of both nurse and patient in the learning activity. In this way, nurses and patients identify measurable behaviors to help each other monitor progress toward the learning goals. For example, a contract might contain these terms:
- "Nursing staff will provide written home bowel prep instructions by 5/12/91."
- "Mr. Franklin will review these instructions and

verbally describe home bowel prep procedure at next office visit on 5/15/91."

### Providing learning opportunity

In providing an environment conducive to learning, it is important for gastroenterology nurses to convey an attitude of support rather than condescension. Finding a room or space where distractions can be kept at a minimum also augments the patient learning opportunity. Adequate preparation for learning activities ensures that the learning content can be delivered in a logical and comprehensive manner. Involving the patient and family members and the patient's significant others also facilitates learning and ensures that proper followup is arranged by the patient and family. Finally, the nurse/teacher who exercises accomplished communication skills ensures not only that information is imparted in a clear, concise, and comprehensive manner but also that comprehension occurs. The learning opportunity may be facilitated by continually reminding the patient about the learning contract.

### Evaluating learning

Methods for evaluating learning correspond to the type of skill learned. Cognitive skills are best evaluated by oral questioning or written questionnaire. Affective skills are better evaluated through observation of behavioral response. Psychomotor skills may be evaluated by return demonstration. Short-term goals (i.e., those that may be attained within 1 week) may often be evaluated during the period of hospitalization, but long-term goal evaluation must be referred to home health nurses, office nurses, or long-term care nurses.

### Counseling

Counseling may be one of the most important gastroenterology nursing activities. Anxiety about hospitalization, the gastroenterology procedure, an outcome of surgery, or the results of laboratory studies can manifest itself in insidious ways that impede learning and healing. Fear, when suppressed, may precipitate a crisis marked by a total breakdown in a patient's coping mechanisms. To reduce fear and anxiety, gastroenterology nurses counsel patients throughout the course of therapy.

**Counseling** is the act of rendering guidance to a patient and/or significant other, an act which sometimes entails assisting the patient in problem solving. Counseling may be short-term, long-term, or motivational.
- Short-term counseling is given when ineffective coping patterns surface that require immediate attention. The severity of the underlying emotional issue may cause disturbance ranging from a minor dilemma to a major crisis.
- Long-term counseling is rendered consistently over a period of weeks or months and involves repeated contact with a nurse via telephone or personal visit.
- Motivational counseling is performed either to

stimulate a patient's inner drive to get well or to enhance motivation to cooperate in performing or learning to perform self-care. Motivational counseling generally requires an exploration of attitudes, values, and feelings underlying the disinterest in or indifference to recovery. To implement motivational counsel, nurses typically design incentives to stimulate drive and ambition.

In the gastroenterology unit, short-term counseling to enable patients to overcome anxiety and fear is an important function. Several factors influence the patient's vulnerability to crisis in the gastroenterology lab, including personality, cultural factors, and availability of support systems.

- Anxiety-prone personalities are more vulnerable to crisis when faced with a physical threat than are persons not identified as anxious personalities.
- Misperceptions related to religious belief or ethnic experiences and misunderstandings because of language barriers predispose patients to psychologic stress.
- Actual lack of supportive family and friends or perceived lack of professional support from a competent, knowledgeable, and willing staff may precipitate crisis.

Wheeler (1988) offers six signs of impending crisis that gastroenterology nurses should be alert for to prevent breakdown of existing coping mechanisms:

- Debilitating fear of impending procedure: what physician will find, pain and anesthesia, lack of control
- Disorganized thought and behavior caused by an inability to use cognitive, judgement, or decision-making abilities
- Regressive dependency marked by helplessness and reduced ability to cope
- Inability to limit emotional reactions in a customary manner in the midst of loss of privacy, control, or both
- Inappropriate response to hospital personnel or family, manifest as withdrawal or isolation
- Maladaptive behavior as the result of intense and uncontrollable feelings: magical thinking, excessive fantasies, regressive behavior (frequently anger), or somatic delusion

Wheeler (1988) suggests a counseling outcome and three criteria, listed as follows, for evaluating nursing intervention when implementing measures to assist a patient in emotional crisis:

Outcome:     Patient will exhibit adaptive behaviors.
Criteria:     1. Patient accepts tasks.
      2. Patient talks openly about impressions and feelings during the experience.
      3. Patient makes predictions and plans concerning recovery.

Wheeler also offers the following suggestions for short-term and long-term counseling intervention in crisis situations:

Short-term
- Acknowledge the crisis: The event is stressful, yet competent personnel are standing by to help. (This supports the patient's right to dignity.)
- Encourage patient to express feelings while listening empathetically.
- Give information in nontechnical terms.
- Explore coping alternatives.

Long-term
- Explore the patient's past in an attempt to identify his or her strengths and similar situations in which the patient coped successfully. Avoid discussion focused on chronic past problems.
- Reframe the situation by restating it in a more meaningful and positive way; for example, "You are angry because you care."
- Consider a referral to a social worker, psychiatrist, or psychologist.

**Advocacy**

In nursing the act of supporting patient rights is receiving greater emphasis by both consumers and nursing professionals. Consumers' expectations and demands have evolved with changes in healthcare delivery. At the same time, nursing professionals have come to value the promotion of individual well-being and to respect the individual's right to self-determination.

**Advocacy** behaviors in nursing exhibit two components: informing patients, and supporting them in their decisions. Informing patients enables them to make educated decisions. Information gastroenterology nurses can impart to help patients make educated decisions should include not only information about patient rights but also information concerning options.

This section elaborates on two areas in which the gastroenterology nurse can act to safeguard patient rights in gastroenterology: informed consent and assisting patients to make informed decisions when confronted by ethical dilemmas.

**Informed consent**

Endoscopic procedures are becoming more varied and technical, and the role of the gastroenterology nurse as an educator and advocate is becoming more important. When gastroenterologists and nurses work together to educate patients, there is no reason why any physically and mentally competent patient should not be totally informed about impending gastrointestinal procedures. Yet nurses in the endoscopy unit frequently encounter circumstances in which they question a patient's comprehension of a proposed procedure or the risks involved. They also witness situations in which a patient's ability to freely consent to treatment is altered.

The effects of anxiety, pain, medication, depression, or temporary or permanent disorientation are among the factors that can influence an individual's normal ability to judge and make decisions about his or her health care.

Although it is common to think of informed consent as a thing (i.e., a legal document), it is actually a process. **Informed consent** is an interaction between physician and patient, in which a meaningful exchange of information concerning an impending healthcare ministration occurs. Only the patient or a legally authorized guardian may give consent, and a legal guardian may give consent only in the event that the patient is incompetent by reason of age (i.e., the patient is a minor and neither married nor self-supporting), physical inability, or legal incompetence (see below).

Informed consent is required on three occasions; on admission, before any diagnostic procedure or medical or surgical treatment is performed, and/or before any human experimentation is enacted. Furthermore, the conditions under which consent can be waived are very specific, as listed in the following explanations:

- Consent is not needed in an emergency if there is immediate threat to life or health; if experts agree that an emergency exists; and/or if the patient is unable to consent and a legally authorized person cannot be reached.
- Consent is not required for an action necessary to treat an unanticipated complication incurred during surgery when a legally authorized person cannot be reached.

A patient's refusal of treatment constitutes a slightly different circumstance. Refusal to consent must be documented and, when appropriate, accompanied by an explanation of consequences that the patient may incur by refusing. A release form should be signed and witnessed, relieving nurses, doctors, and the hospital of all liability for outcome of the treatment refusal.

Failure to obtain consent may result in charges of battery against the nurse, doctor, and hospital caring for the patient. Even when given, consent is legally valid only when the following conditions are met:

- The physician and hospital make full disclosure concerning the proposed treatment or experiment.
- The patient possesses competent judgment and decision-making ability.
- The patient claims to comprehend the procedure and attending risks and aftereffects.
- The patient gives consent voluntarily of his or her own free will.

Responsibility for obtaining consent rests with the person(s) who are to perform the therapeutic or diagnostic procedure, or who are conducting the research study. Gastroenterology nurses may play a role in evaluating comprehension, assessing impediments to comprehension (including deficits in reasoning or judg-

ment processes), or detecting deleterious influences on patient decision making (i.e., force, coercion, and/or manipulation).

### Advocacy in ethical dilemmas

Reeder (1989) has proposed the following model of nursing ethics that upholds four ethical values, including fidelity, accountability, virtues, and caring:

- Fidelity refers to the commitment, covenant, or contract nurses have with patients. It is fostered by accountability, virtues, and caring and it implies a promise of advocacy and alliance in fulfilling patient needs.
- Accountability requires responsibility and being answerable for breach of responsibility.
- The relevant virtues are courage, honesty, and justice (i.e., treating all with equality and openness in the midst of certain risks and possible harms).
- Caring is "a commitment to protecting and enhancing the dignity of patients. . . . It is attending to the 'objectness' of persons without reducing them to the moral status of objects."

There are three circumstances when nurses may experience moral conflict when implementing a plan of care:

- Moral uncertainty, which is an inability to recognize the nature of an ethical problem
- Moral dilemmas, as when a conflict arises between two or more ethical principles with no obvious solution
- Moral distress, which is a conflict between an individual's knowledge of ethically appropriate action and institutional constraints preventing action

One dilemma frequently encountered in the gastroenterology unit concerns whether or not to maintain nutrition of severely debilitated or vegetative patients through percutaneous endoscopic gastrostomy tubes.

McDonald (1986) notes that a nurse's role in facilitating ethical decision making varies between institutions. Nonetheless, he suggests that nurses can be active in professional healthcare dilemmas via decision-making teams. He suggests that the current lack of nursing participation in ethical decision making is to some extent a function of traditional views of the nurse's role as held by physicians. Moreover, MacDonald suggests that the lack of preparation in nursing education systems surrounding ethical decision making causes nurses to shy away from participation. Finally, he suggests that avoidance of ethical decision making is also motivated by fear. Fear of superiors, of coworkers, of emotions, or even fear of greater responsibility can lead to complacency and passivity.

It may help to understand and accept the fact that in ethical dilemmas all participants are "morally equal." McDonald suggests the following ways nursing leaders can implement involvement:

- Leaders must temporarily defer some leadership roles to others.
- Each member must assume equal responsibility and obligation for his or her own views.
- A decision-making mechanism in which each member's opinion is respected must be enacted to handle treatment dilemmas.

In addition, Barnie (1990) offers some basic guidelines to gastroenterology nurses who participate in ethical decision making.

- Teach, clarify, and reinforce medical information.
- Remain as objective as possible, segregating personal opinions from the medical and legal options of the patient and family. Give insight without influence.
- Provide a willing ear and a cautious mouth: listen empathetically; avoid hasty, emotional, and irrational accusations at all cost.
- Approach patients respectfully and provide support for existing coping mechanisms.
- Accept and support the family's legal decisions without imposing personal principles, morality, or religious beliefs.
- Observe and communicate appropriately.
- Work through appropriate channels, providing referrals to such resources as support groups or financial aid advisors when appropriate.

---

**CASE SITUATION**

Bennett Brandish is a 48-year-old executive with rectal polyps who is undergoing a colonoscopic polypectomy. He sought medical attention when he began to notice occasional blood in his stool. He reports having confidence in his physician, Dr. MacElroy, but has also heard "a few horror stories" about hospital care. Mr. Brandish is somewhat edgy, but cooperates in his care. In fact, Mr. Brandish responded favorably to preprocedural teaching, listening carefully to the information given him and asking many questions. He claimed to feel "more in control of the situation."

He is now under conscious sedation for the colonoscopic polypectomy. Dr. MacElroy began to report difficulty maintaining light in the operative field just after the procedure began. The gastroenterology nurse has been attempting to troubleshoot the equipment difficulty when Dr. MacElroy notices that the patient has begun to hemorrhage.

### Points to think about

1. In removing the rectal polyps, Dr. MacElroy has encountered one of the possible complications (he-morrhage) of the procedure and must now treat it. What intervention must the gastroenterology nurse take to help Dr. MacElroy correct the immediate problem?
2. Of the actions identified, which might the gastroenterology nurse be able to delegate?
3. Which of the actions identified are activities the nurse may initiate independently? Which must occur under Dr. MacElroy's direction and supervision?
4. What variables may influence how the nurse implements the actions identified?

### Suggested responses

1. The gastroenterology nurse might identify the following actions to help Dr. MacElroy correct the problem:
   - Call for additional help.
   - Increase the IV flow rate.
   - Place the patient in the Trendelenburg position.
   - Insert a large-bore IV line.
   - Set up cautery equipment.
   - Continue to troubleshoot equipment failure.
   - Type and cross and send for blood (stat).
   - Change the suction canister.
   - Increase frequency of vital sign monitoring.
   - Administer oxygen through nasal cannula.
   - Plan to take further action; for example, to reverse narcotic.
   - Comfort Mr. Brandish as appropriate.
   - Document all actions, observations, patient responses.
2. The following list includes actions the gastroenterology nurse might delegate:
   - Sending for blood
   - Changing the suction canister
   - Setting up the cautery
   - Continuing to troubleshoot equipment failure
3. Actions the gastroenterology nurse might take independently include the following:
   - Increasing the frequency of vital sign monitoring
   - Planning further actions
   - Counseling Mr. Brandish when appropriate
   - Documenting actions, observations, and patient responses

   Actions the nurse might implement, depending on Dr. MacElroy's directions and under his supervision, include the following:
   - Increasing the IV flow rate
   - Placing the patient in the Trendelenburg position

   In this circumstance, the nurse may need to prompt Dr. MacElroy to elicit direction, as he may be preoccupied with the hemorrhaging vessel.
4. Variables that may affect the way the nurse treats this situation may include the following:
   - Mr. Brandish's level of awareness of the problem
   - The patient's coping style

- Rapidity of change in the patient's metabolic condition
- Whether or not the nurse has available support personnel
- Whether or not the nurse has backup equipment
- The nurse's experience in similar situations

---

## REVIEW TERMS

**advocacy, consultations, counseling, dependent intervention, documentation, independent intervention, informed consent, interdependent intervention, liability, nursing care conferences, nursing rounds, referral**

---

## REVIEW QUESTIONS

1. The implementation phase of the nursing process is characterized by all of the following, except that:
   a. Evaluation criteria are developed, against which the effectiveness of nursing intervention can be measured.
   b. The nursing plan of care is put in motion.
   c. The data base is updated as data collection continues.
   d. Nursing care and patient progress are documented and communicated.
2. The act of rendering guidance or assisting a patient with problem solving is:
   a. Referring.
   b. Consulting.
   c. Counseling.
   d. Documenting.
3. Whether or not a nurse allocates time for teaching, counseling, or advocacy behaviors is a function of all of the following, except:
   a. The nurse's ability to manage time.
   b. Whether or not the institution values these activities.
   c. Whether or not the nurse likes patient contact.
   d. Whether or not a doctor has ordered it.
4. A gastroenterology nurse might vary the way he or she comforts an anxious 10-year-old boy based on:
   a. The developmental task of children in the 7- to 11-year-old age group.
   b. His willingness to participate in counseling.
   c. Recent findings concerning the impact of certain words in calming/provoking anxiety.
   d. All of the above.
5. Administering medication is:
   a. An independent nursing activity.
   b. An interdependent task.
   c. A dependent nursing obligation.
   d. A nonnursing chore.
6. Nurses accomplish patient teaching in four phases, including planning the learning activity, providing learning opportunity, evaluating learning, and:
   a. Correcting mistakes.
   b. Developing learning objectives.
   c. Explaining the patient's privacy needs to significant others.
   d. Helping patients make informed decisions.
7. The objective of the Partners in Practice model of professional nursing is to:
   a. Expand the types of actions nurses can take independently.
   b. Involve the patient in self-care.
   c. Increase cooperation between nurses and support services.
   d. Allow RNs to use their time more efficiently and effectively.
8. A research nurse wants a gastroenterology nurse's patient to participate in a research study. Whose responsibility is it to obtain the patient's consent?
   a. The research nurse.
   b. The physician.
   c. The charge nurse.
   d. The gastroenterology nurse.
9. Before implementing any nursing action, the gastroenterology nurse should follow all of these guidelines, except:
   a. Think critically about the plan of care, always questioning whether routines are really the best method of treatment.
   b. Consult immediate colleagues and colleagues in related nursing fields and relevant literature to discover more effective ways of managing health problems.
   c. Before instituting any measure to treat a health problem, assess the patient to be sure that the action is still necessary.
   d. Document his or her action.
10. Nurses participating in ethical decision making are "morally equal" and therefore need not:
    a. Give insight without influence.
    b. Fear the advice and opinions of physicians, hospital risk managers, and ethics committees.
    c. Accept and support the family's legal decisions.
    d. Work through appropriate channels, providing referrals to such resources as support groups or financial aid advisors when appropriate.

## BIBLIOGRAPHY

Barnie, D. "Percutaneous Endoscopic Gastrostomy Tubes: The Nurse's Role in a Moral, Ethical, and Legal Dilemma." *Gastroenterology Nursing* 12(Spring 1990): 250-54.

Black, M. "Documentation in the GI Lab." In *SGA Journal Reprints,* ed. Trivits, S, 275-76. Rochester, N.Y.: Society of Gastrointestinal Assistants, 1988.

Bodinsky, G. *Documentation: Charting to Standardize.* SGNA Monograph Series. Rochester, N.Y.: Society of Gastroenterology Nurses and Associates, 1989.

Carpenito, L. *Nursing Diagnosis: Application to Clinical Practice.* 2nd ed. Philadelphia: J.B. Lippincott, 1987.

Huey, F. "Working Smart." *American Journal of Nursing* 86(1988): 679-84.

Jakobsen, E. "Three New Ways to Deliver Care." *American Journal of Nursing* 90(1990): 24-26.

"Johns Hopkins Nurses Earn Salaries and Pursue Autonomy in New 'Professional Practice' Units." *American Journal of Nursing* 87(1987): 713-14, 730-34.

LaFontaine, P. "Alleviating Patient's Apprehensions and Anxieties." *Gastroenterology Nursing* 11(Spring 1989): 256-57.

McAloose, B, and Gruber, M. "SGNA Standards of Practice for Gastroenterology Nurses and Associates." *Gastroenterology Nursing* 12(1990): 229-31.

McDonald, D. "Nurses on Ethical Teams–Expanding Their Decision-Making Role." *AORN Journal* 44(1986): 83-85.

McGregor, P. "Developing a Patient Questionnaire." *SGA Journal* 10(Summer 1987): 50-51.

McGregor, P. "Your Patient's Escort: Teaching the Significant Other." *SGA Journal* 10(Spring 1988): 234-35.

Mikels, C. "Patient Education for Enhancement of Compliance." *Gastroenterology Nursing* 12(Summer 1989): 60-62.

Mikels, C. "Patient Education Guidelines." *SGA Journal* 11(Summer 1988): 43-44.

Monroe, D. "Patient Teaching for X-ray and Other Diagnostics." *RN* 53(1990): 52-56.

North American Nursing Diagnosis Association. *Taxonomy I with Official Diagnostic Categories.* St. Louis: NANDA, 1989.

Ord, B. "Communication: Care Plan Sharing." *Nursing Times* 86(1990): 40-41.

Plumeri, Peter A. "Informed Consent for Endoscopy." In *Journal Reprints II,* ed. Trivits, S, 329-31. Rochester, N.Y.: Society of Gastroenterology Nurses and Associates, 1990.

Reeder, J. "Secure the Future: A Model for an International Nursing Ethic." Keynote address to the Sixth World Conference of Operating Room Nurses in Vienna, Austria. *AORN Journal* 50(1989): 1298-1307.

Taylor, C, Lillis, C, and LeMone, P. "Implementing/Documenting." In *Fundamentals of Nursing: The Art and Science of Nursing Care,* eds. Cleary, P, Faven, E, and Intenzo, D, 303-36. Philadelphia: J.B. Lippincott, 1989.

Thurlow, J. "Informed Consent: Every Patient's Right." *Gastroenterology Nursing* 12(Fall 1989): 132-34.

Wheeler, B. "Crisis Intervention," *AORN Journal* 47(1988): 1242-48.

# Chapter 13

# EVALUATION

This chapter will acquaint gastroenterology nurses with the evaluation phase of the nursing process. Because the patient is the primary focus during evaluation, the first activities described concern the evaluation of the achievement of patient outcomes and evaluation of the effectiveness of nursing actions in assisting patients toward achieving agreed-upon outcomes. Evaluating overall effectiveness of care through quality assurance (QA) programs is highlighted and ANA and SGNA guidelines for implementing QA programs are detailed.

**Learning objectives**

After reviewing the content of this chapter, the gastroenterology nurse should be able to:
1. Describe evaluation and its purpose and relationship to other steps in the nursing process.
2. List three activities performed when evaluating nursing care.
3. Distinguish a concurrent audit from a retrospective audit.
4. Describe three alternative actions nurses may choose following evaluation of patient progress toward desired outcomes.
5. List one technique each for evaluating cognitive, psychomotor, and affective outcomes.

## JUDGING THE QUALITY OF NURSING CARE

Evaluation is an appraisal of the quality of care based on outcomes of nursing intervention and patient participation in the plan of care. When evaluating patient care, nurses engage in the following three activities:
- They determine whether or not a patient has achieved desired outcomes or is making progress toward outcomes identified in an earlier stage of care.
- They determine whether nursing interventions chosen to treat identified health problems are effective in reducing or resolving identified health problems.
- They examine the overall effectiveness of health care provided in achieving patient outcomes.

The process of evaluation is motivated by the aim of nursing professionals to provide quality nursing care, yet defining *quality* in health care is in itself a challenge. The meaning is so elusive and complex that, in the words of one observer, "it can blur one's vision easily." The earliest definition of quality in health care appears in health literature before 1933, where it is defined as "the application of all necessary services of modern scientific medicine to the needs of all people." More recently, healthcare financiers imposed a new meaning: "Quality of Care [sic] is the degree to which care is available, acceptable, comprehensive, continuous, and documented" (Reerink, 1989). This chapter defines quality of care as "the extent to which actual care is in conformity with preset criteria for good care with a minimum of unnecessary expenditure."

As apparent in the definition above, appraising the quality of care in the evaluation phase is accomplished by comparing actual outcomes with preset criteria. **Criteria** are measurable qualities, attributes, or characteristics that specify skills, knowledge, or health states (Taylor et al, 1989). When they accompany nursing standards of care, they delineate nursing behaviors. Every standard of nursing care is accompanied by one or more criteria to be fulfilled so the standard is met.

| Standards | Criteria |
|---|---|
| The gastroenterology nurse will maintain all equipment and facilities to assure safe, quality care of the patient undergoing an endoscopic procedure. | All endoscopes will be cleaned and disinfected in the scope washer, as per institutional policy. |
| The gastroenterology nurse completes the documentation required for patients undergoing endoscopic procedures. | 1. Vital signs are recorded pre- and post-procedure.<br>2. Times of starting and completing the procedure are documented.<br>3. Patient's tolerance to sedation is recorded. |

In the plan of care, expected patient outcomes represent the core of evaluation because they reflect desired changes in terms of the patient's status or behavior.

| Nursing diagnosis | Expected outcome |
| --- | --- |
| Ineffective airway clearance; potential | The patient is free from respiratory injury related to positioning, extraneous objects, or hypoxia post-procedure. |
| Skin integrity, impaired; actual | Normal wound healing without signs of infection or breakdown by 7/14. |

As illustrated in the examples above, criteria in the plan of care should specify a time frame indicating when evaluation should take place. (Evaluation should occur as early as possible.)

Evaluation of patient care is performed jointly by nurse and patient and sometimes includes family and other members of the nursing or healthcare team. The process involves three activities: evaluating the extent to which the desired outcome is achieved, evaluating effectiveness of nursing interventions, and evaluating overall effectiveness of care.

Evaluating a patient's progress toward or achievement of desired outcomes allows nurse and patient to direct further nurse-patient interaction. Both nurse and patient measure how well the patient has achieved desired outcomes by comparing progress against evaluation criteria developed during planning. (See Chapter 11.)

The following sections examine five steps toward evaluating the effectiveness of planned care:
- Collecting evaluative data
- Analyzing success or failure to achieve outcomes
- Rating effectiveness of nursing intervention
- Choosing a course of action based on evaluation
- Documenting outcomes of postdischarge needs

**Step 1. Collecting evaluative data**

The aim of the first step is to answer the question, "Were predetermined patient outcomes achieved?" The answer can be determined by one of several techniques, depending on whether the outcome is a cognitive, psychomotor, or affective outcome:
- Cognitive outcomes define increases in knowledge. Data are collected by asking the patient to repeat information or to apply information to everyday situations.
- Psychomotor outcomes address achievement of new skills. Demonstration by the patient of the new skill is an effective way of measuring attainment of this type of outcome.
- Affective outcomes are more difficult to evaluate because they define less concrete changes; that is, changes in values, beliefs, and attitudes. Patient

behavior and conversation are observed to determine whether or not affective outcomes have been achieved.

Once the data have been collected, they are compared with standards of nursing care, expected outcomes, and institutional policies.

**Step 2. Analyzing success or failure to achieve outcomes**

Once the nurse has determined whether or not the patient has achieved identified patient outcomes, analyzing the variables contributing to therapeutic success or failure is useful. In doing so, nurses are able to recognize patterns and look for differences in practice that lead to varying results. Moreover, this process prompts nurses to revise or continue planned care as indicated. Factors leading to the patient's success or failure in achieving desired outcomes are numerous and often complex. They may come from the patient, the nurse, the availability or unavailability of resources, ethical or legal dimensions of the patient's clinical situation, and other variables. (See Chapter 12.) By identifying these factors, nurses may reinforce influences that promote outcome achievement and deal directly with hindrances.

**Step 3. Rating the effectiveness of nursing intervention**

The purpose of this step is to determine how effectively nurses help targeted groups of patients achieve specific outcomes. Two component processes are used in evaluating the effectiveness of nursing intervention: evaluating the efficacy of nursing action in resolving a health problem, and evaluating nursing performance in implementing the nursing process.

The usefulness of every modality employed must be evaluated in relation to the individual's needs. Here, nursing research plays an invaluable role because it provides a means of evaluating treatment options implemented in a plan of care. For example, Rothrock (1989) summarizes abounding evidence that psychoeducational preparation of patients before stressful procedures promotes successful coping and speedy recovery. However, she notes that the medium used to provide procedural and sensory information may influence the effectiveness of preprocedural teaching and counseling. She cites a study by Zeimer that found no significant effect on patients' coping responses when preprocedural psychoeducational information was conveyed via tape-recorded messages. She also cites a study by Abrams, who found that children who viewed slides and listened to taped information offered less resistance to care in the operating and recovery rooms than those who only heard tapes. Visual representation of events may enhance the effectiveness of taped presentations of psychoeducational information.

**Step 4. Choosing a course of action based on evaluation**

Following evaluation of the patient's response to nursing intervention and the degree to which expected outcomes have been achieved, a nurse has three options: to terminate the plan of care, to modify the plan of care, or to continue the plan of care.

Planned care may be terminated if each outcome has been achieved. If the patient is having difficulty achieving the outcomes, the plan may require modification. In this event, each step of the nursing process is reviewed. If the patient simply needs more time to achieve the desired outcomes, the plan of care is continued. If it is apparent that care or assistance will be required beyond the hospital stay, discharge planning should occur.

**Discharge planning**

The most common mistake nurses make is to wait until discharge is imminent to evaluate whether or not a patient has achieved the desired outcomes. This is the reason that evaluation should be performed concurrently with implementation before discharge. If evaluation has been delayed, it may be too late to redress failure to achieve desired outcomes. Harris (1988) offers the following guidelines for discharge planning:

- Identify a tentative discharge date.
- Develop a plan that includes teaching needs and an assessment of the patient's ability to provide for basic needs.
- Arrange a discharge planning conference with the entire care team: inpatient staff, outpatient staff, community resource persons, patient, and family/significant others.
- Identify a network of communication within the community.
- Obtain an assigned case manager.
- Develop a clear follow-up plan with appointments and provisions for long-term hospitalization.
- Set a date for the first home visit.
- Agree on patient's prognosis and what constitutes success or failure to meet established outcomes.
- Arrange for equipment and supplies in the home.
- Investigate both reimbursement by third-party payers and other financial concerns raised by patient/family.

In addition, Harris identifies the following resources to look for in the patient's community:

- A home care agency whose staff is available for case management and includes a nurse(s) with skills appropriate to meet the patient's needs, and staff that can provide 24-hour care in the home, if necessary
- Suppliers who will provide equipment and supplies and can respond to emergency replacement requests
- Collaboration, support, and supervision from local physicians

- Family support systems
- Rehabilitation professionals (such as physical therapists, occupational therapists, and speech pathologists)

**Step 5. Documenting outcomes and postdischarge needs**

New **standards** are soon to be applied by the Joint Commission on Accreditation of Healthcare Organizations (JCAHO) indicating that the formal nursing care plan is "expiring, unmourned, as the heart of nursing's method of mapping and delivering care to patients" (Brider, 1991). At many hospitals, the formal nursing care plan has never been made a part of the permanent record. This softening of requirements is an acknowledgement of the need to find more flexible ways of reporting comprehensive care and simultaneously allowing nurses to streamline operations. Nonetheless, JCAHO continues to demand evidence of the nursing process in the patient's medical records. In particular, either directly or by referencing some document or standard of care, the JCAHO wants nurses to note evidence of:

. . . initial assessments and reassessments . . . nursing diagnosis and/or patient care needs . . . interventions identified to meet the patient's nursing care needs . . . nursing care provided . . . *the patient's response to, and the outcomes of, the care provided [and] the abilities of the patient and/or significant others to manage continuing care needs after discharge.*

Documentation of actual outcomes should appear in the patient's record as an evaluative statement. An **evaluative statement** defines whether each outcome was achieved, partially achieved, or not achieved, and summarizes findings in terms of measurable qualities, attributes, or characteristics. It should include all patient data that support the conclusion made. For example, in response to the expected outcome, "Parents will accept community support in caring for their son at home," a nurse might record, "Only mother expresses desire to contact community support group, but both parents report eagerness to care for son at home." Or, in response to the outcome statement, "Patient will perform colostomy care independently," another nurse might write, "Patient remains extremely anxious about colostomy care, refusing to touch stoma and looking away when stoma is exposed." If, in the latter case, the patient's discharge is approaching, this nurse should document her efforts to provide for continued teaching, counseling, and supervision following release from the hospital.

**EVALUATING THE OVERALL EFFECTIVENESS OF CARE**

Monitoring quality of care is the responsibility of all care givers. In many institutions, specially designed programs operate for the sole purpose of quality assurance (QA), an ongoing process of review in which data collected over a period of time are used to compare actual practice against standards of practice. Comparison is made to determine if care actually rendered meets a level of quality deemed acceptable within a practice setting (Cline, 1985). The review may also analyze the degree to which external factors, such as different types of healthcare services, specialized equipment or procedures, and/or socioeconomic factors influence health and wellness (Taylor et al, 1989).

The effectiveness of nursing care and the efficiency with which it is delivered is the concern of nurses, patients, fiscal intermediaries, other health professionals, and the community, which determines allocation of scarce resources to the healthcare delivery system (Taylor et al, 1989). In particular, they are concerned with the following items:

- The kinds of health and wellness problems nurses help patients resolve
- Which nursing interventions are most successful in achieving desired outcomes
- The costs to achieve them
- Whether these are the best interventions, considering the current technology of nursing science and other health or health-related sciences

### Participation in quality assurance programs

Quality assurance programs are designed to promote excellence in nursing. They provide the mechanism by which nurses are accountable to society for the quality of care they provide. These programs may focus narrowly on a single nursing unit or may be broad enough in scope to evaluate an entire institution, state, or country. They may be performed by individuals specially trained, or by staff members who act as quality monitors (Fralic et al, 1991). From a broad perspective, QA programs focus on the following four areas:

- Patient satisfaction with the services provided
- Professional performance (technical quality of services provided)
- Use of resources (efficiency of services provided)
- Risk management (the risk of injury or illness associated with the services provided)

Nursing participation in QA programs is motivated not only by the desire to provide excellent care but also by the desires to be self-regulating and self-correcting, to improve professional performance by identifying deficiencies in care and therefore educational needs, and to analyze and explain the differences in patterns of practice and results of care. Nursing participation is also motivated by the need to be accountable to society for the funds spent to purchase health services, the need to ensure the safety of the public, and the need to protect the public from care that is inappropriate, suboptimal, or harmful (Fralic et al, 1991).

In QA programs, nurses play an important role in assessing structure, process, and outcome standards (Taylor et al, 1989). **Structural standards** are those concerned with the environment in which care is provided. For example, structural standards describe organizational characteristics, policies and procedures, fiscal resources and personnel, and physical facilities and equipment. **Process standards** focus on the nature and sequence of activities carried out by nurses during the nursing process. They describe acceptable performance levels for nursing actions. **Outcome standards** are patient-focused; they address changes in the patient's health status or the results of nursing care. In all cases the method used to fulfill these objectives is the nursing audit.

The **nursing audit** is a method of evaluating the outcome of care or the process by which these outcomes are achieved using a review of patient records. Two distinct types of audits are conducted: the concurrent audit and the retrospective audit.

A **concurrent audit** is a review of nursing care and patient outcomes, and is performed while the patient is receiving care. It is accomplished through direct observation of nursing care, patient interview, and chart review. Concurrent auditing is performed to determine whether or not specific evaluative criteria are being met.

JCAHO requires that a certain number of retrospective chart audits be performed each year by accredited healthcare organizations. A **retrospective audit** is an evaluation of nursing care and patient outcomes, and is performed after the patient is discharged. Postdischarge questionnaires, interviews over the telephone or face-to-face, or chart review are retrospective auditing techniques. In addition, ambulatory surgery units and short-stay units (including endoscopy departments) have found discharge surveys useful in evaluating nursing care and patient outcomes (Williams and Brett, 1989; Dayton, 1988).

### GUIDELINES FOR DEVELOPMENT OF QA PROGRAMS

The American Nursing Association has outlined broad guidelines for instituting QA programs in nursing (Taylor et al, 1989).

1. Identify nursing values.
2. Identify structure, process, and outcome criteria and standards.
3. Measure the degree of attainment of criteria and standards.
4. Make interpretations about strengths and weaknesses based on such measurements.
5. Identify possible courses of action.
6. Choose a course of action.
7. Take action.

SGNA offers similar guidelines for gastroenterology nurses, as outlined in the nine-step process below for implementing QA in an endoscopy department (Mikels et al, 1990).

### Step 1. Develop accepted standards of practice

SGNA recognizes characteristics of nurse practice standards that ensure adherence to the standards. Not only must standards of practice be realistic, they must be tailored to the environment and to the system of health care in which they apply and to the patient population in the environment. Moreover, they should focus on tasks rather than expectations of the person assigned to the task. As standards of practice are developed, levels of performance are identified commensurate with resources available to meet standards (i.e., materials, equipment, and personnel) and existing mechanisms to implement the standards. Once standards are developed, they must be communicated to those delivering care, thereby establishing common ground for understanding a definition of quality of care and each individual's role in providing quality care.

### Step 2. Identify pertinent issues and/or problems

SGNA offers two ways of recognizing pertinent issues and/or problems that would merit a QA study.
- Evaluation of clinical performance against preset criteria is the first method. As described earlier, this method evokes opportunity to improve patient care and clinical performance.
- The second method is retrospective in nature. It entails a review of consequences following substandard practice.

SGNA cautions that abiding issues and problems should be distinguished from isolated incidents or mishaps when identifying issues and problems. Only abiding issues and problems warrant a full QA study. Moreover, some issues and problems are *multidisciplinary,* overlapping departmental boundaries. In this case all departments should agree on a definition of the problem and criteria to be used to evaluate measures taken to resolve the problem.

### Step 3. Prioritize topics

Because resources available to troubleshoot quality problems are limited, problems and issues must be prioritized. The extent to which the patient population is affected by the problem and the severity of the impact should be considered when assigning priority. In addition, the frequency with which the problem occurs and whether or not it can be resolved are factors that must be weighed when deciding whether to commence a full-scale QA effort.

### Step 4. Refine questions and criteria

As is true when defining patient outcomes and criteria for nurse practice standards, QA goals must be well-focused. For example, SGNA suggests that criteria such as "Review patient teaching" or "Review cleaning and disinfection technique" are too general to be monitored. When refined, criteria for resolving quality problems might instead read "Gastroenterology nurse will show the patient education film and record that the patient viewed it" or "Gastroenterology nurse will gas sterilize all endoscopic retrograde cholangiopancreatography (ERCP) cannulas after each use."

### Step 5. Collect data

Retrospective and concurrent auditing are methods of data collection endorsed by SGNA. Data collection by retrospective audit reveals trends in nursing care, but not necessarily why those trends are occurring. This method is less valuable when collecting data on problems that occur less frequently. It is an appropriate tool when collecting data from a large sampling of charts. The concurrent audit offers the advantage of immediate feedback. Collecting data while the problem is occurring enables immediate corrective action and therefore promises improvement in the quality of care while the patient still requires the care and is available. Patient medical records, hospital admission data, medication sheets, incident reports, lab reports, minutes, direct observation of care, questionnaires or patient satisfaction reports, patient interviews, and observer interviews provide information for both retrospective and concurrent audits.

### Step 6. Analyze data

Analysis of data should be performed by gastroenterology nurses who have developed the QA process to this step. Both positive and negative results are significant. In many instances, QA demonstrates what has been done correctly, and when analyzing data, positive findings should be communicated to staff, supervisors, and administrators. When deficits occur, they can be identified in the following four general categories:
- Personnel deficit: time or staffing problems
- Skill deficit: lack of knowledge
- Environmental deficit: lack of equipment
- Supply deficit: lack of materials

Positive and negative results (compliance or noncompliance with standards) should be summarized and documented with alternative conclusions and means of problem resolution.

### Step 7. Communicate results

Each practice setting should develop a format through which QA efforts are documented and communicated. Whatever the format, all gastroenterology nurses and subordinates, supervisors, QA department members, and administrators should be privy to the results. Department staff meeting minutes provide a convenient way of recording QA activities.

## Step 8. Take corrective action

Corrective action or problem resolution should involve personnel in the planning stage and should be directed toward the cause of the problem. If the cause is known, plans should be made to solve the problem. If the cause is unknown, further investigation may be necessary. For example, the following QA study did not result in problem resolution but instead generated a set of possible causes of the problem:

*Problem*   The majority of patients are choking during insertion of the upper endoscope.

*Possible causes*

1. Outdated topical anesthetic
2. Patient noncompliance (i.e., patient not gargling correctly)
3. Gastroenterology nurse error in applying topical anesthetic
4. Excessive time span between topical application and beginning of procedure
5. Unskilled physician

## Step 9. Reevaluate issues and problems

Taking corrective action may not result in problem resolution. The corrective action chosen may not have been appropriate to solve the problem. It may not have been communicated or understood by those involved. Or it may have been appropriate, but personnel may harbor attitudes toward the effort or resist changes for other reasons. Therefore reevaluation following corrective efforts should occur, and if problem resolution cannot be obtained for personnel reasons, individual performance should be dealt with through an employee appraisal process.

Quality care is a concept to which SGNA health professionals are committed. Nursing care documented in procedure manuals, patient education materials, and standards of care used by SGNA members should reflect concern for patients above all other concerns. QA plans are powerful tools to help meet standards for optimal care of gastroenterology patients and to validate that care in an organized and scientific format.

The six stages of the nursing process do not occur in isolation from one another. They are overlapping, sometimes concurrent, always recurrent. Achievement of a desired outcome rarely leaves the nurse and patient free of the task of identifying new outcomes, because the process is never complete. There is always a higher standard, always a greater goal.

---

CASE SITUATION

Last year, St. Vrain Hospital opened an endoscopy unit to serve the needs of its community. Although standards of nursing care have not yet been developed for the unit, nurses in the unit have been

meeting to develop criteria to be used for discharging postendoscopy patients. Following a survey of factors gastroenterology nurses use to evaluate patient fitness for discharge, the nurses at St. Vrain were asked to rank the factors in descending order of importance. Ultimately, they agreed on the rank-ordered list of factors below which they expect to use when developing standards and planning patient care:

| Rank | Item |
|---|---|
| 1 | Stability of vital signs |
| 2 | Level of orientation |
| 3 | Level of alertness |
| 4 | Skin color, warmth, dryness |
| 5 | Oxygen saturation (if oximetry is used) |
| 6 | Ability to ambulate |
| 7 | Clarity of vision |

Gastroenterology nurse Janice Brody monitors Jerald Finebelt as he awaits discharge from the endoscopy unit following a colonoscopic exam with laser therapy for a large, malignant rectal mass. Jerald had been premedicated with meperidine (Demerol) and atropine and received diazepam (Valium) during the procedure. His physician, Dr. Bechtold, has written orders to discharge Mr. Finebelt when stable. Janice overhears Dr. Bechtold instruct Mr. Finebelt to return to the office for a check-up in 3 days.

*Points to think about*

1. Given the list of factors gastroenterology nurses at St. Vrain hospital consider important when judging patient fitness for discharge, how might Janice evaluate Jerald Finebelt's progress after the procedure?
2. Janice notes that preprocedural teaching was documented in the nurse's record, including teaching about expected sensations during and after the colonoscopy, changes in bowel habits, and dietary restrictions. When should evaluation of teaching take place and how might an evaluation be performed?
3. Assuming that Mr. Finebelt achieves all expected outcomes (i.e., criteria for discharge fitness), what evaluative statement might Janice enter in the patient's records?
4. When Janice evaluates Jerald Finebelt's progress 1 hour after the procedure, his vital signs are stable, he is alert and oriented, and he has minimal pain. On the other hand, he complains of nausea and refuses fluids. What course(s) of action may Janice take based on these actual outcomes?
5. Janice will participate in the hospital's QA efforts by conducting a retrospective audit of the overall effectiveness of the admission and discharge systems in her

unit. How does this audit differ from a concurrent audit?

### Suggested responses

1. Evaluation of patient progress is a process of comparing actual outcomes with preset criteria—in this application, expected outcomes in the plan of care. Thus, for example, if the first fitness-for-discharge criterion is "stability of vital signs," then the expected outcome may read, "Vital signs are stable within normal limits." The factor "ability to ambulate" would translate into the expected outcome, "Patient ambulates without assistance." The factor "level of orientation" becomes, "Patient is oriented in space/time." Janice would evaluate Mr. Finebelt's progress by assessing whether actual outcomes at the time of evaluation met, partially met, or did not meet these expectations.

2. Evaluation is concurrent and recurrent, meaning that evaluation of patient teaching should occur during implementation of the teaching plan and during evaluation before discharge. Methods for evaluating patient teaching are related to the type of outcome set forth in the plan. The cognitive outcome, "Patient describes expected changes in bowel habits following colonoscopy," can be evaluated by asking the patient to repeat information; that is, to describe how bowel habits should be altered following colonoscopy. Asking the patient to compare his postprocedural sensation with what his nurse taught him to expect would help to evaluate the patient's expectations and recollection of patient teaching.

3. Janice would document the degree to which all outcomes were achieved, partially achieved, or not achieved. For example, she might write, "Patient is alert, oriented, and describes minimal discomfort. No n/v. Vital signs are stable within normal limits. Taking fluids and voiding in q.s. Ambulatory w/o assistance. Skin is warm, color is good, and skin is dry w/ normal turgor. Able to describe postdischarge care measures and self-evaluation criteria. Plan: D/C plan of care; discharge to home with transportation and assistance by wife. Random control trial (RTC) in 3 days."

4. Following evaluation of the patient's response to nursing intervention and the degree to which expected outcomes have been achieved, a nurse may:
   • Terminate the plan of care
   • Modify the plan of care
   • Continue the plan of care
   Planned care may be terminated if each outcome has been achieved. (For example: Mr. Finebelt is alert and oriented; checking responsiveness may be discontinued.) If the patient is having difficulty achieving the desired outcomes, the plan may require modification. In this event, all six steps in the nursing process are reviewed. (For example: Mr. Finebelt is refusing liquids; nurse may offer ice chips and/or administer antiemetic.) If the patient simply needs more time to achieve the desired outcomes, the plan of care is continued. (For example: as latter; NPO with continued monitoring until cause of nausea is found or symptom subsides.) If it is apparent that care or assistance will be required beyond the hospital stay, discharge planning should occur.

5. A concurrent audit is a review of nursing care and patient outcomes, and is performed while the patient is receiving care. It is accomplished through direct observation of nursing care, patient interview, and chart review. Concurrent auditing is performed to determine whether or not specific evaluative criteria are being met. A retrospective audit is an evaluation of nursing care and patient outcomes, and is performed after the patient is discharged. Postdischarge questionnaires, interviews over the telephone or face-to-face, or chart review are retrospective auditing techniques. Data collection by retrospective audit reveals trends in nursing care, but not necessarily why those trends are occurring. This method is less valuable when collecting data on problems that occur less frequently. It is an appropriate tool when collecting data from a large sampling of charts. The concurrent audit offers the advantage of immediate feedback. Collecting data while the problem is occurring enables immediate corrective action and therefore promises improvement in the quality of care while the patient still requires the care and is available.

---

### REVIEW TERMS

concurrent audit, criteria, evaluative statement, nursing audit, outcome standard, process standard, retrospective audit, standards, structural standards

---

### REVIEW QUESTIONS

1. Motives that nursing professionals have for evaluating the quality of nursing care include all of the following, except:
   a. Nurses recognize that *quality* in health care is elusive and complex.
   b. Nursing professionals aim to promote excellence in nursing care.
   c. Nurses must be accountable to society for the quality of care they provide.
   d. Nurses want to improve professional performance by identifying deficiencies in care provided and therefore educational needs, and to analyze and explain the differences in patterns of practice and results of care.

2. Criteria are:
   a. Standards.
   b. Facts.
   c. Interventions.
   d. Measurable.
3. A nursing audit is:
   a. An acceptable, expected level of performance established by authority, custom, or consent.
   b. An ongoing process of review in which data collected over a period of time are used to compare actual practice against standards of practice to determine if the care actually rendered meets a level of quality deemed acceptable within a practice setting.
   c. A review of documentation for the purpose of determining whether or not specific objectives were met during the period of time outlined.
   d. A statement defining an actual outcome (e.g., skills developed, knowledge obtained, change in health status).
4. Which statement is least accurate concerning QA programs?
   a. They collect data for evaluation by performing retrospective and concurrent audits.
   b. They conduct studies of overall effectiveness of care.
   c. They focus on two general areas of concern: resource allocation and risk management.
   d. They analyze the degree to which external factors, such as different types of health services, specialized equipment or procedures, or socioeconomic factors influence health and wellness.
5. SGNA offers two ways of recognizing pertinent issues and/or problems that would merit a QA study:
   a. Evaluating clinical performance against preset criteria and reviewing of consequences following substandard practice.
   b. Cataloging isolated incidents and differentiating them from actual problems.
   c. Surveying nursing interest in problems and recording the frequency with which these problems occur.
   d. Researching state-of-the-art interventions and comparing actual practice to these.
6. Nurses, patients, fiscal intermediaries, other health professionals, and the community who determines allocation of scarce resources to healthcare delivery systems concerned with the effectiveness of nursing care want to discover:
   a. Whether nurses or doctors are better able to provide specific kinds of care.
   b. Which nursing interventions are most successful in achieving desired outcomes and what it costs to achieve them.

   c. A and B.
   d. A only.
7. Evaluation of nursing care consists of:
   a. Examining the cost effectiveness of nursing actions, the efficiency with which admission and discharge takes place, and the rate of patient readmission.
   b. Determining whether or not a patient has achieved outcomes or is making progress toward goals developed in the outcome identification stage of care, whether nursing interventions chosen to treat identified health problems are effective in reducing or resolving identified health problems, and whether health care provided has been effective overall.
   c. Verifying whether or not policies and procedures are eliminating problems, whether the doctors are practicing according to the dictums of their specialty, and whether administrators are adequately staffing nursing units.
   d. Examining nursing values, identifying structure, process and outcome criteria, and executing performance appraisals to correct individual resistance to quality practices.
8. Evaluative statements:
   a. Must include the patient's response to care provided.
   b. Must describe actual outcomes of care.
   c. May define skills developed, knowledge obtained, or change in health status.
   d. All of the above.
9. The Joint Commission for Accreditation of Healthcare Organizations (JCAHO) requires:
   a. A written care plan for every patient treated.
   b. A written care plan for inpatients only.
   c. Documentation of the patient's and/or significant other's ability to manage continuing care needs after discharge.
   d. B and C.
10. Changes in values, beliefs, and attitudes are difficult to evaluate because:
    a. They are less concrete.
    b. Survey questionnaires used to evaluate them are rarely valid.
    c. There is little value placed on casual conversation with patients.
    d. All of the above.

**BIBLIOGRAPHY**

Brider, P. "Who Killed the Nursing Care Plan?" *American Journal of Nursing* 91(1991): 35-39.

Cleary, B, Faven, E, and Intenzo, D, eds. *Fundamentals of Nursing: The Art and Science of Nursing Care.* Philadelphia: J.B. Lippincott, 1989.

Cline, J. "Quality Assurance." In *SGA Journal Reprints,* ed. Trivits, S, 277-78. Rochester, N.Y.: Society of Gastrointestinal Assistants, 1988.

Dayton, G. "Development, Distribution, and Interpretation of a Patient Survey." *SGA Journal* 11(Summer 1988): 47-49.

Fralic, M, Kowalski, P, and Llewellyn, F. "The Staff Nurse as a Quality Monitor." *American Journal of Nursing* 91(1991): 40-42.

Harris, F. "Sometimes Pediatric Home Care Doesn't Work." *American Journal of Nursing* 88(1988): 851-54.

Kitz, D, Robinson, D, Schiavone, P, Walsh, P, and Conahan, T. "Discharging Outpatients." *AORN Journal* 48(1988): 87-91.

Manuel, B. *The Nursing Process Series V: Evaluation.* Modular Independent Learning Systems for the Association of Operating Room Nurses. Denver: Association of Operating Room Nurses, 1979.

Maradieque, Anne Hurdle. "Quality Assurance as Reflected in Documentation." *Gastroenterology Nursing* 12(Fall 1989): 135-37.

Mikels, C, Calvette, B, and Dahl, C. *Quality Assurance for the Endoscopy Department.* 2nd ed. SGNA Monograph Series. Rochester, N.Y.: Society of Gastroenterology Nurses and Associates, 1990.

Reerink, E. "Defining Quality of Care: Mission Impossible?" *Quality Assurance in Health Care* 2(1990): 197-201.

Rothrock, J. "Perioperative Nursing Research, Part I: Preoperative Psychoeducational Intervention." *AORN Journal* 49(1989): 597-619.

Taylor, C, Lillis, C, and LeMone, P. "Implementing/Documenting." In *Fundamentals of Nursing: The Art and Science of Nursing Care*, eds. Cleary, P, Faven, E, and Intenzo, D, 303–36. Philadelphia: J.B. Lippincott, 1989.

Williams, M, and Brett, S. "Discharge Surveys: A Quality Assurance Method for Ambulatory Surgery." *AORN Journal* 49(1989): 1371-80.

World Health Organization Working Group. "The Principles of Quality Assurance." *Quality Assurance in Health Care* 1(1989): 79-95.

# ANATOMY, PHYSIOLOGY, AND PATHOPHYSIOLOGY

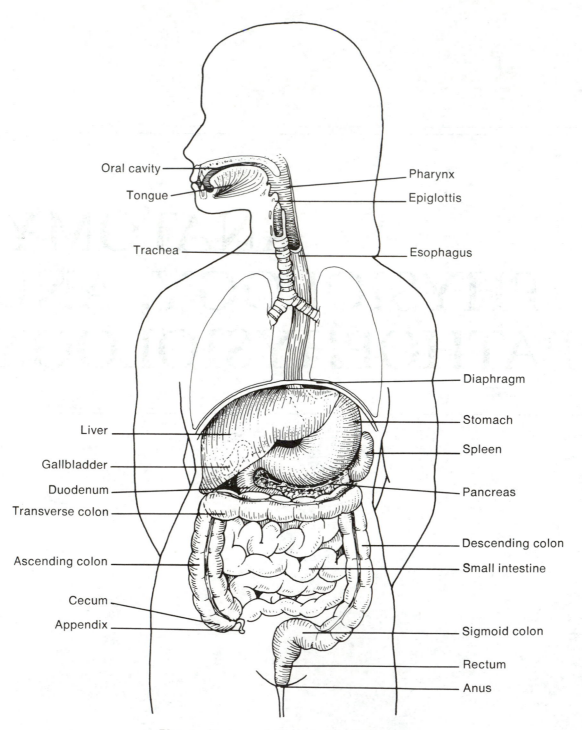

Oral cavity

Tongue

Trachea

Liver

Gallbladder

Duodenum

Transverse colon

Ascending colon

Cecum

Appendix

Pharynx

Epiglottis

Esophagus

Diaphragm

Stomach

Spleen

Pancreas

Descending colon

Small intestine

Sigmoid colon

Rectum

Anus

**Plate 1**. Anatomy of the gastrointestinal system.

## Chapter 14

# ESOPHAGUS

This chapter will acquaint the gastroenterology nurse with the normal anatomy and physiology of the esophagus and the clinical features, diagnosis, and treatment of selected esophageal disorders.

**Learning objectives**

Upon completing study of this chapter, the gastroenterology nurse should be able to:
1. Describe the anatomy of the esophagus, including the upper and lower esophageal sphincters and the esophageal body.
2. Explain the normal motility of the esophagus.
3. Discuss a number of pathologic conditions of the esophagus and the corresponding pathophysiology, diagnosis, and treatment alternatives.

## ANATOMY AND PHYSIOLOGY

The **esophagus** is a hollow, muscular tube, approximately 23 to 25 cm (10 inches) in length and 2 to 3 cm (approximately 1 inch) in diameter, which serves as a channel for food going from the mouth to the stomach (Fig. 14-1). It is considered the third organ of digestion, after the mouth and pharynx. The esophagus is located posterior to the trachea and larynx. It passes through the diaphragm and into the abdomen at an opening called the **diaphragmatic hiatus.** Almost immediately after the esophagus passes through the hiatus, it enters the stomach (Plate 1).

The wall of the esophagus is made up of three layers; the mucosa, submucosa, and muscularis. Unlike most of the rest of the GI tract, the esophagus is not surrounded by serosa.

The inner mucosal layer is covered with a layer of stratified squamous epithelium. Beneath the epithelium is the lamina propria, which consists of loose connective tissue. Extensions of the lamina propria, called the dermal pegs, protrude into the epithelium. Particularly at the upper and lower ends of the esophagus, the mucosa contains well-organized mucus-producing glands. A thin band of smooth muscle, the muscularis mucosae, separates the lamina propria from the underlying submucosa.

The submucosa is the middle layer of the esophagus. It contains loose connective tissue with both fibrous and elastic elements, and blood vessels and nerve fibers.

The outermost layer, or muscularis, consists of an inner layer of circular muscle and an outer layer of longitudinal muscle fibers. Between the two muscular layers is the intramuscular Auerbach's nerve plexus. Approximately the first 5% of the esophagus is made up

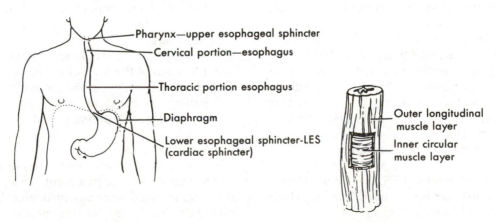

**Fig. 14-1.** Esophageal anatomy. Insert shows muscular layers of esophagus.

Pharynx—upper esophageal sphincter
Cervical portion—esophagus
Thoracic portion esophagus
Diaphragm
Lower esophageal sphincter-LES (cardiac sphincter)
Outer longitudinal muscle layer
Inner circular muscle layer

strictly of striated muscle, and approximately 50% to 60% of the distal esophagus is entirely smooth muscle. A transition zone of both striated and smooth muscles covers as much as 35% to 40% of the length of the esophagus.

At the upper end of the esophagus is the hypopharyngeal, or **upper esophageal, sphincter (UES).** Posteriorly and laterally, the UES is made up of the cricopharyngeal muscle; its anterior border is the cricoid cartilage. At the lower end of the esophagus, directly above the angle of His, which marks the junction between the tubular esophagus and the stomach, is the **lower esophageal sphincter (LES).** The LES is also known as the gastroesophageal sphincter or cardiac sphincter. It controls the passage of ingested food to the stomach. The LES is a physiologic rather than an anatomic sphincter and is 2 to 4 cm in length.

The esophagus receives arterial blood via the esophageal arteries of the aorta, the inferior thyroid artery, and the left gastric artery. The gastroesophageal junction receives arterial blood from branches of the left gastric artery and the inferior phrenic arteries. Blood is returned by way of the azygos, thyroid, and left gastric veins.

The esophagus receives both sympathetic and parasympathetic innervation. The swallowing center in the medulla initiates peristaltic contractions via the vagus nerve, which innervates striated muscle in the upper esophagus. Sympathetic innervation, which controls secondary peristalsis (which arises from within the esophagus), is derived from cervical and thoracic ganglia and from preganglionic fibers of the greater and lesser splanchnic nerves. The LES is believed to receive both sympathetic and parasympathetic innervation.

### Motility

At rest, both the UES and the LES are closed. When a bolus of food is pushed through the pharynx, the UES opens, allowing the bolus to pass into the esophagus. At this point, gravity and peristalsis combine to advance the bolus down through the esophagus.

**Peristalsis** is defined as a distally progressive band of circular muscle contraction. When it is initiated by swallowing, it is known as primary peristalsis. Secondary peristalsis originates below the hypopharynx with no antecedent swallowing movement; it is elicited by esophageal distention. In the esophagus, peristalsis begins in the pharynx and moves distally at a rate of 3 to 5 cm per second, effectively transporting material toward the stomach.

When the bolus reaches the LES, the sphincter opens to allow the bolus to enter the stomach, and then closes to prevent a reflux of food and acid.

## PATHOPHYSIOLOGY

Important disorders of the esophagus include esophageal reflux, varices, tumors, diverticula, and strictures. Other noteworthy pathologic conditions include esophageal rings and webs, foreign-body obstructions, infectious diseases, Mallory–Weiss tears, motility disorders, caustic injuries, Barrett's esophagus, fistulas, and congenital disorders.

### Esophageal reflux

**Esophageal reflux** develops when gastric or duodenal contents flow back into the esophagus without vomiting or belching. All adults and children normally have some amount of reflux, particularly after eating. Esophageal reflux is considered a pathologic condition only when it is excessive or symptomatic. Patients with excessive or symptomatic esophageal reflux have an incompetent LES; that is, the LES does not have sufficient intraluminal pressure to prevent reflux. Esophageal reflux may also occur as a result of pyloric stenosis, intestinal malrotation, or a motility disorder.

The most common symptoms of esophageal reflux are **dyspepsia** (epigastric discomfort or pain), **heartburn** (pyrosis), and **regurgitation.** Other symptoms may include **dysphagia** (a sensation of difficulty in swallowing), **odynophagia** (painful swallowing), bleeding from erosions or **esophagitis,** asthma, and aspiration pneumonia. To diagnose esophageal reflux, the physician may order a barium swallow, 24-hour pH monitoring, manometry, or an esophagoscopy and a tissue biopsy to evaluate the extent of mucosal injury. To confirm a noncardiac source for the patient's chest pain, a Bernstein test may be ordered. This test attempts to reproduce the patient's symptoms by instilling hydrochloric acid through a tube positioned in the esophagus.

The first step in treatment of esophageal reflux is behavior modification by incorporating the following recommendations:

- Dietary adjustment with avoidance of foods and beverages that lower LES pressure, including alcohol, tomatoes, peppermint, and caffeine-containing foods and beverages, such as coffee, tea, chocolate, and colas
- Weight loss and avoidance of tight-fitting garments
- Elevation of the head of the bed on blocks; the use of pillows to elevate the patient's head causes the patient to bend at the waist, thus increasing intraabdominal pressure and thereby increasing reflux
- Smoking cessation
- Avoidance of food or drink 2 hours before bedtime

The next step in the treatment of esophageal reflux is drug therapy, using antacids, histamine-2 (H2) blockers, sucralfate (Carafate), or the proton-pump inhibitor omeprazole (Prilosec). If these drugs are not helpful, the addition of a medication to strengthen the LES, such as metoclopramide (Reglan, a dopamine antagonist) or bethanechol (Urecholine, a cholinergic agent) may be useful.

If patients are debilitated by severe esophagitis, aspiration pneumonia, or other disabling symptoms, antireflux surgery may be needed to provide an artificial closing mechanism. Surgical possibilities include invaginating the esophagus into itself (Belsey's operation), or creating a gastric wraparound with or without fixation (Hill and Nissen procedures).

For patients with gastrostomy tubes, reflux may be prevented by elevating the head of the bed on blocks, slowing the rate of feedings, and checking for gastric emptying.

Complications of esophageal reflux may include esophageal stricture, esophageal ulcer, Barrett's esophagus, pulmonary aspiration, or upper GI bleeding.

One fourth to one half of all infants manifest some symptoms of esophageal reflux up to 6 months of age. In most cases, the condition has a benign course, and symptoms improve by 8 or 9 months of age. The most common symptom in infants is recurrent vomiting, which is frequently effortless in nature, but may be forceful. A differential diagnosis in infants may require a radiographic upper GI series, radionuclide gastroesophageal imaging, esophageal manometry, acid reflux test, sweat test for cystic fibrosis, and/or extended pH monitoring. An upper GI endoscopy is performed if anatomic abnormalities or esophagitis are suspected. Infants who vomit frequently after feeding but have no respiratory symptoms and are growing well may need no testing or treatment.

If symptoms are severe, the following measures may be helpful:
- Limiting the volume of formula
- Thickening feedings with dry rice cereal
- Placing the infant in a 30-degree prone position
- Avoiding active play in the first hour after feeding

The physician may prescribe bethanechol (Urecholine) or metoclopramide (Reglan) to strengthen the LES. Up to 15% of infants with esophageal reflux undergo surgery, most often the Nissen fundoplication, in which the fundus of the stomach is wrapped around the distal esophagus.

### Esophageal varices

Although varices may occur in other parts of the gastrointestinal tract, they develop most commonly in the submucosal veins of the distal esophagus, the stomach, and the hemorrhoidal plexus.

Esophageal **varices** are related to portal hypertension, which is often associated with alcoholic cirrhosis, but may also be seen in patients with cirrhosis resulting from other causes, such as chronic hepatitis. In such cases, fibrotic liver changes and hepatic vein obstruction cause increased pressure within the portal venous system. This pressure is transmitted to preexisting collateral circulation, which results in dilation of submucosal esophageal veins. Although varices may be asymptomatic and variceal bleeding is painless, there is a high risk of rupture of the distal esophageal veins, which causes life-threatening bleeding. In an acute episode, bright red blood gushes from the patient's mouth and the patient shows signs and symptoms of hypovolemia. An upper endoscopy is useful to diagnose esophageal varices and to evaluate the risk of bleeding. Varices can be classified on a scale of I to IV, depending on their size. Larger varices (grade III or IV) carry a higher risk of bleeding. Supportive measures are required for shock. The physician may order replacement of blood volume with packed red blood cells, albumin, and intravenous hydration and correction of concurrent coagulopathy with fresh frozen plasma.

Endoscopic injection of a sclerosing agent is the most effective treatment for acute variceal bleeding. Potential complications of sclerotherapy include inflammation of the mediastinum secondary to extraesophageal injection or perforation; rebleeding; stricture formation; or ulceration. Following sclerotherapy, patients should be observed for any signs of complications.

If bleeding is not controlled with injection sclerotherapy, a trial of intravenous vasopressin (Pitressin) is often the next step. Although vasopressin appears to stop variceal bleeding, it is also associated with serious systemic side effects, including hyponatremia, hypertension, cardiac arrhythmias, and decreased cardiac output.

A newer treatment alternative for variceal bleeding is esophageal variceal ligation (EVL), which involves the endoscopic placement of rubber bands or O-rings on the target vessel(s). A last resort may be balloon tamponade, a procedure that makes use of either a four-lumen Minnesota tube or a triple-lumen Sengstaken-Blakemore tube.

For long-term prevention of recurrent bleeding, a portal-systemic shunt may be used to divert esophageal blood from the portal circulation to the systemic circulation. Because operative morbidity and mortality are high in patients with end-stage liver disease and active variceal bleeding, this type of surgery is most useful as a long-term measure and may not be appropriate in emergency situations.

Overall prognosis for patients with acute variceal bleeding is poor. Approximately one third die during initial hospitalization, one third within the first 6 weeks after hemorrhage, and one third during the first year after bleeding.

## Tumors

The esophagus may develop benign or cancerous tumors. The most common cancer type is squamous cell carcinoma. Adenocarcinoma occurs about 5% of the time in patients with Barrett's esophagus. Chronic irritation of the esophageal mucosa caused by caustic ingestion, chronic or persistent reflux, or excessive smoking or drinking may predispose a patient to esophageal cancer.

The most common indications of an esophageal tumor are dysphagia and odynophagia. A steady pain may be located substernally or occasionally in the back. Other symptoms may include anorexia and weight loss, anemia, hoarseness, and cough. Blood loss is usually slow and steady rather than by acute hemorrhage. The primary diagnostic method is direct-vision esophagogastroduodenoscopy (EGD) with a tissue biopsy and/or cytologic examination. By the time the diagnosis is made, esophageal tumors are usually large.

The overall survival rate for patients with esophageal tumors is only 3%. Because cure is uncommon, surgery is primarily palliative and is intended to restore normal swallowing. Surgical procedures include excision and reconstruction or bypass. Endoscopic prosthetic intubation is another alternative. Radiation therapy or endoscopic laser therapy may be recommended for advanced untreatable tumors. A patient with an obstructing tumor may need dilatation or stent placement to allow limited oral nutrition and to relieve symptoms. If surgery is impossible and palliative care is unsuccessful, a gastrostomy may be initiated to bypass the esophagus and allow the patient to be fed directly into the stomach.

Psychologic care is important for patients who undergo a gastrostomy, or have inoperable cancer or an esophageal obstruction. Such patients may experience feelings of grief and altered body-image and should be encouraged to express them.

## Diverticula

**Diverticula** are outpouchings of one or more layers of the esophageal wall, and probably result from esophageal motor abnormalities. Esophageal diverticula may occur immediately above the UES (Zenker's diverticulum), near the esophageal midpoint (traction diverticulum), immediately above the LES (epiphrenic diverticulum), or intramurally along the body of the esophagus (intramural diverticulosis).

### Zenker's diverticulum

Zenker's diverticulum is associated with a dysfunctioning UES and is usually found in men over 50 years of age. Patients usually present with cervical dysphagia, halitosis, or aspiration pneumonia. Diagnosis is by barium swallow. Except in cases of recurrent disabling aspiration pneumonia, the condition is left untreated. Patients may be encouraged to sleep with the head of the bed elevated on blocks and should not eat or drink within 3 to 4 hours of bedtime.

If surgical intervention is necessary in such cases, small diverticula may be treated simply by cutting the cricopharyngeal muscle under local anesthesia (myotomy alone), by diverticulectomy, or in a two-stage operation involving both myotomy and diverticulectomy. Currently, the most common method is the one-stage diverticulectomy.

Complications of Zenker's diverticulum may include malnourishment caused by poor oral intake, aspiration pneumonia, or perforation of the diverticulum, leading to severe inflammation of the mediastinum with possibly fatal sequelae.

### Traction diverticula

Traction diverticula may cause no signs or symptoms. They are commonly small and nonretentive, and usually do not require therapy. Recent evidence suggests that they may be caused by esophageal motor dysfunction. Occasionally this underlying abnormality requires a long myotomy.

### Epiphrenic diverticula

The patient with epiphrenic diverticula may regurgitate massive amounts of fluid, usually at night when lying down. Incoordination between esophageal contraction and LES relaxation may be the cause of this abnormality. If surgical intervention is indicated, epiphrenic diverticula are best treated with removal and long myotomy.

### Intramural diverticulosis

Intramural diverticulosis is characterized by numerous small intramural outpouchings that probably represent dilated ducts that come from submucosal glands and are often associated with a smooth stricture in the upper esophagus. In rare cases, a *Candida* infection is present. Intramural diverticulosis generally responds to dilatation of the stricture.

## Strictures

An esophageal **stricture** is an abnormal formation of white fibrous tissue that is usually at the lower end of the esophagus and may or may not be circumferential. Esophageal strictures are common complications of caustic injuries or may be the result of candidiasis or of prolonged and severe reflux. Progressive dysphagia is the most common clinical feature. To exclude malignancy as the cause of the stricture, endoscopic exam with multiple biopsies and a brush exfoliative cytologic exam is mandatory.

In treatment of a stricture, the physician may use weighted mercury-filled bougies, also known as Maloney or Hurst dilators; pneumatic balloon dilators; or graduated plastic Savary-Gilliard or American dilators.

Many patients require follow-up with further dilatation at variable intervals, but this is easily accomplished. A long, narrow stricture is seen more often in children and may be treated surgically by colon interposition.

Perforation is the primary complication of dilatation. The most common symptom of esophageal perforation is persistent pain after dilatation; even mild pain is abnormal, although minor bleeding is common. Bacteremia, another complication, is a serious problem only in immunocompromised patients.

**Rings and webs**

**Esophageal rings and webs** are thin, circumferential, mucosal shelves within the esophagus. Webs consist of mucosa and submucosa, while rings, which are usually thicker than webs, consist of mucosa and muscle. Webs generally appear in the upper esophagus, whereas rings usually arise in the lower esophagus at the gastroesophageal junction.

Esophageal webs often present as intermittent dysphagia. Although endoscopic exam can provide the diagnosis, it usually ruptures the web. If the obstruction remains after an endoscopy, bougienage with Maloney dilators may be used. In rare cases a patient may require dilatation with a pneumatic balloon. If symptoms recur, further dilatation may be necessary.

The association of a cervical esophageal web and iron deficiency anemia in middle-aged women is known as Paterson-Kelly or Plummer-Vinson syndrome. In these patients the webs seem to regress spontaneously with treatment of the iron deficiency anemia. This syndrome is also associated with an increased incidence of postcricoid carcinoma.

Lower esophageal rings, also known as **Schatzki's ring** or B-rings, are thin, concentric membranes located at the esophagogastric junction. Rings are more likely to cause symptoms than are esophageal webs. A characteristic symptom is episodic dysphagia, or food impaction, which is often related to eating rapidly. Diagnosis is by barium swallow; endoscopic investigation may also be needed to rule out the presence of a peptic stricture. To relieve symptoms, patients may need one or two esophageal bougienages with a large Maloney dilator. Occasionally, pneumatic dilatation is required.

**Foreign bodies**

The esophagus is the most common site of acute foreign body obstruction. Eighty percent of foreign-body ingestions occur in children, with coins being the most frequently ingested object. In adults, the most frequently observed foreign body is meat. Eighty to ninety percent of ingested foreign bodies pass spontaneously.

Patients with an acute esophageal obstruction usually experience local pain, dysphagia, or odynophagia. Plain x-ray films may be ordered to provide information on the location and size of the obstruction if the object is radiopaque. If barium x-ray films are used to visualize an obstruction, it is important to be aware of the danger that the patient may aspirate the barium.

Larger foreign bodies tend to lodge at the gastroesophageal junction; once objects enter the stomach, most will pass uneventfully.

The treatment method used to remove the obstruction depends on the type of foreign body and the etiology of the obstruction.

- Pharmacologic agents, such as sublingual nitroglycerin or intravenous glucagon may be used to relax the LES and allow passage of the item.
- Endoscopy may be used to extract the foreign body by using a snare or basket, or the object may be crushed and then pushed into the stomach. Elongated forceps are used to extract coins that have been swallowed by pediatric patients.
- Surgery may be indicated for large or long objects that do not clear the stomach in 3 to 5 days, for sharp objects, for bags of illegal narcotics, or when there is perforation or bleeding.

Meat boluses have been dissolved enzymatically using papain. However, the use of papain may be associated with esophageal perforation or pulmonary aspiration and is not recommended.

Potential complications of foreign-body esophageal obstructions include esophageal perforation or penetration of the aorta or its branches, followed by hemorrhage. The risk of perforation can be minimized by the use of overtubes and hoods that cover the object as it is being withdrawn.

It is not uncommon for children to ingest small alkaline batteries, such as those found in electronic equipment. Such batteries must be retrieved as soon as possible and any signs of perforation should be treated surgically, because local corrosive effects may be fatal.

If a pill is swallowed with little or no fluid intake when the patient is in a supine position or just before going to bed, it can remain in the esophagus, thus eroding the esophageal tissue and causing an ulcer. Medications known to damage the esophagus include doxycycline, tetracycline, clindamycin, potassium chloride, ferrous sulfate, quinidine, aspirin, and ibuprofen (Motrin). Treatment involves stopping medication, relieving odynophagia, providing adequate nutrition, and watching for complications. In 3 to 6 weeks, symptoms should be relieved.

**Infectious diseases**

Viruses, bacteria, fungi, and mycobacteria can all cause esophageal infection. The most common causes are *Candida,* herpes simplex virus, and cytomegalovirus (CMV).

### Esophageal candidiasis

Esophageal **candidiasis** rarely develops in patients who do not have an underlying disease, such as diabetes, immune deficiency, or malignancy. The main symptoms are dysphagia and odynophagia. Severe infection can destroy esophageal innervation, thus causing abnormal motility. Serious complications include hemorrhage, yeast dissemination, and, rarely, perforation.

Esophagitis can be diagnosed on barium swallow, but a specific diagnosis of candidiasis is difficult. An endoscopy will reveal whitish plaques with a normal mucosal pattern between the plaques. Definitive diagnosis is by demonstration of mycelial forms in tissue samples obtained from a biopsy or cytology brushings. Therapy consists of a trial of nystatin suspended in water or mixed in methyl cellulose. More severe infections may respond to ketoconazole (Nizoral) or amphotericin B (Fungizone).

### Herpetic esophagitis

Predisposing factors to herpetic esophagitis include lymphoma, leukemia, or any immunocompromised state. Separate ulcers or shallow plaques are visible on endoscopy. Diagnosis is by virus tissue culture or by characteristic cellular changes on cytology or biopsy.

### CMV esophagitis

CMV esophagitis appears as areas of mucosal injury with small ulcerations. Diagnosis is made by viral tissue culture. At present, treatment for CMV esophagitis is only experimental.

## Mallory-Weiss tears

A **Mallory-Weiss tear** is a mucosal tear at the gastroesophageal junction. It is associated with prolonged, forceful vomiting, trauma, childbirth, or complications of EGD. Patients who have a Mallory-Weiss tear often have a history of alcohol abuse. Typically, prolonged emesis, or dry heaves, is followed by vomiting of bright red blood. The amount of blood lost is usually small and these patients are generally treated conservatively because bleeding stops spontaneously. Profuse bleeding may be controlled endoscopically with a coagulating contact probe.

## Motility disorders

Esophageal motility disorders are primary if the etiology of the abnormality is unknown but the esophagus is the site of major involvement, or secondary if the esophageal abnormalities are features of a more generalized disease process. Primary esophageal motility disorders include achalasia, diffuse esophageal spasm, and nutcracker esophagus.

### Achalasia

**Achalasia** is a combined defect of aperistalsis of the esophageal body and elevated LES pressure. Patients with achalasia present with dysphagia to solids and liquids, regurgitation, and weight loss. Diagnostic evaluation procedures may include a radiographic exam, manometric study, and EGD. On x-ray films the esophagus appears dilated, with a narrow "bird beak" at the distal end. Microscopically, a loss of nonargyrophilic ganglion cells in the myenteric plexus is evident.

Symptoms may be relieved by eating slowly, chewing well, drinking fluids with meals, and sitting up while eating. Many patients benefit from pneumatic balloon dilatation. A cardiomyotomy (Heller's operation) may be performed to reduce LES pressure in patients who experience unsuccessful treatment with pneumatic dilatation or who are poor candidates for dilatation. In patients who are not considered suitable for dilatation or surgery, long-acting nitrates such as sublingual isosorbide dinitrate (Isordil), or calcium channel blockers such as nifedipine (Adalat), may be used to reduce LES pressure.

Complications of achalasia are related to retention and stasis in the esophagus. Esophagitis may be evident endoscopically. Aspiration of esophageal contents is a danger and may be followed by bronchopneumonia. The prevalence of esophageal carcinoma is higher than normal in achalasia patients, possibly because it may be precipitated by stasis and mucosal irritation. Regular follow-up care is recommended.

### Diffuse esophageal spasm

**Diffuse esophageal spasm (DES)** is a motility disorder of unknown cause and pathophysiology. It is defined manometrically as repetitive or prolonged simultaneous contractions (nonperistaltic esophageal contractions that occur all at once up and down the length of the esophagus, independent of pharyngeal contractions) with intermittent normal peristalsis. One symptom may be noncardiac substernal chest pain, which may be severe and may closely mimic angina pectoris. Dysphagia may be present with both solids and liquids and is most severe when the patient ingests extremely hot or cold foods. In most cases, the distal two thirds of the esophagus show muscular thickening.

A barium swallow may show isolated, uncoordinated movements of the lower two thirds of the esophagus. The entire two thirds of the esophagus may contract as a unit, propelling barium both retrograde and into the stomach. Manometric examinations may reveal a simultaneous high-amplitude, abnormally long contraction in the lower two thirds of the esophagus.

DES may be relieved by pharmacologic therapy with anticholinergics, nitrates, smooth muscle relaxants such as hydralazine, or calcium channel blockers such as nifedipine (Adalat) or verapamil. When the condition is severe and unresponsive, dilatation may be used to relieve symptoms. Some patients benefit from a long esophagomyotomy, which involves cutting the esophageal muscles to prevent peristalsis.

**Nutcracker esophagus**

**Nutcracker esophagus,** also known as symptomatic esophageal peristalsis, is the most common manometric disorder in patients presenting with noncardiac chest pain. Nutcracker esophagus is defined manometrically as peristalsis with a contractile amplitude that is two to three times the normal value. If treatment is necessary, pharmacologic therapy may be tried, as described for DES.

## Caustic injury

Accidental or suicidal ingestion of highly alkaline or acid compounds may result in injury to the esophagus. The most common symptom is odynophagia, but patients may also complain of dysphagia and chest pain, or may drool profusely. Prognosis depends on the depth and extent of injury. Esophageal burns may be classified as one of the following:

- First degree, characterized by mucosal erythema and edema and generally favorable outcomes
- Second degree, characterized by erythema, blister formation, superficial ulceration, and fibrous exudate and often associated with stricture formation
- Third degree, characterized by deep ulceration and/or eschar formation and possible perforation

Alkaline compounds, such as lye, drain cleaners, and bleaches typically cause more damage than acidic compounds, such as toilet bowl cleaners, soldering fluxes, and battery fluids. In the case of acid ingestion, the physician may order large volumes of milk or water to dilute the acid.

Diagnostic evaluation of caustic injuries involves determining the nature of the ingested agent; radiographic examinations of the neck, chest, and abdomen to exclude perforation or pneumonia; and endoscopic examination to document the extent of injury, unless there is evidence of a perforation or extensive necrosis.

Treatment following caustic injury depends on the extent of the injury, but patients should always be kept NPO. Vital functions should be supported as needed, and intake and output should be carefully documented. To maintain the esophageal lumen and gastric access, a nasogastric tube should be placed. If the patient shows evidence of laryngeal involvement or respiratory difficulties, endotracheal intubation or tracheostomy may be required. The physician may also order parenteral corticosteroids and broad-spectrum antibiotics, but this type of treatment is controversial. Dilatation may be required for second-degree injury and surgery is indicated for patients who deteriorate despite intensive medical management.

Complications of caustic ingestion may include formation of strictures or squamous cell carcinoma.

## Barrett's esophagus

**Barrett's esophagus** is defined as epithelial metaplasia in which normal squamous epithelium is replaced by one or more of the following types of columnar epithelium: a distinctive, specialized columnar epithelium; a junctional type of epithelium; and/or a gastric fundus type of epithelium. Barrett's esophagus occurs in up to 10% of patients with chronic esophageal reflux.

Diagnosis of Barrett's esophagus is by endoscopic visualization of the mucosa, supported by examination of tissue biopsy. There is no effective medical or surgical treatment for Barrett's esophagus. Treatment is directed at the underlying reflux esophagitis and may include stricture dilatation.

The prevalence of adenocarcinoma in patients with Barrett's esophagus has been reported to be about 30 to 40 times that of the general population. Although the actual frequency with which dysplasia progresses to cancer is not known, some endoscopists continue to recommend annual screening with endoscopy and biopsy to identify early neoplastic changes.

## Congenital defects

In embryonic development, the esophagus and trachea begin as one tube. If the two do not separate completely, or if they retain a communication channel, atresia and/or a fistula may develop. The most common abnormality is a tracheoesophageal **fistula,** where the esophagus closes to form a blind sac (**atresia**) and either the upper or lower esophagus links with the trachea through a fistula (a tubelike passage between the two cavities). In another type of tracheoesophageal fistula, a normal trachea and esophagus attach to form an H-type fistula.

These anomalies become apparent shortly after birth when the infant regurgitates mucus and fluid. Atresia without tracheal involvement causes cyanotic coughing or other signs of aspiration during feeding. Fistulas may be located by cinematoradiography, which is performed during feeding.

To ensure the infant's survival, prompt surgical closure of the fistula at the communication point and anastomosis to correct atresia are required. As the child grows, stricturing of the esophageal anastomosis may occur but can be resolved with simple dilatation.

## Fistulas in adults

Bronchoesophageal or tracheoesophageal fistulas in adults are usually caused by cancer but may also be caused by a benign inflammatory process or trauma. Symptoms include chronic cough, fever, and recurrent pulmonary infections, with or without dysphagia. Diagnosis is by barium swallow. The treatment of choice for a benign fistula is surgery to remove necrotic and irreversibly damaged tissue and to close the fistula. Fistulas related to cancer cause acute episodes of coughing after eating. Surgical procedures are purely palliative in such cases.

Aortoesophageal fistulas may develop if an ingested foreign object lodges in the region above the aortic arch or if a tumor extends through the wall of the esophagus. Minor bleeding usually occurs as erosion connects the aorta and esophagus. Massive bleeding may begin at any time and almost always causes death.

---

CASE SITUATION

Doris Johnson is a 51-year-old woman who lives with her husband and four grown, unmarried sons on a large dairy farm in Wisconsin.

For the past 4 years Mrs. Johnson has been experiencing increasing amounts of retrosternal discomfort or a burning sensation shortly after eating or on sudden bending. Recently, the discomfort, described as "heartburn," has progressed to a painful ache that radiates to her neck, shoulders, and upper arms. Because both gallbladder and coronary artery disease are in her family history, Mrs. Johnson has become concerned enough to seek medical assistance. Her physician has made a tentative diagnosis of esophageal reflux and has referred her for diagnostic workup before prescribing treatment.

Mrs. Johnson is 5' 7" tall and weighs 186 pounds. Her admitting vital signs are as follows: blood pressure 170/90; pulse 90; respiration 22; temperature 99.2 degrees F. She denies use of all habit-forming substances, including tobacco, although she admits she may have a small amount of alcohol on festive occasions. She takes no prescribed drugs regularly, but has used an antacid to help the "burning" sensation. She is scheduled for a complete cardiac workup, barium swallow, esophageal function studies, and an EGD.

*Points to think about*

1. Mrs. Johnson comes to the endoscopy unit for her EGD. Besides the information on the normal assessment form, what other information would be helpful to the gastroenterology nurse?

2. What finding during EGD would help make Mrs. Johnson's diagnosis?
3. What nursing diagnosis would fit this case?
4. How might a nurse assist Mrs. Johnson in managing the stress associated with EGD?
5. What can the nurse teach Mrs. Johnson?

*Suggested responses*

1. Additional data about Mrs. Johnson that might be helpful would include:
   - Whether the other studies in her recent workup were normal, including cardiac workup and upper GI studies
   - Whether Mrs. Johnson is currently taking any medications other than the antacid; whether she is allergic to any medications; the effectiveness of the antacid she is using, length and frequency of use, and name of drug
   - The presence of symptoms specific to reflux, such as regurgitation, dysphagia, or odynophagia; duration, time, and other factors associated with discomfort/pain episodes (e.g., eating, bending over, exercise, tight clothing, pregnancy, or sleeping)

2. A finding of gross esophagitis would give a definitive diagnosis of esophageal reflux; however, 40% of symptomatic patients may not have this finding with endoscopic examination.

3. An appropriate nursing diagnosis might be "altered nutrition: more than body requirements, related to caloric intake exceeding metabolic need." It is important to note that excessive weight gain can increase intraabdominal pressure and exacerbate reflux. Furthermore, eating the wrong foods can add calories, decrease LES tone, exacerbate pain, and increase gastric acid secretion rate. If a full nutritional assessment seems warranted, an appropriate referral should be provided.

4. Measures by which a nurse can help Mrs. Johnson manage stress during EGD might include:
   - Reiteration of the procedural process, focusing on Mrs. Johnson's questions and concerns
   - Reexplanation of the method and type of anesthetic to be used, rationale for its use, its duration, and related postprocedural nursing precautions and measures
   - Periodic reassurance before and during the procedure that she will be able to breathe normally
   - Teaching and practicing basic muscle relaxation techniques so that she can recognize tense muscles and relax them voluntarily or on request during the procedure
   - Reassurance that salivary secretion can be managed and an explanation of how this is accomplished without swallowing or speaking
   - Assignment of a nurse who can support Mrs.

Johnson throughout the procedure both verbally and through touch

5. To be sure that Mrs. Johnson has adequate knowledge about her condition and proposed treatment, the gastroenterology nurse might:
   - Use anatomic drawings to describe the physical process involved, such as LES area, hiatal hernia, location of inflammation or strictures
   - Explain how to use gravity to decrease reflux, by not lying down after meals and elevating the head of the bed on 6-inch blocks to decrease acid reflux at night
   - Explain the medications the physician has prescribed for this problem, how they work, when to take them, and any side effects to watch for.
   - Review any medications Mrs. Johnson is already taking to avoid those that are potentially harmful to this condition; for example, anticholinergics, sedatives, tranquilizers, theophylline, or calcium channel blockers
   - Explain dietary modifications that may be helpful.
   - Suggest other lifestyle modifications that may be helpful, such as cessation of smoking (cigarette smoking reduces LES tone); avoidance of clothing that is tight around the abdomen; if overweight, initiation of a supervised diet; use of proper body mechanics to avoid bending
   - Advise Mrs. Johnson that chronic irritation of the esophagus can lead to complications, such as ulceration, stricture formation, Barrett's esophagus, and pulmonary problems
   - Encourage her to follow the prescribed treatment regimen carefully and to seek follow-up care

---

## REVIEW TERMS

achalasia, atresia, Barrett's esophagus, candidiasis, diaphragmatic hiatus, diffuse esophageal spasm (DES), diverticula, dyspepsia, dysphagia, esophageal reflux, esophageal rings and webs, esophagitis, esophagus, fistula, heartburn, lower esophageal sphincter (LES), Mallory-Weiss tear, nutcracker esophagus, odynophagia, peristalsis, regurgitation, Schatzki's ring, stricture, upper esophageal sphincter (UES), varices

---

## REVIEW QUESTIONS

1. In adults, the approximate length of the esophagus is:
   a. 15 cm.
   b. 25 cm.
   c. 35 cm.
   d. 45 cm.

2. The outermost layer of the esophagus is made up of:
   a. Mucosa.
   b. Submucosa.
   c. Muscularis.
   d. Serosa.

3. The progressive circular muscle contraction initiated by esophageal distention is known as:
   a. Achalasia.
   b. Diffuse esophageal spasm.
   c. Primary peristalsis.
   d. Secondary peristalsis.

4. The first step in the treatment of esophageal reflux disease is:
   a. Behavior modification.
   b. Drug therapy.
   c. Dilatation.
   d. Antireflux surgery.

5. Life-threatening bleeding is a frequent complication of:
   a. Esophageal varices.
   b. Esophageal reflux.
   c. Esophageal tumors.
   d. Zenker's diverticulum.

6. Outpouchings of the esophageal wall located immediately above the lower esophageal sphincter are known as:
   a. Zenker's diverticula.
   b. Traction diverticula.
   c. Epiphrenic diverticula.
   d. Intramural diverticulosis.

7. The most frequently observed foreign-body obstructions in the esophagus of adults are:
   a. Coins.
   b. Pieces of bone.
   c. Hard candy.
   d. Pieces of meat.

8. The infectious disease found most often in the esophagus is:
   a. Cytomegalovirus.
   b. Herpes simplex virus.
   c. Candidiasis.
   d. Giardiasis.

9. A patient's radiographic exams show a dilated esophageal body with a narrow "bird beak" at the end. The most likely diagnosis is:
   a. Achalasia.
   b. Diffuse esophageal spasm.
   c. Nutcracker esophagus.
   d. Caustic ingestion.

10. Esophageal fistulas in adults are most often caused by:
    a. Trauma.
    b. Foreign-body obstruction.
    c. Cancer.
    d. Congenital defects.

## BIBLIOGRAPHY

Bongiovanni, G, ed. *Essentials of Clinical Gastroenterology.* 2nd ed. New York: McGraw–Hill, 1988.

Ellett, M. "Pediatric Gastroesophageal Reflux: A Nursing Perspective." *SGA Journal* 11(Summer 1988): 3-10.

Given, B, and Simmons, S. *Gastroenterology in Clinical Nursing.* 4th ed. St. Louis: Mosby–Year Book, 1984.

Goldberg, K, ed. *Gastrointestinal Problems.* Nurse Review Series. Springhouse, Pa.: Springhouse Corporation, 1986.

Lencki, B. "The Esophagus." *SGA Journal* 10(Fall 1987): 117–19.

Misiewicz, J, Bartram, C, Cotton, P, Mee, A, Price, A, and Thompson, R. *Atlas of Clinical Gastroenterology.* Vol. 1. London: Gower Medical Publishing, 1985.

Nastasi, A. "Zenker's Diverticulum: A Cause for Complete Esophageal Obstruction and Its Management." *Gastroenterology Nursing* 12(Summer 1989): 25-27.

Sachar, D, Waye, J, and Lewis, B, eds. *Gastroenterology for the House Officer.* Baltimore: Williams & Wilkins, 1989.

Silverman, A, and Roy, C. *Pediatric Clinical Gastroenterology.* 3rd ed. St. Louis: Mosby–Year Book, 1983.

Silvis, S, ed. *Therapeutic Gastrointestinal Endoscopy.* New York: Igaku-Shoin, 1985.

Sleisenger, M, and Fordtran, J, eds. *Gastrointestinal Disease: Pathophysiology, Diagnosis, Management.* 4th ed. Philadelphia: W.B. Saunders, 1989.

# Chapter 15

# STOMACH

This chapter will acquaint the gastroenterology nurse with the normal anatomy and physiology of the stomach. The symptoms, diagnosis, and treatment options for selected gastric ailments will be reviewed.

**Learning objectives**

After completing study of the content of this chapter, the gastroenterology nurse should be able to:
1. Describe the anatomy of the stomach, including both macroanatomy and microanatomy.
2. Explain the normal motor and secretory functions of the stomach.
3. Discuss the pathophysiology, diagnosis, and treatment of certain pathologic conditions that affect the stomach, including peptic ulcer disease, gastric cancer, and gastritis.

**ANATOMY AND PHYSIOLOGY**

The stomach is a J-shaped, collapsible organ located just below the diaphragm, between the esophagus and the duodenum (see Plate 1). It is approximately 25 to 30 cm (10 to 12 inches) long and 10 to 15 cm (4 to 6 inches) wide at its widest point. The portion of the stomach that immediately adjoins the esophagus is the **cardia.** The gastric **fundus** is the dome-shaped part of the stomach that extends to the left above the cardia. Below the fundus is the gastric **body,** which extends to the incisura angularis, a notchlike indentation located on the upper lateral border of the stomach. Below the incisura angularis and extending to the narrow, tubular pylorus is the **antrum.** The upper lateral border of the stomach is called the **lesser curvature** and the lower lateral border is called the **greater curvature** (Fig. 15-1).

The entry of food into the stomach is controlled by the lower esophageal, or cardiac, sphincter (LES), which comprises a group of thickened circular muscles at the distal end of the esophagus. The LES regulates the opening and closing of the esophageal lumen. At the distal end of the stomach is the **pylorus,** which has a thick, muscular wall that forms the **pyloric sphincter.**

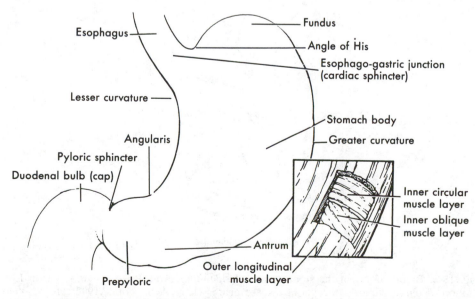

**Fig. 15-1.** Gastric anatomy. Insert shows muscular layers of stomach.

The pyloric sphincter controls the movement of stomach contents into the duodenum.

The stomach wall consists of the following four layers: an outer serosa, a three-tiered muscular layer (muscularis propria), a submucosa, and a mucosa. The outer serous layer of visceral peritoneum that covers the exterior of the stomach includes both the **greater omentum,** which hangs in a double layer from the greater curvature over the anterior side of the abdominal viscera, and the **lesser omentum,** which connects the lesser curvature to the underside of the liver.

The muscularis propria consists of an outer layer of longitudinal muscle fibers, a middle layer of circular fibers, and an inner layer of transverse fibers. These three muscle layers contract to produce the peristaltic motion of the stomach while it churns and compresses the food during digestion.

Below the muscular layers of the stomach lies the submucosa. The submucosa is composed mainly of areolar connective tissue. It contains the blood vessels, lymph channels, and nerve plexuses.

The gastric mucosa lines the interior of the stomach. When it is not filled, the stomach interior has a series of wrinkled ridges called **rugae.** The rugae allow the stomach to distend to hold a large quantity of food without any substantial increase in pressure, thus helping to control the rate at which food enters the duodenum.

The stomach receives arterial blood from the celiac axis, which sends branches to the lesser and greater curvatures. Along the lesser curvature the left gastric artery flows down from the cardia. At this point it joins with the right gastric artery, which is a branch of the hepatic artery. The greater curvature receives blood from the gastroepiploic artery, which runs from the fundus to the pylorus. In addition, short gastric arteries derived from the splenic artery supply blood to the fundus of the stomach (Fig. 15-2). Blood is drained from the stomach via the portal vein. The greater curvature is drained by the right and left gastroepiploic veins and the lesser curvature is drained by both the right gastric vein and the coronary vein.

Parasympathetic innervation of the stomach is via branches of the vagus nerve. Over the lower esophagus, the vagus nerves split. The anterior vagus divides into anterior gastric and hepatic branches. The posterior vagus also divides into two branches, one that supplies the posterior wall of the fundus and the body of the stomach, and another that supplies the posterior wall of the antrum.

Sympathetic innervation of the stomach is derived from the greater splanchnic nerves and the celiac ganglia. The afferent fibers conduct visceral gastric pain impulses and the efferent fibers inhibit gastric secretion and motility. Intrinsic innervation of the stomach involves Auerbach's and Meissner's plexuses. Auerbach's plexus influences gastric motility and Meissner's plexus is believed to be involved in gastrin release.

The primary function of the stomach is to initiate digestion by using both chemical secretions and mechan-

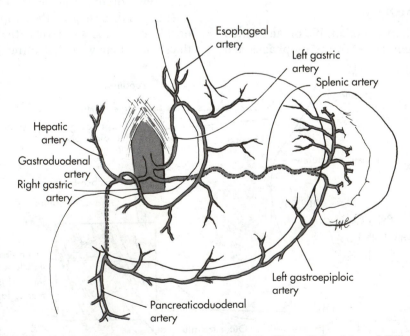

**Fig. 15-2.** Blood supply of the stomach and duodenum. (From Price SA and Wilson LM: Pathophysiology: clinical concepts of disease processes, ed 4, St. Louis, 1992, Mosby–Year Book.)

ical movements. Gastric secretions also promote the absorption of vitamin B12. In addition the stomach serves as a reservoir for ingested food and liquid and regulates their entry into the duodenum.

### Secretion

The mucosa contains three types of glands, which differ from one region of the stomach to another. **Cardiac glands** are located just distal to the esophagogastric junction. These glands secrete mucus and pepsinogens, which are converted by hydrochloric acid to pepsin.

The proximal two thirds of the stomach is the **oxyntic gland** area. At least four types of cells have been identified in these glands: zymogen or **chief cells,** oxyntic (parietal) cells, mucous neck cells, and endocrine or endocrine-like cells. **Parietal cells** secrete hydrochloric acid and intrinsic factor, which is a glycoprotein necessary for the absorption of vitamin B12. The chief cells secrete pepsinogens.

The antrum and pylorus contain the **pyloric glands;** these glands contain mucous cells, which secrete mucus and pepsinogens, and **G-cells,** which secrete gastrin. The pyloric and oxyntic glands also have **enterochromaffin cells,** which secrete serotonin. In addition, the cardiac, oxyntic, and pyloric glandular mucosae contain at least nine different types of endocrine cells, which secrete hormonal products such as somatostatin and glucagon. In addition, the parietal and pyloric glands both secrete bicarbonate.

When the stomach is at rest, normal secretions occur at a rate of about 0.5 ml/min. With food in the stomach, secretions increase to about 3.0 ml/min. The stomach secretes approximately 1,500 to 3000 ml of gastric juice daily.

### Motility

The movements of the stomach serve the following two functions: mixing and grinding of food, which takes place in the distal areas; and the controlled emptying of the gastric contents into the duodenum.

The peristaltic movement of the stomach combines each bolus of food with a mixture of digestive juices to form a relatively homogeneous, semiliquid mass called **chyme.** Normally, peristalsis moves the chyme slowly toward the pylorus at a rate of about three waves per minute, as regulated by a small region in the middle of the gastric body known as the gastric pacemaker. Before the chyme is ready to enter the duodenum, it must be of the proper consistency and acidity and the duodenum must be receptive. When these conditions are present, antral peristaltic contractions force the chyme through the pyloric sphincter and into the duodenum.

Only a portion of the chyme that is advanced toward the pylorus actually moves through the pyloric sphincter and into the duodenum. The rest is propelled backward, colliding with and further breaking down larger food particles in the antrum and body. Normally, particles passing into the duodenum have a diameter of 1 mm or less.

The gastric emptying rate is controlled by neural impulses, by the composition of the chyme, and by hormones secreted by the small intestine.

### PATHOPHYSIOLOGY

Pathologic conditions that are frequently seen in the stomach include gastric ulcer disease, gastric cancer, and gastritis. Other important gastric disorders include hiatus hernia, gastric outlet obstruction, congenital anomalies, gastric motor disorders, and bezoars.

### Gastric ulcer disease

When the normal balance between factors that promote mucosal injury (such as gastric acid, pepsin, bile acids, and ingested substances) and those that protect the mucosa (such as an intact epithelium, mucus, and bicarbonate secretion) is upset, inflammation or **ulcers** may arise. In the case of **gastric ulcers** a variety of irritants can initially disrupt the gastric mucosa. In some patients, decreased pyloric sphincter pressure may permit an increased reflux of duodenal material into the stomach, which disrupts the gastric mucosal barrier and leads to an increased back-diffusion of acid into the mucosa. Subsequent histamine release may cause mucosal damage and edema. Continued erosion may damage mucosal capillaries and submucosal blood vessels, thus leading to hemorrhage and shock. If erosion continues through the serosa, perforation and peritonitis may result.

Risk factors for gastric ulcer disease include the following:

- Family history of gastric ulcers
- Chronic use of salicylates or nonsteroidal antiinflammatory drugs (NSAIDs), such as indomethacin (Indocin) or ibuprofen (Motrin)
- Bile reflux with pyloric sphincter incompetence
- Delayed or abnormal gastric emptying
- *Helicobacter* infection
- Cigarette smoking

The roles that stress and personality type play in the development of gastric ulcers remain controversial.

Symptoms of gastric ulcers may include epigastric pain, which is often temporarily relieved by food. Some patients experience nausea and/or vomiting and weight loss. Others may gain weight because the pain is relieved by food so they eat more. Most patients with uncomplicated gastric ulcers will have epigastric tenderness, but no other remarkable symptoms. Patients who experience these symptoms without an ulcer are said to have Moynihan's syndrome, which may be caused by duodenitis, gastritis, spasm, or rarely, no detectable lesion.

To diagnose peptic ulcer disease, the physician may order an upper GI series, upper GI endoscopy, gastric acid secretion test, and/or a serum gastrin level. Upper endoscopy is the diagnostic procedure of choice for patients with active bleeding. Unlike duodenal ulcers, gastric ulcers may be malignant; cytologic brushings and multiple tissue biopsies are mandatory to exclude the possibility of malignancy.

If bleeding ceases spontaneously, air-contrast upper GI studies may show the ulcer crater. Gastric ulcers are most often seen on the lesser curvature of the stomach, but they are also found in the antrum and occasionally on the greater curvature. Prepyloric ulcers are invariably benign and are best diagnosed endoscopically. Ulcers along the greater curvature are more often malignant and must be screened for the presence of carcinoma. Complications of gastric ulcers may include hemorrhage, perforation, penetration, and/or obstruction.

Upper GI bleeding is experienced by approximately 12% of patients with gastric ulcers. Hemorrhage that results from diffuse mucosal inflammation or ulceration may cause the patient to vomit red blood or material resembling coffee grounds. Less active bleeding may result in melenic stools. In some cases, life-threatening hemorrhage is the first indication of an active ulcer.

Perforation is an extension of the ulceration through the serosa and into the peritoneal cavity. It occurs most often along the lesser curvature of the stomach. Patients who have a perforation frequently experience upper abdominal pain, guarding, rebound tenderness, or absent bowel sounds. Most patients need surgery to close the perforation.

Penetration is an extension of the ulceration through the serosa and into an adjacent structure, most frequently the pancreas. Secondary sites are the biliary tract, the gastrohepatic omentum, and the liver. Symptoms include back pain, night distress, shift or spread of epigastric pain, and refractoriness to agents that previously provided relief. Most patients need surgical correction of the penetration.

Inflammatory edema, chronic scarring or fibrosis, and/or spasm may cause an obstruction in the pylorus or proximal duodenum, or rarely, in the body of the stomach. Symptoms of obstruction include abdominal distention, tympany, or a succussion splash, which is a splashing sound heard on abdominal palpation. The patient may vomit after meals or report a feeling of fullness. Vague abdominal pain and early satiety may be symptoms of a partial obstruction. Diagnosis is by testing for gastric emptying or performing radiographic exams or endoscopy. Obstructions are treated by decompressing the stomach by using nasogastric aspiration, restoring fluid and electrolyte balance, and giving intravenous H2 blockers. Surgery is indicated for patients with repeated episodes of complications and/or failure of other types of therapy.

Depending on the patient's needs, treatment for gastric ulcers may include dietary therapy, drug therapy, or surgery. With regard to diet, patients should be counseled to avoid foods that are known to cause gastric discomfort or increase acid secretion, such as alcoholic beverages, colas, tea, or caffeinated or decaffeinated coffee. Patients on bland diets, however, do not seem to heal any more quickly than those on a more liberal diet. Experts no longer consider milk and milk products appropriate for ulcer treatment. In fact, milk can lead to marked increases in gastric acid secretion.

Drug therapy for ulcer patients centers on the following agents:

- Histamine-2 (H2) blockers, such as cimetidine (Tagamet), famotidine (Pepcid), or ranitidine (Zantac), all of which reduce the amount of acid produced by the stomach by binding to the histamine receptor on parietal cells and blocking histamine-stimulated acid production.
- Sucralfate (Carafate), which is a complex of aluminum hydroxide and sulfated sucrose that forms a protective gel at the site of disrupted mucosa, thus providing a protective covering for the ulcer.
- Antacids, which act to neutralize gastric acid, strengthen the gastric mucosal barrier, and heighten the tone of the LES. Optimally, antacids should be taken 1 and 3 hours after meals and before sleep. Most antacids contain either magnesium hydroxide (Milk of Magnesia), aluminum hydroxide (Gaviscon), or calcium carbonate (Tums). They are not recommended for maintenance treatment of gastric ulcer disease.
- Prostaglandins (Cytotec) and omeprazole (Prilosec), which are new agents, are now available for treatment of peptic ulcers. Prostaglandins have antisecretory and cytoprotective effects, whereas omeprazole acts as a hydrogen pump inhibitor. It blocks all three direct acid secretagogues (gastrin, histamine, and acetylcholine), thus promoting rapid healing of ulcers.
- Investigational drugs include both tricyclic compounds, which block acid production by interfering with acetylcholine-stimulated acid secretion, and colloidal bismuth compounds, which act by coating the ulcer crater.

Surgery may be indicated for refractory ulcers that fail to heal despite prolonged treatment and changes in medication. Emergency gastric surgery may be needed for uncontrolled hemorrhage. Surgery for benign peptic ulcer disease usually involves an acid-reducing procedure combined with a drainage procedure. The surgical procedure depends on the nature and extent of the patient's problem. Alternatives include truncal or partial vagotomy with pyloroplasty, Billroth I (gastroduodenostomy and hemigastrectomy), Billroth II (gastrojejunostomy), total gastrectomy (esophagojejunostomy), or gastric resection (antrectomy).

Complications of gastric surgery may include dumping syndrome, hypoglycemic symptoms, nutrient deficiency states, weight loss, diarrhea, and recurrent ulceration. In addition, the risk of gastric carcinoma may be increased after certain types of surgery for peptic ulcer disease.

### Gastric cancer

Gastric cancer tends to be hereditary and occurs more frequently in individuals with type A blood and lower socioeconomic status. Its incidence is higher in blacks than in whites, in the northern United States than the southern United States, and in men as compared to women. The incidence of gastric cancer increases with age, and among those who eat foods high in starch, nitrates, pickled vegetables, and salted fish and meat. Gastric ulcers, previous gastric surgery, achlorhydria, pernicious anemia, gastric atrophy, intestinal metaplasia, and **adenomatous polyps** may also increase the risk of gastric cancer.

Ninety-seven percent of gastric cancers are adenocarcinomas; the remaining three percent are lymphomas, leiomyosarcomas, carcinoid tumors, or sarcomas.

Most gastric carcinomas develop in the antrum or along the lesser curvature, although cancer stemming from gastric atrophy tends to affect the upper portion of the stomach. Metastatic disease usually spreads to the liver and lungs, but may spread to any organ. Benign lesions on the greater curvature are rare; therefore, all lesions in this area should be considered malignant until proven otherwise.

Signs and symptoms of gastric cancer include weight loss, epigastric discomfort, vomiting, and occult blood. Gross hematemesis is rare. Depending on the location of the lesion, patients may also present with the following symptoms:
- Dysphagia to solid foods
- Unexplained weight loss, early satiety, or anorexia
- Anemia
- Abdominal mass
- Gastric outlet obstruction
- Epigastric mass
- Ascites
- Enlarged liver nodes in the supraclavicular areas

Palpation of a mass in the rectum's pelvic cul-de-sac (Blumer's shelf) confirms cancer and tumor spread. Cancer may also infiltrate the umbilicus.

Gastric cancer may be revealed in plain stomach x-ray or chest x-ray films, upper GI series, CT scan, or endoscopy with biopsy specimen and cytologic examination. Patients may also have a low hematocrit, occult blood, or **hypoalbuminemia.** An air-contrast upper GI series is about 90% sensitive, but a gastroscopy with multiple tissue biopsies and cytologic exam is needed to make a definitive diagnosis. An abdominal CT scan may be ordered to determine the spread of the tumor.

The 5-year survival rate for patients with early gastric cancer that is limited to the mucosa or submucosa is 95%. This survival rate is most common in Japan, where mass screening programs make early detection more likely.

Another variation is superficial-spreading cancer, where the cancer spreads laterally within the mucosa and submucosa without deep invasion. The 5-year survival rate for patients who have these tumors is also 95%.

Surgery is the treatment of choice for curable lesions. Patients without metastatic disease who undergo partial gastrectomy with local lymphadenectomy have a 50% or greater 5-year survival rate if lymph nodes test negative. Unfortunately, in the United States, gastric cancer is frequently diagnosed at an advanced stage and therefore prognosis is poor. Most patients survive less than 5 years.

The worst prognosis is for patients with linitis plastica or "leather bottle stomach," which is a submucosal tumor that spreads diffusely and is associated with the formation and development of fibrous tissue. In this condition, the stomach becomes narrowed and nondistensible.

Treatment for advanced gastric cancer is largely palliative. It involves tumor resection to relieve obstruction or dysphagia or to control chronic bleeding, or gastrojejunostomy to provide temporary relief or to prevent obstruction. Following surgery, combination chemotherapy may be used alone or with local radiation therapy. Complications of metastasis, such as perforation and obstruction, should be managed as they develop. Primary nursing responsibilities are to meet the patient's emotional needs, to provide adequate nutrition, and to help with pain management.

### Polyps

Gastric **polyps** are defined as any circumscribed, discrete stomach tumor and are relatively uncommon. Single polyps appear more often than multiple polyps and frequently arise in the antrum and along the lesser curvature. Polyps most often develop after the age of 55; they are seldom found in young people. Types of gastric polyps include the following:
- Hyperplastic (regenerative) polyps, which consist of normal gastric epithelium, are the most common type of gastric polyp and are always benign
- Adenomas
- Leiomyomas, or smooth muscle tumors
- Adenomyomas (hamartomas), which are abnormal admixtures of tissue indigenous to the organ

Generally speaking, polyps that are more than 2 cm in diameter are more likely to be malignant.

Gastric polyps are more common in patients with **achlorhydria,** atrophic gastritis, pernicious anemia, and gastric cancer, or in patients who have undergone gastric resection.

Gastric polyps are usually detected by an upper GI series or endoscopy with a tissue biopsy and a cytology. Unless a polyp bleeds, it usually causes no symptoms. Endoscopic polypectomy or partial gastrectomy may be used to remove polyps.

### Gastritis

**Gastritis** is an inflammation of the gastric mucosa. It is caused by an irritant material, such as gastric acid, bile reflux, medications, or toxins, and is often combined with an impairment of natural protective mechanisms.

Gastritis may be classified according to the inflammatory pattern as acute (erosive, hemorrhagic gastritis) or chronic (nonerosive gastritis). There are also specific forms of gastritis, including Menetrier's disease, eosinophilic gastritis, and certain infections, but they are less common (e.g., *Helicobacter*).

In acute gastritis, erosive mucosal damage occurs. Acute gastritis may be associated with serious illness, alcoholism, localized gastric trauma, and gastrectomy.

Chronic gastritis (also known as nonerosive, nonspecific gastritis or NNG) is common in adults, and may be associated with normal aging, gastric ulcers, pernicious anemia, gastric cancer, or *Helicobacter*. The types of NNG are superficial gastritis, atrophic gastritis, or gastric atrophy.

- In superficial gastritis, pathologic changes are limited to the upper one third of the mucosa.
- Atrophic gastritis involves the full thickness of the mucosa, producing atrophy of gastric glands with loss of chief and parietal cells.
- In gastric atrophy, there is marked or total gland loss but little inflammation and the mucosa is thinned.

Severe atrophic gastritis and gastric atrophy may be seen endoscopically as a thinned mucosa with prominent submucosal vessels.

NNG is a histologic, rather than clinical, diagnosis. It has never been proved to be a cause of pain or other symptoms. It is possible that no specific treatment is necessary, except for vitamin B12 in cases of **pernicious anemia.**

In both acute and chronic gastritis, patients may have a gradual blood loss that goes unnoticed for years. Patients may test positive for occult blood, may have flecks of blood in vomitus, or may exhibit chronic anemia.

In patients with acute gastrointestinal bleeding the most effective tool for diagnosing gastritis is an upper endoscopy. Serum gastrin and a gastric analysis may also be ordered to determine the cause of gastritis.

Treatment for gastritis without bleeding depends on the patient's signs and symptoms. Pharmacologic treatment may involve the use of antacids, sucralfate (Carafate), H2 blockers, or prostaglandins. Most patients who bleed from diffuse gastritis cease bleeding spontaneously. Contributing pathogenetic factors must be eliminated, including medications, sepsis, and/or diabetic ketoacidosis.

### Stress ulcers

**Stress ulcers** are gastric mucosal stress erosions that are associated with serious illness. They seem to arise in four different situations, which are listed as follows:

- In patients who have sustained severe trauma, who have ongoing sepsis, or are being treated for serious illness
- In patients who have significant burn injuries **(Curling's ulcer)**
- In patients who sustain intracranial trauma, such as craniotomy or traumatic head injuries **(Cushing's ulcer)**
- In patients who chronically ingest drugs that have adverse effects on the gastric mucosa, such as NSAIDs or alcohol

Cushing's ulcers may be located in the esophagus, stomach, or duodenum. They tend to be deep and of full-thickness and therefore are more prone to perforation than gastric mucosal ulcerations induced by trauma or sepsis.

The most common symptom of a stress ulcer is massive upper GI bleeding. Bleeding usually occurs within 3 to 7 days, but occasionally as many as 21 days, after the initial injury. Stress ulcers rarely cause classic ulcer signs and symptoms before bleeding begins. Once hemorrhage is apparent, the mortality rate is about 50%. Treatment is focused on controlling bleeding, correcting shock, and treating the underlying disorder.

### Gastric varices

Portal hypertension, which is most often the result of alcoholic cirrhosis, may lead to the development of collateral circulation with formation of varices that carry blood away from the portal circulation. Esophageal varices are by far the most clinically significant type; however, two thirds of patients with esophageal varices also have gastric varices. Other less common sites of varices are the duodenum, ileum, and colon.

Upper GI bleeding from esophagogastric varices is potentially lethal. Approximately one third of the deaths in cirrhotic patients are caused by variceal hemorrhage. The chances of recurrent variceal bleeding are about 9 in 10. Reducing variceal pressure by pharmacologic or other means may decrease the risk of bleeding in early cirrhosis. A complete upper endoscopy is needed to diagnose variceal bleeding.

The objectives for managing gastric varices are listed as follows:

- To hemodynamically stabilize the patient
- To stop acute variceal bleeding by using vasopressin or a Sengstaken-Blakemore tube
- To prevent recurrent bleeding by using sclerotherapy, or if all else fails, surgical insertion of a shunt between the portal and systemic circulations

## Hiatus hernia

In normal subjects, the muscle structure at the diaphragmatic hiatus anchors the stomach under the diaphragm. A **hiatus hernia** occurs when part of the stomach protrudes through the diaphragm and into the thoracic cavity. Such hernias are extremely common in older people and more common in women than in men. Most are sliding hernias, in which a portion of the stomach slides up through the opening so the gastroesophageal junction lies above the level of the diaphragm. A sliding hiatus hernia is often associated with a weakening of the LES and esophageal reflux.

In the less common rolling hiatus hernia, the gastroesophageal junction is located below the level of the diaphragm, but a part of the greater curvature of the stomach herniates through the diaphragm and into the thoracic cavity. Patients may have a feeling of fullness and discomfort after meals, but reflux is not common. Strangulation and infarction are potential complications of a rolling hiatus hernia. Ulceration may occur with either type of hiatus hernia.

Diagnostic tests for hiatus hernia include a chest x-ray exam, barium swallow, and endoscopic examination. The condition is treated in much the same way as esophageal reflux.

Complications of hiatus hernias include reflux esophagitis, heartburn, acid regurgitation, water brash, and dysphagia.

## Congenital abnormalities

After inguinal hernia, the most common disorder requiring surgery in the first few months of life is **infantile hypertrophic pyloric stenosis,** which affects approximately 1 in 500 births. Boys are affected four to five times as often as girls and the disorder seems to occur in family clusters. Patients have a history of progressive nonbilious vomiting, which becomes projectile. They may become dehydrated, have electrolyte disturbances, and commonly are in metabolic alkalosis with hypokalemia. An upper GI series demonstrates an unchanging elongation and narrowing of the antrum and pylorus. The treatment of choice is pyloromyotomy.

Other congenital abnormalities of the stomach include the following:

- Gastric, antral, and pyloric atresias, in which the stomach ends blindly or is totally occluded by two apparent membranes connected by a strand each of mucosa and submucosa
- Pyloric or antral membranes, which may produce no obstructive symptoms until late in life
- Microgastria or hypoplasia, a rare condition with limited life expectancy, in which the stomach never becomes differentiated from the primitive foregut into a true fundus, body, and pylorus
- Gastric duplication, a rare condition in which a distinct mass lesion that contains all layers of the gastric wall develops in the stomach
- Neonatal perforations of the gastric wall, a rare condition associated with prematurity, peptic ulceration, and distal small intestinal obstruction

Most gastric diverticula are also congenital and are located high on the posterior wall of the stomach, below the gastroesophageal junction. Prepyloric diverticula, which are relatively rare, are usually associated with previous peptic ulceration. Occasionally, gastric diverticula may cause dyspepsia or symptoms of postprandial vomiting and nausea.

## Motor dysfunctions

A number of gastric motor abnormalities have been identified, ranging from conditions that are of little or no clinical importance to those that result in severe or chronic disability. Both excessively slow and excessively rapid gastric emptying can produce disabling symptoms. Symptomatic gastric motor abnormalities may be seen after vagotomy and pyloroplasty, or in patients with mechanical obstructions, acute metabolic disorders and inflammatory diseases, or long-standing diabetes mellitus. Serious gastric motor dysfunction may also be idiopathic, as in antral tachygastria, where an aberrant pacemaker in the antrum cycles three to four times faster than the usual pacemaker area in the gastric body.

Management of acute gastric retention is directed at the underlying cause, if known. Gastric muscle stimulants such as metoclopramide (Reglan) or bethanechol (Urecholine) may be of benefit.

Gastric surgery that alters gastroduodenal anatomy (e.g., gastroenterostomy, gastrojejunostomy, or Billroth II) may lead to rapid gastric emptying and a group of disabling symptoms known as **dumping syndrome.** Early symptoms appear 15 to 30 minutes after the start of a meal and include anxiety, weakness, dizziness, tachycardia with a pounding pulse, sweating, flushing, abdominal cramps, and diarrhea. Approximately 90 to 120 minutes after a meal, symptoms mimic **hypoglycemia;** weakness, sweating, tachycardia, and sometimes a decreased level of consciousness may be experienced.

Dumping syndrome may be related to rapid fluid shifts from plasma to intestinal lumen as a result of the rapid introduction of hyperosmolar solutions into the jejunum. This complication may be managed by providing liquids 1 hour before or after meals, but not during meals; giving six small, high-protein, high-fat, low-carbohydrate meals daily; and administering anticholinergic drugs to suppress gastrointestinal activity and antispasmodic drugs to slow the passage of food into the intestine.

### Infectious diseases

The number of cases of infectious gastritis has increased in recent years. Immunocompromised patients are particularly at risk, including those with AIDS or those who have undergone transplantation or chemotherapy for cancer.

The agents implicated in infectious gastritis may be bacterial, fungal, or viral. Bacterial inflammations are relatively rare, but may include phlegmonous and emphysematous gastritis, tuberculosis, *Helicobacter,* and syphilis. Fungal infections, such as *Candida albicans* or *Torulopsis glabrata,* may be found in gastric ulcer or erosion beds in immunocompromised hosts. Gastric cytomegalovirus has been observed in transplant patients, in cytomegalovirus mononucleosis, in children, and in AIDS patients. Parasitic infestations that have been found in the stomach include cryptosporidiasis, anisakiasis, and strongyloides.

### Gastric outlet obstruction

Obstruction of the pyloric sphincter at the outlet of the stomach blocks the flow of gastric contents into the duodenum. Patients may vomit partially digested gastric contents and may complain of gastric pain or a feeling of fullness that is relieved only by vomiting. The pain is aggravated by eating, and as many as two thirds of patients with gastric outlet obstruction may become anorexic. Prolonged vomiting may lead to metabolic alkalosis and the patient may complain of abdominal tenderness; a succussion splash may be noted. Abdominal x-ray films, nasogastric tube placement, an upper GI series, barium burger test, nuclear scanning, endoscopic exam, or a saline load test may be ordered to confirm gastric retention and to rule out atony as the cause.

Treatment begins with restoration of fluid and electrolyte balance, decompression of the stomach, and correction of nutritional deficiencies. To eliminate the obstruction, the physician may use an endoscope to dilate the pylorus with a balloon. If surgery is indicated, the procedure used depends on the cause of the obstruction.

### Caustic injury

The ingestion of acid or alkaline chemicals may cause tissue injury on contact with the oropharynx, esophagus, stomach, or duodenum. The severity of the tissue injury after caustic ingestion depends on the nature, concentration, and quantity of the caustic agent ingested and the duration of tissue contact. Contact with strong alkaline agents causes liquefactive necrosis, which is the complete destruction of entire cells and their membranes. In contrast, contact with strong acids promotes coagulation necrosis and the formation of a firm, protective eschar, which limits the depth, penetration, and injury produced by the acid.

The oropharynx and esophagus are most frequently injured by ingestion of alkaline agents, but 20% to 30% of patients with esophageal injury also have some extent of gastric injury. In the case of acid ingestion, the caustic agent tends to pass rapidly through the esophagus, thus producing shallow burns. In the stomach, acids usually collect in the antrum, where the most severe damage occurs. The severity of tissue injury ranges from diffuse gastritis to hemorrhagic ulceration and necrosis, thus leading to perforation of the stomach. Gastric perforation, in turn, may lead to mediastinitis, peritonitis, and shock. Patients with severe gastric injury may present with epigastric pain, retching, or emesis of tissue, blood, or material resembling coffee grounds. There is no definitive evidence of an increased risk of gastric carcinoma in patients with a history of caustic ingestion.

Stricture formation is a common late complication of caustic ingestion, and is usually apparent by the eighth week following injury. Strictures in the stomach may cause gastric outlet obstruction, which leads to early satiety and postprandial vomiting and weight loss.

Management of caustic injuries includes determining the type of agent ingested, keeping the patient NPO, performing x-ray examinations to assess signs of aspiration pneumonia or perforation, and performing cautious endoscopy to establish the extent and severity of tissue damage. Emergency surgery may be necessary in the event of perforation, peritonitis, or severe hemorrhage. If strictures develop, they may be treated by dilatation. In the case of severe gastric burns, antral and pyloric stenosis may require partial or total gastrectomy.

### Bezoars

**Bezoars** are concretions of foreign material that build up in the stomach. They are usually composed of either vegetable and plant material (phytobezoars) or hair that has been chewed (trichobezoars).

Phytobezoars, which are more common, are composed of partially digested fibers, leaves, roots, and skins of almost any plant matter. Excessive ingestion of rinds from melons and oranges is a frequent cause of phytobezoars. They are most commonly seen in men over the age of 30 and may be associated with hypochlorhydria, diminished antral motility, and incomplete mastication. Recent reports describe a link between phytobezoars and partial gastrectomy, especially when accompanied by vagotomy.

Trichobezoars are hairballs composed of decaying foodstuff enmeshed in a large amount of hair. They are most commonly seen in females under the age of 30 and are caused by trichophagia (hair ingestion), which may represent a neuropsychiatric disturbance.

Patients with bezoars may present with dragging or fullness in the upper quadrants, epigastric pain, and periodic attacks of nausea and vomiting. A palpable mass is evident in 57% of phytobezoars and 88% of trichobezoars.

Gastroscopy is the best technique for diagnosing and classifying bezoars, although plain films of the abdomen or an upper GI series may show evidence of an abdominal mass.

Bezoars can result in anorexia and vomiting, ulceration and bleeding, perforation, or small bowel obstruction. Phytobezoars may be disrupted endoscopically or enzymatically by using papain, acetylcysteine, or cellulase. If these methods fail, a gastrotomy may be necessary. The surgical mortality is minimal; however, the mortality of untreated bezoars is significant, although much less than the oft-quoted 60%. To prevent postgastrectomy phytobezoars, it may be helpful to improve dentition and to counsel the patient to avoid pulpy, fibrous fruits (especially oranges) and vegetables. Trichobezoars must be treated surgically, because there is no way to dissolve the matted hair in vivo.

Lactobezoars, also known as milk curd bezoars, have been reported in infants as a result of ingesting a powdered formula diluted with an inadequate amount of water. Continuous-drip feeding of preterm infants seems to be the most important predisposing factor. Symptoms may be resolved by withholding feedings for 48 hours, implementing gastric lavage with saline solution, and using proper hydration.

---

**CASE SITUATION**

Mr. Williams, age 74, passed out during his daily walk and the paramedics brought him to the emergency room (ER). His doctor is perplexed because 2 months previously Mr. Williams passed his annual physical with flying colors. His only complaint had been right arm and shoulder pain, which he attributed to the exertion of building a fence, and for which his physician prescribed an NSAID. Mr. Williams stopped smoking 10 years ago and drinks alcohol only at occasional social functions. He does drink two to three cups of coffee daily.

In the ER, Mr. Williams' chest x-ray films and ECG are normal. His CBC shows hemoglobin, 9 grams,

but he denies any abdominal pain. Mr. Williams reports having had occasional black-looking bowel movements for the last 6 weeks, but attributes them to something in his diet. A rectal exam in the ER confirms that there is blood in his stool.

*Points to think about*

1. Because Mr. Williams denies abdominal pain, is there any easy way to identify upper GI bleeding?
2. Mr. Williams is admitted. Before going to his room he is taken to the GI Endoscopy Unit for a gastroscopy. What has the nurse learned that will help in evaluating Mr. Williams?
3. Mr. Williams is found at endoscopy to have acute erosive hemorrhagic gastritis. What two nursing diagnoses might apply?
4. How might the defining characteristics of the two nursing diagnoses stated above be identified?
5. What are specific expected outcomes and associated nursing interventions for each of these nursing diagnoses?
6. What else can the gastroenterology nurse tell Mr. Williams about treatment and follow-up care?

*Suggested responses*

1. In the ER, aspiration of gastric contents through a nasogastric tube reveals coffee-ground appearing material that tests positive for occult blood. Blood in the nasogastric aspirate is good evidence of an upper source of gastrointestinal bleeding, but a negative test does not rule it out. Care must be taken to avoid trauma to the nares or to the esophageal or gastric mucosa because it might cause bleeding and obscure the diagnosis.
2. Some things the gastroenterology nurse has learned about Mr. Williams that will help with the evaluation are listed as follows:
   - Mr. Williams was taking an NSAID, which is known to be a gastric mucosal irritant and may cause gastritis or a gastric ulcer. Older patients are more likely to bleed from NSAID use and are more likely to suffer upper GI tract perforations.
   - Gastritis or gastric erosions may heal very quickly when offending mucosal irritants are discontinued, often within 48 hours, so early endoscopy is important.
   - Mr. Williams had noticed occasional black stools, which may indicate gradual blood loss, leading to anemia, which is even more indicative of gastritis.
   - Gastritis is an inflammation of the gastric mucosa caused by an irritant material, such as gastric acid, bile reflux, medications, or toxins, and is often combined with an impairment of natural protective mechanisms.

3. Two nursing diagnoses that might be applicable in Mr. Williams' case are:
   - Fluid volume deficit related to active blood loss
   - Altered tissue perfusion: gastrointestinal
4. The defining characteristics of these nursing diagnoses include the following:
   a. Fluid volume deficit related to active blood loss
      - Decreased urine output
      - Output greater than intake
      - Decreased venous filling
      - Increased serum sodium
      - Thirst
      - Increased pulse rate
      - Decreased pulse amplitude
      - Increased body temperature
      - Dry mucous membranes
      - Concentrated urine
      - Sudden weight loss
      - Hemoconcentration
      - Hypotension
      - Narrowed pulse pressure
      - Decreased skin turgor
      - Change in mental status
      - Dry skin
      - Weakness
   b. Altered tissue perfusion: gastrointestinal
      - Nausea and/or vomiting
      - Lack of bowel sounds
      - Abdominal pain that increases after meals
      - Constipation
      - Diarrhea
      - Abdominal distention

(Note: Critical defining characteristics have not yet been defined for these two diagnoses.)

5. Some, but not necessarily all, expected outcomes and nursing interventions for the two nursing diagnoses might be as follows:
   a. Fluid volume deficit related to active blood loss

| Expected outcomes | Nursing interventions |
| --- | --- |
| There will be an adequate fluid volume | Monitor and record vital signs and central venous pressure (CVP) |
| | Weigh daily |
| | Monitor intake and output |
| | Assess for signs and symptoms of dehydration |
| | Administer drugs and IV/oral fluids as ordered |
| Laboratory values will be within normal limits | Monitor laboratory values pertinent to fluid volume deficit and hemoconcentration |

b. Altered tissue perfusion: gastrointestinal

| Expected outcomes | Nursing interventions |
| --- | --- |
| There will be adequate tissue perfusion and cellular oxygenation of the GI system | Assess blood pressure |
| | Record any nausea/vomiting |
| | Monitor bowel sounds (four quadrants) and record |
| | Maintain gastric decompression |
| | Maintain and record intake and output |
| There will be control of metabolic needs of the GI system | Encourage rest periods after meals |
| | Provide small, easily digestible meals |
| | Use elemental product for tube feedings |
| | Assess medications for damaging effects on gastrointestinal function |
| | Administer IV fluids |
| | Check secretions and excretions for blood |

6. Because Mr. Williams' gastric mucosa is sensitive to injury, he should discontinue use of NSAIDs and aspirin-containing products. Caffeine and alcohol are also recognized as gastric irritants and should be discontinued, at least during treatment. Depending on what medication is prescribed, the gastroenterology nurse should inform Mr. Williams of the following:
   - Antacids are usually taken between meals and at bedtime to neutralize gastric acid. It is sometimes difficult to adhere to this regimen; if so, the patient should ask the physician for an alternative treatment. Liquid antacids should be shaken well and should be taken with a little water to ensure passage to the stomach. Some antacids can cause diarrhea or constipation and may need to be alternated. In older patients it is best to use low-sodium antacids.
   - H2 blockers inhibit the action of histamine at receptor sites in gastric parietal cells, which inhibits the production of gastric acid, thus decreasing further mucosal injury by acid contact. Tablets should be taken with meals or at bedtime if the patient is on once-daily therapy. Some H2 blockers interact with other medications, so it is important to know all medications the patient is taking and to choose an H2 blocker accordingly.
   - Sucralfate (Carafate) is an oral medication that adheres to the gastric mucosa to form a protective barrier against further damage, particularly where cell protein is exposed because irritants have

eroded the protective mucosa. The medication should be taken on an empty stomach for best results, one hour before meals and at bedtime. Since sucralfate is not readily absorbed systemically, there are few side effects. Occasionally, patients experience constipation.

- Misoprostol (Cytotec) is a synthetic prostaglandin E, which replaces prostaglandins that are depleted by NSAIDs, and may be given concomitantly with NSAIDs to help prevent gastric mucosal damage. (This drug is strictly contraindicated in pregnant women because it can cause abortion.)

In addition, the gastroenterology nurse should teach Mr. Williams how to use slides to test for occult blood in his stool at home. He should be told to report any further signs of bleeding and/or epigastric pain to his physician. The nurse should provide a list of foods high in iron to help raise hemoglobin levels to normal.

## REVIEW TERMS

achlorhydria, adenomatous polyp, antrum, bezoars, body, cardia, cardiac glands, chief cells, chyme, Curling's ulcer, Cushing's ulcer, dumping syndrome, enterochromaffin cells, fundus, G-cells, gastric ulcers, gastritis, greater curvature, greater omentum, Helicobacter, hiatus hernia, hypoalbuminemia, hypoglycemia, infantile hypertrophic pyloric stenosis, lesser curvature, lesser omentum, oxyntic gland, parietal cells, pernicious anemia, polyps, pyloric glands, pyloric sphincter, pylorus, rugae, stress ulcer, ulcers

## REVIEW QUESTIONS

1. Entry of food into the stomach is controlled by the:
   a. Lower esophageal sphincter.
   b. Fundus.
   c. Pyloric sphincter.
   d. Antrum.
2. The stomach wall has four layers, the mucosa, submucosa, the muscularis, and the:
   a. Rugae.
   b. Cardia.
   c. Serosa.
   d. Connective tissue.
3. The parietal cells secrete:
   a. Mucus.
   b. Hydrochloric acid and intrinsic factor.
   c. Pepsinogens.
   d. Gastrin.
4. Intrinsic factor is necessary for the:
   a. Conversion of pepsinogens to pepsin.
   b. Secretion of mucus.
   c. Absorption of vitamin B12.
   d. Secretion of hormones.
5. The gastric emptying rate is controlled by neural impulses, hormones secreted by the small intestine, and:
   a. The amount of food ingested.
   b. The composition of the chyme.
   c. The amount of gastric secretions.
   d. Vitamin B12 absorption.
6. Gastric ulcers are most often treated by:
   a. Drug therapy.
   b. A bland diet.
   c. Surgery.
   d. Drinking milk before meals.
7. Most gastric cancers are of which of the following types:
   a. Adenocarcinomas.
   b. Leiomyosarcomas.
   c. Sarcomas.
   d. Lymphomas.
8. Cushing's ulcers are a form of:
   a. Specific gastritis.
   b. Nonerosive, nonspecific gastritis.
   c. Peptic ulcers.
   d. Stress ulcers.
9. Gastric surgery may lead to rapid gastric emptying and a group of disabling symptoms that mimic hypoglycemia. This syndrome is called:
   a. Moynihan's syndrome.
   b. Paterson-Kelly syndrome.
   c. Dumping syndrome.
   d. Cushing's syndrome.
10. The best technique for diagnosing bezoars is:
    a. Plain X-rays.
    b. Palpation.
    c. Gastroscopy.
    d. Upper GI series.

## BIBLIOGRAPHY

Beare, P, and Meyers, J. "Nursing Management of Adults with Disorders of the Stomach and Duodenum." In *Principles and Practice of Adult Health Nursing,* 1561-82. St. Louis: Mosby–Year Book, 1990.

Bongiovanni, G, ed. *Essentials of Clinical Gastroenterology.* 2nd ed. New York: McGraw-Hill, 1988.

Chopra, S, and May, R, eds. *Pathophysiology of Gastrointestinal Diseases.* Boston: Little, Brown & Co, 1989.

Eastwood, G, and Avunduk, C. *Manual of Gastroenterology: Diagnosis and Therapy.* Boston: Little, Brown & Co, 1988.

Given, B, and Simmons, S. *Gastroenterology in Clinical Nursing.* 4th ed. St. Louis: Mosby–Year Book, 1984.

Goldberg, K, ed. *Gastrointestinal Problems.* Nurse Review Series. Springhouse, Pa.: Springhouse Corporation, 1986.

Lencki, B. "Certification Review: The Stomach—Anatomy and Physiology." In *SGA Journal Reprints,* ed. Trivits, S, 61-63. Rochester, N.Y.: Society of Gastrointestinal Assistants, 1988.

McFarland, G, and McFarlane, E. "Activity-Exercise Pattern— Altered Tissue Perfusion (Gastrointestinal)." In *Nursing Diagnoses and Intervention: Planning for Patient Care,* 444-73. St. Louis: Mosby–Year Book, 1989.

McFarland, G, and McFarlane, E. "Nutritional and Metabolic Pattern—Fluid Volume Deficit (2)." In *Nursing Diagnoses and Intervention: Planning for Patient Care,* 186-91. St. Louis: Mosby-–Year Book, 1989.

Misiewicz, J, Bartram, C, Cotton, P, Mee, A, Price, A, and Thompson, R. *Atlas of Clinical Gastroenterology,* Vol 1. London: Gower Medical Publishing, 1985.

Sachar, D, Waye, J, and Lewis, B, eds. *Gastroenterology for the House Officer.* Baltimore: Williams & Wilkins, 1989.

Silverman, A, and Roy, C. *Pediatric Clinical Gastroenterology.* 3rd ed. St. Louis: Mosby–Year Book, 1983.

Sleisenger, M, and Fordtran, J, eds. *Gastrointestinal Disease: Pathophysiology, Diagnosis, Management.* 4th ed. Philadelphia: W.B. Saunders, 1989.

# Chapter 16

# SMALL INTESTINE

This chapter will acquaint the gastroenterology nurse with the normal anatomy and physiology of the small bowel (small intestine). In addition, a number of pathologic conditions of the small bowel are described in terms of their pathophysiology, diagnosis, and treatment alternatives.

**Learning objectives**

Upon completing study of the content of this chapter, the gastroenterology nurse should be able to:
1. Describe the normal macroanatomy and microanatomy of the small bowel.
2. Discuss the physiology of intestinal absorption, secretion, and motility.
3. Explain the pathophysiology, diagnosis, and treatment of a number of important disorders of the small bowel.

## ANATOMY AND PHYSIOLOGY

The **small bowel** (small intestine) is a tubular structure with two concentric layers of smooth muscle that extends from the pyloric sphincter to the cecum (see Plate 1). It is approximately 6.7 to 7.0 m (22 to 23 feet) in length, with a diameter of about 1.9 to 3.8 cm (¾ to 1½ inches). The first 30 cm (12 inches) of the small intestine is the C-shaped, muscular **duodenum,** which begins at the pyloric sphincter and ends at the **ligament of Treitz.** The common bile duct empties into the duodenum at the **ampulla of Vater** (Fig. 16-1). After the duodenum, the proximal two fifths of the small bowel is known as the **jejunum.** The distal three fifths of the small bowel, known as the **ileum,** extends from the jejunum to the **ileocecal valve.** This valve controls the flow of chyme into the large intestine and prevents reflux into the ileum.

The small intestinal wall consists of the following layers:
- An outer serous layer (serosa) composed of peritoneum and connective tissue

- A muscular layer (muscularis) containing outer longitudinal and inner circular muscles, separated by a nerve network called the myenteric plexus
- A submucous layer (submucosa) of areolar connective tissue containing blood vessels, lymphatics, and a submucosal nerve plexus
- An inner mucous layer (mucosa) containing simple columnar epithelium, a layer of connective tissue known as the **lamina propria,** and a thin sheet of smooth muscle, which separates the mucosa from the submucosa.

The mucosa and submucosa are arranged in circular folds called the plicae circulares, which provide a greater surface area for secretion and absorption during the 3 to

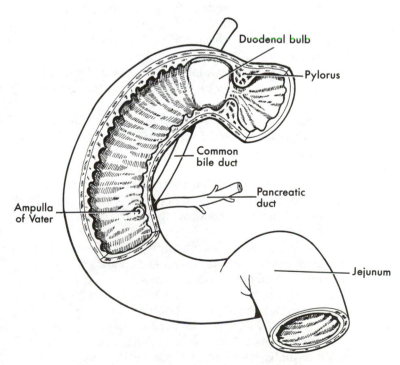

**Fig. 16-1.** Duodenal anatomy.

133

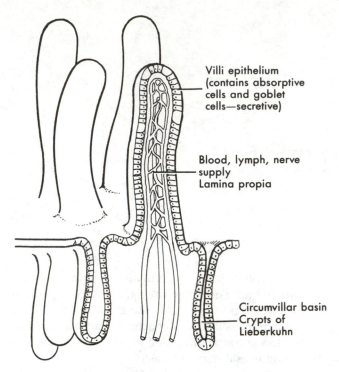

Villi epithelium
(contains absorptive
cells and goblet
cells—secretive)

Blood, lymph, nerve
supply
Lamina propia

Circumvillar basin
Crypts of
Lieberkuhn

**Fig. 16-2.** Small bowel villi anatomy.

6 hours the chyme remains in the small intestine.

In addition, the mucosa forms an estimated 4 to 5 million small, fingerlike villi, which project into the intestinal lumen (Fig. 16-2). Each **villus** is lined with simple columnar epithelial cells. Below the epithelium, the lamina propria contains nerve fibers, smooth muscle, lymphatic vessels or lacteals, blood vessels, and connective tissue. A brush border consisting of multiple **microvilli** covers the surface of each columnar cell.

The presence of the mucosal folds, the villi, and the microvilli increases the total surface area and therefore the absorptive capacity of the small bowel by approximately 600-fold.

Between the villi are small, tubular glands known as the **crypts of Lieberkühn.** The entire intestinal epithelial surface is replaced every 32 hours. Extremely mitotic undifferentiated cells that lie deep in the crypts serve to replace the epithelium. **Paneth's cells** are also located at the base of the crypts. The function of Paneth's cells is uncertain but it is possible that they regulate the intestinal flora.

In the proximal duodenum, the normal villous pattern is interrupted at intervals by **Brunner's glands,** which are elaborately branched acinar glands that contain both mucous cells and serous secretory cells. Brunner's glands empty into the crypts of Lieberkühn.

Lymphoid tissue makes up approximately 25% of the intestinal mucosa. The gastrointestinal-associated lymphoid tissue is made up of three distinct populations, which are listed as follows:

- **Peyer's patches** are circular, aggregated lymph nodes that lie in the mucosa and submucosa of the ileum. They participate in antibody synthesis and in the body's immune response.
- Lymphocytes and plasma cells are located in the lamina propria. Approximately 70% to 80% of these cells produce immunoglobin A (IgA), which is the major immunoglobulin in intestinal secretions. This secretory IgA plays an important role in the resistance of the mucous membranes to pathologic microorganisms and dietary antigens.
- A third population of lymphocytes, known as the intraepithelial lymphocytes, lies between the intestinal epithelial cells. A large proportion of these intraepithelial lymphocytes are T-cells.

The duodenum receives arterial blood from the hepatic artery, whereas the rest of the small bowel derives its blood supply from the superior mesenteric artery. Blood from the entire small bowel drains through the superior mesenteric vein.

The wall of the digestive tract is innervated by the **enteric plexus,** which is an autonomic nerve plexus made up of the submucosal plexus (**Meissner's plexus),** myenteric plexus (**Auerbach's plexus),** and the subserosal plexus. Parasympathetic stimulation by way of the vagus nerve increases the tone of the small bowel and the frequency, strength, and velocity of smooth muscle contractions. Vagal stimulation also enhances motor and secretory activities. Sympathetic stimulation via spinal nerves from levels T6 to T12 reduces peristalsis and inhibits gastrointestinal activity. The intrinsic nerve supply, which initiates motor function, passes through Auerbach's and Meissner's plexuses.

### Absorption

The primary function of the small intestine is to absorb nutrients from the chyme. The small intestine receives up to 8 L of fluid per day and passes only 500 to 1000 ml to the large intestine. The rest is absorbed by the columnar cells of the villous epithelium.

Absorption of different nutrients takes place at different locations in the small intestine. The duodenum is the primary site of iron and calcium absorption, and the jejunum is the site of absorption of fats, proteins, and carbohydrates. The ileum absorbs vitamin B12 and bile acids.

There are five basic mechanisms for absorption in the small intestine: hydrolysis, nonionic movement, passive diffusion, facilitated diffusion, and active transport. Water, for instance, diffuses passively across the wall of the small intestine, with only a small portion left unabsorbed.

Sodium is absorbed in the jejunum through active transport. Magnesium, phosphate, and potassium are absorbed throughout the small intestine. Chloride diffuses with sodium in the jejunum; in the ileum, it is actively transported. Dietary iron is absorbed predominantly by the duodenum and proximal jejunum.

Calcium absorption occurs by each of the following mechanisms: a transcellular route that takes place largely in the duodenum and proximal jejunum, and a concentration-dependent process that occurs along the length of the small bowel.

Absorption of most water-soluble vitamins takes place by diffusion. The exception is vitamin B12, which combines with intrinsic factor for active transport and is absorbed in the ileum.

Carbohydrates are hydrolyzed by intestinal enzymes into simple sugars (glucose, fructose, and galactose), which are then absorbed into the bloodstream via the intestinal mucosa, using either active transport or facilitated diffusion. Proteins are hydrolyzed into amino acids, which are absorbed by active transport.

Fats are emulsified and then broken down primarily by the enzyme pancreatic lipase into glycerides, fatty acids, and glycerol. Fatty acids and monoglycerides are made water-soluble by the formation of micelles with bile acids. Fat-soluble vitamins also combine briefly with bile salts to form water-soluble micelles.

### Secretion

In addition to their absorptive function, cells located in the small bowel secrete digestive juices, mucus, and a variety of hormones. The small bowel also receives secretions from the liver and pancreas.

The microvilli contain the peptidases and disaccharidases that are required for digestion of proteins and carbohydrates.

Brunner's glands, which are located in the proximal duodenum, secrete a clear, alkaline (pH 8.2 to 9.3), viscous fluid that protects the duodenal mucosa from gastric acid secretions. **Goblet cells** located on and between the villi on the mucosa secrete a protective mucus.

The crypts of Lieberkühn secrete 2 to 3 L of succus entericus per day. This watery fluid supplies a carrier substance for absorption of nutrients when the villi come in contact with the chyme.

There are ten different types of endocrine cells located in the crypts that produce a number of peptides and hormones, including secretin, cholecystokinin, gastrin, somatostatin, enteroglucagon, motilin, neurotensin, gastrin inhibitory peptide, vasoactive intestinal peptide, and serotonin.

### Motility

Within the small bowel, three types of movement contribute to the mixing of the chyme. They are listed as follows:

- Concentric, segmenting contractions, which normally take place in the jejunum, give the small intestine the look of a chain of sausage links. The concentric movement helps to mix secretions of the small intestine with the chyme particles.
- Short, propulsive contractions or peristaltic waves slowly push the chyme in the direction of the colon. Peristaltic contractions are found predominantly in the first portions of the duodenum and jejunum.
- The continuous shortening and lengthening of the villi constantly stirs the intestinal contents.

As the chyme nears the large intestine, contractions in the ileum increase. After a meal the ileocecal sphincter relaxes, allowing the chyme to move from the ileum into the cecum.

### PATHOPHYSIOLOGY

Important pathologic conditions of the small bowel include duodenal ulcer disease, parasitic infestations, bacterial and viral infections, Crohn's disease, Meckel's diverticulum, vitamin B12 deficiency, and small bowel tumors. A variety of malabsorption syndromes also affect the small bowel, such as celiac sprue, tropical sprue, Whipple's disease, short bowel syndrome, and lactose intolerance.

#### Duodenal ulcers

**Peptic ulcers** can develop in the lower esophagus, stomach, pylorus, duodenum, or jejunum. About 80% of all peptic ulcers are duodenal ulcers. They occur when the protective mucosa of the duodenum cannot resist corrosion by above-normal hydrochloric acid levels.

Duodenal ulcers are most common in men who are between the ages of 20 and 50 and in persons with Type O blood. The sequence of events is the same as that observed with gastric ulcers; that is, erosion of the abdominal wall and histamine release, followed by further stimulation of acid secretion and mucosal edema; damage to mucosal capillaries and submucosal blood vessels, leading to hemorrhage and shock; and erosion through the serosa, causing possible perforation and peritonitis.

Symptoms of duodenal ulcers include gnawing or burning epigastric pain occurring 1 to 3 hours after meals, heartburn, and intermittent nighttime pain or discomfort, which is localized in the epigastrium. Pain is exacerbated by fatty foods but may be relieved by other foods. Attacks usually occur about 2 hours after meals, when the stomach is empty, or after consumption of orange juice, coffee, aspirin, or alcohol. Many patients report symptoms that are at odds with those expected from the classic presentation.

Diagnosis is by upper GI radiographic exam and/or upper GI endoscopy. The sensitivity of individual radiologists in detecting ulcers varies between 44% and 80%, with a double-contrast technique being somewhat more sensitive than a single-contrast technique. Endoscopy may be more sensitive than radiography, with experienced endoscopists detecting 85% to 95% of gastroduodenal lesions. Duodenal ulcers frequently follow a chronic course, with remissions and exacerbations. Treatment is basically symptomatic and includes antacids to reduce gastric acidity; short-term treatment with H2 blockers, such as cimetidine (Tagamet) or ranitidine (Zantac) to reduce gastric secretion; and physical rest. If gastrointestinal bleeding occurs, intraarterial infusion of vasopressin (Pitressin) may be necessary.

A small percentage of patients with duodenal ulcer disease requires surgical intervention because of hemorrhage, obstruction, perforation, or intractability. There are four surgical procedures in use today. The choice of procedure depends on the needs of the individual patient, the indication for the operation, and the experience of the surgeon. Surgical procedures include the following:

- Subtotal gastric resection without vagotomy, which is seldom used now because of the high incidence of side effects
- Truncal vagotomy with a drainage procedure (pyloroplasty), which is preferred in very elderly or very ill patients with hemorrhage
- Truncal vagotomy and antrectomy (Billroth I or II), which is preferred in patients with recurrent hemorrhage because of the low incidence of rebleeding; also it may offer better long-term results in patients presenting with obstructions
- Highly selective vagotomy, which is preferred for patients with intractable ulcers because of its low mortality and morbidity and fewer postoperative side effects

Patients with perforations may undergo a simple closure or closure combined with one of the definitive operations described above.

### Bacterial and viral infections

Gastrointestinal tract infections are a major cause of morbidity and mortality throughout the world. The small bowel may become infected by any of the following types of agents:

- Enterotoxigenic bacteria produce enterotoxins that stimulate the active secretion of electrolytes into the lumen of the proximal small bowel. The watery, voluminous diarrhea caused by these bacteria is not usually accompanied by fever, and fecal leukocytes are seldom present. Examples are toxigenic *Escherichia coli, Vibrio cholerae, Bacillus cereus, Clostridium perfringens,* and *Staphylococcus aureus.*
- Invasive bacteria invade and damage the intestinal mucosa of the distal small bowel and colon, often producing scant, bloody, mucoid stools; fever; and fecal polymorphonuclear leukocytes. Examples are

*Salmonella* species, *Shigella* species, *E. coli, Vibrio parahaemolyticus, V. cholerae, Clostridium difficile,* and *S. aureus.*

- Penetrating bacteria invade the mucosa, usually in the distal small intestine, but do not produce extensive mucosal ulcerations. They often cause extraintestinal disease (such as sepsis), fever, and fecal leukocytes. *Yersinia enterocolitica* and *Salmonella typhi* are examples of penetrating bacteria.
- Viruses, such as rotavirus, Norwalk virus, and adenovirus, may also invade the small bowel mucosa, resulting in malabsorption and diarrhea.

Identification of the etiologic agent in gastrointestinal infections requires taking a careful history to obtain information on the symptom pattern, any recent exposure to infected individuals or contaminated food or water, or any recent history of foreign travel. Patients should be evaluated for fluid status and abdominal tenderness, and stools should be examined for the presence of fecal leukocytes.

In most cases, infectious diarrhea can be treated with rest and fluid replacement. Intravenous fluids may be needed for patients with severe dehydration. Antidiarrheal agents may be prescribed before a specific diagnosis is made, and once the etiologic agent is identified, specific antibiotics may be indicated. Table 16-1 lists some of the causes of infectious diarrhea and the antibiotics used in their treatment.

### Parasitic diseases

There are a number of parasitic diseases that affect the small intestine, including giardiasis, coccidiosis,

**Table 16-1.** Antibiotics used to treat infectious diarrhea

| Infectious agent | Antibiotic(s) used |
| --- | --- |
| *Staphylococcus aureus* | None; self-limited |
| toxigenic *Escherichia coli* | Trimethoprim-sulfamethoxazole (Septra) |
| *Vibrio cholerae* | Tetracycline (Achromycin) or chloramphenicol (Chloromycetin) |
| *Clostridium botulinum* | Polyvalent antitoxin, penicillin, and colonic lavage |
| *Clostridium perfringens* | None |
| *Vibrio parahaemolyticus* | Tetracycline |
| *Shigella* | For severe infection, ampicillin or trimethoprim-sulfamethoxazole |
| *Salmonella* | For debilitated patient, ampicillin, chloramphenicol, amoxicillin, or trimethoprim-sulfamethoxazole |
| *Clostridium difficile* | Metronidazole (Flagyl) or vancomycin (Vancocin) |

cryptosporidiosis, strongyloidiasis, ascariasis, and diphyllobothriasis.

**Giardiasis**

**Giardiasis** is caused by the protozoan *Giardia lamblia* and is most often associated with ingestion of contaminated food or water. Overall prevalence of giardiasis in the United States is 7% to 10%. Endemic areas include upstate New York and the Rocky Mountain region, especially Colorado.

The two forms of the parasite are cysts and trophozoites. After the cyst is ingested orally or nasally it matures, and once in the stomach, releases four trophozoites. These trophozoites adhere to the wall of the proximal small intestine, thus causing an inflammatory response.

Most adults with giardiasis are asymptomatic, although nonbloody diarrhea and even malabsorption may occur. Clinical symptoms exhibited by children range from none at all to acute illness characterized by abdominal discomfort and distention, nonbloody diarrhea, headaches, nausea, and vomiting. Diagnosis is by examination of multiple fresh stool specimens, or by duodenal aspiration and small intestinal biopsy examination.

If treatment is necessary, the drug of choice is metronidazole (Flagyl), which is administered in 3 divided doses for 1 week. Pediatric patients may be treated with furazolidone (Furoxone). Stools and/or duodenal aspirate should be rechecked 2 weeks after treatment, and a second course of treatment instituted if necessary. For patients who are resistant to metronidazole alone, a combined regimen of quinacrine (Atabrine) and metronidazole for 2 weeks may be effective.

**Coccidiosis**

Coccidiosis is caused by the intracytoplasmic protozoans *Isospora belli*, *Isospora hominis*, and *Isospora natelensis*. It is endemic throughout the world but is rarely seen in the United States. The parasite multiplies in the small bowel, thus causing mucosal damage. Clinical features include acute fulminant diarrhea, continuous or intermittent chronic diarrhea, and steatorrhea (fatty stools). Diagnosis is by stool examination, small intestinal biopsy examination, and blood tests for eosinophilia.

Most patients have a benign, self-limited course that lasts from a few days to 6 months. Adult patients with a mild case may be treated with fluid and electrolyte replacement only. In children, severe diarrhea and malabsorption may require temporary parenteral nutrition. For severe cases, the drug of choice is furazolidone (Furoxone).

**Cryptosporidiosis**

Cryptosporidiosis is caused by the coccidial sporozoa *Cryptosporidium*. The colon and small bowel are the most common sites of infection, but *Cryptosporidium* has been reported in all parts of the GI and respiratory tracts.

Transmission is fecal-oral; it may be transmitted between animals and humans, but is rarely transmitted from human to human. Water-borne transmission has also been reported. After the oocysts are ingested they embed in the surface of the bowel, where they complete their entire life cycle. After about 12 days, oocysts are passed in the stools.

Before 1981, only eight cases had been reported in humans. However, because immunocompromised patients are particularly susceptible to *Cryptosporidium*, the beginning of the AIDS epidemic marked a noteworthy increase in its prevalence in humans. Recent evidence indicates that it may be more common than was previously supposed.

The severity of the illness ranges from self-limited diarrheal episodes lasting from 3 days to 4 weeks in immunocompetent hosts, to death in immunocompromised individuals. Onset is acute, with malaise and fever, followed by abdominal pain, diarrhea, vomiting, steatorrhea, and occasionally mild rectal bleeding and nonspecific proctitis.

The diagnosis may be made by serial stool examinations or intestinal biopsy examination. The most accurate staining method for identification of the parasite is a three-step procedure that involves concentration evaluation using a sugar flotation technique, iodine staining, and a modified acid-fast stain.

Therapy focuses on correction of severe fluid and electrolyte imbalance. In complicated, life-threatening cases, conventional antiparasitics, such as metronidazole (Flagyl) or thiabendazole (Mintezol) may be effective.

**Strongyloidiasis**

This infection occurs in warm, moist climates and is caused by the helminth *Strongyloides stercoralis*. Filariform larvae are the infectious form; rhabditiform larvae are noninfectious. Multiple cycles of the parasite may occur in a single host, thereby allowing some patients to harbor *S. stercoralis* for 30 to 50 years. In some patients, repeated autoinfection may produce an overwhelming fatal hyperinfective syndrome.

Early symptoms of strongyloidiasis include fever; migratory, erythematous, macular eruptions over the distal extremities; and productive or nonproductive cough. Later, gastrointestinal symptoms predominate. Patients with hyperinfective syndrome may have heavy worm burdens, which are manifested by esophagitis, pneumonitis, gastritis, enterocolitis, hepatitis, myocarditis, intestinal obstruction or perforation, shock, or meningitis.

Diagnosis is by blood tests, stool examination, duodenal aspirate, chest x-ray, or upper GI series with small bowel follow-through.

For both symptomatic and asymptomatic patients, the drug of choice is thiabendazole (Mintezol). Patients with hyperinfective syndrome also require fluid and electrolyte maintenance and appropriate bacterial cultures. Stools and/or duodenal aspirate should be rechecked 1 to 2 weeks after completion of appropriate therapy, with a second course of treatment initiated if necessary.

With treatment, most patients with mild to moderate cases have an excellent prognosis. In patients with hyperinfective syndrome, however, the mortality rate approaches 50%.

### Ascariasis

Ascariasis is caused by the roundworm *Ascaris lumbricoides,* which is the largest intestinal nematode. Endemic areas in the United States include the southeastern Appalachian range and the Southern states, with prevalence rates approaching 90% in some areas.

Transmission is by ingestion of eggs that are passed in the stool. The adult worms live in the small bowel for 6 months or longer and then penetrate intestinal blood vessels and lymphatics. At this point they are carried through the portal circulation and pass through the liver into the lungs.

Reactions to the larvae include high fever, frequent spasmodic coughing, and hemoptysis. Reactions to the adult worms include colicky midepigastric pain, abdominal distention, vomiting, and constipation. The most frequent complication is partial or complete intestinal obstruction.

Definitive diagnosis requires that the egg or the adult worm be identified in the stool. Uncomplicated ascariasis may be treated with mebendazole (Vermox). For patients with complete obstruction, surgical intervention may be necessary. Prognosis is usually good, but is dependent on the worm burden and the presence of complications.

### Diphyllobothriasis

Diphyllobothriasis is caused by the fish tapeworm *Diphyllobothrium latum.* Infection results from ingestion of infected, raw fish. Endemic areas in the United States include northern Wisconsin, Michigan, and Minnesota. The tapeworm lives with its head attached to the small intestinal mucosa and may reach 10 mm in length. Although the effects on the intestinal mucosa are minimal, profound vitamin B12 deficiency may develop. The majority of patients with this infection are asymptomatic. When symptoms do develop, those most often seen are abdominal pain, ataxia and paresthesia, nausea, vomiting, diarrhea, and weight loss.

Definitive diagnosis requires finding the operculated egg in the stool. Diphyllobothriasis is most often treated with niclosamide (Nicloside). With proper treatment, prognosis is excellent.

## Crohn's disease

**Crohn's disease,** also known as **regional enteritis,** granulomatous colitis, or transmural colitis, is a transmural, predominantly submucosal inflammation that may affect any part of the GI tract, but occurs most commonly in the terminal ileum. Crohn's disease and ulcerative colitis, the latter of which is discussed in Chapter 17, are both chronic intestinal disorders. The two are often grouped together under the term *inflammatory bowel disease,* and differential diagnosis may be difficult in some cases.

The incidence of Crohn's disease is higher in persons of Jewish descent than in the general population. It most commonly occurs between the ages of 15 and 30. In some surveys, males and females are equally afflicted; in others, females predominate by as much as 1.6 to 1. The cause of Crohn's disease remains unknown, but possibilities include allergies and other immune disorders, abnormal response to some dietary or bacterial antigen, lymphatic obstruction, infection, and/or genetic factors.

Inflammation spreads slowly and progressively, with periods of remission often alternating with exacerbations. Segmental inflammation and rectal sparing are features that distinguish Crohn's from ulcerative colitis.

The disease process begins with lacteal blockage and lymphedema in the submucosa. Peyer's patches appear in the intestinal mucous membrane. Lymphatic obstruction causes edema, with inflammation, mucosal ulceration, stenosis, and development of fissures, abscesses, and possibly granulomas. Typically, deep longitudinal "rake ulcers" appear in the bowel. If deep ulcers appear between islands of edematous inflamed mucosa, the bowel wall takes on a "cobblestone" appearance. As the disease progresses, fibrosis occurs and serositis develops, causing diseased bowel loops to adhere to other normal or diseased loops.

During periods of acute inflammation, patients with Crohn's disease may report lower right quadrant pain, cramping, abdominal tenderness, spasms, increased flatulence, nausea, low-grade fever, diarrhea, and **borborygmi** (abnormally loud bowel sounds). Diarrhea may worsen during periods of emotional upset or following ingestion of such foods as milk, fatty foods, and spices. Stools typically appear to be soft or semiliquid; they may also be foul-smelling and fatty.

Chronic symptoms are more persistent, but less severe. They include diarrhea, lower right-quadrant pain, steatorrhea, anorexia and weight loss and nutritional deficiencies. Extraintestinal symptoms may include arthritis, spondylitis, iritis, skin involvement, renal disease, liver disease, and clubbing of the fingers.

Upper GI series and small bowel x-ray are the mainstays of diagnosing Crohn's disease in the small intestine. When the colon is involved, colonoscopy is the most effective means of diagnosis. An intestinal biopsy exam may be used for confirmation of Crohn's disease. The typical mucosal biopsy exam shows a focal ulcerative and inflammatory process, rather than the diffuse abnormality seen with ulcerative colitis.

Dietary and drug therapy aim to reduce inflammation, maintain fluid and electrolyte balance, and relieve symptoms. Therapeutic measures may include the following:

- A bland diet that is high in protein, calories, vitamins, and minerals and low in fats and fiber to maintain nutrition and to control pain, diarrhea, and flatulence
- Small, frequent meals, with avoidance of lactose by some patients
- Total parenteral nutrition for patients with severe disease or short bowel syndrome refractory to oral therapy
- Drug therapy, including corticosteroids, sulfasalazine (Azulfidine) for Crohn's colitis, antidiarrheal medications, vitamin supplementation, immunosuppressive agents, and/or antibiotics.

Potential complications of Crohn's disease include intestinal obstruction, fistula formation between the small bowel and the bladder, perianal and perirectal abscesses and fistulas, intraabdominal abscesses, and perforation. Malabsorption of bile acids and vitamin B12 is not uncommon.

More than half of all patients with Crohn's disease eventually need surgery because the disease progression has caused permanent structural changes. Surgery may be needed to correct bowel perforation, massive hemorrhage, fistulas, or acute intestinal obstruction. The most common type of surgery performed is bowel resection with restoration of bowel continuity. Although surgery may successfully alleviate acute complications, the rate of recurrence is high.

Patients with Crohn's disease should be encouraged to rest, to reduce the tension in their lives, and to communicate their feelings about this chronic and often disabling disorder. They should be educated about the disease, its process, and its treatment and should be told how to contact community agencies and support groups that can help them adjust. Depression is a common emotion experienced by patients with Crohn's disease; therefore, the provision of emotional support is an important part of the treatment process.

**Meckel's diverticulum**

**Meckel's diverticulum,** or diverticular disease of the ileum, is the most common congenital anomaly of the intestinal tract. In these cases, a blind tube, like the appendix, opens into the distal ileum, near the ileocecal valve. The lining of the diverticulum may be either gastric mucosa or pancreatic tissue.

Meckel's diverticulum results from failure of the intraabdominal portion of the yolk sac to close completely during fetal development. It is more common in male infants than in females, occurring in approximately 2% of the male population.

The majority of cases of Meckel's diverticulum are uncomplicated and asymptomatic. The first clinical sign in symptomatic patients is often painless rectal bleeding, frequently accompanied by severe **anemia** or shock. Intestinal obstruction is the mode of presentation in 25% to 40% of cases. Such obstruction may be caused by **intussusception** (a prolapse of one part of the intestine into the lumen of an immediately adjoining part), **volvulus** (a knotting or twisting of the bowel), or herniation of a loop of the intestine through an abnormal opening. Diverticulitis may also occur and be mistaken for acute appendicitis.

Not infrequently, the apex of Meckel's diverticulum is connected to the umbilicus by a fibrous band or cord. If this band snares a loop of the intestine, bowel obstruction may result.

Meckel's diverticulum should be considered in cases of gastrointestinal obstruction or hemorrhage, especially when routine GI radiographic exams are negative. Diagnosis is by radionuclide imaging with pertechnetate scan. Treatment involves correction of hypovolemic shock and control of infection, if present, followed by diverticulectomy.

**Vitamin B12 deficiency**

In the stomach, protein-bound vitamin B12 is freed by the action of gastric pepsin. The free B12 binds to two molecules of intrinsic factor, which is a glycoprotein secreted by gastric parietal cells. This complex protects vitamin B12 from use by bacteria and from the formation of unabsorbable aggregates while it is in the small bowel. In the ileum the complex of B12 and intrinsic factor binds to receptor sites on the brush border, thus facilitating B12 entry into the enterocytes. After passage through the enterocytes, B12 is transported in the blood bound to transcobalamins, which deliver the vitamin to the tissue. Intrinsic factor remains bound to the receptor site, where it may promote the uptake of more B12. When the amount of ingested B12 is very large, absorption also occurs by diffusion, probably at all levels of the intestine.

Vitamin B12 deficiency may occur if any one of these steps is impaired. Disorders or conditions that may result in B12 deficiency include gastrectomy, pernicious anemia, pancreatic insufficiency, Zollinger-Ellison syndrome, Crohn's disease, bacterial overgrowth, ileal disease or resection, familial cobalamin malabsorption, or transcobalamin deficiency.

The source of vitamin B12 malabsorption may be pinpointed by using the three-part Schilling test, which traces the excretion of radiolabeled B12 in the urine with or without the addition of intrinsic factor or a broad-spectrum antibiotic. Treatment is directed at the underlying disease state.

### Malabsorption syndromes

Malabsorption syndromes include abnormalities of mucosal transport and/or intraluminal digestion of one or more dietary constituents. Because all nutrients are absorbed across the mucosa of the small bowel, disorders that affect the mucosa may affect the absorption of fat, protein, carbohydrates, and vitamins and/or minerals. The clinical significance of malabsorption depends on the site and extent of involvement.

The primary symptom of **malabsorption** is **steatorrhea,** with an increased number of bulky, gray, foul-smelling stools. (The strict definition of steatorrhea is excretion of more than 7 g of fat in 24 hours, on a diet of 80 to 100 g of fat per day.) Other symptoms include weight loss and anorexia despite normal or high caloric intake, physical weakness, abdominal distention and cramping, and malaise.

A wide variety of disorders of the digestive organs may cause malabsorption or **maldigestion,** including pancreatic exocrine deficiency; bile acid insufficiency; lymphatic disorders; gastric hypersecretory states; postgastrectomy disorders, especially following a Billroth II operation; small bowel resection; and small bowel disease, such as celiac sprue, tropical sprue, Whipple's disease, lactase deficiency, or abetalipoproteinemia.

To pinpoint the cause of malabsorption, the physician may order laboratory blood tests and specific absorption tests. Small bowel x-ray may be used to detect mucosal disease. A small bowel biopsy may be ordered to diagnose celiac sprue, Whipple's disease, abetalipoproteinemia, or agammaglobulinemia.

Treatment of most malabsorption conditions is directed at the underlying disease.

#### Celiac sprue

**Celiac sprue** is characterized by poor food absorption and intolerance of gluten, which is a protein found in wheat and wheat products. Malabsorption in the proximal small bowel results from atrophy of the villi and a decrease in the activity and amount of enzymes in the surface epithelium.

Celiac sprue is also known as idiopathic steatorrhea, nontropical sprue, gluten-induced enteropathy, and celiac disease. The exact cause is unknown, but it probably results from a combination of environmental factors and genetic predisposition. Risk factors for celiac sprue include female sex, family history, and northwestern European ancestry.

Together with cystic fibrosis, celiac sprue is the most common cause of malabsorption in infants and children. The typical age of onset is between 8 and 24 months, after the child has been receiving gluten in his or her diet for at least 3 to 6 months. In some cases, clinical signs disappear during adolescence and reappear in adulthood. The second peak age of presentation is in the twenties, in adults who have been previously asymptomatic.

Symptoms of celiac sprue may include the following:
- Recurrent attacks of diarrhea, vomiting, steatorrhea, abdominal distention, flatulence, stomach cramps, and weakness
- Anorexia and occasionally increased appetite without weight gain
- Irritability, uncooperativeness and/or apathy
- Growth failure, muscle wasting, delayed development, and/or anemia

Diagnosis is by small bowel biopsy examination, absorption and tolerance studies, and barium x-rays. Definitive diagnosis requires an initial biopsy examination that shows typical characteristics of celiac disease (severe flattening or complete absence of intestinal villi and hypertrophied crypts), followed by a second biopsy examination after strict adherence to a gluten-free diet, and a third biopsy examination after gluten challenge to demonstrate a recurrence of the disease.

Treatment of celiac sprue involves *lifelong* elimination of gluten from the patient's diet, which means avoidance of all wheat, barley, rye, and oats. It is important that the patient also avoid meats containing wheat fillers and certain commercially prepared foods that may use wheat as an extender, such as ice cream and candy bars. Rice, corn, soy, and the flours of these grains are acceptable. Parents and children require continuing education and support to maintain compliance with a gluten-free diet, even when overt symptoms disappear.

In addition to diet, supportive therapy may include supplemental iron, vitamin B12, and folic acid; reversal of electrolyte imbalance; intravenous fluid replacement for dehydration; corticosteroids to treat accompanying adrenal insufficiency; and vitamin K for hypoprothrombinemia. The clinical response to treatment is often dramatic, beginning with an improved disposition and general appearance. In adults, potential complications include an increased risk of malignant small bowel lymphoma and carcinoma of the esophagus and stomach.

#### Tropical Sprue

Celiac sprue is not to be confused with **tropical sprue,** which is a chronic disorder acquired in endemic tropical areas and is characterized by progressively more severe alterations of the jejunum and ileum.

Histologic changes associated with tropical sprue consist of lengthening of the crypt area, broadening and shortening of the villi, epithelial cell changes, and infiltration by chronic inflammatory cells. Resulting nutritional deficiencies, notably megaloblastic anemia, may be ameliorated by treatment with a 2- to 6-month course of folic acid and tetracycline (Achromycin).

### Whipple's disease

**Whipple's disease** is a rare disorder characterized by chronic diarrhea and progressive wasting. Only about 200 cases have been reported, primarily in the United States, England, continental Europe, and South America. It is also known as intestinal lipodystrophy and lipophagia granulomatosis. The cause is unknown, but it may be caused by an infection.

Whipple's disease most often affects Caucasian men between the ages of 20 and 67. Signs and symptoms include arthralgia; vague abdominal pain; diarrhea; steatorrhea; impaired intestinal absorption; progressive weight loss; slight fever; hyperpigmentation; peripheral, mesenteric, periaortic, and celiac lymphadenopathy; and occasional splenomegaly.

Diagnosis is by biopsy examination of the small intestine, which shows macrophages and large cytoplasmic granules that stain a brilliant magenta with the periodic acid-Schiff stain.

Treatment consists of hospitalization and a 14-day course of therapy with penicillin G procaine (Bicillin) and streptomycin, followed by daily administration of tetracycline (Achromycin) for 10 to 12 months. During the acute phase, corticosteroids may be administered. Patients with iron deficiency anemia need iron supplements.

### Short bowel syndrome

**Short bowel syndrome** is a condition of malabsorption and **malnutrition** that follows a major small bowel resection. The severity of the symptoms depends on the extent and the level of the resection. Massive resection causes reduced absorption of water, electrolytes, fat, protein, carbohydrate, vitamins, and trace elements. Unless vigorous fluid and electrolyte replacement is instituted promptly, life-threatening dehydration and electrolyte imbalance may develop.

If the patient survives the first few weeks after massive resection, adaptation occurs in three stages.

- Stage 1 consists of 1 to 3 months of massive diarrhea, requiring parenteral replacement of fluids and electrolytes. During this stage, codeine may help to control diarrhea, and antacids and cimetidine (Tagamet) may be used to control gastric hypersecretion.
- During Stage 2, which may last from a a few months to more than a year, limited oral intake is begun. Oral feedings should be initiated as soon as possible, although intravenous hyperalimentation is usually continued until the oral intake exceeds 2,000 calories per day. Osteomalacia and anemia may appear during this time.

- In Stage 3, the patient resumes a relatively normal nutritional intake. Small, frequent meals are best, beginning with carbohydrates and proteins. Fats and milk products should be initiated slowly. Oral antibiotics, anticholinergics, or opiate-like drugs may be helpful. Potassium, calcium, magnesium, and vitamin supplements are necessary.

The transient gastric hypersecretion that occurs in 50% of patients subjected to massive small bowel resection may result in complicating peptic ulcer disease, diffuse mucosal damage, and/or impaired intraluminal lipid digestion.

Patients who still have 25% or more of morphologically and functionally normal small bowel have a good prognosis, particularly if the remaining intestine includes duodenum, proximal jejunum, and distal ileum.

### Lactase deficiency

The most common disorder of carbohydrate absorption is acquired **lactase deficiency,** in which a deficiency in the brush-border enzyme lactase causes malabsorption of the disaccharide lactose (hence the phrase lactose intolerance). Secondary lactase deficiency can result from diseases that damage the small bowel mucosa, such as celiac disease, tropical sprue, and radiation enteritis. Congenital lactase deficiency is a rare disorder in which mucosal lactase levels are low at birth.

Patients with lactase deficiency typically experience distention, flatulence, abdominal cramps, and watery diarrhea within minutes of ingesting milk. The diagnosis is suggested by relief of symptoms on a lactose-free diet and reappearance of symptoms upon reintroduction of lactose. Definitive diagnosis may be made by a breath hydrogen test, a lactose tolerance test, or by biochemically assaying the lactase content of the small bowel mucosa obtained by peroral biopsy examination. Treatment consists of restricting milk and milk products or use of lactose enzyme supplements.

### Abetalipoproteinemia

**Abetalipoproteinemia** is another absorption defect. Lack of betalipoproteins causes accumulation of fat and consequent malabsorption, resulting in increased stool fat. A small bowel biopsy examination will show villous epithelial cells distended with fat. Fat malabsorption lessens by restricting dietary long-chain triglycerides and administering medium-chain triglycerides.

## Small bowel tumors

Benign or malignant neoplasms of the small bowel make up less than 5% of gastrointestinal tumors. Small bowel neoplasms may be hamartomas, lymphomas, alpha heavy chain disease, primary or secondary carcinoma, or carcinoid tumors.

- **Peutz-Jeghers syndrome** is characterized by mucocutaneous pigmentation on the face, hands and feet, and in the perianal and genital areas. Gastrointestinal hamartomas may appear anywhere from the cardiac sphincter to the anus, but are regularly present in the small bowel.

- Lymphomas of the GI tract may be primary, with or without involvement of the adjacent mesenteric nodes, or secondary, having spread from elsewhere. In primary small bowel lymphomas, patients present with abdominal pain or obstruction. In secondary lymphomas, nonalimentary complaints usually precede involvement of the gut.
- Alpha heavy chain disease is a proliferation of lymphoid tissue that involves the IgA secretory system, thus leading to the production of incomplete immunoglobulin molecules made up of IgA heavy chains. Clinical features of alpha heavy chain disease include severe malabsorption syndrome and, frequently, finger clubbing. Histopathologic features include plasma cell proliferation in the small intestinal mucosa and in the nodes, followed by the development of overt malignant lymphoma in most cases.
- Primary carcinomas of the small bowel are most likely to occur in the duodenum; virtually all are adenocarcinomas. Symptoms include pain, vomiting, anorexia, malaise, and/or nausea. Diagnosis is by barium x-ray. Small bowel carcinomas are usually flat, stenosing, ulcerative or polypoid.
- Secondary carcinomas of the small bowel are relatively common. They most often arise from the breast or bronchus or are metastatic malignant melanomas.
- Carcinoid tumors are often found by chance during appendectomy and occur most frequently in the ileum and appendix. Carcinoid tumors that metastasize to the liver may be associated with carcinoid syndrome, which includes watery diarrhea, abdominal cramps, borborygmi, episodic flushing and lacrimation, pellagra-like skin lesions, bronchospasm, and valvular lesions of the right side of the heart.

Small bowel tumors usually only occur in patients who are over the age of 50. Presenting symptoms may include small bowel obstruction; abdominal pain and/or vomiting; gastrointestinal bleeding; weight loss; distended, tympanitic abdomen; and high-pitched bowel sounds. The patient's stool may contain occult blood. The physician may order blood studies, an upright plain x-ray of the abdomen, barium contrast x-rays, endoscopy and biopsy exam for lesions in the proximal duodenum, ultrasonography or computed tomography (CT) scan, or selective arteriography of the celiac axis and superior mesenteric artery.

Most small bowel tumors are treated surgically. Even metastatic tumors may require palliative surgery to relieve obstruction or bleeding. Institutional protocols for treatment of lymphomas may include surgical resection in addition to radiotherapy and chemotherapy. Radiation and chemotherapy of other malignant small bowel tumors have been largely ineffective. In Peutz-Jeghers syndrome, multiple enterotomies are usually required over the lifetime of the patient to remove large polyps that may be responsible for severe colicky pain.

---

**CASE SITUATION**

Mrs. O'Malley, age 43, was referred to a gastroenterologist after a 2-year history of diarrhea, abdominal distention with increased flatulence, stomach cramps, and fatigue. She has experienced two to four daily stools that are usually soft and bulky, and a 15-pound weight loss. She describes herself as "tense and nervous" because of family problems. Her referring physician has treated her for IBS with antispasmodics and sedatives without improvement in her symptoms. She had upper and lower GI barium studies 18 months ago, which were negative. Her blood work shows she is anemic and hypoalbuminemic, but her stool is negative for occult blood.

*Points to think about*

1. Given Mrs. O'Malley's symptoms, what might be possible medical diagnoses?
2. What factors point to a diagnosis of celiac sprue?
3. Mrs. O'Malley had normal upper and lower GI barium studies; would further barium studies be helpful?
4. It would also be necessary to obtain stool specimens for ova and parasites to rule out infectious or parasitic causes for Mrs. O'Malley's symptoms. What should the gastroenterology nurse tell the patient about collecting stool specimens?
5. The gastroenterology nurse knows that small bowel biopsy examination of the distal duodenum/proximal jejunum is the most definitive test for celiac disease. It will show that the mucosal surface is flat with shortened villi and elongated crypts, with changes in surface epithelial cells from tall columnar to cuboidal. What can he or she tell Mrs. O'Malley to expect when she goes for her biopsy examination?
6. What is one nursing diagnosis the nurse might consider for a patient with celiac sprue?
7. What might the nurse teach Mrs. O'Malley about her follow-up care?

*Suggested responses*

1. Possible medical diagnoses in Mrs. O'Malley's case might include the following:

- Irritable bowel syndrome (IBS) might explain her symptoms, but weight loss, anemia, and hypoalbuminemia are not usually seen in IBS. Also, her primary physician has tried treating her for IBS without success.
- An inflammatory bowel disease could cause these symptoms, particularly Crohn's disease.
- Lymphoma of the small bowel can cause obstruction of lymphatic drainage necessary for fat absorption.
- Chronic pancreatitis causing pancreatic insufficiency and inadequate amounts of lipase for fat digestion might account for steatorrhea.
- Tropical sprue or some parasitic disorders can cause these symptoms, but Mrs. O'Malley denies any travel history.
- Nontropical or celiac sprue with malabsorption in the proximal small bowel and intolerance of gluten could cause these symptoms, but her age may extend beyond the typical range.

2. Factors that point to a diagnosis of celiac sprue include the following:
   - Female sex
   - Presentation of features of malabsorption syndrome, including anemia (iron deficiency), protein deficiency (hypoalbuminemia), and steatorrhea (excessive fat in stool)
   - Age factor: while celiac sprue is often diagnosed by 2 years of age, many patients experience the onset of this disease beginning in the third or fourth decade.

3. Because celiac sprue affects the small bowel, an upper GI series with small bowel follow-through should be done. This may show excessive secretions and dilatation of mucosal folds in the proximal small bowel.

4. Regarding collection of stool specimens, Mrs. O'Malley should receive the following instructions:
   - Obtain stool specimens before barium x-ray because barium interferes with microscopic examination.
   - Use a clean, dry container.
   - Do not use stool that has been in contact with toilet-bowl water or urine.
   - Take the specimen to the laboratory immediately to ensure accurate results.
   - It is often necessary to test several specimens; for example, the first morning stool each day for 3 days.

5. Regarding her upcoming small bowel biopsy examination, Mrs. O'Malley should be told that:
   - The physician may try to get a large enough biopsy specimen by doing a standard esophagogastroduodenoscopy (EGD). Mrs. O'Malley may have this done in the hospital endoscopy unit or in the office endoscopy setting. The gastroenterology nurse should explain this procedure to the patient, with reassurance that he or she will be there to assist her through all phases of the procedure.
   - Large submucosal biopsy specimens may be obtained by suction capsules that are guided under fluoroscopic control to the proper location in the proximal jejunum. The patient is attended during the procedure by the gastroenterologist and the gastroenterology nurse. Full explanation of the procedure and complications should be provided by the physician and may be reinforced by the nurse during the procedure.
   - Normally, a submucosal biopsy exam is done as an outpatient procedure; therefore, Mrs. O'Malley will not be admitted to the hospital. The nurse should instruct her to immediately report any severe abdominal pain or distention, nausea, vomiting, or bleeding.

6. The nurse might consider the nursing diagnosis "knowledge deficit related to necessary dietary modifications for celiac sprue." A nurse can begin her intervention predicated on such a diagnosis in many instances; however, it is important to recognize that the act of acquiring and recalling new information does not necessarily mean that the learner will change his or her behavior as a consequence.

   The "knowledge deficit" diagnosis is broad and involves three learning domains: receiving/retaining new information; responding emotionally by personalizing the information; and changing behavior by alteration in neuromuscular pathways. There may be a deficit or deficits in any one or more of these learning dimensions, although most deficits occur in the cognitive or psychomotor areas.

   Other factors that might influence the patient's response to nursing interventions based on this diagnosis include intellectual limitations, lack of exposure to information, memory loss, visual or auditory sensory deficits, pathophysiologic states or conditions, lack of motivation or readiness to learn, cultural or language barriers, or interfering coping strategies (e.g., denial or anxiety).

7. Regarding her follow-up care, the nurse should explain the following to Mrs. O'Malley:
   - That it will be necessary for her to make permanent, lifelong adjustments in her diet based on written gluten-free diet instructions that the nurse will provide
   - That it will be necessary to keep a dietary log that the nurse will review at intervals
   - That fecal fat studies and laboratory blood studies will be required at specified intervals
   - That foods containing lactose may not be tolerated well (because they may cause diarrhea and flatulence) and often must be eliminated from the diet also

- That the response to dietary changes can be dramatic; within a few days or weeks general appearance will improve and fatigue will lessen, stools will be more formed and less frequent, and abdominal distention will decrease
- That lost weight is usually recovered within several months
- That the villous architecture in the small bowel should return to normal and that a follow-up biopsy exam might be done to confirm improvement
- That there are several support groups for families with celiac disease and that several companies produce gluten-free products

## REVIEW TERMS

abetalipoproteinemia, ampulla of Vater, anemia, Auerbach's plexus, borborygmi, Brunner's glands, celiac sprue, Crohn's disease, crypts of Lieberkühn, duodenum, enteric plexus, giardiasis, goblet cells, ileocecal valve, ileum, inflammatory bowel disease, intussusception, jejunum, lactase deficiency, lamina propria, ligament of Treitz, malabsorption, maldigestion, malnutrition, Meckel's diverticulum, Meissner's plexus, microvilli, Paneth's cells, peptic ulcers, Peutz-Jegher's syndrome, Peyer's patches, regional enteritis, short bowel syndrome, small bowel, steatorrhea, tropical sprue, villus, volvulus, Whipple's disease

## REVIEW QUESTIONS

1. The proximal two fifths of the small bowel is known as the:
   a. Duodenum.
   b. Ileum.
   c. Jejunum.
   d. Cecum.
2. The mucous layer of the small bowel is lined with:
   a. Squamous epithelium.
   b. Columnar epithelium.
   c. Connective tissue.
   d. Peritoneum.
3. The principal function of Brunner's glands is to:
   a. Synthesize antibodies.
   b. Absorb nutrients.
   c. Secrete a viscous, alkaline fluid.
   d. Secrete hormones.
4. The primary site of absorption for vitamin B12 and bile acids is the:
   a. Duodenum.
   b. Jejunum.
   c. Ileum.
   d. Stomach.
5. The intestinal contents are constantly being stirred by:
   a. Active transport.
   b. Segmenting contractions.
   c. Peristalsis.
   d. Shortening and lengthening of the villi.
6. Segmental submucosal inflammation and a cobble-stoned appearance of the bowel wall are associated with:
   a. Ulcerative colitis.
   b. Crohn's disease.
   c. Duodenal ulcers.
   d. Celiac sprue.
7. The most effective treatment for symptomatic Meckel's diverticulum is:
   a. Diverticulectomy.
   b. Antibiotic therapy.
   c. Bowel resection.
   d. Dietary modification.
8. About 80% of all peptic ulcers occur in the:
   a. Stomach.
   b. Duodenum.
   c. Ileum.
   d. Jejunum.
9. A malabsorption syndrome characterized by gluten intolerance is:
   a. Cystic fibrosis.
   b. Whipple's disease.
   c. Tropical sprue.
   d. Celiac sprue.
10. Primary carcinomas of the proximal small bowel are virtually all:
    a. Lymphomas.
    b. Melanomas.
    c. Adenocarcinomas.
    d. Sarcomas.

## BIBLIOGRAPHY

Beare, P, and Myers, J. "Nursing Management of Adults with Intestinal Disorders." In *Principles and Practice of Adult Health Nursing*, 1583-86. St. Louis: Mosby–Year Book, 1990.

Black, M. "Crohn's Disease: Pathophysiology, Diagnosis and Management." *Gastroenterology Nursing* 11 (Spring 1989): 259-63.

Bongiovanni, G, ed. *Essentials of Clinical Gastroenterology*. 2nd ed. New York: McGraw–Hill, 1988.

Coleman, D. "Anatomy and Physiology of the Small Bowel." *SGA Journal* 10 (Summer 1987): 44-45.

Eastwood, G, and Avunduk, C. *Manual of Gastroenterology: Diagnosis and Therapy*. Boston: Little, Brown, & Co., 1988.

Given, B, and Simmons, S. *Gastroenterology in Clinical Nursing*. 4th ed. St. Louis: Mosby–Year Book, 1984.

Goldberg, K, ed. *Gastrointestinal Problems*. Nurse Review Series. Springhouse, Pa.: Springhouse Corporation, 1986.

Hamilton, H, editorial director. *Diseases*. Nurse's Reference Library Series. Springhouse, Pa.: Springhouse Corporation, 1985.

McFarland, G, and McFarlane, E. "Cognitive-Perceptual Pattern-Knowledge Deficit (Specify)." In *Nursing Diagnosis and Intervention*, 549-56. St. Louis: Mosby–Year Book, 1989.

Misiewicz, J, Bartram, C, Cotton, P, Mee, A, Price, A, and Thompson, R. *Atlas of Clinical Gastroenterology.* Vol 1. London: Gower Medical Publishing, 1985.

Phaosawasdi, K, Lee, B, Tyler, C, and Rice, P. "Cryptosporidiosis in the immunocompetent host: a case report and an examination of an increasingly important parasite." *SGA Journal* 11 (Fall 1988): 80-84.

Sachar, D, Waye, J, and Lewis B, eds. *Gastroenterology for the House Officer.* Baltimore: Williams & Wilkins, 1989.

Silverman, A, and Roy, C. *Pediatric Clinical Gastroenterology.* 3rd ed. St. Louis: Mosby–Year Book, 1983.

Sleisenger, M, and Fordtran, J, eds. *Gastrointestinal Disease: Pathophysiology, Diagnosis, Management.* 4th ed. Philadelphia: W.B. Saunders, 1989.

# Chapter 17

# LARGE INTESTINE

This chapter will acquaint the gastroenterology nurse with the normal anatomy and physiology of the large intestine. Selected diseases and disorders of the large intestine in terms of pathophysiology, diagnosis, and treatment are discussed.

**Learning objectives**

After completing study of this chapter, the gastroenterology nurse should be able to:

1. Explain the normal macroanatomy and microanatomy of the large intestine.
2. Outline the physiology of absorption, secretion, and motility in the large intestine.
3. Discuss the pathophysiology, diagnosis, and treatment of a number of diseases and disorders of the large intestine, including intestinal polyps; inflamma-

tory, parasitic and diverticular diseases; cancer; and anorectal disorders.

**ANATOMY AND PHYSIOLOGY**

The large intestine is 90 to 150 cm (4 to 5 feet) long and approximately 4 to 6 cm (2 inches) in diameter (see Plate 1). It extends from the ileocecal valve to the anus and is divided into the following five sections: the ascending, transverse, descending, and sigmoid colon, and the rectum (Fig. 17-1 and Plate 1).

At the distal end of the small intestine, a flap valve known as the ileocecal valve acts as a sphincter both to control the passage of intestinal contents from the ileum to the **colon** and to prevent the reflux of bacteria from the colon back into the small bowel, thus preserving the relative sterility of the small bowel.

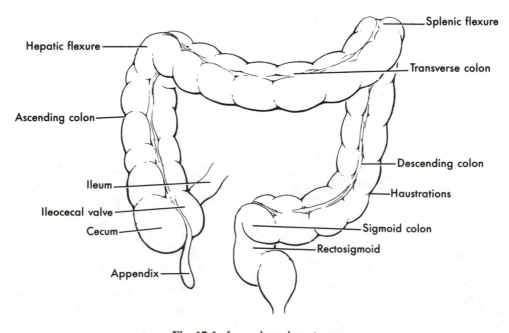

**Fig. 17-1.** Large bowel anatomy.

The first section of the large intestine to receive material from the small bowel is the **cecum,** a short blind sac to which the **vermiform appendix** is attached. The appendix itself is a thin, tubular structure that ranges from 2 to 20 cm in length and is about 8 mm in diameter. It has no known digestive role.

Immediately above the cecum is the **ascending** (right) **colon,** which passes up the right side of the abdomen to the lower border of the liver, where it bends to the left at the right colic, or **hepatic, flexure.** The **transverse colon** is the portion of the bowel that crosses the abdomen from right to left, from the hepatic flexure to the left colic, or **splenic, flexure.** The **descending** (left) **colon** runs down the left side of the abdomen from the spleen to the iliac crest, where it makes an S-curve at midline to form the **sigmoid colon.**

The last major portion of the large intestine is the rectum, which follows the curvature of the lower sacrum and coccyx. The **rectum** is about 13 cm (5 inches) long. The distal portion forms the anal canal. Movement of feces through the anal canal is controlled by an inch-wide internal sphincter composed of involuntary smooth muscle and an external sphincter made up of voluntary striated muscle. Levator ani muscles surrounding the rectum also help keep defecation under voluntary control. The actual opening is called the **anus.**

The wall of the large intestine has four layers: the serosa, the muscularis, the submucosa, and the mucosa. The outer serous layer is formed by the visceral peritoneum. The rectum does not have a serous layer.

The second layer, or muscularis, includes an inner circular layer and an outer longitudinal layer that is composed of three heavy longitudinal bands (**tenia coli**). The tenia coli are shorter than the intestine, thus causing it to pucker and form small sacs called **haustra.** The size and shape of the haustra vary with the state of contraction of the circular and longitudinal muscle layers. Auerbach's nerve plexus is located between the circular and longitudinal muscle layers.

The third layer of the large intestine is the submucosa, which contains small arteries, veins, and lymphatic vessels and the nerve fibers and ganglion cells that form Meissner's plexus. The submucosa is separated from the mucosa by the muscularis mucosae, a layer of smooth muscle cells.

The mucosa itself is smooth-surfaced and is arranged in folds called the plicae semilunares. As in the small bowel, the tubular crypts of Lieberkühn open into the lumen of the large intestine. Intestinal villi, however, are absent in the large bowel; the absorptive surface is flat and is lined by columnar epithelial cells and a number of goblet cells. There are fewer microvilli on the colonic columnar cells than in the small intestine. The epithelium in the lower half of the crypts is composed of proliferating undifferentiated columnar cells, mucus-secreting goblet cells, and a few endocrine cells.

The mucous membrane that lines the rectum is arranged in longitudinal rows called rectal or anal columns. Each rectal column contains an artery and a vein. These rectal columns end about 2 cm from the anal orifice, where they join transverse tissue folds. At the anorectal line, also known as the mucocutaneous border, the colonic mucosa meets the external anal canal. The anorectal line also marks a change in nerve supply and venous drainage.

The right half of the large intestine receives arterial blood from the branches of the superior mesenteric artery, and the left or lower portion receives arterial blood from branches of the inferior mesenteric artery. Venous blood from the colon is drained mainly through the inferior and superior mesenteric veins (Fig. 17-2).

The rectum and anal canal receive arterial blood from the hemorrhoidal artery, which is a branch of the inferior mesenteric artery. The rectum is also supplied by branches of the hypogastric artery. Above the anorectal line, venous blood drains upward to the superior hemorrhoidal veins and from there to the portal veins. Below the anorectal line, venous blood drains downward to the inferior hemorrhoidal veins.

Parasympathetic innervation of the right portion of the colon is derived from the vagus nerve. The remaining portion receives parasympathetic innervation through branches of the sacral nerves and sympathetic innervation through the spinal nerves. In general, stimulation of the parasympathetic nerves increases intestinal contraction and mucus secretion and inhibits the rectal sphincter, whereas stimulation of sympathetic fibers inhibits colonic motility and secretions and stimulates the rectal sphincter.

The main functions of the large intestine are the storage and movement of intestinal contents; absorption of water, some electrolytes, and bile acids; and to a minor extent, the excretion of mucus, potassium, and bicarbonate.

**Motility**

The colon has three basic patterns of movement, which are explained as follows:

- Periodic, uncoordinated tonic contractions or segmentations of both the longitudinal and circular muscles bunch up the folds of the mucosa, thus forming the haustra.
- Phasic, random, nonpropulsive contractions last 30 seconds to 2 minutes and include peristalsis and retrograde peristalsis, which mix the stool material and help absorb its liquid contents without advancing the material toward the anus.
- Spontaneous mass movements occur three or four times a day when the colon becomes filled and distended. When mass movements of the sigmoid

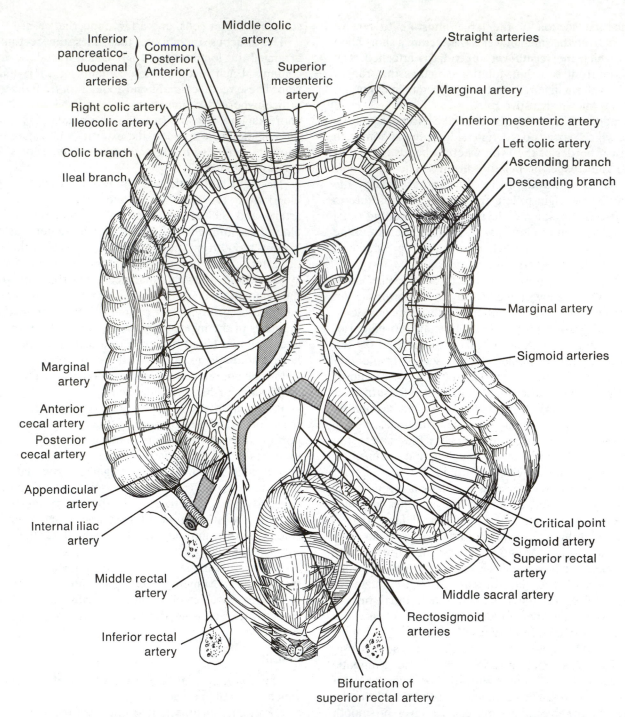

**Fig. 17-2.** Arterial and venous blood supplies to primary and accessory organs of the gastrointestinal tract. (From Broadwell DC and Jackson BS: Principles of ostomy care, St. Louis, 1982, Mosby–Year Book.)

colon move feces into the rectum, the urge to defecate is stimulated, causing peristaltic waves in the rectum and relaxation of the internal and then the external anal sphincter.

If relaxation of the internal and external sphincters is not enough to provide for defecation, a **Valsalva maneuver** assists in the process. Through the Valsalva maneuver, the involuntary movement of the bowel wall and the relaxation of the external sphincter are assisted by contraction of the diaphragm and the thoracic and abdominal muscles. This strain and downward push lasts approximately 8 seconds, thus increasing the intraabdominal pressure and frequently emptying the colon from as high as the splenic flexure.

Under normal conditions, gas moves down the colon at a rate of about 1 to 4 inches per second. Liquids are moved by gravity and peristalsis and by mass movements, but solid materials move primarily by mass movements.

## Secretion

Colonic secretion is scanty and consists primarily of water, mucus, potassium, and bicarbonate. The alkaline mucus secreted by goblet cells in the crypts lubricates the intestinal walls, protects the mucosa from acidic bacterial action, and helps lubricate the passage of stool.

## Absorption and elimination

Of the 1000 to 2000 ml of liquid chyme that enter the colon daily, only 150 to 250 ml of fluid are evacuated in the stool. The colon absorbs sodium, chloride, and water, with most absorption being accomplished in the ascending colon.

Normal feces contain intestinal bacteria that help break down and putrefy body wastes, trace fluids, mucus, indigestible cellulose, undigested connective tissue and toxins from meat proteins, undigested fats, and bile pigments. Feces are normally brown in color because of the metabolism of bile pigments to stercobilin. Odor is the result of indole and skatole, both of which are products of protein catabolism.

## Indigenous bacteria

The colon is sterile at birth, but rapidly becomes colonized by swallowed bacteria. The normal adult colon contains approximately $10^9$ to $10^{11}$ organisms per g of stool, which consist primarily of gram-negative anaerobic bacteria, such as *Bacteroides, Lactobacillus,* and *Clostridium.* The positive effects of these resident bacteria include; breaking down cellulose and other waste material; deconjugating bile salts; synthesizing vitamin K; controlling the overgrowth of harmful bacteria; thickening the mucosal lining of the bowel; and destroying pancreatic enzymes that are harmful to the skin and other structures.

Indigenous bacteria also have a number of potentially harmful effects, including the manufacture of gas; production of the toxins or chemicals that produce colitis or diarrhea; invasion of the bowel wall, thereby producing infectious colitis; and the production of ammonia, which can cause hepatic encephalopathy in patients with hepatic cirrhosis.

## PATHOPHYSIOLOGY

Among the diseases and disorders that affect the large intestine are intestinal polyps, angiodysplasia, colitis, irritable bowel syndrome, parasitic infestations, diverticular disease, tumors, obstructions, and anorectal disorders.

## Polyps

Colonic polyps are discrete tissue masses that protrude into the lumen of the bowel. Pedunculated polyps are attached to the intestinal wall by a stem. Broad-based, sessile polyps attach directly to the intestinal wall. **Polyps** may be adenomatous or hyperplastic. Diagnosis is by colonoscopy or proctosigmoidoscopy and air-contrast barium enema.

Most polyps are asymptomatic, but some patients experience bleeding. Research shows that removal of rectal polyps dramatically reduces the incidence of subsequent rectal cancer.

### Familial polyposis

In **familial polyposis,** which is inherited as an autosomal dominant trait, hundreds of adenomatous polyps develop throughout the colon. Familial polyposis is diagnosed by digital rectal examination, colonoscopy or proctosigmoidoscopy, and barium enema. Patients may also present with nonspecific symptoms, such as **hematochezia** (passage of bloody stools), **diarrhea,** and abdominal pain. Because these polyps may become cancerous, surgery is strongly recommended; most likely total proctocolectomy with ileostomy.

### Gardner's syndrome

In **Gardner's syndrome,** multiple adenomatous polyps appear along the colon or other parts of the GI tract, and osteomas appear on the mandible, skull, and long bones. Like familial polyposis, Gardner's syndrome is familial. Symptoms of both diseases are similar and some sources suggest that the two may be variable expressions of a single disease. Because the polyps associated with Gardner's syndrome tend to become cancerous in 10 to 15 years, surgical treatment is recommended.

## Angiodysplasia

Angiodysplasias are vascular dilatations in the submucosa that consist of arterial, venous, and capillary elements. They are often multiple and occur most frequently in the cecum and right colon, but may be found throughout the GI tract. Most are associated with normal aging, but their etiology remains uncertain. In the hereditary disorder Osler-Weber-Rendu disease, also known as hereditary hemorrhagic telangiectasia, angiodysplasias occur throughout the GI tract and on the skin, in the nail beds, and in the mucosa of the mouth and nasopharynx.

As many as 25% of individuals over the age of 60 with no history of gastrointestinal bleeding may have vascular ectasias of the colon. Asymptomatic individuals require no treatment. In symptomatic individuals, the usual presentation is acute lower gastrointestinal bleeding, which may be attributed to another coexisting disorder. It is not uncommon for a patient to experience several bleeding episodes before the proper diagnosis is made. Diagnosis of angiodysplasias (arteriovenous malformations) is by colonoscopy or angiography. Treatment is by resection of the bowel segment that contains the lesion. Bleeding recurs in 15% to 37% of patients who are treated surgically. Alternative treatment methods include endoscopic treatment with a laser, heater probe, or bipolar electrocoagulation.

### Colitis

**Colitis** is broadly defined as an inflammation of the colon. Several different forms of this disorder are recognized, including ischemic colitis, ulcerative colitis, pseudomembranous colitis, Crohn's colitis, and radiation enteritis.

#### Ischemic colitis

**Ischemic colitis** is an acute vascular insufficiency of the colon. It may occur in any portion of the small or large bowel, but usually affects the descending colon (most often in the region of the splenic flexure) or the sigmoid colon, which are the portions of the colon that are supplied by the inferior mesenteric artery.

Ischemic colitis may be either occlusive or nonocclusive. Occlusive ischemic disease represents a mechanical obstruction in the blood vessels that supply the bowel. It can often be traced to emboli from an artificial mitral valve or a fibrillating atrium or to surgical bypass, especially vascular surgery involving the distal aorta. Nonocclusive ischemia is usually related to a severe derangement in the central circulation consequent to such conditions as congestive heart failure, myocardial infarction, major hemorrhage, sepsis, or cardiac arrhythmia.

Symptoms of ischemic colitis include abrupt onset of pain at the left iliac fossa, bloody diarrhea, low-grade fever, abdominal distention, and minor abdominal tenderness. The classic radiologic sign is *thumbprinting* in the affected area of the bowel, resulting from localized elevation of the mucosa by submucosal hemorrhage or edema. Sigmoidoscopy may reveal nonspecific colitis, ulcerations, and/or bluish soft nodules.

Most patients recover spontaneously, although a minority develop peritoneal signs and absent bowel sounds, signifying bowel infarction and peritonitis. Such patients require surgical intervention consisting of segmental resection and either primary anastomosis or temporary colostomy. Follow-up barium enema x-rays or colonoscopy should be done 6 to 8 weeks after recovery to rule out ischemic strictures.

#### Ulcerative colitis

**Ulcerative colitis (UC)** is a chronic, recurrent inflammation that affects the mucosa and submucosa of the large intestine. Inflammation often originates in the lower colon and then spreads proximally. The mucosa develops diffuse ulceration and hemorrhage, with congestion, edema, and exudative inflammation in the lamina propria and submucosa. Crypt abscesses form

and become necrotic, leading to bloody, mucoid stools. Periods of remission often alternate with exacerbations. As crypt abscesses heal, granulation tissue forms, causing the colon to narrow, shorten, and lose its haustra. The cause of UC is unknown.

UC and Crohn's disease (see Chapter 16) are often described together as inflammatory bowel disease; signs and symptoms of the two disorders are similar. Crohn's disease, however, typically affects all layers of the bowel wall, not just the mucosa. In addition, UC is usually continuous from the rectum and is limited to the large intestine; Crohn's disease is often segmental and most often involves the small bowel, particularly the terminal ileum, but may affect any area of the GI tract.

Symptoms of UC may begin abruptly. They include the following:

* Bloody, mucopurulent diarrhea and cramping
* Nausea, vomiting, and lethargy
* Fever, dehydration, and anemia in severe cases
* Decreased appetite, leading to nutritional deficiencies
* Lower left quadrant tenderness, guarding, and abdominal distention, although abdominal findings may be absent even in the presence of total colonic involvement
* Extraintestinal symptoms involving the liver, skin, eyes, or joints

Following a thorough history and physical examination, diagnostic sigmoidoscopy is usually performed. Findings consistent with UC include granularity and increased friability of the mucosa when wiped with a cotton swab, ulceration, and pseudopolyps. A rectal biopsy examination may provide additional histologic evidence, and colonoscopy may be necessary. The physician may also order a stool analysis, stool cultures, and blood studies. A barium enema may be ordered, but is contraindicated in patients with very active or fulminant colitis.

Dietary and drug therapy may be ordered to reduce inflammation, maintain fluid and electrolyte balance, and relieve symptoms. The ultimate goal is to enable the patient to return to a normal, active lifestyle. Treatment methods may include the following:

* A bland, nonlaxative diet with small, frequent feedings and possibly avoidance of lactose
* Sulfasalazine (Azulfidine), antidiarrheal medications, immunosuppressive agents, and/or antibiotics
* Corticosteroid therapy, administered topically (rectally), orally, or intravenously
* Bed rest, possibly in the hospital
* Surgery in 20% to 25% of patients, including unresponsive patients or those with complications such as perforation and hemorrhage. If surgery is required, the physician may perform a total proctocolectomy with ileostomy.

Potential minor local complications of UC include pseudopolyps, hemorrhoids, anal fissures, perianal or ischiorectal abscess, and rectal prolapse. More serious local complications may include massive colonic hemorrhage, colonic strictures, colonic perforation, and toxic megacolon.

**Toxic megacolon** is an acute dilatation of the colon that is associated with systemic toxicity. It is the most severe, life-threatening complication of UC, but may also be associated with any severe inflammatory condition of the bowel, including Crohn's disease, bacterial colitis, and amebiasis. In some patients with UC, toxic megacolon represents the first attack.

Prominent symptoms of toxic megacolon are fever, abdominal pain and distention, vomiting, and fatigue. The patient may experience a progressive decrease in the frequency of stools resulting from loss of colonic propulsive activity. Leukocytosis, anemia, and hypoalbuminemia are common laboratory findings. Plain films of the abdomen will reveal dilatation of the entire colon or only the transverse colon. Perforation of the transverse and sigmoid colon is a common and often catastrophic complication.

Treatment of toxic megacolon includes NPO status, nasogastric suction, and intravenous fluids, electrolytes, steroids, and broad-spectrum antibiotics. If toxic megacolon does not improve within 48 to 72 hours, total colectomy is indicated. UC patients are also at increased risk of developing adenocarcinoma of the colon. The risk of cancer is directly related to the extent of colon involvement and duration of disease. For surveillance purposes, it is recommended that colonoscopy be performed yearly after 7 to 10 years of pancolitis and after 12 to 15 years of left-sided colitis. Other complications may include liver disease, hematologic abnormalities, thromboembolic disease, arthritis, ocular lesions, dermatologic disease, renal disease, and sclerosing cholangitis.

### Pseudomembranous colitis

**Pseudomembranous colitis** is defined as an acute inflammation of the bowel mucosa, with the formation of pseudomembranous plaques overlying an area of superficial ulceration. It is also called necrotizing enteritis, pseudomembranous **enterocolitis,** or pseudomembranous enteritis. The preferred method of diagnosis of pseudomembranous colitis is endoscopy to detect typical yellow-white raised plaques that may extend from the rectosigmoid area to the proximal colon. Sigmoidoscopy is usually adequate, but up to one third of patients have lesions restricted to the right colon, thus necessitating colonoscopy.

The great majority of cases of pseudomembranous colitis involve a toxin or toxins produced by *Clostridium difficile,* which is a spore-forming, gram-positive, anaerobic rod capable of producing a cytopathic toxin. One diagnostic test is the demonstration of this toxin in the stool, using either enzyme-linked immunosorbent assay (ELISA) or counterimmunoelectrophoresis. Pseudomembranous colitis is commonly associated with oral or intravenous antibiotic therapy and, less often, with chemotherapeutic agents. It should be suspected in any patient who develops diarrhea during or within 10 weeks of antibiotic therapy.

Symptoms of pseudomembranous colitis include nonbloody, watery diarrhea; crampy abdominal pain; fever; and leukocytosis. Complications may include toxic megacolon, pneumoperitoneum, severe electrolyte imbalance, hypoalbuminemia, and acute migratory polyarthritis.

Pseudomembranous colitis is usually self-limited, although one third of patients require hospitalization. It is treated by discontinuing antibiotics and administering an agent that binds the *C. difficile* toxin, such as cholestyramine (Questran) or colestipol (Colestid), or one that eradicates the organism altogether, such as vancomycin (Vancocin), metronidazole (Flagyl), or bacitracin.

### Crohn's colitis

Crohn's disease may be confined to the colon (hence **Crohn's colitis**) or may be associated with small bowel disease. Clinically, Crohn's colitis may resemble UC, but the ulceration is often longitudinal and involves the full thickness of the bowel. The disease is often segmental. Stricture formation is common, and fistulas are a frequent complication, especially in the perineum. Crohn's colitis is most often diagnosed by colonoscopy. Treatment options are discussed in Chapter 16.

### Radiation enteritis

When radiation injury occurs to the GI tract, it is usually a result of radiotherapy for pelvic, intraabdominal, or retroperitoneal malignancies, such as carcinoma of the cervix, prostate, bladder, testicle, or ovary. Many patients experience mild acute symptoms during treatment, but approximately 5% to 15% experience severe, chronic damage.

The acute phase of **radiation enteritis** occurs during treatment and is related to alterations in epithelial cell function. It is characterized by nausea, cramping, and altered bowel habits. If the colon is involved, there may be acute proctocolitis with diarrhea, tenesmus, and rectal bleeding. The extent of injury can be controlled by altering the size and timing of radiation dosage and by using antiemetics, bulk-forming agents, and antidiarrheal agents.

The chronic phase of radiation enteritis results from abnormalities in vascular and connective tissues. Symptoms may appear 3 months to 30 years after radiation treatment. When the colon and rectum are involved, proctocolitis, bleeding, strictures, perforation, and fistula formation may result. Chronic enteritis is often an intractable and progressive disease associated with significant morbidity and mortality. Medical management consists of administration of steroid enemas and sulfasalazine (Azulfidine), and transfusions for chronic bleeding. Strictures can be dilated manually or by using a colonoscope. Surgery may be used selectively in patients with complete obstruction, uncontrolled bleeding, perforation, or fistulas. Complications and disease progression following surgery are common. Resection is recommended for localized disease, but bypass is preferred for more extensive disease.

### Irritable bowel syndrome

**Irritable bowel syndrome (IBS)** is the most common gastrointestinal disorder in the United States and is the most frequent reason for outpatient visits to gastroenterologists. Synonyms for IBS include irritable colon and spastic colon.

IBS is characterized by motility disorders of the large and small intestine, without evidence of anatomic abnormality or organic illness. Patients with IBS present with complaints of abdominal discomfort, pain, and constipation and/or diarrhea. Symptoms vary in pattern and intensity, but usually can be traced to periods of emotional stress. Although it is associated with severe discomfort, IBS is not related to other chronic or life-threatening conditions, nor with decreased longevity.

The anatomic cause of IBS is unknown, but the most commonly accepted etiologic theory is that the behavioral tendencies of these patients cause exaggerated colonic motility in response to environmental stress.

Diagnosis is by identification of the characteristic symptom complex and by careful exclusion of other, organic gastrointestinal disorders.

The usual treatment for IBS involves the following regimen:
- Sympathetic diagnosis and reassurance that organic causes have been ruled out
- A high-fiber diet
- Anticholinergic agents to decrease abdominal pain
- Psychologic support aimed at decreasing stress

In 75% of children with IBS, at least one parent or sibling has a functional gastrointestinal disorder. Irritable bowel syndrome is more common in Jewish and white children, but the female predominance that is found in adults does not exist in children. In three fourths of school-age children with IBS, the onset of symptoms can be traced to stress-associated school problems or parental marital problems. In treating children with IBS, medications should be prescribed sparingly.

### Parasitic infestations

There are a number of parasitic diseases that affect the large intestine, including amebiasis, trypanosomiasis, and trichuriasis.

### Amebiasis

**Amebiasis** is a form of colitis caused by the protozoan *Entamoeba histolytica*. It is transmitted primarily by fecal contamination of food or water, but other modes of transmission include close interpersonal contact, venereal spread, and houseflies and cockroaches. Ingested cysts form trophozoites in the small bowel. The amebas penetrate host tissues, causing necrosis without inflammation. Lesions are located throughout the colon, most often in the cecum, ascending, and rectosigmoid colon areas.

Carriers of *E. histolytica* are often asymptomatic, but may suffer from amebic diarrhea, amebic dysentery, amebic appendicitis, ameboma (a large, masslike lesion in the wall of the intestine, most often in the cecum), or visceral abscess, particularly a single abscess in the right lobe of the liver. Amebic diarrhea is an afebrile illness that is usually intermittent and followed by constipation. Amebic dysentery, on the other hand, is associated with headache, nausea and vomiting, fever and chills, **tenesmus** (a felt need to urinate or defecate, combined with an ineffectual straining to do so), abdominal cramps, and stools with a large amount of blood-tinged mucus.

Diagnosis of amebiasis requires demonstration of *E. histolytica* in the stool. Sigmoidoscopy and indirect hemagglutination titers may be useful, and a barium enema may be helpful in diagnosing amebomas. In cases of suspected liver abscess, liver-spleen scan, abdominal ultrasonography or CT scan, or percutaneous needle aspiration may be used.

Amebiasis is treated with oral antibiotics, most often diiodohydroxyquin (Yodoxin) with or without metronidazole (Flagyl). With appropriate treatment, response to therapy is often dramatic and prognosis is excellent.

### Trypanosomiasis

Trypanosomiasis is a chronic illness caused by the protozoan *Trypanosoma*. *T. cruzi* causes Chagas' disease, also known as South American trypanosomiasis, which is transmitted primarily by the bite of the reduviid bug, but may also be transmitted by blood transfusions, damage to the placenta during delivery, or contaminated food. The parasite multiplies rapidly at the site of inoculation, producing a severe inflammatory reaction. It may be disseminated through the bloodstream to any organ, particularly the heart, esophagus, or colon. At the site of infection, the parasite causes degeneration of the intramuscular autonomic nerve plexuses, resulting in megaesophagus, **megacolon,** or dilatation of other tubular organs.

Symptomatic Chagas' disease has been confined largely to rural areas of South and Central America, but it has been found in all Western Hemisphere countries except Guyana, Surinam, and Canada. Acute Chagas' disease is most often seen in children who are under the age of 2. Symptoms include anorexia, nausea, and vomiting; generalized lymphadenopathy; diarrhea; unilateral conjunctivitis; edema of the face and eyelids; swelling of lacrimal and submaxillary glands; hepatosplenomegaly; cardiac arrhythmias; congestive heart failure; and frequently death.

Diagnosis requires identification of *T. cruzi* in blood or tissue. For active infections, prolonged oral administration of Lampit (nifurtimox) is 70% to 95% effective.

**Trichuriasis**

Trichuriasis is caused by the nematode *Trichuris trichiura*. It is also known as whipworm because of the whip-like appearance of the parasite. Whipworm is most often found in tropical areas or in areas of poor sanitation. Transmission is fecal-oral. The ingested eggs hatch in the duodenum. When the larvae mature into adult worms, they migrate down the GI tract and accumulate in the cecum and ascending colon.

The majority of patients are asymptomatic. Heavy infestations may cause dehydration, weakness, abdominal distention and cramping, acute and chronic diarrhea, bloody mucoid stools, anemia, and occasionally rectal prolapse.

Diagnosis requires identification of the characteristic eggs in the stools or, rarely, detection of the worms by sigmoidoscopy or colonoscopy. After treatment with mebendazole (Vermox), prognosis is excellent.

## Diverticular disease

Diverticular disease affects 30% of all adults over the age of 60. It is characterized by herniation at weak points on the intestinal mucosa and submucosa, most often in the descending and sigmoid colon. A diverticulum typically has a narrow neck that contains all four mucosal layers and a spherical sac that contains intestinal serosa and mucosa only.

Contributing factors for diverticular disease include the following:

* Hypertrophy of segments of the colon's circular muscle
* Increased intracolonic pressure
* Age-related atrophy or weakness in the bowel muscles
* Chronic constipation and straining
* Irregular, uncoordinated bowel contractions
* Lack of dietary fiber
* Obesity

Diverticular disease is found in approximately 10% of the population in the United States, the United Kingdom, Australia, and other developed nations. In contrast, it affects only about 1% of the population in Asian countries. In migrants from low-prevalence areas to westernized countries, diverticular disease increases within 10 years. Prevalence is strongly correlated with advancing age.

Diverticular disease may take the form of diverticulosis or diverticulitis.

**Diverticulosis**

**Diverticulosis** is uncomplicated diverticular disease. Patients with diverticulosis show no signs of infection; in fact, most are asymptomatic. When symptoms are reported, they may include pain, usually in the left lower quadrant; diffuse abdominal pain that may be chronic or intermittent and is affected by eating or bowel evacuation; constipation alternating with diarrhea; and possibly lower quadrant tenderness and hypertrophic sigmoid colon. Diagnosis of diverticulosis is confirmed by barium enema or colonoscopy.

**Diverticulitis**

**Diverticulitis** is an inflammation in the wall of the diverticulum at its apex and, rarely, at its neck. It occurs most often in the sigmoid colon and adjacent structures and may last for several weeks.

The most common symptoms of diverticulitis are fever and left lower quadrant pain. Other symptoms include nausea and vomiting, constipation, left lower quadrant tenderness, and palpable sigmoid. Diagnosis is by abdominal pain x-ray films and proctosigmoidoscopy. Repeated attacks of diverticulitis may cause pericolic abscesses.

Possible complications of diverticular disease include rupture of an inflamed diverticulum, with localized or generalized peritonitis; abscess formation around the diverticulum; edema or spasm related to inflammation; vesicolonic fistula formation; erosion of an artery or vein; and colonic fibrosis and narrowing, possibly leading to obstruction.

Treatment of mildly symptomatic diverticular disease usually involves dietary management, most often in the form of a high-fiber diet, and use of hydrophilic colloids or bulk-forming laxatives to help maintain a regular, soft stool. Bed rest, antibiotics, and analgesics may be prescribed for acute attacks. For patients with colonic strictures or peritonitis or septicemia, surgical intervention may be necessary, in the form of a colon resection or a temporary diverting colostomy.

## Colorectal cancer

Colorectal cancer is the second most common cancer type in adults, after lung cancer in men and breast cancer in women. It occurs most frequently in persons who are between the ages of 50 and 80. Approximately 95% of intestinal cancers are adenocarcinomas. The highest percentage of colorectal cancers in U.S. whites are currently located in the cecum and ascending colon (22% in males, 27% in females) and sigmoid colon (25% in males and 23% in females). Metastasis usually involves the liver.

Risk factors for colorectal cancer include the following:

- A diet high in fat, protein, and beef and low in fiber
- Increasing age
- A family history of colon or rectal cancer
- Previous colon cancer
- A personal history of adenomatous polyps
- Familial polyposis or Gardner's syndrome
- UC for more than 7 years
- Genital cancer or breast cancer (in women)

Early detection of colon cancer is of primary importance, because for patients with carcinoma limited to the bowel wall, the 5-year survival rate is 75%, compared to only 5% for patients with disseminated disease. Unfortunately, large bowel tumors often exhibit no signs or symptoms until they become rather large, thereby reducing the likelihood of early diagnosis and making surgical cure difficult.

Periodic serial stool screening for occult blood is important to detect colorectal lesions before metastasis occurs. The American Cancer Society recommends annual digital rectal examinations after age 40, annual serial stool screening for occult blood for all persons over age 50, and sigmoidoscopy every 3 to 5 years from age 50 on, after two initial negative sigmoidoscopies 1 year apart. Patients with predisposing factors for colorectal cancer should receive more frequent and lifelong surveillance, beginning at an earlier age.

Signs and symptoms of a right-sided tumor may include melenic stools, dull abdominal pain referred to the upper abdomen and back, anorexia and weight loss, malaise, lethargy, weakness, and indigestion. Left-sided tumors frequently cause a distinct change in bowel habits, including difficulty passing stools, abdominal distention, ribbon- or pencil-shaped stools, constipation, cramping, flatulence, and a feeling of rectal pressure or incomplete stool evacuation.

To diagnose colorectal cancer, the physician may order a stool test for occult blood; sigmoidoscopy or colonoscopy with biopsy exam and brush cytology; barium enema, usually with air contrast; upper GI series if small intestine involvement is suspected; and possibly a serum carcinoembryonic antigen test.

Treatment of colorectal cancer depends on the stage of the disease. Two different methods are used to stage colon cancer: Duke's classification and the TNM classification. Duke's classification recognizes four stages of tumor involvement.

- Class A—limited to the mucosa and submucosa
- Class B—penetration of the entire bowel wall and serosa or pericolic fat
- Class C—Class A and B, plus invasion of the regional draining lymph node system
- Class D—advanced and widespread regional metastasis

TNM is an abbreviation for tumor, nodal involve-ment, and metastasis. The TNM classification describes the anatomic extent of the primary tumor depending on its size, invasion depth, and surface spread; the extent of nodal involvement; and the presence or absence of metastasis.

Most patients with colon cancer require either curative or palliative surgery, such as bowel resection and anastomosis or stoma formation. Surgery involves resection of the tumor and associated blood vessels, lymphatic channels, and affected structures as a unit. In some cases, the physician will irrigate the peritoneum with an antineoplastic agent and will do a biopsy examination of the liver and abdominal lymph nodes.

Many patients with intestinal cancer or other intestinal disorders require formation of a permanent or temporary colostomy. Formation of a colostomy involves making an outside opening, or **stoma,** on the abdomen using a section of the colon. There are three types of stomas, which are listed as follows

- A single-barrel stoma, in which the functioning proximal end of the bowel is brought through the abdominal wall, and then folded in on itself and sutured to form a cuff.
- A double-barrel stoma, in which both the active and inactive bowel ends are temporarily brought through the abdominal wall, thereby creating two stomas.
- A loop stoma, which is also a temporary procedure, and is formed by bringing an intact bowel loop through the abdominal wall and making an incision in the top of the loop.

Such patients require conscientious ostomy care, with priority given to protecting the skin from corrosive enzymes and to controlling odor and fecal drainage, and emotional support and encouragement.

Additional interventions for patients with colorectal cancer may include radiation therapy, chemotherapy, and/or immunotherapy.

### Intestinal obstruction

Congenital or acquired intestinal obstructions may occur in either the large or small intestine. The source of an obstruction may be mechanical, neurogenic, or vascular.

#### Mechanical obstruction

Mechanical obstructions that are related to congenital defects include atresia, stenosis, hernia, **malrotation,** meconium ileus, or aganglionic megacolon (Hirschsprung's disease).

**Hirschsprung's disease** is the congenital absence of intramural ganglia of the anorectum and variable lengths of the distal colon, resulting in failure of relaxation of the internal sphincter, followed by severe constipation and dilatation of the more proximal normal colon. It occurs in 1 of each 5000 live births and is familial. Approximately 2% of these patients have Down's syndrome.

Hirschsprung's disease becomes apparent shortly after birth when the infant passes little meconium and develops a distended colon. It is diagnosed by barium enema and anorectal manometry and confirmed by a full-thickness biopsy examination of the rectal mucosa. Surgical treatment is required and a number of operations have been proposed to remove or to counterbalance the obstructing effect of the aganglionic segment. One surgical method involves excision of the aganglionic rectum and colon and creation of a *neoanorectum* by pulling normal colon through the anal canal.

Acquired mechanical obstructions may develop secondary to adhesions from previous surgery, hernias, tumors, intussusception, volvulus, foreign objects, fecal impaction, or masses outside the intestine.

### Neurogenic obstruction (intestinal pseudoobstruction)

In neurogenic obstruction, there is no mechanical blockage, instead, this anomaly results from ineffective intestinal peristalsis. Paralysis in such patients is usually incomplete. Pain results from abdominal distention and heightens with increasing distention.

Chronic **intestinal pseudoobstruction** may be primary, associated with generalized visceral neuropathy, or secondary, associated with identifiable smooth muscle, endocrine, neurologic, or pharmacologic causes. Esophageal manometry has shown many of these patients to have poor peristalsis of the esophagus and incomplete relaxation of the LES.

Abdominal surgery may be a cause of neurologic impairment of peristalsis (adynamic or paralytic ileus), which is a reversible, self-limited form of pseudoobstruction that usually disappears 2 to 3 days after surgery. Diagnosis is made by observation of abdominal distention, gastric aspiration, lack of flatus, and **constipation.** **Paralytic ileus** may be prevented by maintaining fluid and electrolyte balance and by handling the bowel gently during surgery. It is treated by nasogastric suction and intravenous fluid administration to correct electrolyte imbalance. In some cases, rectal tube decompression or colonoscopic decompression may be performed.

### Vascular obstruction

Vascular obstructions occur when emboli or atherosclerotic narrowing interrupt the blood supply to the bowel. This type of obstruction inhibits peristalsis and can lead to life-threatening intestinal ischemia in as little as 40 minutes.

Another source of vascular obstruction is telangiectasia, in which capillaries and venules are dilated in the mucous membranes throughout the gastrointestinal system.

Symptoms of intestinal obstruction include abdominal pain, vomiting, **obstipation** (intractable constipation), failure to pass flatus, and abdominal distention. Diagnosis can be made by taking a careful history and conducting a thorough physical examination, but the physician may also order abdominal radiographic exams, a barium enema or swallow, and blood tests to detect dehydration, tissue necrosis, and electrolyte imbalance.

Intervention strategies for patients with intestinal obstructions involve the following:
- Restoring bowel patency
- Regulating fluids and electrolytes, often intravenously
- Administration of medications to control pain and nausea
- Administration of antibiotics to treat bacterial growth
- Use of a nasogastric or intestinal tube to relieve abdominal distention

After abdominal distention and compression have been controlled, surgical intervention is usually necessary. The type of surgery performed depends on the source of the obstruction, but may include hernia reduction, adhesion division, intestinal bypass, lesion excision, or a diverting colostomy.

After surgery the patient should be monitored for signs of recurrent obstruction or paralytic ileus. Any abdominal drain should be monitored for patency and drainage amount.

### Anorectal disorders

Anorectal disorders typically cause rectal pain, rectal bleeding, and/or a change in bowel habits. The cause may be hemorrhoids, fecal incontinence or impaction, rectal cancer, trauma, anorectal abscess, fissure, or fistula.

#### Hemorrhoids

Hemorrhoids are vascular masses in the anal canal. Internal hemorrhoids bulge into the rectal lumen above the internal sphincter and the anorectal line. External hemorrhoids are dilations of the inferior hemorrhoidal plexus; they lie below the anorectal line and protrude below the external sphincter. Symptoms include bright red rectal bleeding, occasionally leading to iron deficiency anemia; rectal pain, which may be severe; and in the case of external hemorrhoids, a sensation of a bulging mass upon exertion. Diagnosis is by proctoscopy or anoscopy.

Medical interventions for patients with hemorrhoids may include the following:
- A high-fiber diet and adequate fluid intake
- Warm compresses, analgesic ointments, and sitz baths
- Surgical intervention, such as rubber band ligation,

hemorrhoidectomy, cryosurgery, or infrared photocoagulation

### Fecal impaction

Fecal impaction is the formation of a large, firm, immovable mass of stool that occurs when normal movement of the feces is impaired. This allows the bowel to absorb more water than usual, thereby hardening the fecal matter and making it difficult to pass. Fecal impaction may be caused by dehydration, chronic constipation, inactivity, medications, anal disease that causes painful defecation, neurologic problems, or barium retention after radiologic studies. It is relatively common in children, resulting from voluntary withholding of stool subsequent to a painful bowel movement.

Symptoms of fecal impaction are abdominal discomfort; a sensation of rectal fullness; nausea, vomiting, and headache; passing small amounts of watery, malformed stool; or a large firm mass in the left lower quadrant. Treatment options include breakup of low-lying impactions digitally or administration of enemas and/or fluids or drugs to soften the stool and encourage its passage.

Possible complications of an untreated impaction include intestinal or urinary tract obstruction or spontaneous perforation.

### Anorectal abscess

Anorectal abscess occurs when infection causes localized accumulation of pus in the tissue spaces around the anorectum. Patients with Crohn's disease are particularly susceptible. One symptom may be throbbing pain in the anorectum, which worsens when the patient walks or sits. Typically, the physician will drain the abscess surgically and prescribe followup treatment of antibiotics and analgesics, sitz baths, and stool softeners. Complications of untreated abscess may include abscess extension or anorectal fistula.

### Anorectal fistula

An anorectal fistula is a hollow, fibrous tract leading from the anal canal or rectum to the perianal skin. The two main types of anorectal fistulas are an intersphincteric fistula and a transsphincteric fistula, which extends through the external sphincter muscles.

Usually, a primary drainage port drains into an anal crypt while a secondary port drains into the perianal skin or rectal mucous membrane. The primary symptom of anorectal fistula is a purulent drainage of pus, blood, mucus, or less commonly, stool. Females may complain of passage of flatus or feces through the vagina. Other symptoms may include pruritus, pain, or odor and the presence of a palpable tract on rectal examination. Anoscopy or sigmoidoscopy may locate the source of the fistula or abscess.

Anal fistulae are treated by fistulectomy to repair superficial, straight fistulas or fistulotomy to correct deep fistulas.

### Anal fissure

An anal fissure is a thin tear of the superficial anal mucosa. It occurs most commonly along the midline of the posterior anal canal. The most common cause is trauma following passage of a large, firm stool. If the fissure's edges adhere immediately after defecation, thereby preventing pus drainage, the resulting edema and fibrosis of adjacent tissue may cause the development of a sentinel pile or tag at the lower end of the fissure.

Symptoms of anal fissures include severe tearing or burning sensations after defecation, anal itching, and discharge of bright red blood. Diagnosis is by digital rectal exam, anoscopy, or sigmoidoscopy.

Most fissures can be treated with analgesic ointments, sitz baths, and bulk agents or laxatives. Surgical excision or lateral subcutaneous sphincterotomy may be required for chronic fissures.

### Rectal prolapse

Rectal prolapse occurs when rectal mucosa bulges through the anus, often as a result of increased intraabdominal pressure when straining. Prolapse may also result from relaxed anal sphincters and weak pelvic muscles. Symptoms are a protruding rectal mass that is apparent on defecation or other exertion, mucus discharge, rectal bleeding, and fecal incontinence.

Rectal prolapse may be prevented by avoiding constipation and prolonged straining. Primary treatment involves reduction of the prolapse.

---

**CASE SITUATION**

David Rosenstein, age 24, is a medical student who has been doing an internship rotation in pediatrics. In the last few months he has experienced fatigue and aching joints. Feeling overworked and stressed, he took a week off to go camping with his wife. During the following month he began to notice frequent episodes of bloody, mucopurulent diarrhea. He then began having abdominal cramps and more joint tenderness. He thought he must have gotten "a bug" and visited a gastroenterologist because his symptoms seemed to be getting worse. After a battery of tests and colonoscopic examination with biopsy exam, Mr. Rosenstein was diagnosed as having UC and was placed in the hospital for treatment because of his debilitated condition.

*Points to think about*

1. After learning of Mr. Rosenstein's diagnosis and history, what physical findings might the gastroenterology nurse expect?

2. The nurse knows that colonic biopsy exam can differentiate UC from Crohn's disease by showing submucosal inflammatory reactions and granuloma; what else differentiates these two types of inflammatory bowel disease?

3. Initial planning and nursing intervention for Mr. Rosenstein would, of necessity, focus on restoration of his physiologic equilibrium. The nurse's data search and assessment could substantiate at least four possible nursing diagnoses in the physiologic realm. What are they?

4. UC requires a great deal of reorganization of the victim's life. Establishing a trusting relationship with Mr. Rosenstein and his wife is critical if the gastroenterology nurse is to help them in these efforts. Once such a relationship is tentatively established, what is the most important psychologic area to which assessment should be directed?

5. Because it is quite likely that Mr. Rosenstein is anxious, substantiation of the nursing diagnosis *anxiety,* possibly related to threats to bodily health, self-concept, and altered role performance and lack of control over events is necessary. What are the defining characteristics of this diagnosis?

6. There are three general goals for the nursing care of a patient with the nursing diagnosis *anxiety.* What are they?

### Suggested responses

1. Physical findings that might be expected in a patient with UC include the following:
   - Fever, tachycardia, signs of dehydration and hypovolemia; imminent cardiovascular collapse in severe abrupt-onset cases
   - Pallor, secondary to anemia
   - Tenderness on abdominal palpation and increased bowel sounds on auscultation
   - Redness, swelling, and tenderness in large joints
   - Abdominal distention and profuse bloody mucopurulent diarrhea, vomiting, and debilitation in severe cases with toxic megacolon
   - Skin manifestations on the arms and legs, such as erythema nodosum or pyoderma gangrenosum
   - Ankylosing spondylitis (occuring in 6% of patients with UC), defined as an inflammation of one or more vertebrae and the sacroiliac joint
   - Conjunctivitis or uveitis (inflammation of the vascular middle coat of the eye) in the early course of UC

2. Factors that differentiate UC from Crohn's disease are as follows:

| Ulcerative colitis | Crohn's disease |
| --- | --- |
| Continuous inflammation | "Skip areas" or segmental areas of ulceration, with normal tissue between ulcerations |
| Mucosal ulceration only | Ulcerations typically affect all layers of the bowel wall |
| Most often seen in the left colon and rectosigmoid areas, but at times may involve the entire colon | Usually seen in the right colon and involving the terminal ileum, but may involve any area of the GI tract |
| Characterized by exacerbations and remissions | Often slow and progressive |
| May cause a shortening effect on the bowel | Can narrow the lumen, with stricture formation |
| Cobblestoning effect less consistent | More consistent mucosal "cobblestoning" effect seen on radiographic examination |
| Diarrhea is bloody and mucopurulent | Diarrhea is watery and sometimes associated with steatorrhea |
| Pseudopolyps common | Pseudopolyps rare |
| Inflammatory masses rare | Inflammatory masses common |

3. Possible nursing diagnoses in the physiologic realm include the following:
   - Altered nutrition: less than body requirements
   - Diarrhea related to bowel irritability
   - Fluid volume deficit
   - Acute pain related to bowel irritability
   - activity intolerance related to weakness, debilitated condition, and joint swelling

4. The most important psychologic priority toward which assessment should be directed is determining Mr. Rosenstein's coping mechanisms and skills. Without knowing the mechanisms by which he commonly manages problems and stresses in his daily life, a nurse cannot initiate a plan to aid him in adapting his life.

5. The defining characteristics* of the nursing diagnosis *anxiety* are as follows:
   - Reported apprehension, nervousness
   - Escape/avoidance behavior
   - Physiologic arousal
   - Narrowed perceptual field; difficulty concentrating; self-focusing
   - Inappropriate behaviors, such as anger, fear, guilt, and regression
   - Denial
   - Withdrawal
   - Increased wariness

6. Three general goals for the nursing care of a patient with the nursing diagnosis *anxiety* are: prevention of severe anxiety or panic status, elimination or reduction of incapacitating anxiety status, and use of effective coping skills.

---

* Critical indicators have not been identified.

The nurse must realize that specific, concrete, personalized patient outcomes within these broad goals may be multiple and may be based on a variety of factors and possible patient responses.

---

## REVIEW TERMS

**amebiasis, anus, ascending colon, cecum, colitis, Crohn's colitis, colon, constipation, descending colon, diarrhea, diverticulitis, diverticulosis, enterocolitis, familial polyposis, Gardner's syndrome, haustra, hematochezia, hepatic flexure, Hirschsprung's disease, intestinal pseudoobstruction, irritable bowel syndrome (IBS), ischemic colitis, malrotation, megacolon, obstipation, paralytic ileus, polyps, pseudomembranous colitis, radiation enteritis, rectum, sigmoid colon, splenic flexure, stoma, tenesmus, tenia coli, toxic megacolon, transverse colon, ulcerative colitis (UC), Valsalva maneuver, vermiform appendix**

---

## REVIEW QUESTIONS

1. The first portion of the large intestine to receive material from the small bowel is the:
   a. Ileum.
   b. Cecum.
   c. Appendix.
   d. Ascending colon.
2. The small sacculations in the large intestinal wall that are formed by the tenia coli are called the:
   a. Haustra.
   b. Diverticula.
   c. Crypts of Lieberkühn.
   d. Plicae semilunares.
3. The colonic mucosa is:
   a. Made up of thousands of fingerlike projections called villi.
   b. Covered with a layer of squamous epithelium.
   c. Arranged in folds called the plicae circulares.
   d. Smooth-surfaced.
4. Colonic secretion consists primarily of:
   a. Sodium, chloride, and water.
   b. Water, mucus, potassium, and bicarbonate.
   c. Mucus and hormones.
   d. Bile pigments and toxins.
5. The appearance of multiple adenomatous polyps in the GI tract and osteomas of the mandible, skull, and long bones is symptomatic of:
   a. Osler-Weber-Rendu disease.
   b. Colorectal cancer.
   c. Familial polyposis.
   d. Gardner's syndrome.
6. Toxic megacolon is a potentially serious complication of:
   a. Ischemic colitis.
   b. Ulcerative colitis.
   c. Pseudomembranous colitis.
   d. Transmural colitis.
7. The most commonly accepted cause of irritable bowel syndrome is:
   a. An anatomic abnormality.
   b. A high-fat, low-fiber diet.
   c. An exaggerated motility response to environmental stress.
   d. A parasitic infestation.
8. Mildly symptomatic diverticular disease is most often treated by:
   a. Diverticulectomy.
   b. Colon resection.
   c. Dietary management and hydrophilic colloids or bulk-forming laxatives.
   d. Colostomy.
9. Metastatic colorectal cancer most often involves the:
   a. Small bowel.
   b. Liver.
   c. Pancreas.
   d. Stomach.
10. A hollow, fibrous tract leading from the anal canal or rectum to the perianal skin is called a(n):
    a. Hemorrhoid.
    b. Anorectal fissure.
    c. Anorectal abscess.
    d. Anorectal fistula.

## BIBLIOGRAPHY

Bahr, A. "The Large Intestine." In *SGA Journal Reprints,* ed. Trivits, S, 143-44. Rochester, N.Y.: Society of Gastrointestinal Assistants, 1988.

Bongiovanni, G, ed. *Essentials of Clinical Gastroenterology.* 2nd ed. New York: McGraw–Hill, 1988.

Chobanian, S, and Van Ness, M, eds. *Manual of Clinical Problems in Gastroenterology.* Boston: Little, Brown & Co., 1988.

Chopra, S, and May, R, eds. *Pathophysiology of Gastrointestinal Diseases.* Boston: Little, Brown & Co., 1989.

Eastwood, G, and Avunduk, C. *Manual of Gastroenterology: Diagnosis and Therapy.* Boston: Little, Brown & Co., 1988.

Gardner, S. "Colorectal Cancer." In *SGA Journal Reprints,* ed. Trivits, S, 159-60. Rochester, N.Y.: Society of Gastrointestinal Assistants, 1988.

Given, B, and Simmons, S. *Gastroenterology in Clinical Nursing.* 4th ed. St. Louis: Mosby–Year Book, 1984.

Goldberg, K, ed. *Gastrointestinal Problems.* Nurse Review Series. Springhouse, Pa.: Springhouse Corporation, 1986.

Kraft, S. "Ulcerative Colitis." In *SGA Journal Reprints,* ed. Trivits, S, 145-48. Rochester, N.Y.: Society of Gastrointestinal Assistants, 1988.

Larson, D. "Advanced Anatomy and Physiology of the Colon." *SGA Journal* 10(Fall 1987): 92-97.

Sleisenger, M, and Fordtran, J, eds. *Gastrointestinal Disease: Pathophysiology, Diagnosis, Management.* 4th ed. Philadelphia: W.B. Saunders, 1989.

Swartz, M. "Beyond the Scope: A Nursing View of the Extraintestinal Manifestations of Inflammatory Bowel Disease." *Gastroenterology Nursing* 12(Summer 1989): 172-78.

# Chapter 18

# BILIARY SYSTEM

This chapter will acquaint the gastroenterology nurse with the normal anatomy and physiology of the biliary system. In addition, selected pathologic conditions of the gallbladder and its associated duct system are described with respect to pathophysiology, diagnosis, and treatment.

**Learning objectives**

After reviewing the content of this chapter, the gastroenterology nurse should be able to:
1. Describe the normal gross structure and histology of the biliary system, including the gallbladder and its associated duct system.
2. Explain the motility and secretory functions of the gallbladder.
3. Discuss a number of pathologic conditions that

affect the biliary system in terms of pathophysiology, diagnosis, and treatment.

**ANATOMY**

The biliary system consists of the gallbladder and its associated duct system; that is, the hepatic, cystic, and common bile ducts (Fig. 18-1). The **gallbladder** itself is a pear-shaped, saclike bile storage structure. It is attached to the undersurface of the liver by connective tissue, peritoneum, and blood vessels (see Plate 1). The gallbladder is approximately 7 to 10 cm (3 inches) long and 2.5 to 3.5 cm (about 1 inch) wide and is capable of holding up to 50 ml of bile.

The four anatomic divisions of the gallbladder are as follows:
• The distal blind sac, or fundus

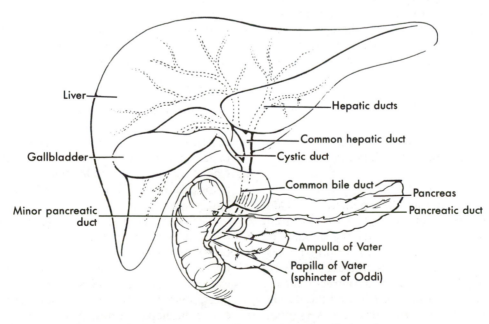

**Fig. 18-1**. Anatomy of liver, biliary, and pancreatic ductal systems.

- The funnel-shaped body, which connects the fundus and the infundibulum
- The infundibulum, which connects the body to the neck
- The neck, which narrows into the cystic duct

As it emerges from the gallbladder, the **cystic duct** combines with the **hepatic duct** to form the **common bile duct,** which joins with the main pancreatic duct to form the ampulla of Vater. The ampulla empties into the duodenum at an orifice called the papilla of Vater, or major papilla. During their passage through the duodenal wall, the common bile duct, the pancreatic duct, and the ampulla of Vater are surrounded by a complex arrangement of smooth muscles called the **sphincter of Oddi.**

The functions of the sphincter of Oddi are to regulate the flow of bile and pancreatic juices into the intestine, inhibit entry of bile into the pancreatic duct, and prevent reflux of intestinal contents into the ducts. The gallbladder is not an essential organ; if it is removed, bile flow continues to be regulated by the sphincter of Oddi.

The walls of the gallbladder have three layers, which are listed as follows:

- An outer serosa that is derived from the peritoneum
- A fibromuscular layer that contains longitudinal and spiral smooth muscle and fibrous tissue
- An inner mucosa that is made up of simple columnar epithelium and is arranged in folds or rugae similar to those of the stomach

Blood supply to the biliary system is delivered by the hepatic artery and is drained through the cystic vein. Sympathetic innervation is derived from the splanchnic nerve and the seventh through tenth thoracic segments. Sympathetic stimulation inhibits smooth muscle gallbladder contraction. Parasympathetic innervation is derived from the right branch of the vagus nerve. Mild parasympathetic stimulation causes the gallbladder to contract and relaxes the sphincter of Oddi at the duodenal junction.

## PHYSIOLOGY

The functions of the biliary system are to collect, concentrate, and store bile and to release it into the duodenum when it is needed for digestion.

### Motility

Under normal conditions the sphincter of Oddi remains slightly opened, thereby allowing for a constant but miniscule amount of bile to enter the duodenum. When food enters the duodenum during normal digestion, the hormone cholecystokinin-pancreozymin is released, thus causing the gallbladder to contract, which in turn pushes increased amounts of bile into the duodenum. Other factors, such as certain drugs, sensory input, disease, and emotional states may also affect the filling and contracting of the gallbladder.

### Secretion

**Bile** is an alkaline, greenish yellow fluid that is secreted continuously by the liver. Its major components are water, which makes up 97% of hepatic bile; bile salts; fatty acids; lipids, mainly cholesterol and lecithin; inorganic electrolytes; conjugated bilirubin; and other organic substances. When bile flows from the liver, through the cystic duct, and into the gallbladder for storage, up to 90% of the water is removed.

Bile has a variety of functions, which include the emulsification of undigested fats; the facilitation of the absorption of fat-soluble vitamins; the activation of intestinal and pancreatic enzymes; and the provision of a route for the excretion of bilirubin, cholesterol, and certain sex, thyroid, and adrenal hormones. Bile also affects the absorption of certain minerals and helps to neutralize gastric acid in the duodenum.

If the flow of bile through the common bile duct or hepatic ducts is obstructed by gallstones or other abnormalities, bile builds up in the blood, resulting in hyperbilirubinemia. Bile pigments, mainly bilirubin, are deposited in the skin, mucous membranes, and sclera, causing a yellow discoloration of these areas that is commonly known as **jaundice.** Jaundice may also result from destruction of red blood cells or from liver cell dysfunction.

## PATHOPHYSIOLOGY

Gallbladder and duct diseases may be short-term and easily correctable or may be long-term and debilitating. Generally, they present during middle age and incidence increases with age. In persons who are between the ages of 20 and 50, gallbladder and duct diseases are 6 times more common in women than in men, but after age 50 the incidence in men and women becomes equal.

Biliary tract disorders include cholelithiasis, choledocholithiasis, cholecystitis, cholangitis, carcinoma, and various congenital anomalies.

### Cholelithiasis

**Cholelithiasis** is the presence of stones or calculi in the gallbladder. As many as 1 million new cases of cholelithiasis are diagnosed each year and approximately half of those patients undergo biliary surgery. Cholelithiasis is the fifth leading cause of hospitalization among adults and accounts for 90% of all diseases of the biliary system.

The two types of gallstones are cholesterol stones and pigment stones. Cholesterol stones, including both pure cholesterol stones and mixed stones, make up three fourths of all gallstones. They contain cholesterol, calcium salts, bile acids, fatty acids, protein, and phospholipids. Cholesterol stones are associated with either the hepatic production of bile that is supersaturated with cholesterol, or with reduced bile-salt secretion. When cholesterol is no longer soluble in this supersaturated system, it forms crystal nucleates, which grow and cluster with each other and with other bile constituents to form recognizable stones in the gallbladder.

Pigment stones are less common than cholesterol stones. They include black pigment stones, which are made up of bilirubin polymers and inorganic calcium salts, and brown pigment stones, which are composed principally of calcium bilirubinate and organic fatty-acid salts of calcium. Black, radiopaque stones are seen more frequently in the West, while brown, radiolucent stones are more common in the Orient.

Risk factors for the formation of cholesterol gallstones include the following:

- Increasing age
- Female sex
- Pregnancy or use of oral contraceptives
- Estrogen therapy
- Ethnicity, particularly specific nonobese European and Chilean patients; obese American Indian females
- Ileal disease, resection, or bypass
- Certain forms of hyperlipidemia
- Obesity
- Weight reduction diets
- Use of certain drugs, such as clofibrate (Atromid-S)
- Gallbladder stasis
- Spinal cord injury

The prevalence of pigment stones is not influenced by gender. Risk factors for the formation of pigment stones include the following:

- Increasing age
- Chronic hemolysis, such as sickle cell disease or thalassemia
- Alcoholism or alcoholic cirrhosis
- Biliary infection, usually *Escherichia coli,* or parasitic infestation, such as *Clonorchis sinensis, Ascaris lumbricoides*
- Total parenteral nutrition
- Vagotomy
- Periampullary diverticula
- Gallbladder stasis

Gallstones may move around in the gallbladder as it empties and refills. If they remain in one place they may be asymptomatic. However, stones that move to the neck, cystic duct, or common duct may obstruct those passages, thus resulting in mucosal irritation and subsequent bacterial invasion. Stones may also pass through the biliary ducts, causing pain, or they may obstruct the flow of bile if they become lodged there. It is possible for small stones to be located in any part of the biliary system without causing distress or even to pass into the duodenum and be discharged in the stool.

Gallstones are asymptomatic in at least 50% of patients. Even in symptomatic patients, the severity, extent, and nature of the symptoms vary considerably depending on the movement of the stones, the degree of obstruction, if any, and the presence or absence of inflammation.

Symptomatic patients usually complain of a steady pain, which often stems from gallbladder distention or spasm of the sphincter of Oddi or ductal muscles. This pain is referred to as **biliary colic.** Pain most often occurs 3 to 6 hours after the heaviest meal of the day, frequently during the early hours of the night. Pain often radiates to other parts of the abdomen or back, and sometimes to the scapula, the middle of the back, or the tip of the right shoulder. Nausea and vomiting may occur and pain may be relieved by vomiting. Patients may have vague symptoms of upper abdominal discomfort, increased eructation, and dyspepsia. Some patients also have fever and chills resulting from a common duct stone, acute cholecystitis, or associated pancreatitis.

In children, mild to moderate jaundice is a common symptom, but gallbladder enlargement is infrequent. Because the diagnosis of cholelithiasis is seldom considered in children, the delay between onset of symptoms and diagnosis in this age group may be from 1 to 5 years. Stones are generally found in the gallbladder, and seldom occlude either the cystic or the common bile duct. Most children have a specific etiologic factor, such as prolonged total parenteral nutrition, congenital hemolytic disease, or ileal disease.

Ultrasonography is the most effective diagnostic technique for cholelithiasis; it can identify stones that are as small as 2 mm. Oral cholecystography or cholangiography may also be ordered. If both oral cholecystography and ultrasonography are negative and symptoms are suggestive of cholelithiasis, the next test should be endoscopic retrograde cholangiopancreatography (ERCP) and/or examination of duodenal bile for cholesterol crystals or bilirubinate granules.

Noninterventional "expectant" management is preferred for asymptomatic patients because neither medical dissolution therapy nor elective cholecystectomy is warranted in such cases. Management of patients with minor symptoms may include pain relief and dietary control to reduce fat intake. Small, frequent meals can sometimes help to prevent future attacks. In children, cholecystectomy is probably indicated, regardless of the severity of symptoms.

Surgery is the treatment of choice for most symptomatic patients. Typically, a cholecystectomy is used to excise the gallbladder and ligate the cystic duct. Prognosis is generally good, but may vary depending on the patient's age, sex, and the presence of complicating conditions, such as cholecystitis, cholangitis, or pancreatitis.

In addition to cholecystectomy, a variety of newer techniques exist for the dissolution or removal of cholesterol stones, including the following:

- Dissolution of gallstones using chenodeoxycholic

acid (CDCA, Chenix) or ursodeoxycholic acid (UDCA, Actigall), both of which are naturally occurring bile salts. This alternative is successful in 50% of patients. Patients who are considered for medical dissolution therapy must have patent cystic ducts and radiolucent stones; be postmenopausal or be using mechanical contraceptive methods; and have small stones. Notable adverse reactions to CDCA therapy include both dose-related serum aminotransferase elevations and diarrhea. Diarrhea is a less frequent adverse effect of UDCA.

• Continuous infusion of methyl tert-butyl ether into the gallbladder to dissolve stones.
• Infusion of substances such as cholate sodium and heparin through a T-tube to dissolve stones.
• Biliary lithotripsy, which involves fragmentation of gallstones by use of extracorporeal acoustic shock waves, and is often combined with dissolution therapy. This experimental treatment method can be used on an outpatient basis. Patients have less pain, a shorter recovery period, and less chance of infection than those who have cholecystectomies.

The disadvantages of all of these medical therapies are the probability of recurrence of cholelithiasis after cessation of the therapeutic modality and concerns regarding the effects of long-term use.

No medical intervention options exist for pigment stones. Surgery is the only alternative for symptomatic patients with stones of this type.

Approximately 5% to 8% of cholecystectomy patients later exhibit postcholecystectomy syndrome, defined as abdominal pain or dyspepsia in patients who have had a cholecystectomy. Postcholecystectomy syndrome is most often seen in women who are between the ages of 40 and 49. Their distress cannot be attributed to the surgical procedure itself. Potential causes include residual biliary tract disease, nonbiliary digestive disease, nonspecific digestion dysfunction, and psychiatric disorders. Treatment is determined by the specific diagnosis. Retained common bile duct stones, for example, are not uncommon following cholecystectomy. These stones may be removed by endoscopic introduction of a basket or balloon into the common bile duct, by a second surgical procedure, or through nonoperative manipulation of a basket inserted through a T-tube.

Potential complications of cholelithiasis include cholecystitis, cholangitis, abscess or fistula formation, perforation of the gallbladder, gangrene, and hepatic damage. Cholelithiasis has also been linked to gallbladder cancer.

### Choledocholithiasis

The presence of gallstones in the common bile duct or the hepatic duct is called **choledocholithiasis.** This problem occurs when stones passed out of the gallbladder lodge in the hepatic duct or the common bile duct and obstruct the flow of bile into the duodenum. In about 5% of cases, common duct stones are primary stones that form in the common bile duct. Such stones are always pigment stones; in fact, about 40% of common bile duct stones are pigment stones. The available evidence suggests that cholesterol stones in the duct are always secondary stones that were formed in the gallbladder, while pigment stones can be either primary or secondary.

Patients with choledocholithiasis may have no symptoms or may present with any combination of the following:

• Biliary colic, with constant epigastric or right upper quadrant pain or tenderness
• Obstructive jaundice and pruritus
• Cholangitis, with fever, right upper quadrant pain, jaundice, and often, rigor
• Acute gallstone pancreatitis, manifested by severe abdominal pain that radiates into the back

Differential diagnosis may require laboratory blood and liver function tests, ultrasonography, radioisotope imaging, oral cholecystography, ERCP, or percutaneous transhepatic cholangiography (PTC).

Patients with choledocholithiasis should be kept NPO. They should be stabilized by intravenous maintenance of fluid and electrolyte balance. Continuous nasogastric suction and analgesia should be provided and antibiotics may be prescribed if there is evidence of sepsis or cholangitis. The preferred method of treatment is an endoscopic sphincterotomy, which involves cutting the fibers of the sphincter of Oddi during ERCP. Alternatively, the common bile duct may be explored surgically, through a choledochotomy.

If the common bile duct is explored surgically to remove retained stones, a T-tube is inserted to provide a means of decompressing the biliary ducts. The tube can be removed in the clinician's office 3 weeks after surgery. Before postoperative extraction of the T-tube, a cholangiogram should be performed to detect residual stones. About 2% of patients undergoing choledochotomy have residual stones.

Retained common bile duct stones can be removed by inserting a basket through the T-tube or by endoscopically introducing a basket or balloon for extraction. Large stones that are difficult to remove may be fragmented by a mechanical lithotripter basket and the fragments pulled out by a balloon. Another alternative is to place a nasobiliary catheter into the duct and infuse a cholesterol solvent to dissolve the stone or shrink its size for easier mechanical removal. Attempted dissolution of retained common duct stones with T-tube infusion of other cholesterol solvents is not recommended.

Complications of choledocholithiasis may include cholangitis, cirrhosis with hepatic failure, portal hypertension, or hepatic abscess formation.

## Cholecystitis

**Cholecystitis** is an acute or chronic inflammation that causes painful distention of the gallbladder. Ten to twenty-five percent of patients who require surgery for gallbladder disease have cholecystitis.

### Acute calculous cholecystitis

More than 90% of the time, cholecystitis is associated with a gallstone that is impacted in the cystic duct, hence acute calculous cholecystitis. The obstructed gallbladder becomes distended, and the walls become edematous, ischemic, and inflamed. Secondary infections with enteric organisms may compound the inflammation, leading to cholangitis and sepsis.

Predisposing factors to acute cholecystitis include older age, ethnicity (especially persons of Italian, Jewish, or Chinese descent), obesity, a sedentary lifestyle, pregnancy, hemolytic anemias, and insulin-dependent diabetes mellitus.

Acute cholecystitis produces the following symptoms, which are similar to those of cholelithiasis:

- Acute abdominal pain, usually midepigastric or localized to the right upper quadrant, with radiation to the shoulders and back
- Nausea, vomiting, and anorexia
- Fever, headache, leukocytosis
- Tachycardia and tachypnea
- Tenderness, guarding, and rebound tenderness in the right upper quadrant
- Intolerance of fatty foods and heavy meals

To confirm the diagnosis, the physician may order blood tests, ultrasonography, and radioisotope imaging.

Patients with cholecystitis should be stabilized with nasogastric suctioning, intravenous fluid and electrolyte replacement, and analgesia. Antibiotics should be given in cases of severe illness, sepsis, or complications. Early cholecystectomy is the preferred treatment approach.

If cholecystectomy is contraindicated by the patient's condition, an operative or percutaneous cholecystostomy may be performed. In this procedure the gallbladder is evacuated of stones and infected bile, and a Foley catheter drains to the outside. Temporary or short-term biliary decompression can also be accomplished by using ERCP to place a nasobiliary catheter (NBC) above the impacted stone. An NBC catheter consists of a long polyethylene tube, one end of which is placed inside the biliary tree with the other end exiting through the nostril and connecting to a bile drainage bag, thereby allowing the NBC to function as a T-tube.

Potential complications of acute cholecystitis include perforation with subsequent peritonitis or cholecystenteric fistula, or gallstone ileus, which is a form of intermittent or permanent intestinal obstruction that is caused by the impaction of a large gallstone that has entered the intestine through a cholecystenteric fistula. Such obstructions are most often found in the ileum because of its relatively small diameter compared to the rest of the intestine. Gallstone ileus requires an emergency laparotomy.

### Acalculous cholecystitis

Acute cholecystitis in the absence of stones is relatively rare and usually occurs in otherwise severely ill hospitalized patients. Intercurrent illnesses include bacterial enteric infections, such as typhoid fever, shigellosis, or *E. coli;* viral gastroenteritis; scarlet fever; respiratory infections; or pneumonia. Parasitic infestations with *Giardia* or *Ascaris* have also been found in the gallbladders of some patients. Acalculous cholecystitis also occurs in patients who have been hospitalized for burns, trauma, or severe cardiovascular disease. Most of these patients have been receiving total parenteral nutrition. Absence of oral intake associated with gallbladder stasis, sludge formation, and increased biliary pressure caused by narcotic drugs that increase the tone at the sphincter of Oddi may contribute to its pathogenesis.

Symptoms of acute acalculous cholecystitis include an acute onset of abdominal pain on the right side, abdominal tenderness and guarding, vomiting, and nausea. Usually, the diagnosis is made by abdominal ultrasonography. The incidence of gangrene, necrosis, and perforation is high in this group of patients, and mortality may be as high as 50%. Because of the high incidence of complications, the treatment of choice for acalculous cholecystitis is urgent cholecystectomy or cholecystostomy. Patients should also be treated with antibiotics to cover enteric organisms and enterococcus, and other supportive measures should be taken as needed.

### Emphysematous cholecystitis

In emphysematous cholecystitis, the gallbladder walls and bile ducts contain gas that has been produced by infective organisms such as *E. coli, Clostridium,* and other anaerobes. Acute cholecystectomy is performed in these cases.

## Cholangitis

**Cholangitis** is a rare bacterial infection of the bile duct that is often associated with choledocholithiasis or with obstruction of the bile duct by strictures, cysts, fistulas, or neoplasms. Widespread inflammation may cause fibrosis and stenosis of the common bile duct. Most patients experience a transient, self-limited illness that is characterized by a fever spike, chills, dark urine, and abdominal pain. In other patients, however, the illness is devastating, consistent with profound toxic sepsis with shock and impaired mental function. Prognosis for these patients is poor.

Bacteremia is present in 40% of these patients. The organisms responsible are most often *E. coli* and *Klebsiella.* When bacterial infection is severe, invasion of the liver parenchyma may occur, resulting in abscess formation.

Cholangitis is a medical and surgical emergency. The patient should be stabilized with intravenous hydration and antibiotics, which should be followed by prompt surgical or endoscopic decompression of the common bile duct. Drainage of the biliary tree should produce immediately beneficial results.

### Primary sclerosing cholangitis

**Primary sclerosing cholangitis (PSC)** is a rare inflammatory process that results in multiple strictures of the bile ducts. Its etiology is unknown. Sixty to seventy percent of patients with PSC have ulcerative colitis (UC) or have had it in the past.

Clinical manifestations of PSC are jaundice, pruritus, portal hypertension, abdominal pain, and elevated serum alkaline phosphatase. Diagnosis is by ultrasonography, ERCP or PTC, and liver biopsy examination. ERCP might show strictured areas in the intrahepatic and extrahepatic ducts with areas of dilatation between the strictures, thus producing a beaded appearance to the ducts.

Subclinical PSC requires no treatment. If pruritus occurs, it can be treated with bile-salt binding agents, such as cholestyramine (Questran). To bypass tight strictures, surgery or endoscopic placement of biliary stents may be required. Liver transplant may be the only viable treatment in the advanced stages of the disease. Progression to cirrhosis and portal hypertension is expected; most deaths occur 5 to 7 years after the onset of symptoms.

## Carcinoma

Cancer of the biliary system may involve the gallbladder or, less often, the bile ducts.

### Gallbladder cancer

Carcinoma of the gallbladder accounts for approximately 3% of all cancers. It occurs more frequently in women than in men and incidence peaks at age 70. Approximately 80% of patients with gallbladder carcinoma also have gallstones.

Patients with gallbladder cancer usually present with vague abdominal symptoms, including nausea, vomiting, substantial weight loss, anorexia, fat intolerance, and right upper quadrant pain. If a palpable right upper quadrant mass can be felt, the lesion is almost always incurable.

Diagnostic tests that are used include cholecystograms, cholangiograms, PTC, and ERCP. Scanning and ultrasonography may also be done. In practice, cancer of the gallbladder is rarely diagnosed preoperatively because signs and symptoms are similar to those for cancer of the liver or pancreas or for obstructive cholelithiasis.

Approximately 80% of gallbladder cancers are adenocarcinomas. The remainder are squamous cell carcinomas, adenocanthomas, and others. Benign tumors are rare. Most patients have evidence of local or metastatic spread, often through the lymph nodes, at the time of diagnosis. The majority survive less than 1 year following diagnosis; the 5-year survival rate is approximately 5%, and in most of these patients the tumor was discovered incidentally.

Medical treatment should be supportive and symptomatic, with the goals of comfort and short-term rehabilitation. For most patients, neither resection, radiotherapy, nor chemotherapy seems to prolong survival. If surgery is performed, the average postoperative survival time is only 8 months. Cholecystectomy is indicated only for patients with small, localized tumors. If the lesion is inoperable, an internal bile drainage system may be inserted to permit the flow of bile directly from the liver into the intestine. The objectives of this procedure are to relieve symptoms and to prolong the quality and length of life.

To minimize malnutrition and dehydration problems, the patient may be given antiemetics or small sips of carbonated beverages to control nausea; vitamin and mineral replacements; frequent small meals; small amounts of pain medication before meals; and, if necessary, tube feeding. In the terminal stages of the disease, skin care, pain relief, and emotional support are of vital importance.

### Bile duct cancers

Cancer of the extrahepatic biliary tree is associated with gallstones in only 30% of patients. It may also be associated with long-standing UC, PSC, and/or congenital dilatations of the bile ducts (e.g., choledochal cysts). Often, the patient presents with painless obstructive jaundice. Later, pruritus, nausea, vomiting, weight loss, and intermittent or steady right upper quadrant pain may develop. Serum alkaline phosphatase is always elevated.

Adenocarcinoma is the most common form of cancer in the biliary tree. Benign neoplasms are relatively rare. This type of cancer is most often diagnosed at the time of laparotomy for other biliary tract disease. Most patients have localized extension or metastatic disease at the time of diagnosis.

Ultrasonography or CT scan may be used to visualize dilated intrahepatic bile ducts, and PTC or ERCP should be used preoperatively to define the level and cause of the obstruction.

The treatment of choice for patients with localized carcinoma of the proximal biliary tree is surgery, consisting of pancreaticoduodenectomy. Five-year survival rates are less than 20%. For distal common duct or hepatic duct carcinomas, treatment is basically palliative. These patients often survive less than 1 year.

The most common pediatric neoplasm of the biliary tract is botryoid embryonal rhabdomyosarcoma. Symptoms include pruritus, jaundice, right upper quadrant and epigastric abdominal pain, and sometimes a palpable mass. The tumor is usually locally invasive. Even with a large surgical resection and radiation and drug therapy, prognosis is extremely poor.

### Congenital abnormalities

Congenital anomalies may occur in either the gallbladder or the bile ducts.

#### Gallbladder anomalies

Congenital anomalies of the gallbladder include the following:

- Agenesis, or congenital absence of the gallbladder, which most likely occurs as a result of embryonic maldevelopment.
- Anomalies of location (ectopic gallbladder), which may occur anywhere in the abdomen, and often require cholecystectomy.
- Anomalies of form, in which more than one cystic structure is found in the gallbladder fossa, suggesting either double gallbladder, bilobed gallbladder, folded fundus, or Ladd's bands across a normal gallbladder. If one of the two organs is found to be diseased at the time of surgery, both should be removed.
- Anomalies of fixation, which occur when the mesenteric supporting structures of the gallbladder are elongated, leaving a normally functioning gallbladder to "float" below the inferior surface of the liver and occasionally into the pelvis. If this floating gallbladder twists, vascular occlusion, ischemic necrosis, or perforation may occur, requiring cholecystectomy.

#### Bile duct anomalies

Congenital anomalies of the bile ducts include the following:

- Anomalies of extrahepatic duct configuration, such as atresia, accessory ducts, abnormal lengths of ducts, and variations in the junction of the cystic and hepatic ducts. Liver transplantation has greatly improved the survival rate of children with biliary atresia.
- Cystic anomalies of the common bile duct, including cystic dilatation of the common bile duct (choledochal cyst), which makes up 85% of these anomalies; congenital choledochocele; and congenital diverticulum of the common bile duct. In patients with choledochal cyst, symptoms generally appear after age 17. Diagnosis is by ultrasonography, and the recommended treatment is Roux-en-Y choledochocystojejunostomy with cholecystotomy. Complete excision of the cyst is recommended.
- Cystic dilatation of the intrahepatic ducts, or Caroli's disease, which is a rare disorder that most

often presents in young adults. Symptoms include bile stasis, cholangitis, and intrahepatic stone or abscess formation.

Anomalies of either the gallbladder or the bile ducts may impair the normal flow of bile, resulting in **cholestasis**, which leads to sludging—the formation in the gallbladder of an amorphous material consisting of cholesterol monohydrate crystals and bilirubin granules embedded in a matrix of mucous gel.

Congenital anomalies of the bile ducts often present in infancy, whereas congenital gallbladder anomalies are rarely of clinical significance until adulthood. Biliary anomalies do not follow recognizable patterns of genetic inheritance, nor are they associated with other developmental abnormalities, which suggests that they may be caused by pathogenic factors, such as viruses, drugs, or toxins transmitted by the mother.

---

**CASE SITUATION**

---

Dr. David Rosenstein, a pediatrician, was diagnosed with UC at age 24. In the following 5 years, he had two exacerbations of the disease that required medication, but they were not as serious as his first attack. For the last 13 years, the disease has been in remission and Dr. Rosenstein has required no medication.

Now, at age 42, Dr. Rosenstein has experienced fatigue and pruritus for several months. Last week, he began to notice yellowing of his skin and eyes and sought out the gastroenterologist again. He says he has been feeling fine for the last 13 years, except for the recent fatigue and itching. He denies any pain, gallbladder disease, hepatitis, IV drug use, or alcohol abuse. He has had no blood transfusions. His blood work shows elevated total bilirubin and alkaline phosphatase, with normal serum transaminases. His hepatitis panel is all negative. Ultrasonography shows that the biliary system and pancreas are normal.

#### Points to think about

1. Because of the negative hepatitis panel and normal ultrasonography, and given the past history of UC, what might be the diagnosis for Dr. Rosenstein?
2. Dr. Rosenstein will undergo an ERCP to visualize the biliary tree. The ERCP should show strictured areas in the intrahepatic and extrahepatic ducts, with areas of dilatation between the strictures, which can produce a beaded appearance to the ducts. How can the gastroenterology nurse help Dr. Rosenstein through this procedure?

3. What data are available in relation to the nursing diagnosis "alteration in comfort?"
4. What outcome criteria and associated nursing interventions may be devised for this diagnosis?

### Suggested responses

1. Based on Dr. Rosenstein's negative hepatitis panel, normal ultrasound examination, and past history of UC, PSC might be the diagnosis. Up to 5% of patients with UC develop PSC, but PSC has no correlation with UC exacerbations or remissions. Males who are under the age of 45 account for 60% to 70% of patients with PSC. It can be diagnosed before or after a diagnosis of UC and can occur even after a total colectomy.

2. Educational endeavors by nurses must take into account an individual patient's current level of understanding and his or her readiness to learn. In this example, there are two possible inferences about Dr. Rosenstein's level of understanding:
   * Dr. Rosenstein has the usual medical school foundation in reference to UC and its accompanying problems and diagnostic procedures.
   * Because he has lived with the diagnosis of UC for many years, Dr. Rosenstein has a near-exhaustive knowledge of UC and its accompanying problems and diagnostic tests. (He had probably already made a tentative diagnosis of PSC before he consulted the gastroenterologist.)

Although the second inference would seem the most likely, it should not be assumed without testing its truth. In regard to the ERCP procedure, testing can be conducted through the use of straightforward or open-ended questions, such as those that follow:
   * Do you have any questions about the ERCP procedure?
   * Are you aware of what happens during the ERCP procedure . . . ?

If responses do not elicit sufficient details, leading statements and other open-ended questions can focus on specific aspects of the procedure. The nurse must be aware that Dr. Rosenstein may choose not to respond.

For a patient who does not have a medical background, the nurse might consider the following preprocedural activities:
   * Assess the patient's knowledge and offer any necessary explanations of what will happen during the procedure.
   * Encourage questions.
   * Explain the duration of the procedure.
   * Explain about the x-ray room and that radiographic exams will be taken during the procedure.
   * Explain the medications given and their expected effects.

   * Reinforce awareness that he or she will be with the patient during the entire procedure and will be monitoring his or her response to sedative drugs and to the procedure itself and will be taking vital signs regularly.
   * Review the record before the procedure to refresh recall of laboratory data so he or she will be aware of incipient problems during the procedure.
   * Review probable postprocedural events with the patient.

3. Data are available to indicate that Dr. Rosenstein is still experiencing pruritus. The gastroenterology nurse does not know whether it is severe nor whether it is confined to limited skin areas or more widespread. Furthermore, Dr. Rosenstein may have open lesions that are associated with severe scratching on areas of his skin. The nursing diagnosis "alteration in comfort* related to pruritus caused by PSC" seems applicable.

4. Outcome criteria and associated nursing interventions for the diagnosis "alteration in comfort related to pruritus caused by PSC" are as follows:

| Outcome criteria | Nursing interventions |
| --- | --- |
| Patient will experience some relief from pruritus | Cool skin with wet compresses or baths<br>Pat skin dry after bathing<br>Apply prescribed antipruritic drugs<br>Apply pressure to itchy areas instead of scratching<br>Implement sensory distraction techniques |
| Patient will sleep for at least 2- to 3-hour intervals during night | Encourage therapeutic bath before retiring<br>Have patient keep a log of sleeping/waking periods<br>Place a clock and writing material at bedside |

NOTE: If patient has excoriation or open wounds from scratching, additional criteria would be added.

### REVIEW TERMS

**bile, biliary colic, cholangitis, cholecystitis, choledocholithiasis, cholelithiasis, cholestasis, common bile duct, cystic duct, gallbladder, hepatic duct, jaundice, primary sclerosing cholangitis (PSC), sphincter of Oddi**

### REVIEW QUESTIONS

1. The gallbladder wall is made up of:
   a. Serosa, muscularis, submucosa, and mucosa.

* NANDA does not list this diagnosis among those currently on the approved list.

b. Serosa, a fibromuscular layer, and mucosa.

c. Muscularis, submucosa, and mucosa.

d. Serosa, a fibromuscular layer, submucosa, and mucosa.

2. Blood is supplied to the gallbladder by the:
   a. Superior mesenteric artery.
   b. Hepatic artery.
   c. Celiac artery.
   d. Inferior phrenic artery.

3. What is the maximum amount of bile that can be stored in the gallbladder?
   a. 5 ml
   b. 10 ml
   c. 50 ml
   d. 500 ml

4. What is the major component of the bile that is produced by the liver?
   a. Cholesterol
   b. Bilirubin
   c. Bile salts
   d. Water

5. By far the most common disease affecting the biliary system is:
   a. Choledocholithiasis.
   b. Cholecystitis.
   c. Cholelithiasis.
   d. Cholangitis.

6. Chronic hemolytic disease, total parenteral nutrition, and alcoholism are among the risk factors for the formation of:
   a. Cholesterol gallstones.
   b. Pigment gallstones.
   c. Cholangitis.
   d. Gallbladder cancer.

7. The primary disadvantage of most nonsurgical treatment alternatives to cholecystectomy is:
   a. Potential recurrence of cholelithiasis after cessation of treatment.
   b. Unpleasant side-effects.
   c. The need for specialized equipment.
   d. The need for specially trained personnel.

8. For most patients, the treatment of choice for choledocholithiasis is:

a. Sphincteroplasty.

b. Cholecystectomy.

c. Endoscopic papillotomy.

d. Endoscopic retrograde cholangiopancreatography.

9. The most common cause of cholecystitis is:
   a. Cholecystenteric fistula.
   b. Bacterial infection.
   c. A gallstone impacted in the cystic duct.
   d. Gallstone ileus.

10. Treatment for cancer of the gallbladder most often involves:
    a. Supportive and symptomatic measures only.
    b. Cholecystectomy.
    c. Pancreaticoduodenectomy.
    d. Insertion of an internal drainage system.

**BIBLIOGRAPHY**

Bongiovanni, G, ed. *Essentials of Clinical Gastroenterology.* 2nd ed. New York: McGraw–Hill, 1988.

Briem, F. "Review of the Anatomy and Physiology of the Gallbladder." In *SGA Journal Reprints,* ed. Trivits, S, 105-06. Rochester, N.Y.: Society of Gastrointestinal Assistants, 1988.

Calvette, B. "Biliary Pathophysiology." In *SGA Journal Reprints,* ed. Trivits, S, 107-08. Rochester, N.Y.: Society of Gastrointestinal Assistants, 1988.

Chobanian, S, and Van Ness, M, eds. *Manual of Clinical Problems in Gastroenterology.* Boston: Little, Brown & Co., 1988.

Chopra, S, and May, R, eds. *Pathophysiology of Gastrointestinal Diseases.* Boston: Little, Brown & Co., 1988.

Eastwood, G, and Avunduk, C. *Manual of Gastroenterology: Diagnosis and Therapy.* Boston: Little, Brown & Co., 1988.

Given, B, and Simmons, S. *Gastroenterology in Clinical Nursing.* 4th ed. St. Louis: Mosby–Year Book, 1984.

Goldberg, K, ed. *Gastrointestinal Problems.* Nurse Review Series. Springhouse, Pa.: Springhouse Corporation, 1986.

Hamilton, H, editorial director. *Diseases.* Nurse's Reference Library Series. Springhouse, Pa.: Springhouse Corporation, 1985.

Silverman, A, and Roy, C. *Pediatric Clinical Gastroenterology.* 3rd ed. St. Louis: Mosby–Year Book, 1983.

Sleisenger, M, and Fordtran, J, eds. *Gastrointestinal Disease: Pathophysiology, Diagnosis, Management.* 4th ed. Philadelphia: W.B. Saunders, 1989.

Waye, J, Geenen, J, Fleischer, D, and Venu, R. *Techniques in Therapeutic Endoscopy.* Philadelphia: W.B. Saunders, 1987.

# Chapter 19

# PANCREAS

This chapter will acquaint the gastroenterology nurse with the normal anatomy and physiology of the pancreas and will discuss selected pancreatic disorders in terms of pathophysiology, diagnosis, and treatment.

**Learning objectives**

Upon completing study of this chapter, the gastroenterology nurse should be able to:

1. Describe the normal gross structure and histology of the pancreas.
2. Explain the normal physiologic functions of the pancreas, including both endocrine and exocrine secretions.
3. Discuss pathologic conditions of the pancreas, including selected diseases, disorders, and congenital anomalies.

## ANATOMY

The **pancreas** is a fish-shaped, lobulated gland that lies behind the stomach (see Plate 1). It is approximately 15 to 20 cm (6 to 8 inches) long and 5 cm (2 inches) wide, and has an average weight of less than 110 g (about 4 ounces). The pancreas has three segments, the head, which lies over the vena cava in the C-shaped curve of the duodenum; the body, which lies behind the duodenum and extends across the abdomen and behind the stomach; and the thin, narrow tail, which is situated under the spleen.

The pancreas contains two basic cell types, exocrine cells and endocrine cells. The pyramidal acinar cells are exocrine cells that make up the majority of the pancreatic tissue. Groups of acinar cells form an **acinus** and groups of acini form grapelike lobules. The lobules, in turn, are joined together by connective tissue into lobes, which unite to form the entire gland.

The acini are arranged around a small, central lumen into which they drain their enzymes. The central lumina

are drained by means of ductules, the most proximal portion of which is lined by clear, cuboidal cells called centroacinar cells. The ductules drain into multiple intralobular ducts; these join the interlobular ducts, which in turn drain into the **duct of Wirsung,** the main pancreatic duct. The duct of Wirsung runs the whole length of the pancreas from left to right and joins the common bile duct, emptying into the duodenum at the papilla of Vater. Most individuals have an accessory duct called the **duct of Santorini,** which leads from the head of the pancreas and drains into the duodenum at an accessory or minor papilla that lies just above the papilla of Vater.

Endocrine cells make up the remaining 1% of the pancreatic cells. They are located in the **islets of Langerhans,** which are embedded in the loose connective tissue between the lobules, mainly in the tail.

Branches of the splenic, superior mesenteric, and celiac arteries supply blood to the pancreas. Blood is drained away from the pancreas into the portal or splenic circulation by the superior mesenteric and splenic veins.

Sympathetic nerve fibers control pain sensations, vascular flow, and enzyme secretion in the pancreas. Parasympathetic fibers control exocrine and endocrine function.

## PHYSIOLOGY

The pancreas is both an exocrine and an endocrine organ. The three types of endocrine cells in the pancreas are alpha cells, which produce glucagon; beta cells, which produce insulin; and delta cells, which produce somatostatin. These endocrine products are released directly into the circulation. When the blood sugar level falls below normal, the alpha cells are stimulated to secrete glucagon, which accelerates the conversion of glycogen to glucose in the liver. When the blood sugar level is above normal, the beta cells secrete insulin, which promotes both the metabolism of glucose by the tissue cells and the conversion of glucose to glycogen, which is then stored in the liver and muscles.

The exocrine acinar cells secrete 500 to 1,000 ml of pancreatic juice daily. This colorless fluid has a pH of 8.3 and consists of water, bicarbonate, enzymes, potassium, sodium, chloride, and calcium. The three major types of enzymes secreted by the pancreas include the following:

- Amylases (predominantly α-amylase), which hydrolyze carbohydrates into glucose and maltose
- Lipases (including pancreatic lipase and phospholipase A), which are important in early stages of fat digestion
- Proteases (including trypsinogen, the precursor of trypsin), which break amino acid bonds of protein chains and also converts other proenzymes to their active forms

Pancreatic secretions are controlled by the hormones **secretin** and **cholecystokinin-pancreozymin (CCK-PCZ).** When the chyme is made up predominantly of undigested proteins and fats, the duodenum releases CCK-PCZ, which stimulates the release of enzyme-rich pancreatic juice. When the chyme is mainly acidic, secretin stimulates the release of pancreatic juice that is rich in bicarbonates and water. These pancreatic juices enter the duodenum with the biliary system secretions at the papilla of Vater.

Pancreatic secretion occurs in the following four phases:

- At rest, the pancreas secretes bicarbonate at about 2% of the maximal rate and enzymes at about 15% of the maximal rate.
- The cephalic phase of pancreatic secretion occurs when the sight and smell of food stimulates a modest output of enzyme-rich pancreatic juice.
- In the gastric phase, distention of the stomach stimulates secretion of a moderate amount of pancreatic juice that is rich in enzymes but low in bicarbonate.
- In the intestinal phase, the delivery of food into the proximal intestine evokes secretion of pancreatic enzymes at about 70% of the maximal rate. The volume of pancreatic juice and bicarbonate output increases as the pH of the meal decreases and the acid load increases.

In the absence of pancreatic enzymes, up to 40% of dietary fat and protein may be assimilated using other, less efficient pathways of digestion, such as salivary amylase, pharyngeal lipase, and peptidases from the brush borders of the gut mucosa. It has been estimated that pancreatic enzyme secretion must fall below 10% of normal before maldigestion or malabsorption occurs.

## PATHOPHYSIOLOGY

Noteworthy pathologic conditions that affect the pancreas include acute and chronic pancreatitis, Zollinger-Ellison syndrome, malignant and benign tumors, congenital defects, and cystic fibrosis.

### Pancreatitis

**Pancreatitis** is an inflammation of the pancreas that generally results from obstruction of a pancreatic duct. It may be acute or chronic. The cause of the inflammation may be chemical, anatomic, or traumatic.

#### Acute pancreatitis

Acute pancreatitis is most commonly caused by chronic, heavy alcohol abuse; abdominal trauma; peptic ulcer disease with penetration; cholelithiasis; hyperparathyroidism; hyperlipidemia; and hypercalcemia. It occurs in less than 1% of cases after endoscopic retrograde cholangiopancreatography (ERCP). An association between pancreatitis and α1-antitrypsin deficiency has been reported, but its significance is not known. The characteristic anatomic changes associated with acute pancreatitis are results of enzymatic digestion of the pancreatic parenchyma and peripancreatic tissues by enzymes that are normally present in the pancreas in their inactive proenzyme form. The results are varying degrees of edema, necrosis, and hemorrhage.

The most severe form of acute pancreatitis is hemorrhagic pancreatitis. Morphologic findings associated with hemorrhagic pancreatitis include proteolytic destruction of pancreatic tissue, necrosis of blood vessels with subsequent hemorrhage, fat necrosis, and accompanying inflammation. The mass of inflamed pancreas containing necrotic tissue is called a phlegmon. Massive necrosis frequently leads to the formation of pseudocysts, which are loculated collections of fluid, blood, and necrotic debris that have been walled off to form a saclike structure. Overall mortality in patients with hemorrhagic pancreatitis is 50%.

Edematous pancreatitis, on the other hand, is a more mild form of acute pancreatitis that is characterized by interstitial edema, mild polymorphonuclear leukocyte or lymphocyte response, and intact pancreatic acini and ducts. Interstitial fibrosis is rare and fat necrosis is infrequent. Histopathologic examination shows no apparent changes in the acini or ductules.

Symptoms of acute pancreatitis include the following:
- Pain in the midepigastrium, left chest, shoulder, and back
- Abdominal swelling and tenderness
- Anorexia and weight loss
- Low-grade fever
- Shock, hypovolemia, and hypotension
- Hypocalcemia
- Hypoxia
- Nausea and vomiting

- Elevated levels of serum amylase, serum lipase, and urine amylase; transient elevation of serum bilirubin, alkaline phosphatase, and aminotransferase
- Leukocytosis, hematocrit elevation, and hyperglycemia

Patients with hemorrhagic pancreatitis may also develop Grey Turner's sign, which is a bluish flank discoloration, or Cullen's sign, which is a bluish periumbilical discoloration.

There is no specific test for acute pancreatitis; a combination of laboratory tests and diagnostic procedures is used, which may include radiologic evaluations, percutaneous transhepatic cholangiography (PTC), and ERCP.

Treatment of acute pancreatitis is aimed at hemodynamic stabilization, correction of metabolic abnormalities, and resting the pancreas. Medical treatment methods may include the following:

- Administration of colloids and crystalloids to increase blood volume and to maintain osmotic pressure
- Blood transfusions if the patient hemorrhages
- Electrolyte replacement
- Pain relief
- Withholding of foods and fluids and nasogastric suctioning to allow the GI tract to rest
- Bed rest and temperature control measures to reduce the patient's metabolic rate and therefore the amount of pancreatic enzyme secretion
- Peritoneal lavage, in severe cases
- Enzyme and vitamin supplements
- Insulin for patients with impaired islet cell function

To correct the underlying problem, surgery may be recommended, including cholecystectomy or choledochojejunostomy to correct biliary obstruction, vagotomy to decrease pancreatic stimulation, or surgical repair of a traumatic injury. Pancreatitis secondary to biliary tract obstruction may also be relieved by endoscopic placement of a stent for biliary drainage.

Complications of pancreatitis may include secondary infection, especially potentially fatal pulmonary infections; pleural effusion; respiratory distress; pseudocyst; abscess; or fistula formation.

Experimental techniques for the replacement of the endocrine function of the pancreas include total pancreas transplantation, and islet cell transplantation using an autotransfusion technique.

### Chronic pancreatitis

Most chronic pancreatitis is associated with long-term, heavy alcohol abuse; it may also be the result of protein caloric malnutrition, cystic fibrosis, or obstruction of the pancreatic excretory ducts by carcinoma or anatomic malformations. It is generally found in male patients who are between the ages of 40 and 60.

In such cases, persistent inflammation produces irreversible morphologic changes and functional loss. Fibrotic changes develop throughout much of the organ, along with focal fat necrosis and chronic inflammation. Exocrine function is gradually lost, but the islet cells are not affected until the disease reaches an advanced stage.

Symptoms of chronic pancreatitis may include the following:

- Epigastric, subcostal, or umbilical pain
- Weight loss and debilitation related to malabsorption
- Steatorrhea
- Possibly diabetes and/or obstructive jaundice, depending on the progression of pancreatic damage.

To confirm the diagnosis, the physician may order blood tests, malabsorption tests, tests of pancreatic function, and radiologic examinations. ERCP may be used to explore the extent of ductal involvement.

Treatment for chronic pancreatitis is usually nonsurgical and includes abstaining from alcohol, acute and chronic pain relief, nutritional support, and oral replacement of missing digestive enzymes. Surgical intervention may be necessary in certain situations. A sphincterotomy may be performed to relieve calcium stone obstruction. Patients with pancreatic fibrosis may need a pancreaticojejunostomy, or Roux-en-Y procedure, to relieve ductal obstruction. In this procedure the duct of Wirsung is anastomosed to the side or end of the jejunum. To relieve pain the physician may resect up to 80% of the pancreas. The other alternative is to perform a subtotal pancreatectomy, removing 95% of the organ and leaving a small remnant of the head of the gland attached to the duodenum.

### Pseudocysts

A **pseudocyst** is an encapsulated sac that is lined by inflammatory cells and is filled with fluid, pancreatic enzymes, and blood. Pseudocysts may be single or multiple and are most often associated with alcoholic pancreatitis. Symptoms include epigastric pain, persistent nausea and vomiting, weight loss, jaundice, and low-grade fever. In 30% to 40% of patients, the cyst may be palpated. Abdominal ultrasonography and computed tomography (CT scan) are the best methods of identifying a pancreatic pseudocyst or abscess that is greater than 1 to 2 cm in size.

Many pseudocysts resolve spontaneously. If medical treatment for pancreatitis does not resolve symptoms, a drainage procedure may be required. Urgent surgical intervention is recommended if there is bacterial infection of a pseudocyst, free pseudocyst rupture into the peritoneal cavity, or massive pseudocyst hemorrhage from intracystic bleeding or erosion into an adjacent organ or vessel. Analgesics may be given for pain and antibiotics may be ordered in case of an abscess or surgical drainage.

## Pancreatic fistulas

The majority of clinically significant **pancreatic fistulas** are external. Possible causes of pancreatic fistulas include the following:

- Trauma, usually pancreatic duct injury that was overlooked or inadequately treated
- External drainage of a pseudocyst
- Pancreatic surgery, usually pancreaticoduodenectomy for pancreatic cancer

About 75% of pancreatic fistulas close spontaneously within 5 months, but some persist for over a year. Of those requiring surgical repair, about 90% remain permanently closed.

## Carcinoma

Most pancreatic tumors are malignant and involve the exocrine portion of the pancreas. Benign endocrine tumors that involve the islet cells are discussed separately.

Pancreatic carcinoma most often develops in persons who are between the ages of 30 and 50. It is more common in men than in women. Potential risk factors include chronic pancreatitis or diabetes mellitus, exposure to industrial carcinogens, a high-fat diet, and heavy cigarette smoking. Metastasis generally involves the duodenum, stomach, lymph nodes, liver, gallbladder, and the vascular and nervous systems. Ninety percent of pancreatic carcinomas are adenocarcinomas, with duct cell adenocarcinoma predominating.

Symptoms of pancreatic cancer depend on the site of the tumor. Tumors of the head of the pancreas typically result in dull midepigastric pain, weight loss, and possibly progressive obstructive jaundice with pruritus. Tumors of the pancreatic body or tail appear later in the disease and may include steady pain that is often experienced as back or spinal pain, anorexia, weight loss, and jaundice. Obstruction and/or metastasis may also cause signs and symptoms of liver involvement. Dark urine and light-colored stools appear in about 75% of patients with pancreatic carcinoma and mental depression is found in 50% to 75% of these patients.

ERCP has been found to be the most specific test for pancreatic cancer. Ultrasonography, radiography, nuclear scanning, and angiography may also be helpful.

Therapy for pancreatic cancer is primarily palliative and supportive. Most patients present with locally invasive or metastatic disease and are not candidates for curative surgery; only about 10% to 15% of patients with pancreatic cancer can benefit from potentially curative surgery. In operable cases, pancreaticoduodenectomy may be performed. Palliative surgery may relieve symptoms for patients with inoperable cancer.

## Zollinger-Ellison syndrome

In **Zollinger-Ellison syndrome (ZES),** gastrinomas, or nonbeta islet cell tumors of the pancreas, release gastrin into the circulation, which stimulates gastric acid hypersecretion and, in turn, leads to severe ulcers in the upper GI tract, predominantly in the proximal duodenum. The disease has two common variants, a sporadic type, which is usually malignant and is seen later in life; and a genetic type, which is associated with multiple endocrine neoplasia type 1 (MEN1) and causes tumors or hyperplasia of the parathyroid, pancreatic islet, and pituitary glands.

Patients with ZES have signs and symptoms of peptic ulcer disease, and sometimes diarrhea and steatorrhea. An increased serum gastrin level is the most specific and reliable test for ZES, although this finding also occurs in pernicious anemia and other diseases. Other diagnostic tests may include secretin infusion, calcium infusion, and/or standard test meal ingestion, gastric analysis, and an upper GI series. The best methods for finding tumor localization are CT scans, ultrasonography, and visceral angiography.

Medical treatment of ZES involves long-term administration of histamine blockers, such as cimetidine (Tagamet) or ranitidine (Zantac). For metastatic disease, preliminary results of chemotherapy have been promising. When medical treatment fails, surgery may be recommended. In patients who do not have MEN1, approximately 25% of gastrinomas can be completely resected with resultant cure; if resection is possible, this is the optimal treatment. Surgical treatment may also include total gastrectomy or proximal gastric vagotomy.

The extent of morbidity and mortality in patients with ZES is related principally to ulcer complications, fistulae, hemorrhage, or perforation.

## Endocrine tumors

Islet cell tumors are classified on the basis of the predominant hormone they secrete, although most secrete more than one hormone. Types of islet cell tumors include insulinomas, glucagonomas, somatostatinomas, and VIPomas (see pp. 171-172). Most are benign.

### Insulinomas

The most common type of islet cell tumor is an insulinoma, which arises from the beta cells. The tumor is typically round, firm, and encapsulated and is most frequently located in the body or tail of the pancreas. Seventy to eighty percent are solitary benign tumors. Patients with insulinomas present with symptoms of hypoglycemia on fasting or after exercise. These patients may also exhibit neuropsychiatric manifestations, ranging from subtle personality changes to confusion, coma, or seizure disorders. Insulin to glucose ratio is also elevated in these patients.

### Glucagonomas

Glucagon-secreting tumors of the alpha islet cells are called glucagonomas. They are far less common than insulinomas or gastrinomas. The most distinctive feature is a skin disorder, necrolytic migratory erythema, which appears as an erythematous area that develops a central blister and is followed by crusting, healing, and sometimes bronze hyperpigmentation. Most patients also have diabetes mellitus. Because of the catabolic activity of glucagon, patients with glucagonomas often exhibit profound weight loss and anemia. More than 50% of patients have metastases at the time of diagnosis.

### Somatostatinomas

Patients with somatostatinomas may present with steatorrhea, mild diabetes mellitus, and/or cholelithiasis. These symptoms are consistent with somatostatin's inhibitory effect on the secretion of gastrin, secretin, insulin, glucagon, and cholecystokinin.

### VIPomas

Patients with tumors that produce vasoactive intestinal peptide (VIPomas) generally experience profuse watery diarrhea, hypokalemia, and hypochlorhydria or achlorhydria, also known as the pancreatic cholera syndrome.

The treatment of choice for most islet cell tumors is surgical excision. Patients with metastatic disease may improve after surgical reduction of the tumor mass. Streptozocin has been shown to decrease tumor size and prolong survival. A long-acting analog of somatostatin effectively controls symptoms in patients with several types of islet cell tumors.

## Pancreatic enzyme insufficiency

**Pancreatic exocrine insufficiency** generally results from chronic inflammation of the pancreas. Because pancreatic enzymes are necessary for the digestion of fat, protein, and carbohydrates, pancreatic insufficiency leads to panmalabsorption. Weight loss is a common symptom. Plain x-ray films commonly show calcification of the pancreatic ducts. Other expected diagnostic findings include abnormal small bowel upon radiographic exam, severe steatorrhea, and possibly an abnormal Schilling test, indicating mild malabsorption of vitamin B12. Fat malabsorption also may be quantified by using a 72-hour fecal fat analysis.

Exocrine insufficiency is treated with oral enzyme preparations and supplemental antacids or bicarbonate. Severe steatorrhea may be controlled by a low-fat diet and oral pancreatic enzyme preparations. In some patients, supplemental calcium, vitamin D, and other fat-soluble vitamins may be needed.

## Cystic fibrosis

**Cystic fibrosis** is the most common lethal genetic defect in Caucasian populations, occurring in 1 out of every 2000 live births. It is an autosomal recessive disease of the exocrine glands that affects not only the pancreas but also the respiratory system, the sweat glands, and the reproductive system. The dysfunction of pancreatic exocrine function forces the patient to rely on oral pancreatic enzymes. The disease also affects the mucus-producing organs, making their secretions excessively viscous. Mucus may block the bronchi, small intestine, bile ducts, and pancreas.

Conflicting pathogenetic mechanisms for cystic fibrosis have been suggested, but none of these theories satisfactorily reconcile the unique sweat gland defect with the abnormal characteristics of mucus secretion. The most promising avenue of research centers on electrolyte secretion and chloride channel regulation. Elevation of sodium and chloride concentrations in the sweat is the most characteristic finding in cystic fibrosis. It is possible that in affected tissues of cystic fibrosis patients, alteration in a common intracellular mediator or inhibitor protein distal to the site of generation of cyclic adenosine monophosphate is likely to be the underlying abnormality.

Cystic fibrosis is easily recognized in the first year of life; about 90% of affected children have obvious clinical signs and symptoms resulting from both pulmonary and pancreatic involvement. Symptoms of cystic fibrosis include poor fat and protein digestion, leading to oily and foul-smelling stools; weight loss despite an increased appetite; repeated episodes of pneumonia and bronchitis; diminished or absent pancreatic enzymes; and pulmonary changes. The infant's production of thick, sticky, dry mucus leads to noisy respirations, intermittent wheezing, and coughing, particularly when lying down.

Approximately 80% of patients with cystic fibrosis have pancreatic insufficiency at birth, although the extent of pancreatic involvement is highly variable. The definitive diagnostic test for cystic fibrosis is the sweat electrolyte test where quantitative pilocarpine iontophoresis shows elevated sodium and chloride levels in affected patients.

Cystic fibrosis is managed by controlling respiratory complications and by aiding digestion through dietary regulation and pancreatic enzyme replacement.

Much of the morbidity and virtually all of the mortality beyond the neonatal period in cystic fibrosis patients is attributable to chronic obstructive pulmonary disease. In 1960, the mean survival age after diagnosis was less than 5 years. Since then it has increased to 20 years. This prolongation of life can be attributed largely to the development of pancreatic replacement therapy, use of antibiotics, and vigorous pulmonary hygiene.

## Congenital anomalies

Congenital anomalies of the pancreas may include pancreatic rest, pancreas divisum, and annular pancreas.

### Pancreatic rest

A **pancreatic rest** is a rare condition that is defined as the presence of ectopic pancreatic tissue in the stomach. A pancreatic rest is usually an incidental finding of an upper GI series or gastroscopy. When symptomatic, it may produce obstruction, ulceration, and/or bleeding, or may be associated with clinical pancreatitis. Symptomatic lesions are treated with simple excision.

### Pancreas divisum

**Pancreas divisum** is a congenital anomaly that occurs when the two embryonic duct systems fail to fuse, thereby resulting in a dorsal and ventral pancreas. The dorsal gland is drained by the duct of Santorini and through an accessory papilla into the duodenum, whereas the ventral gland is drained by the duct of Wirsung and enters the duodenum through the papilla of Vater. Pancreas divisum has been observed in about 5% to 10% of autopsy series and in about 2% to 7% of patients undergoing ERCP.

Clinical pancreatic disease is an uncommon sequela of this anomaly, although the risk of developing acute pancreatitis is increased. It may be that both pancreas divisum and a stenotic accessory papilla must be present for clinically evident pancreatic disease to occur. In most cases, the patient presents with recurrent acute pancreatitis, but some patients present with chronic pancreatitis.

For patients with frequent episodes of recurrent acute pancreatitis or disabling pain without other apparent cause, surgical intervention may be indicated. Surgical alternatives include sphincteroplasty of the accessory papilla alone or in combination with the duodenal papilla, pancreaticoduodenectomy, endoscopic sphincterotomy of the accessory papilla, and endoscopic placement of stents through the accessory papilla. Accessory sphincteroplasty seems to be the most successful technique.

### Annular pancreas

**Annular pancreas** occurs when the embryonic dorsal and ventral glands fail to fuse and part of the ventral pancreas encircles the duodenum, often resulting in duodenal obstruction. Annular pancreas is the most common anomaly obstructing the duodenum in infancy and may also be associated with other congenital anomalies, such as atresia of the duodenum and Down's syndrome. Histologically, there may be penetration of the duodenal wall by pancreatic tissue.

Annular pancreas may not cause any symptoms until adulthood. At that time, presenting complaints include intermittent epigastric discomfort, which is relieved by vomiting. Upper GI x-ray films show a narrowing of the second portion of the duodenum. Symptomatic cases are best treated by surgical bypass using a duodenostomy or a duodenojejunostomy, rather than by division of the pancreatic tissue.

---

**CASE SITUATION**

---

Carolyn Jones, age 55, went to her doctor because of severe epigastric pain. She had endured the pain, along with nausea and vomiting, for 3 days, thinking she had "stomach flu." Her doctor noted that she was dehydrated and put her in the hospital for a further workup. He suspects she has pancreatitis.

*Points to think about*

1. In making a nursing assessment, what questions might the gastroenterology nurse ask Mrs. Jones about her pain to support the physician's tentative diagnosis of pancreatitis?
2. Mrs. Jones is scheduled for an ultrasonogram, a CT scan, and a gastroscopic exam. What might be found on these tests?
3. Under what circumstances might the nurse expect to do an ERCP on Mrs. Jones?
4. What nursing interventions would be appropriate for the desired outcome "Mrs. Jones will have no increase in pain or fever after the ERCP?"
5. What can the nurse teach Mrs. Jones that will help her avoid future attacks of pancreatitis?

*Suggested responses*

1. In performing a nursing assessment, the gastroenterology nurse might ask Mrs. Jones the following questions about her epigastric pain:
   - "How long have you had the pain? Can you describe it?" Onset, duration, and character of pain is always an important factor. The pain of pancreatitis can be gradual or sudden and usually becomes severe, constant, and boring.
   - "Can you point to where the pain is?" Pancreatic pain usually localizes in the left epigastric area and often radiates to the back and left shoulder. The pancreas is located in the left epigastric area and lies posterior to the stomach, which accounts for radiation of pain to the back and left shoulder.
   - "Does it hurt to touch there?" The inflamed pancreas is often tender to palpation.
   - "Does the pain come and go or is it there all the time; do you notice that it is worse at certain times?" Pain is usually constant and is worse several hours after eating a large meal or ingesting alcohol.
   - "Is the pain better after you vomit?" Vomiting does

not relieve the pain of pancreatitis as it might for patients with intestinal obstruction.

- "Is there anything you do that helps relieve the pain?" Patients with pancreatitis often assume a characteristic position of bending over at the torso with hands over the left epigastric area.

2. Most of the time, pancreatitis in women of this age group is a result of gallstones. The second leading cause of pancreatitis is alcohol abuse. You might expect the following findings when Mrs. Jones undergoes ultrasonography, CT scan, and gastroscopy:

- Ultrasonography would be a first-line test for choledocholithiasis. It may also identify pseudocysts, abscesses, common duct dilatation, and calcifications.
- CT scan may further define and evaluate the above findings and may also evaluate the architecture of the liver, biliary tree, and pancreas.
- Gastroscopy may confirm or rule out the presence of ulcer disease as a cause of Mrs. Jones' epigastric pain. Posterior gastric or duodenal ulcers may penetrate or perforate into the pancreatic tissue, thus causing pancreatitis.

3. At present the only indication for ERCP in acute pancreatitis is relief of gallstone-related pancreatitis in selected patients. In such cases, a sphincterotomy may be done to drain the common bile duct and remove any stones that may be causing an obstruction. This allows drainage of the pancreatic duct to resume and pancreatitis will usually subside uneventfully. Care must be taken not to inject dye into the pancreatic duct, which may cause further inflammation of the gland.

   In patients who have had two or more attacks of acute pancreatitis, ERCP should be considered when looking for potentially surgically correctable lesions, such as strictures, obstructions of the main duct, or pseudocysts.

   In 60% of patients with abdominal pain and history of excessive alcohol ingestion, ERCP shows evidence of pancreatic duct abnormality.

4. To ensure that Mrs. Jones will have no increase in pain or fever after ERCP, appropriate nursing interventions might include the following:

- Be aware of the increased risk of causing pancreatitis during ERCP.
- Watch the x-ray monitor while injecting dye to confirm cannulation of the pancreatic duct.
- Slowly and carefully inject the minimal amount of dye, taking care not to produce acinar filling of the pancreas.
- Use sterile accessory equipment.
- Instruct the patient to report any chills, fever, or increase in pain.

5. To avoid future attacks of pancreatitis, Mrs. Jones should be instructed to follow the ensuing instructions:

- Avoid alcohol completely.
- Follow a diet that is low in fat and high in proteins and carbohydrates, and avoid large meals. Replacement of vitamin B12 and fat-soluble vitamins (A, D, E, and K) may be needed.
- Avoid drugs that are known to cause pancreatitis, including estrogens, birth control pills, tetracycline, furosemide, thiazide diuretics, azathioprine, and sulfonamides.
- Use relaxation techniques for pain control.

---

### REVIEW TERMS

acinus, annular pancreas, cholecystokinin-pancreozymin (CCK-PCZ), cystic fibrosis, duct of Santorini, duct of Wirsung, islets of Langerhans, pancreas, pancreas divisum, pancreatic exocrine insufficiency, pancreatic fistulas, pancreatic rest, pancreatitis, pseudocyst, secretin, Zollinger-Ellison syndrome (ZES)

---

### REVIEW QUESTIONS

1. The majority of the pancreatic tissue is made up of:
   a. Acinar cells.
   b. Alpha cells.
   c. Beta cells.
   d. Delta cells.
2. The endocrine cells of the pancreas are located in the:
   a. Crypts of Lieberkuhn.
   b. Islets of Langerhans.
   c. Duct of Wirsung.
   d. Pancreatic lobules.
3. The beta cells secrete:
   a. Somatostatin.
   b. Glucagon.
   c. Vasoactive intestinal peptide.
   d. Insulin.
4. The cephalic phase of pancreatic secretion is stimulated by:
   a. Gastric distention.
   b. The sight and smell of food.
   c. The presence of acidic chyme in the small intestine.
   d. The presence of alkaline chyme in the small intestine.
5. The most severe form of pancreatitis is:
   a. Chronic pancreatitis.
   b. Hemorrhagic pancreatitis.
   c. Edematous pancreatitis.
   d. Alcoholic pancreatitis.

6. A sac-like structure in the pancreas that is filled with fluid, blood, and pancreatic enzymes is called a:
   a. Pancreatic rest.
   b. Pancreas divisum.
   c. Annular pancreas.
   d. Pseudocyst.

7. The most specific test for pancreatic cancer is:
   a. ERCP.
   b. PTC.
   c. Ultrasound.
   d. Plain X-rays.

8. Zollinger-Ellison syndrome often results in what clinical manifestation?
   a. Peptic ulcer disease.
   b. Steatorrhea.
   c. Necrolytic migratory erythema.
   d. Pancreatic cholera syndrome.

9. The preferred treatment for most islet-cell tumors is:
   a. Supportive and palliative measures only.
   b. Radiotherapy.
   c. Chemotherapy.
   d. Surgical excision.

10. The definitive diagnostic test for cystic fibrosis is the:
    a. Sweat electrolyte test.
    b. Schilling test.
    c. Bernstein test.
    d. Serum amylase and lipase level.

## BIBLIOGRAPHY

Bongiovanni, G, ed. *Essentials of Clinical Gastroenterology.* 2nd ed. New York: McGraw–Hill, 1988.

Brewer, J. "The Anatomy and Physiology of the Pancreas." In *SGA Journal Reprints,* ed. Trivits, S, 75-76. Rochester, N.Y.: Society of Gastrointestinal Assistants, 1988.

Chobanian, S, and Van Ness, M, eds. *Manual of Clinical Problems in Gastroenterology.* Boston: Little, Brown & Co., 1988.

Chopra, S, and May, R, eds. *Pathophysiology of Gastrointestinal Diseases.* Boston: Little, Brown & Co., 1989.

Damsgard, C. "Pancreatic Disorders: An Overview." *SGA Journal* 11(Fall 1988): 117-19.

Eastwood, G, and Avunduk, C. *Manual of Gastroenterology: Diagnosis and Therapy.* Boston: Little, Brown & Co., 1988.

Goldberg, K, ed. *Gastrointestinal Problems.* Nurse Review Series. Springhouse, Pa.: Springhouse Corporation, 1986.

Haught, J. "Zollinger Ellison Syndrome: An Overview." In *SGA Journal Reprints,* ed. Trivits, S, 81-84. Rochester, N.Y.: Society of Gastrointestinal Assistants, 1988.

Matthews, J, Maher, K, and Cattau, E, Jr. "The Role of Endoscopic Retrograde Cholangiopancreatography Injection Training Sessions for the Gastroenterology Nurse and Associate." In *Journal Reprints II,* ed. Trivits, S, 120-22. Rochester, N.Y.: Society of Gastroenterology Nurses and Associates, 1990.

Mills, A. "Pancreatitis: Disruption in Structure and Function." *Gastroenterology Nursing* 12(Summer 1989): 63-65.

Palmieri, M. "Pathophysiology of the Pancreas." In *SGA Journal Reprints,* ed. Trivits, S, 77-79. Rochester, N.Y.: Society of Gastrointestinal Assistants, 1988.

Silverman, A, and Roy, C. *Pediatric Clinical Gastroenterology.* 3rd ed. St. Louis: Mosby–Year Book, 1983.

Sleisenger, M, and Fordtran, J, eds. *Gastrointestinal Disease: Pathophysiology, Diagnosis, Management.* 4th ed. Philadelphia: W.B. Saunders, 1989.

Waye, J, Geenen, J, Fleischer, D, and Venu, R. *Techniques in Therapeutic Endoscopy.* Philadelphia: W.B. Saunders, 1987.

# Chapter 20

# LIVER

This chapter will acquaint the gastroenterology nurse with the normal anatomy and physiology of the liver and with certain pathologic conditions that affect this organ.

**Learning objectives**

After reviewing the content of this chapter, the gastroenterology nurse should be able to:

1. Describe the normal anatomy and histology of the liver.
2. Explain the normal physiologic functions of the liver, including its role in bile formation and secretion, metabolism, vitamin storage, coagulation, and detoxification.
3. Discuss the pathophysiology, diagnosis, and treatment of a number of pathologic conditions that affect the liver, including cirrhosis, hepatitis, carcinoma, Wilson's disease, porphyria, and intrahepatic biliary dysplasia.

**ANATOMY**

The liver is the single largest organ in the body, weighing from 1,200 to 1,600 g (3 to 4 pounds). It is located in the right upper quadrant of the abdomen, immediately below the diaphragm (see Plate 1). The normal liver extends from the right fifth intercostal space in the midclavicular line down to the right costal margin.

The entire surface of the liver is covered by a thick capsule of connective tissue called Glisson's capsule, which contains blood vessels and lymphatics. The capsule is covered by a layer of serosa.

The liver is divided into a right and a left lobe by the falciform ligament. This ligament also attaches the liver to the abdominal wall and to the diaphragm. The right lobe is six times larger than the left and may be further divided into the right lobe proper, the caudate lobe, and the quadrate lobe. Each lobe is further divided into lobules that are approximately 2 mm high and 1 mm in circumference.

The hepatic lobule is the functioning unit of the liver. Approximately 1 million lobules form the principal mass of the liver parenchyma. Each lobule consists of a hexagonal row of hepatic cells called **hepatocytes.** The hepatocytes secrete bile into the bile canaliculi and also perform a number of metabolic functions. In the surrounding connective tissue, each lobule has a hepatic artery, a portal vein, and a bile duct, which are known collectively as the **portal triad.**

Between each row of cells are intralobular cavities called **sinusoids.** Each sinusoid is lined with **Kupffer cells,** which are phagocytic cells that belong to the reticuloendothelial system. The Kupffer cells remove amino acids, nutrients, sugars, old erythrocytes, bacteria, and debris from the blood that is flowing through the sinusoids. The main functions of the sinusoids are to destroy old or defective red blood cells, to remove bacteria and foreign particles from the blood, and to detoxify harmful substances.

As much as 1500 ml of blood enter the liver each minute, making the liver one of the most vascular organs in the body (Fig. 20-1). The portal vein supplies about 75% of this blood, bringing in nutrients that are absorbed from the gastrointestinal system. The hepatic artery supplies the other 25% as oxygenated blood.

Because of this large volume of blood supply, the liver can regenerate itself within 3 weeks, and normal function can be restored within 4 months. It is possible for the liver to function even with damage to 90% of its mass, but liver removal or total destruction leads to death within about 10 hours.

Blood leaves the sinusoids by entering the central lobule vein. It then enters the hepatic veins and follows the normal venous circuit into the inferior vena cava.

Nerve fibers to the liver come from the vagus nerve and the thoracolumbar system. Sympathetic nervous stimulation may cause hepatic artery and portal vein vasoconstriction and a dull pain over the area of the liver.

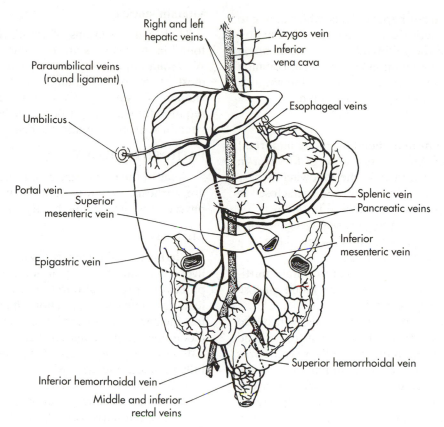

**Fig. 20-1**. Hepatic portal system. Blood is carried from the stomach, intestines, spleen, and pancreas into the liver sinusoids. Hepatic veins convey it to the inferior vena cava. Clinically significant sites of anastomosis between the hepatic and systemic circulations are (1) the esophageal veins (portal tributary), which anastomose with the azygos veins; (2) the paraumbilical veins in the round ligament originate in the left branch of the portal vein and connect with the superficial veins of the anterior abdominal wall (systemic tributaries) in the area of the umbilicus; (3) the superior rectal or hemorrhoidal veins (portal tributary), which anastomose with the middle and inferior rectal veins; (4) the portal tributaries to the intestines, pancreas, and liver, which anastomose with the phrenic, renal, and lumbar veins (systemic tributaries not shown). In portal hypertension and chronic liver disease, blood may be backed up in these veins and shunted around the liver through the points of anastomosis. (From Price SA and Wilson LM: Pathophysiology: clinical concepts of disease processes, ed 4, St. Louis, 1992, Mosby–Year Book.)

Bile ducts receive both sympathetic and parasympathetic innervation.

## PHYSIOLOGY

Following are the major physiologic functions of the liver:

- Bile formation and secretion
- Metabolism of carbohydrates, proteins, fats, and steroids
- Vitamin storage
- Coagulation
- Detoxification of foreign and toxic substances

### Bile formation and secretion

The liver synthesizes and transports the bile pigments and bile salts that are necessary for fat digestion. Bile is a combination of water, bile acids, bile pigments, cholesterol, bilirubin, phospholipids, potassium, sodium, and chloride. Primary bile acids are produced from cholesterol. When bile acids are conjugated in the liver, they become bile salts. Bile pigments are formed from the breakdown of erythrocytes by the cells of the reticuloendothelial system. In this process, heme is converted to biliverdin and then to bilirubin, the main bile pigment. The water-insoluble, indirect (unconjugated) bilirubin formed in this manner is released into the blood, where it is bound to albumin. In the hepatocytes, indirect bilirubin is conjugated with glucuronic acid to form water-soluble, direct (conjugated) bilirubin, which is secreted into the bile canaliculi and excreted in bile.

The bile canaliculi branch and combine and eventually form the right and left hepatic ducts, which merge to form the common hepatic duct. As described in Chapter 18, the cystic duct of the gallbladder joins the common hepatic duct to form the common bile duct. The common bile duct then joins the duct of Wirsung at the ampulla of Vater just before entering the duodenum.

### Metabolism

Carbohydrate and protein metabolism are important functions of the liver. Specific functions of the liver in carbohydrate metabolism include the following:

- Converting glucose, fructose, and galactose to glycogen (glycogenesis) for storage in the liver
- Breaking down glycogen to glucose (glycogenolysis) to maintain blood glucose levels when there is a decrease in carbohydrate intake
- Synthesizing glucose from noncarbohydrate nutrients (gluconeogenesis) to maintain blood glucose levels (e.g., proteins or fats)

Liver cells also deaminate amino acids to produce ketoacids and ammonia, from which urea is formed and excreted in the urine. In addition, the liver synthesizes about 50 g of new protein daily, including most of the plasma proteins, such as albumin, fibrinogen, transferrin, ceruloplasmin, haptoglobin, and the lipoproteins.

Digested fat is converted in the intestine to triglycerides, cholesterol, phospholipids, and lipoproteins. These substances are then taken up by the liver and hydrolyzed to glycerol and fatty acids, through a process known as ketogenesis.

The liver also metabolizes adrenocortical steroids, glucocorticoids, estrogens, testosterone, progesterones, and aldosterone.

### Coagulation

Prothrombin and fibrinogen, which are needed to clot blood, are both produced by the liver. The liver also produces the anticoagulant heparin and releases vasopressor substances after hemorrhage.

### Detoxification

Detoxification is another unique function of the liver. The hepatocytes attempt to make foreign and toxic substances and certain endogenous substances more water-soluble so they can be eliminated in the urine or in bile. Mechanisms of detoxification include reduction, hydrolysis, conjugation, oxidation, excretion in bile, degradation, and storage of certain substances, such as morphine, curare, and strychnine, to be released at a later time into the circulation. In this way, the hepatocytes protect the body from drug-related hepatic injury. The reticuloendothelial system also protects the body by phagocytosis of viruses, bacteria, dyes, and foreign proteins.

### Vitamin storage

High concentrations of riboflavin (vitamin B2) are found in the liver, as are nicotinic acid and pyridoxine. Also found in the liver are small amounts of vitamin C, most of the body's vitamin D stores, vitamin E, and vitamin K. Vitamin E is excreted in bile, which is required for vitamin K absorption. Ninety-five percent of vitamin A stores are also concentrated in the liver.

## PATHOPHYSIOLOGY

Some of the pathologic conditions that affect the liver are cirrhosis, hepatitis, tumors, Wilson's disease, porphyria, and intrahepatic biliary dysplasia.

### Cirrhosis

**Cirrhosis** of the liver is associated with the death of liver cells and subsequent fibrotic regeneration. The process of regeneration alters the normal vasculature, leading to impaired blood flow and ultimately to hepatic insufficiency. One of the key changes is the diversion of blood flow from the hepatic parenchyma. The anatomic hallmarks of this disorder are hepatic parenchymal inflammation and necrosis, nodular regeneration, and formation of new connective tissue (fibrosis).

There are three major etiologic types of cirrhosis.

- Alcoholic cirrhosis, also known as micronodular, portal, or Laennec's cirrhosis, accounts for up to 50% of patients with cirrhosis. In these patients the liver becomes enlarged and greasy as altered lipid metabolism leads to fatty infiltrates. Prognosis depends largely on the patient's ability to abstain from alcohol.
- Primary biliary cirrhosis is a disease of uncertain etiology that primarily affects middle-age women. Liver disease in this case is primarily cholestatic, which leads to jaundice, pruritus, steatorrhea, and death from hepatic failure. Fibrosis, ductal cell destruction, and inflammation make the liver enlarged, firm, and green. The disease usually follows a slow, steady downhill course.
- Postnecrotic cirrhosis is caused by hepatic necrosis and may be related to hepatitis, infection, metabolic liver disease, or exposure to hepatotoxins or industrial chemicals. In patients with this type of cirrhosis, the liver becomes small and distorted.

Cirrhosis may also be classified on the basis of morphology into the following three categories: micronodular cirrhosis, in which regenerative nodules are uniform in size and less than 3 mm in diameter; macronodular cirrhosis, in which the regenerative nodules are variable in size but greater than 3 mm in diameter; or mixed cirrhosis, in which both types of nodules are present in approximately equal proportions.

Signs and symptoms of cirrhosis include weight loss,

**Table 20-1.** Child's classification of liver failure

| Group designation | A | B | C |
|---|---|---|---|
| Serum bilirubin (mg/100ml) | Below 2.0 | 2.0-3.0 | Over 3.0 |
| Serum albumin (g/100ml) | Over 3.5 | 3.0-3.5 | Under 3.0 |
| Ascites | None | Easily controlled | Poorly controlled |
| Neurologic disorder | None | Minimal | Advanced |
| Nutrition | Excellent | Good | Poor |

anorexia, abdominal pain, jaundice, and bruising. Definitive diagnosis requires histologic confirmation of altered hepatic architecture, which is obtained at biopsy examination of the liver.

Most well-established cases of cirrhosis are irreversible, but the progress of the disease may be halted by managing its cause and any complications. Prognosis is grave for cirrhotic patients with persistent jaundice, intractable ascites, coagulopathy, bleeding esophageal varices, or hypoalbuminemia.

Child devised a system that is useful when assessing the severity and prognosis of patients with cirrhosis or other forms of chronic liver disease. This system of classification is detailed in Table 20-1.

### Complications of cirrhosis

Complications of cirrhosis may include portal hypertension, varices, ascites, hepatorenal syndrome, or hepatic encephalopathy. Many of these complications can also be seen with other forms of severe hepatic injury.

In addition, cirrhosis, regardless of cause, is associated with an increased risk of primary hepatocellular carcinoma (PHCC). The mechanism of development of PHCC in patients with cirrhotic livers is unknown, but geographic factors may be important. In South Africa, PHCC is found in more than 30% of cirrhotic livers, while in southern California it is found in only 10%.

#### Portal hypertension

When liver blockage leads to increased portal vein resistance and backflow, portal vein pressure increases. To redirect blood flow and relieve hypertension, collateral circulation channels may develop (Fig. 20-2). Symptoms of **portal hypertension** include splenomegaly, varices, hemorrhoids, and caput medusae (dilated cutaneous veins in the umbilical area). Physical findings may include jaundice, bleeding tendencies, peripheral edema, palmar erythema, fetor hepaticus (a sweet, fetid breath odor), and symptoms of increased estrogen levels, such as spider nevi, altered hair distribution, gyneco-

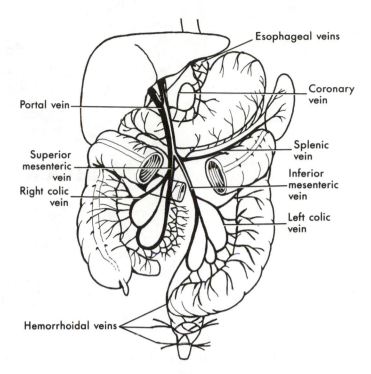

**Fig. 20-2.** Portal circulation showing collateral circulation.

mastia in men, testicular atrophy, or menstrual disorders.

The best way of assessing portal hypertension in cirrhosis of the liver is to measure the portal vein pressure gradient (PVPG). To measure PVPG it is necessary to do simultaneous invasive procedures that measure both the portal pressure and the pressure in the inferior vena cava.

Portal hypertension may be treated by surgery that diverts blood flow around the liver and away from collateral vessels, but allows some blood into the liver. Several types of shunt procedures are available, including the following:

- Portacaval shunt, the most common shunt procedure, which joins the portal vein and inferior vena cava by using either an end-to-side or side-to-side technique
- Splenorenal shunt, which joins the splenic vein and left renal vein by using either an end-to-side or side-to-side technique
- Mesocaval shunt, which joins the superior mesenteric vein to the inferior vena cava

#### Varices

As blood enters the liver through the portal vein, the connective tissue and liver nodules compressing the blood vessels cause resistance, thereby forcing the blood back into collateral vessels that may be formed in the esophagus, umbilical area, duodenum, abdomen, or rectum, thus producing varices (Fig. 20-3). The diagnosis

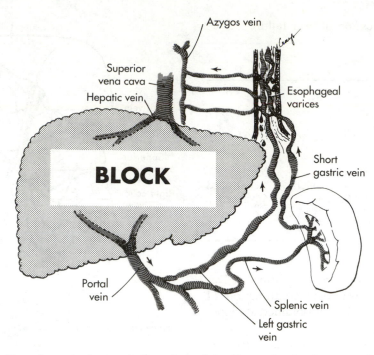

**Fig. 20-3**. Hemodynamic changes in liver cirrhosis leading to the development of esophageal varices. (From Price SA and Wilson LM: Pathophysiology: clinical concepts of disease processes, ed 4, St. Louis, 1992, Mosby–Year Book.)

and treatment of esophageal varices is discussed in Chapter 14.

### Ascites

When fibrotic tissue prohibits blood from leaving the liver via the vena cava, the liver begins to expand beyond its normal capacity. When this happens, fluid (mostly plasma) leaks through the surface of the liver into the peritoneal cavity, thus causing an accumulation of serous fluid that is known as **ascites.**

In some cases, ascites may be controlled by salt restriction, administration of diuretics, and bed rest. Occasionally, a peritoneojugular venous (LaVeen) shunt is inserted to divert ascitic fluid from the abdominal cavity into the superior vena cava. However, successful use of this procedure requires the patient's cooperation, and complications are not uncommon. Paracentesis is done only to relieve acute respiratory or abdominal distress or for diagnostic purposes.

### Hepatorenal syndrome

**Hepatorenal syndrome** is a progressive, functional form of renal failure that occurs in patients with severe liver disease, in the absence of clinical or anatomic evidence of other causes to explain the degree or persistence of renal failure. Most of these patients have cirrhosis, tense ascites, and encephalopathy. It seems most likely that hepatorenal syndrome starts with subclinical renal dysfunction caused by decreased or unstable perfusion of the kidneys in patients with severe liver disease. There is no evidence of renal parenchymal damage.

Hepatorenal syndrome is characterized by progressive azotemia, urine volume less than 500 ml/day, concentrated urine, and urinary sodium concentration less than 10 mEq/l. Urinalysis may show a few hyaline or granular casts, minimal proteinuria, and microscopic hematuria. Hyponatremia, hyperkalemia, hepatic encephalopathy, and coma frequently precede or accompany the renal functional deterioration. Prognosis is very poor, with an associated mortality greater than 90%. Most patients die of hemorrhage, infection, hypotension, or hepatic failure.

Treatment is primarily supportive, but management should include the identification, removal, and treatment of any factors known to precipitate renal failure. A high-calorie, low-protein, low-sodium diet is advisable. All patients should undergo a trial of fluid challenge using saline with salt-poor albumin or plasma to increase the effective plasma volume. Dialysis may be helpful in patients with reversible forms of liver disease. Liver transplantation will cure hepatorenal syndrome in appropriate candidates.

### Hepatic encephalopathy

**Hepatic encephalopathy,** or hepatic coma, is a major neuropsychiatric complication of chronic liver disease. It is conceivably related to the accumulation of large amounts of ammonia within the brain tissue. Ammonia is normally produced by the breakdown of protein in the bowel and in healthy individuals it is metabolized by the liver to form urea. In patients with portal hypertension, the blood cannot pass into the liver and the ammonia enters the systemic circulation and flows to the brain.

Symptoms of hepatic encephalopathy usually progress in the following four stages:

- Stage 1. Mild confusion, mood changes, inability to concentrate, sleep disturbances, and mild asterixis (rapid wrist flapping or liver flap)
- Stage 2. Confusion, apathy, aberrant behavior, asterixis, and apraxia (loss of ability to carry out familiar, purposeful movements)
- Stage 3. Severe confusion, incoherence, diminished responsiveness to verbal stimuli, hyperactive deep-tendon reflexes
- Stage 4. No reaction to stimuli, no corneal reflex, dilated pupils, flexion or extension posture

Hepatic encephalopathy is treated by correcting pH and electrolyte disturbances, restricting dietary protein, preventing constipation, and taking measures to prevent gastrointestinal bleeding, because intestinal blood breakdown also results in ammonia production. Administration of neomycin sulfate (Mycifradin) may decrease the number of bacteria that break down amino acids. Lactulose (Cephulac) may be given to promote ammonia retention and excretion through the intestinal tract.

### Hepatitis

**Hepatitis** is defined as an inflammation of the liver that may be accompanied by parenchymal liver damage. It may be acute or chronic. Signs and symptoms vary depending on etiology. The most prevalent type of hepatitis is viral hepatitis, which may be caused by many different viruses, including Epstein-Barr virus (EBV), cytomegalovirus (CMV), rubella, herpes simplex, varicella, and others. Viral forms of hepatitis include hepatitis A (infectious hepatitis), hepatitis B (serum hepatitis), hepatitis C (parenterally transmitted non-A, non-B hepatitis), hepatitis D (delta hepatitis), and hepatitis E (epidemic or enterically transmitted, non-A, non-B hepatitis). In addition to these viral forms, other types of hepatitis include alcoholic hepatitis, drug-induced hepatitis, and autoimmune hepatitis.

#### Hepatitis A

Hepatitis A virus (HAV) is the most common type of hepatitis. The virus involved is an RNA virus of the enterovirus family. HAV is usually a mild disease and is spread by the fecal-oral route, either through oral-anal sexual practices or by contaminated food, water, or shellfish. Exposed household or sexual contacts should receive prophylactic doses of immune globulin (formerly called ISG or gammaglobulin), which provide passive immunity for 2 to 3 months.

Most HAV infections, especially those acquired during childhood, are subclinical. Symptomatic patients experience early low-grade fever, fatigue, nausea, anorexia, myalgia, and malaise, followed by dark urine, light stools, and right upper quadrant discomfort.

Physical findings include jaundice, tender hepatomegaly and, rarely, splenomegaly.

Most patients with HAV recover uneventfully after a period of rest from strenuous activity. HAV does not progress to chronic hepatitis, although 3% to 5% of patients with HAV infections develop a protracted cholestatic hepatitis characterized by elevated alkaline phosphatase and jaundice. In certain high-risk patients, particularly those over 60 years of age, fulminant hepatic failure is possible, but rare.

#### Hepatitis B

The hepatitis B virus (HBV) is a DNA virus that consists of an inner core and a surrounding envelope. It is transmitted via serum, but can also be transmitted by semen or saliva. A major route of transmission is through perinatal infection of infants born to women who are carriers of the virus.

Individuals at high risk for exposure to HBV should receive the hepatitis B vaccine, which provides active immunity for up to 5 years or longer. Persons who should be vaccinated include healthcare workers; hemodialysis patients; homosexually active men; intravenous drug users; household, sexual, or other contacts of HBV carriers or IV drug users; and refugees from endemic areas, prison inmates, and infants born to women who are carriers of HBV.

In uncomplicated cases, hepatitis B begins with a prodrome, followed by a period of jaundice, which may last from 1 week to 1 month, and then a period of recovery. Common symptoms include dark urine, pale stools, malaise, nausea, fever, headache, anorexia, vomiting, and abdominal pain. Physical signs include jaundice and hepatomegaly with some tenderness. Some patients exhibit splenomegaly, diffuse adenopathy, and/or a maculopapular rash. Diagnosis is usually by finding HBsAg in serum.

Most patients recover uneventfully. Treatment entails 1 to 2 weeks of rest from strenuous physical activity. In-hospital management may be required for elderly patients and for patients who develop ascites or encephalopathy. In-hospital treatment should include a nutritionally balanced diet, intravenous hydration and electrolyte management if necessary, and in some cases, subcutaneous vitamin K and fresh frozen plasma. Medications should be used sparingly and alcohol should be avoided.

Complications of HBV may include chronic hepatitis, which develops in about 10% of HBV patients, and fulminant hepatic failure, which occurs in only 0.1% of these patients. By definition, chronic hepatitis is an inflammatory reaction of the liver that lasts for more than 6 months. Chronic hepatitis may manifest itself in several different ways.

- Chronic persistent hepatitis has a protracted course. Cirrhosis is rare in patients with chronic hepatitis, but the incidence of hepatocellular carcinoma is increased. Symptoms are usually mild, if any. No therapy is needed and prognosis is generally good.

- In chronic lobular hepatitis, there is a more pronounced inflammatory process that resembles protracted acute hepatitis. In addition to the portal and periportal inflammation observed in chronic persistent hepatitis, there is increased lobular activity without erosion of the limiting plate of the hepatocytes.
- Up to 3% of patients with HBV progress to chronic aggressive or chronic active hepatitis (CAH). Compared to chronic persistent or lobular hepatitis, CAH is associated with higher levels of serum transaminases, along with mild hyperbilirubinemia and more severe portal and periportal inflammation with erosion of the limiting plate of peripheral hepatocytes (piecemeal necrosis). In more severe cases, necrosis may span the lobules (bridging necrosis) or multilobular collapse may be seen, thus starting a progressive process that leads to fibrosis, scar formation, and cirrhosis.

**Fulminant hepatic failure** is defined as massive liver cell death within 2 months of the development of acute hepatitis. Patients with fulminant hepatic failure are confused, somnolent, or comatose and usually have ascites, edema, coagulopathy, and a shrinking liver. Death occurs in 80% of these patients as a result of gastrointestinal bleeding, sepsis, brainstem compression from cerebral edema, or multisystem failure. There is no specific therapy for fulminant hepatic failure, but the high mortality rate can be decreased with continuous supportive therapy administered in an intensive care unit.

### Hepatitis C

Hepatitis that could not be classified by etiologic agent was formerly referred to as non-A, non-B (NANB) hepatitis. Recently a serologic test was developed that makes it possible to distinguish parenterally transmitted NANB (hepatitis C virus, or HCV) from other forms of liver inflammation. Hemophiliacs and patients undergoing surgery with high transfusion requirements are at particular risk for developing HCV. Non–transfusion-related transmission accounts for approximately 50% of detected anti-HCV antibody. The mechanism of community-acquired transmission is believed to be IV drug use.

Acute HCV is often subclinical. Approximately 50% of patients with HCV, however, progress to chronic disease; of those, 20% develop cirrhosis. Hepatocellular carcinoma is also associated with HCV, but it is not known whether this association is directly related to the virus or if it is a consequence of chronic liver disease.

Recombinant interferon alfa-2b (Intron) is now available for the treatment of chronic cases. Steroids are sometimes given to enhance the patient's energy and well-being, but they may not alter the clinical course of the disease.

### Hepatitis D

The delta agent, hepatitis D virus (HDV), is a simple parasite, a single stranded RNA virus without enzymes or protein coat, that preys on the hepatitis B virus. HDV is endemic in Italy and other Mediterranean countries and several regions of South America. In nonendemic areas, such as North America and northern Europe, HDV is transmitted primarily by serum and is found primarily in polytransfused children, homosexual men, and IV drug users.

Delta infections can occur only in patients with HBV infection, as either a coinfection or a superinfection. As a coinfection, the HBV is usually eliminated and chronic hepatitis does not ensue. Superinfection with HDV, however, often leads to rapidly progressive liver damage and a more serious prognosis. In general, HDV tends to increase the virulence and severity of HBV infection. The only promising therapeutic approach in chronic hepatitis D has been the use of α-interferon, which has been beneficial in approximately 50% of treated patients.

### Hepatitis E

Hepatitis E is an epidemic or enterically transmitted form of HCV that was first identified in early 1988. It is transmitted by fecal-oral contact or contaminated food and water and is most prevalent in regions with poor sanitation systems. In India, hepatitis E is the leading cause of acute viral hepatitis in young and middle-age adults. The incubation period is 6 to 8 weeks.

### Alcoholic hepatitis

Biopsy of the liver in patients with a history of alcoholism may show scattered fatty deposition, hepatocyte degeneration and necrosis, pericellular fibrosis and inflammation, cholestasis, and cirrhosis. Hepatitis is considered a precirrhotic lesion.

Symptoms of alcoholic hepatitis include right upper quadrant abdominal pain, fever, vomiting, anorexia, and dark urine. Unlike other forms of hepatitis, patients do not present with jaundice. Physical signs include an enlarged and tender liver, splenomegaly, signs of chronic alcohol abuse and cirrhosis, and mental status abnormalities.

Treatment is based on supportive care, identification and correction of metabolic abnormalities, and avoidance of factors that are known to worsen hepatic function. It is reversible with abstinence from alcohol.

### Drug-induced hepatitis

Drugs can cause a wide range of hepatic injuries, including the following:

- A predictable dose-related hepatotoxic reaction, such as that produced by acetaminophen (Tylenol), carbon tetrachloride, and methotrexate
- An unpredictable, non–dose-related viral-like hepatitis, with or without cholestasis, which is produced by such drugs as isoniazid, flurazepam, methyldopa, and intravenous tetracycline (Achromycin)
- Cholestasis, related to the use of anabolic steroids, birth control pills, and haloperidol (Haldol)

The clinical presentation ranges from asymptomatic persons with transaminase elevations to patients who develop fulminant hepatic failure. Most patients recover within 1 to 2 weeks of discontinuing the offending agent.

Patients who ingest massive doses of acetaminophen (Tylenol) are at risk for fulminant hepatic failure. Appropriate therapy must be instituted within 24 hours of ingestion, including ipecac-induced emesis and administration of N-acetylcysteine in a loading dose, followed by maintenance doses until plasma acetaminophen falls below hepatotoxic levels.

### Autoimmune hepatitis

Patients with autoimmune chronic active hepatitis (CAH) demonstrate a predominantly non–T-cell cytotoxicity against autologous hepatocytes. Before the advent of corticosteroid therapy, 80% of patients with autoimmune CAH died of rapidly progressive liver disease within 3 years of diagnosis. Now, patients with autoimmune CAH are treated with daily doses of prednisone or prednisolone (Hydeltrasol), which are gradually reduced and finally withdrawn altogether. Prognosis is generally favorable with treatment, and patients may pursue a nearly normal lifestyle, although frequent relapses are possible.

## Tumors

Most benign liver tumors are hemangiomas that consist of blood vessels. Diagnosis is by ultrasonography, computed tomography (CT) scan, or arteriography. Treatment involves tumor excision to reduce the risk of tumor rupture and hemorrhage.

Primary cancerous liver tumors originate in either the hepatocytes or bile duct cells. Predisposing factors include a history of cirrhosis, hepatitis B, androgen therapy, and exposure to hepatotoxic chemicals. Metastasis is generally to the regional lymph nodes, lungs, and peritoneum. Metastatic or secondary liver tumors are far more common than primary liver tumors, often spreading from the lungs, breasts, GI tract, thyroid, prostate, or skin.

Most patients with liver cancer are asymptomatic until the disease is well advanced. Presenting complaints include right upper quadrant pain, weight loss, and weakness. Physical signs include an enlarged and tender liver and a bruit, or friction rub, over the liver.

Diagnosis is by scans, angiography, and needle biopsy examination. Large elevations in serum α-fetoprotein (AFP) are virtually diagnostic for primary hepatocellular carcinoma. Prognosis is grim. For patients with a localized mass without lymph node, bile duct, or blood vessel involvement or distal metastases, up to 80% of the liver may be resected. Pain may be relieved with chemotherapeutic liver perfusion via the hepatic artery. Ligation or occlusion of the hepatic artery may temporarily slow cell growth and activity.

If the tumor obstructs the bile duct, endoscopic or transhepatic insertion of a biliary decompression catheter or stent may provide some relief.

### Wilson's disease

**Wilson's disease** is a rare autosomal recessive disorder that is characterized by defective excretion of copper into bile, thus leading to excessive amounts of copper accumulating in the brain, liver, kidneys, and cornea. This accumulation of copper causes tissue necrosis, hepatic disease, and potential hepatic failure. Fifty percent of all patients have symptoms before the age of 15.

Patients with Wilson's disease have a characteristic rusty brown ring of pigment, called a Kayser-Fleischer ring, around the periphery of the cornea. Kayser-Fleischer rings may be accompanied by neurologic signs, such as prominent dysarthria, dystonia, and ataxia, emotional change, tremors, and/or seizures. Hepatic involvement may be minor or may be manifested by acute or chronic hepatitis, sometimes progressing to cirrhosis.

Once the diagnosis is confirmed, all family members should be screened for the disease. Treatment of Wilson's disease involves lifelong therapy with D-penicillamine (Cuprimine). Therapy has been most successful in precirrhotic asymptomatic siblings. Without treatment, patients invariably succumb to liver disease or neurologic complications.

### Porphyria

**Porphyria** is defined as a hereditary or acquired enzyme defect in which the biosynthesis of heme, in either the bone marrow or liver, leads to an overproduction of porphyrins or their precursors. Porphyrias are classified as either erythropoietic, hepatic, or erythrohepatic. The four hepatic porphyrias are listed as follows:

- Acute intermittent porphyria
- Hereditary coproporphyria, which is characterized by large amounts of coproporphyrin III in the feces and lesser amounts in urine
- Variegate porphyria, which is characterized by large amounts of protoporphyrin in the feces, with

smaller amounts of coproporphyrin in feces and in urine

- Porphyria cutanea tarda (PCT), which is the most common form of hepatic porphyria and is characterized by chronic skin lesions with fragility, blistering, poor healing, and scar formation, especially on light-exposed skin; increased hair growth, especially on the face; and mild liver disease with fatty infiltration, focal necrosis, or hepatic siderosis

The first three hepatic porphyrias are similar clinically, with acute attacks of abdominal pain, peripheral neuropathy, and psychiatric symptoms. Attacks may be precipitated by drugs, alcohol, fasting, or infection. Inheritance is autosomal dominant. Urinary porphobilinogen and δ-aminolevulinic acid are elevated in acute attacks and can be measured using the Watson-Schwartz test. Treatment consists of intravenous glucose and/or hematin, and supportive care with avoidance of precipitating factors.

PCT may be hereditary or acquired. Acquired PCT may be associated with alcohol abuse, estrogen, or polychlorinated hydrocarbons. Urinary uroporphyrin and urinary coproporphyrin are elevated. No acute abdominal or neuropsychiatric attacks are apparent.

Protoporphyria is an autosomal dominant erythrohepatic porphyria that is characterized by solar urticaria, which is burning and tingling on exposure to light, and solar eczema, which is cutaneous thickening on repeated exposure. Liver involvement may progress to fibrosis or cirrhosis. Free erythrocyte protoporphyrin is elevated. Birefringent protoporphyrin pigment deposits are present in hepatocytes, Kupffer cells, and bile canaliculi.

Cholestyramine (Questran) has been used to reduce the protoporphyrin pool and thereby halt the progression of liver disease or even reverse the process. Patients are also treated with β-carotene.

Patients with PCT or protoporphyria should avoid porphyrin-stimulating agents, such as estrogen containing oral contraceptives, chloroquine (Aralen, an antimalarial amebicidal agent), griseofulvin (Fulvicin, a fungicide), iron compounds, and alcohol.

### Hemochromatosis

**Hemochromatosis** is a recessively inherited disorder of iron metabolism and is characterized by excessive tissue iron deposition. It is the third most common inherited disorder of metabolism in whites, after cystic fibrosis and α1-antitrypsin deficiency.

Hemochromatosis usually occurs in patients who are in middle age. Complaints of weakness, malaise, loss of libido, weight loss, change in skin color, abdominal pain, joint pain, or symptoms related to diabetes mellitus are presenting symptoms. Males are 10 times more likely to be diagnosed than females. Hepatomegaly is found in 95% of symptomatic patients. Skin pigmentation, testicular atrophy, loss of body hair, arthropathy, and congestive heart failure are other prominent physical signs. Hepatocellular carcinoma develops in approximately 30% of symptomatic patients.

In diagnosing hemochromatosis, a high index of suspicion is required. Serum ferritin is usually grossly elevated, and serum iron concentration is usually elevated. Plain x-ray films of the hands may show chondrocalcinosis, sclerosis of subchondral bone, loss of articular cartilage, and subchondral cyst formation. Computed tomography scans of the liver show marked increases in density, but needle biopsy examination of the liver is needed to confirm the diagnosis. Biopsy of the liver permits estimation of tissue irons by histochemical staining, chemical analysis of hepatic iron concentration, and histologic assessment of liver damage.

All first-generation relatives should be screened for iron overload. The mainstay of therapy is removal of iron from the body by phlebotomy. Phlebotomy should be performed weekly or biweekly for approximately 2 years until hemoglobin, ferritin, and iron levels become normal, at which time the frequency of phlebotomy can be reduced to every 1 to 3 months.

### α1-Antitrypsin deficiency

**α1-Antitrypsin (AAT)** is an α1-globulin found in serum, various body fluids, and tissues. It is a potent protease inhibitor and is synthesized in the hepatocytes for protection against tissue injury that results from proteases. At least 26 genetic variants have been identified, designated by different letters of the alphabet. The most common phenotype of AAT deficiency is PiMM, which is associated with normal circulating levels of AAT. The homozygous PiZZ phenotype and most likely the heterozygous PiMZ are both important with regard to liver disease.

The genetic association of AAT deficiency with liver disease and cirrhosis has been confirmed in children and in adults. Its relation to hepatic cancer remains controversial. The incidence of AAT deficiency is similar to that of cystic fibrosis, but early death occurs only in a small percentage of patients. No medical therapy is beneficial to these patients; treatment is primarily supportive. Liver transplantation can confer the donor phenotype in suitable patients, which often results in long-term survival.

### Intrahepatic biliary dysplasia

**Intrahepatic biliary dysplasia (IHBD),** also known as Alagille's syndrome, is a unique, autosomal dominant liver disease that appears in approximately 1 in 100,000 live births. It incorporates a combination of anomalies that occur in conjunction with chronic cholestasis. Patients with IHBD display characteristic facial features, vertebral malformations, and retarded physical, mental, and sexual development, and various cardiac anomalies, most often peripheral pulmonic stenosis. Liver changes progress from a decrease in the number of portal zones to bile plugging small interlobular bile ducts, hepatocytes, and small canaliculi; absence or decrease in portal bile ducts; and collapsed portal bile ducts.

Children with IHBD frequently have cholestatic jaundice in the neonatal period, often accompanied by failure to thrive, prematurity, or small size for gestational age. The liver is enlarged and firm or hard on palpation. Most infants and children with IHBD are more affected by their cardiac abnormalities than by their liver disease.

Treatment of IHBD involves symptomatic and supportive care, including good nutrition and fat-soluble vitamin supplementation. Cholestyramine (Questran) and phenobarbital may be given to relieve pruritus.

The only surgical alternative is liver transplantation, which involves removal of the diseased liver and transplantation of a donor liver. Postoperatively, the patient has a T-tube in the common bile duct anastomosis and Jackson-Pratt drains above and below the new liver. Lifelong cyclosporin (Sandimmune) and prednisone therapy are needed to prevent organ rejection. The patient should be observed for signs of infection, hemorrhage or hypovolemia, pleural effusion, liver function problems, and organ rejection. Other potential complications include disseminated intravascular coagulation, renal failure, vascular graft obstruction, anastomosis leakage, peritonitis, cholangitis, pneumonitis, and gastrointestinal bleeding.

Quality of life and life expectancy for patients with IHBD depend primarily on the degree of heart disease and on long-term liver status. Some patients experience a gradual remission of cholestasis, while others progress to cirrhosis.

---

**CASE SITUATION**

Mr. Rudy Stern, age 34, was admitted to the emergency room for gastrointestinal bleeding. His routine blood work showed a prolonged prothrombin time and elevated transaminase values. A hepatitis screen and an emergency gastroscopy are ordered to determine the cause of his gastrointestinal bleeding. He has a large-bore nasogastric tube in place, which is draining copious amounts of dark red blood. In the endoscopy room, the gastroenterology nurse sets up equipment for gastric lavage and proceeds to lavage Mr. Stern's stomach until the return is clear enough to begin the endoscopy.

Mr. Stern is found to have a large gastric ulcer with an oozing visible vessel, which the physician cauterizes with a bipolar probe. The bleeding stops and Mr. Stern is moved to the intensive care unit. The next day, however, he shows signs of rebleeding. He is taken to surgery and a partial gastrectomy is performed.

When Mr. Stern's hepatitis screen comes back, it is positive for HBsAg, hepatitis B core antibody (anti-HBc), and hepatitis A IgG antibody (IgG-anti-HAV).

*Points to think about*

1. Before the nurse was able to don gloves, she had significant contact with Mr. Stern's blood when he vomited before the lavage. Because the nurse had severe dermatitis on her hands, would she have been exposed to HAV or HBV?
2. Healthcare personnel in high-risk areas for HBV (i.e., those personnel who are in frequent contact with blood and body fluids) should be vaccinated against HBV. However, if a nurse has put off this important vaccination, what prophylaxis is available?
3. It is possible the nurse may never have been informed of Mr. Stern's hepatitis and subsequent possible exposure. What symptoms would alert the nurse to HBV infection?
4. The law requires that certain communicable diseases be reported. The nurse should determine who in the institution is responsible for reporting a communicable disease, to whom it should be reported, and what information is required in the report.
5. Although precise data are not available, the prolonged prothrombin time, Mr. Stern's tendency to bleed, and his diagnosis of viral hepatitis would lead the nurse to tentatively consider what nursing diagnosis?
6. What is an appropriate outcome criterion for this diagnosis? What nursing interventions will lead to this outcome?
7. What special infection-control precautions should the nurse take in the endoscopy setting?

*Suggested responses*

1. The nurse has been exposed to HBV, which is a major nosocomial problem that can have serious sequelae. Finding HBsAg in the blood is diagnostic of HBV infection. HBsAg is first detectable in serum 30 to 60 days after exposure, during the incubation period. This marker will usually be present in the blood until the end of the acute phase of the illness, or longer. Patients are considered infectious as long as HBsAg is detectable in serum. HBV is transmitted via serum,

semen, and saliva. Anti-HBc appears in the blood about the same time as serum transaminase levels rise.

The presence of IgG-anti-HAV is indicative of prior infection with HAV and a naturally acquired immunity. Mr. Stern had HAV in the past and is now immune, so this is not a contagious disease. HAV is transmitted by the fecal-oral route and not in the blood, although dirty needles can serve as a means of transmission.

2. If the nurse has not been vaccinated against HBV, the treatment of choice is hepatitis B immune globulin (HBIG), given within one week of exposure for passive immunity. It is recommended that HBV vaccine (Heptavax-B or Recombivax HB) be given in conjunction with the HBIG. The injections are given at different sites. Either HBV vaccine is safe in healthy adults and is given in three serial intramuscular doses of 1.0 ml within 1 week of exposure, 1 month later, and 6 months later.

3. If the nurse has been infected with HBV, the incubation period is 6 weeks to 6 months, with an average of 12 weeks. Symptoms may be relatively mild or quite severe. If symptoms are mild they can mimic a flulike syndrome. Symptoms may include fatigue, malaise, joint or muscle pain, anorexia, nausea, vomiting, fever and chills, jaundice, clay-colored stools, dark urine, and pruritus. There may be abdominal pain and tenderness in the right upper quadrant. Even though signs and symptoms may be absent during the incubation period, the person with hepatitis is contagious.

4. Ordinarily, the patient's physician is responsible for reporting both HAV and HBV infections to the state health department. The Centers for Disease Control (CDC) will include the case in its national statistics.

The gastroenterology nurse should know what diseases are required by law to be reported. Such cases should be reported to the infection control nurse in the hospital (or a counterpart) and that person can make certain the state health department has been informed. The health department may refer the case to its nursing division for postdischarge follow-up, or the gastroenterology nurse may refer the patient to the visiting nurse service of a local health department, if available.

The information to be reported may vary from state to state. Usually a health department will want, at a minimum, the patient's name, age, address, any possible contacts, the diagnosis, and the physician treating the patient.

5. These data would permit the nurse to consider the nursing diagnosis "potential for injury: bleeding, related to altered clotting mechanisms."

6. An appropriate outcome in relation to this nursing diagnosis would be "Mr. Stern will experience a resolution of bleeding episodes." Related nursing interventions would include the following:
   - Administer prescribed drugs
   - Observe incision and nasogastric drainage every 2 hrs
   - Take vital signs every hour
   - Check the IV site for bleeding, proper cannulation, and flow every 2 hours
   - Monitor neurologic vital signs every 4 hours

7. Special infection-control practices that should be used by gastroenterology nurses in the endoscopy setting include the following:
   - Taking Universal Precautions with *all* patients. When there is a potential for coming in contact with the blood or body fluids of any patient, the nurse should wear gloves, protective gowns, masks, and eyewear.
   - Cleaning and disinfecting equipment following accepted hospital policy. (Also refer to the SGNA monograph, *Recommended Guidelines for Infection Control in Gastrointestinal Endoscopy Settings.*)
   - Using information obtained in the nursing assessment to help identify patients at risk for hepatitis. High-risk patients include those who have recently had procedures using piercing instruments, such as ear piercing, tattooing, acupuncture, dental work, or blood transfusions. HBV is also common among dialysis patients, drug abusers, male homosexuals, AIDS patients, retarded people, and those with Hodgkin's disease, leukemia, or hemophilia.

---

### REVIEW TERMS

$\alpha$1-antitrypsin (AAT) deficiency, ascites, cirrhosis, fulminant hepatic failure, hemochromatosis, hepatic encephalopathy, hepatitis, hepatocytes, hepatorenal syndrome, intrahepatic biliary dysplasia (IHBD), Kupffer cells, porphyria, portal hypertension, portal triad, sinusoids, Wilson's disease

---

### REVIEW QUESTIONS

1. In the liver, bile is produced and secreted by:
   a. Sinusoids.
   b. Hepatocytes.
   c. Glisson's capsule.
   d. Kupffer cells.

2. Seventy-five percent of the blood that flows into the liver is delivered via the:
   a. Inferior vena cava.
   b. Hepatic artery.
   c. Portal vein.
   d. Splenic artery.

3. In the liver, carbohydrates are metabolized to:
   a. Glycogen.
   b. Amino acids.
   c. Ammonia.
   d. Glycerol.
4. The primary physiologic function of the Kupffer cells is:
   a. Metabolism.
   b. Production of prothrombin and fibrinogen.
   c. Vitamin storage.
   d. Phagocytosis of harmful substances.
5. A definitive diagnosis of cirrhosis is obtained through:
   a. Observation of a Kayser-Fleischer ring on the cornea.
   b. Ultrasonography or CT scan.
   c. Palpation of the liver.
   d. Biopsy of the liver.
6. The first line of treatment for ascites is:
   a. Dietary restrictions, diuretics, and bed rest.
   b. Shunt placement.
   c. Paracentesis.
   d. Liver transplantation.
7. The most common form of hepatitis is:
   a. Hepatitis A virus.
   b. Hepatitis B virus.
   c. Non-A, Non-B hepatitis.
   d. Alcoholic hepatitis.
8. Most patients with HBV are treated with:
   a. α-Interferon.
   b. Rest from strenuous physical activity.
   c. The hepatitis B vaccine.
   d. Intravenous hydration and electrolyte management.
9. Accumulation of excessive amounts of copper in certain body tissues is characteristic of:
   a. Alagille's syndrome.
   b. Primary liver cancer.
   c. Wilson's disease.
   d. Porphyria.
10. Chronic skin lesions, increased hair growth, mild liver disease, and a lack of neuropsychiatric manifestations are characteristic of:
    a. Acute intermittent porphyria.
    b. Hereditary coproporphyria.
    c. Variegate porphyria.
    d. Porphyria cutanea tarda.

## BIBLIOGRAPHY

Bongiovanni, G, ed. *Essentials of Clinical Gastroenterology.* 2nd ed. New York: McGraw–Hill, 1988.

Calvette, B. "Biliary Pathophysiology." In *SGA Journal Reprints,* ed. Trivits, S, 107-08. Rochester, N.Y.: Society of Gastrointestinal Assistants, 1988.

Chobanian, S, and Van Ness, M, eds. *Manual of Clinical Problems in Gastroenterology.* Boston: Little, Brown & Co., 1988.

Chopra, S, and May, R, eds. *Pathophysiology of Gastrointestinal Diseases.* Boston: Little, Brown & Co., 1989.

Davis, G, et al. "Treatment of Chronic Hepatitis C with Recombinant Interferon Alfa: A Multi-Center Randomized, Controlled Trial." *New England Journal of Medicine* 321 (November 30, 1989): 1501-06.

Eastwood, G, and Avunduk, C. *Manual of Gastroenterology: Diagnosis and Therapy.* Boston: Little, Brown & Co., 1988.

Eddy, M. *Hepatitis A Through E.* Paper presented at the 17th National Meeting of the Society of Gastroenterology Nurses and Associates, San Antonio, Tex., 16 May 1990.

Ellett, M. "Living with Chronic Hepatitis." *Gastroenterology Nursing* 12 (Fall 1989): 125-30.

Given, B, and Simmons, S. *Gastroenterology in Clinical Nursing.* 4th ed. St. Louis: Mosby–Year Book, 1984.

Goldberg, K, ed. *Gastrointestinal Problems.* Nurse Review Series. Springhouse, Pa.: Springhouse Corporation, 1986.

Newton, M, and Andrews, L. "The Anatomy and Physiology of the Liver." *SGA Journal Reprints,* ed. Trivits, S, 113-15. Rochester, N.Y.: Society of Gastrointestinal Assistants, 1988.

Sachar, D, Waye, J, and Lewis, B, eds. *Gastroenterology for the House Officer.* Baltimore: Williams & Wilkins, 1989.

Silverman, A, and Roy, C. *Pediatric Clinical Gastroenterology.* 3rd ed. St. Louis: Mosby–Year Book, 1983.

Waldecker, C. "Understanding Intrahepatic Biliary Dysplasia." *SGA Journal* 12 (Winter 1989): 174-78.

# PHARMACOLOGY, INTRAVENOUS THERAPY, AND NUTRITION

# Chapter 21

# PHARMACOLOGY

This chapter will acquaint the gastroenterology nurse with diagnostic and therapeutic medications that are administered to gastroenterology patients. General information is provided on techniques and routes of drug administration, dosage calculations, patient education, and documentation. The classes of drugs that are used most often in gastroenterology practice are described in general terms, including indications, contraindications, and possible side effects. An extended table is provided with the generic and trade names of representative medications, including primary use, usual adult dosage, and potential adverse effects.

## Learning objectives

After reviewing the content of this chapter, the gastroenterology nurse should be able to:
1. Discuss general aspects of drug therapy that are relevant to nursing practice, including techniques and routes of administration, dosage calculations and conversions, patient education, and documentation.
2. Describe the general classes of medications that are important in gastroenterology, including general indications, contraindications, and potential adverse effects.
3. Identify representative drugs used in gastroenterology practice, their respective generic and trade names, indications, usual adult dosages, and possible side effects.

## BASIC PRINCIPLES

Gastroenterology nurses should be able to recognize the expected actions of the drugs prescribed, be confident that ordered dosages are within the safe range for a particular patient, and be alert to the possibility of adverse effects or undesirable drug interactions. If, based on knowledge and experience, nurses have any questions about medication or dosage ordered, or if

serious adverse effects are noted, the physician should be consulted immediately.

Before administering any medication, it is important that the nurse compare the physician's order with the patient's medication record. There should be a written order for every medication given. If the medication order is verbal, institutional policies and state laws will determine the time frame in which verbal orders must be signed by the physician. Verification of the patient's identity, the drug to be administered, the dose, the route, and the time of administration is essential. It is also important to check that the label on the medication matches the medication order. Privacy should be provided as needed for injections and for application of topical drugs. The procedure should be explained to the patient. Regardless of the route of administration, prior handwashing is essential.

## Techniques and routes of administration

Medications may be administered orally, parenterally, or topically. The route of administration is determined by the required speed of onset of the drug's effect, patient comfort and safety considerations, and the organ or system targeted by the drug. Intramuscular injections, for example, take effect quickly because they are immediately accessible in the bloodstream, whereas drugs administered by topical routes must be absorbed before they can be effective. However, injections are more uncomfortable for the patient than oral or topical drugs and carry a greater risk of side effects. When the gastrointestinal system is the target of drug therapy, oral administration is usually the most effective.

The **oral** route is the most common route of drug administration. Oral medications may take the form of tablets, capsules, syrups, elixirs, oils, liquids, suspensions, powders, or granules. Most oral medications are swallowed by mouth, but may also be given through a nasogastric or gastrostomy tube, or may be dissolved between the cheek and gum or under the tongue. Nausea, vomiting, inability to swallow, or unconsciousness may contraindicate oral administration of medications.

**Parenteral** medications are administered by injection, using a subcutaneous (SC), intramuscular (IM), or intravenous (IV) route. Subcutaneous injections are administered into the adipose tissue (the fatty layer) beneath the skin. The SC route is faster than oral administration, but allows slower, more sustained drug action than an IM injection. Subcutaneous injections also cause minimal tissue trauma and carry little risk of striking large blood vessels and nerves. The most common SC injection sites are the outer aspect of the upper arm, anterior thigh, buttocks, upper back, and loose tissue of the lower abdomen.

Intramuscular injections deposit medication deep into muscle tissue, where it can be readily absorbed. Muscles used for IM injections include the deltoids, dorsogluteal and ventrogluteal areas, and vastus lateralis (lateral muscle of the quadriceps group). The addition of drugs to IV solutions, and IV push administration are discussed in Chapter 22.

If the volume of medication to be injected is not excessive, the combination of two drugs in one syringe avoids the discomfort of two separate injections. Drugs can be combined from two multidose vials, from one multidose vial and one ampul, or from two ampuls. Drugs may be combined only if their compatibility has been documented. Rarely are more than two drugs combined in one syringe. One exception is the administration of sedative medications in younger pediatric patients. To avoid giving two injections, meperidine (Demerol), promethazine (Phenergan), and chlorpromazine (Thorazine) are routinely combined in one syringe.

Depending on their purpose, **topical** drugs may be administered to gastroenterology patients in the form of ointments or sprays (e.g., antiseptics or anesthetics), transdermal patches (e.g., motion sickness preventives), or rectal suppositories (e.g., antiemetics). Medicated shampoos, eye medications, ear drops, nasal sprays and drops, vaginal medications, and inhaled products are also considered topical medications. The site of topical drug application should be inspected frequently for side effects, such as skin irritation or an allergic reaction.

### Calculations and conversions

To administer the correct dose of a medication, it may be necessary for the nurse to convert the physician's order to a different unit of measure or to dilute available doses. Usually, physicians order medications in grains, grams, milligrams, or other units of *weight*. Before the

**Table 21-1.** Abbreviations used in drug administration

| | |
|---|---|
| ac | Before meals |
| ad lib | As desired |
| bid | Twice a day |
| caps | Capsules |
| fld or fl | Fluid |
| g, gm | Gram |
| gr | Grain |
| gtt | Drop |
| h or hr | Hour |
| hs | At bedtime |
| IM | intramuscular |
| IV | Intravenous |
| kg | Kilogram |
| μg, ug, mcg | Microgram |
| mEq | Milliequivalent |
| mg | Milligram |
| m | Minim |
| pc | After meals |
| per os, po | By mouth |
| prn | When required |
| qd | Every day |
| qh | Every hour |
| q2h | Every 2 hours |
| qid | Four times/day |
| SC | Subcutaneous |
| SL | Sublingual |
| tab | Pill |
| tid | Three times/day |
| U | Units |

medication can be administered to the patient, the order may need to be converted to the corresponding number of tablets, capsules, minims, drams, ounces, milliliters, or other units of *volume*. Abbreviations for these units and for other terms used in drug administration are given in Table 21-1.

Doses may be specified in any one of three different systems of measurement:
- Metric units (e.g., milliliters or grams)
- Apothecaries' units (e.g., ounces, drams, or minims)
- Household units (e.g., teaspoons, drops, cups)

Some of the more common equivalents are contained in Table 21-2. It is important that nurses memorize the equivalents necessary to convert between these three systems of measurement. By applying these conversion factors to simple arithmetic calculations involving ratios and proportions, any dosage problem can be easily solved.

In addition to the metric, apothecaries', or household systems of measurement, some drugs are measured in milliequivalents (mEq) or units (U). A milliequivalent refers to the number of ionic charges of an element or a compound. It is a measure of the chemical combining power of a substance. Units mean something different for every drug. One United States Pharmacopeia (USP)

**Table 21-2.** Approximate equivalents

| Weight units | | | Fluid units | | |
| --- | --- | --- | --- | --- | --- |
| Metric | Apothecaries' | Household | Metric | Apothecaries' | Household |
| 1 gram | 15-16 grains | | 1 ml or 1 cc | 15-16 minims | 15-16 drops |
| 30-32 grams | 1 ounce | 2 tablespoons | 30-32 ml | 1 fluid ounce | 2 tablespoon |
| | 8 drams | 8 teaspoons | | 8 fluid drams | 8 teaspoons |
| 1 kilogram | 2.2 pounds | | 1 liter | 8 ounces | 1 cup |
| | (avoirdupois) | | 1000 ml | 1 quart | 4 cups |
| | | | 4000 ml | 1 gallon | |

unit of insulin, for example, is defined as the quantity that promotes the metabolism of about 1.5 g of dextrose. Labels on drugs that are measured in this way indicate the number of milliequivalents or units in a particular volume measure (e.g., 400,000 U/ml or 20 mEq/15 ml).

When administering medications in tablet or capsule form, it is important to remember that only scored or marked tablets can be divided accurately; capsules cannot be divided. It is best to look for tablets or capsules of the desired dose.

Most volume doses of oral medications can be measured out in medicine cups, which are frequently marked in drams, ounces, milliliters (or cubic centimeters), teaspoons, and tablespoons. Smaller volume amounts, such as minims and drops, must be measured by using droppers or calibrated pipettes or syringes. Drops are an approximate household unit of measure that can be safely measured by using a medicine dropper. A minim is a more accurate, apothecaries' unit of measure and must be measured by using a minim pipette or syringe.

Solutions for parenteral administration may be ordered in units of volume, but are more frequently ordered in units of weight, such as grams or milligrams. The nurse must then convert the weight ordered to a unit of volume, such as drams, ounces, or milliliters. In many cases, labels on drugs in solution indicate a certain weight measure in a particular volume (e.g., 500 mg/5 ml). Labels may also state a percentage or a ratio strength of the solution (e.g., a 5% or 1:20 solution).

Occasionally it may be necessary to prepare oral or topical solutions from crystals, powder, or stock solutions or to prepare children's doses from adult dose tablets. Preparation of solutions is a simple problem in proportions. For pediatric doses, tablets that are soluble in water can be dissolved in a specified amount of water and the ordered dose measured by using a syringe.

Pediatric dosages are usually calculated based on the child's weight in kilograms, although consideration of body surface area is probably the most accurate method. Use of surface area requires consultation of one of the various charts or nomograms used to determine body surface area from height and weight. If surface area can be determined, the following formulas are used to calculate the pediatric dosage from the usual adult dosage:

- (Surface area in m$^2$ × Adult dose)/1.7 = Child's dose
- Surface area in m$^2$ × 60 = Percentage of adult dose

If surface area is not known, the most commonly used procedures for determining approximate pediatric dosages include the following:

- Young's rule (children from 1 or 2 to 12 years)
  **(Age in years/age + 12) × Adult dose = Child's dose**
- Fried's rule (infants and children up to 1 or 2 years)
  **(Age in months/150) × Adult dose = Child's dose**
- Clark's rule (infants or children)
  **(Weight in pounds/150) × Adult dose = Child's dose**

Again, if there is any question about the appropriateness of the ordered dosage for any patient, the physician should be consulted.

**Documentation**

Whenever medications are given, the name of the drug administered, the person administering the drug, the dose and route of administration, the date and time, and the patient's response or adverse reaction, if any, must be noted. For parenteral medications, the site of injection should also be noted.

If the patient refuses a drug, the refusal should be documented, and the charge nurse and the patient's doctor should be notified. If a drug is omitted or withheld for other reasons, such as radiology or laboratory tests, that omission and the reason should be documented according to institutional policy. Narcotics should be signed out on the appropriate narcotics control record.

If the patient's intake and output are being monitored, the fluid volume of any medications administered orally or through a nasogastric or gastrostomy tube should be noted on the intake and output sheet. In the case of topical administration, the nurse should note the condition of the skin at the time of application.

### Patient education

Patient education is another important aspect of drug therapy. The patient and/or the responsible party should understand the purpose of any medication that is ordered. If there is a change in medication or dosage, the patient should be informed. He or she should be instructed, as appropriate, about possible side effects and should be encouraged to report any symptoms that may indicate adverse effects.

Patient education should also encompass drug-diet and drug-drug interaction. Unless gastric irritation is a problem, it is usually best for the patient to take medications on an empty stomach because food can interfere with drug absorption. In addition, most drugs are more efficiently absorbed if taken with 100 to 250 ml of fluid. Antacids, on the other hand, should not be taken with water. It is important that the patient be aware of these considerations to maximize the effectiveness of drug therapy.

The issue of drug-drug interactions is another significant and increasingly complex area of concern. Generally speaking, drugs that increase gastrointestinal motility, such as stimulant cathartics, decrease the rate and extent of absorption of time-released drugs and drugs that require prolonged intestinal contact. Drugs that decrease motility, such as anticholinergics, may alter the absorption of certain drugs. Medications that alter gastric pH, such as antacids, decrease the absorption of some weakly acidic drugs, such as phenobarbital and aspirin. Patients must be cautioned to report all of the prescription and over-the-counter medications they are taking to their physician, and should be informed of any potentially problematic interactions. They should also be encouraged to report any known drug allergies.

### MAJOR GASTROINTESTINAL DRUG CLASSES

It is important that the gastroenterology nurse has a working knowledge of the various classes of drugs used in the practice of gastroenterology/endoscopy. Some of the medications prescribed for gastroenterology patients are intended to alter gastrointestinal secretions and/or motility, including anticholinergics and cholinergics, some laxatives, and certain antiulcer agents. Others are prescribed for their antacid, antiinflammatory, antiemetic, or antidiarrheal effects. Still other medications are used in diagnostic testing or to facilitate endoscopic or invasive procedures, which often require the use of topical anesthetics, sedatives, and/or narcotics. In addition, prophylactic antibiotics and therapeutic antiparasitic agents may be prescribed.

The following pages outline the general characteris-

tics of various drug classifications that should be familiar to gastroenterology nurses. Table 21-3 lists specific medications from these categories, with their respective trade names, indications, adult dosages, and adverse effects.

### Antacids

**Antacids** usually contain combinations of aluminum, calcium, and magnesium salts. Unlike other antiulcer agents, they have no direct effect on gastric acid secretion and they do not coat or protect the mucous lining. Instead they reduce the total acid load in the GI tract by buffering the acid that is being produced, thereby raising the gastric pH and reducing peptic activity. They also strengthen the gastric mucosal barrier.

Antacids are used in the treatment of patients with gastrointestinal disorders such as peptic ulcer disease, esophageal reflux, and hiatus hernia, and for symptomatic treatment of dyspepsia, heartburn, and acid indigestion. Antacids are clearly superior to placebo in healing duodenal ulcers, but studies of their efficacy in healing gastric ulcers are equivocal. Antacids may also be used to reduce gastric acidity in patients with upper GI bleeding that stems from a peptic ulcer.

Because they leave the stomach rapidly, antacids are best used for intermittent symptoms. Taken on an empty stomach, the effects of antacids last less than 1 hour; after meals, the buffering effect may last as long as 3 hours. For optimal effect, antacids should be given about 1 hour after meals or feedings and during periods of acid rebound. Their effect can be enhanced if the patient remains recumbent after eating.

Antacid suspensions have a longer action than tablets or solutions. Tablets should be chewed and followed with a glass of water to help them dissolve.

Prolonged use of magnesium- or calcium-containing antacids may cause systemic absorption of toxic quantities of magnesium or calcium ions. Excessive use of aluminum-containing antacids may lead to hypophosphatemia. Antacids containing sodium can precipitate edema in patients with cirrhosis, hypertension, or renal or congestive heart failure. Aluminum and calcium preparations may be constipating, whereas magnesium preparations produce a laxative effect.

### Antibiotics

**Antibiotics** may be prescribed for gastroenterology patients with severe cases of infectious diarrhea. Infectious organisms that respond to antibiotics include enterotoxigenic and enteropathogenic *Escherichia coli*, *Shigella*, *Helicobacter*, *Vibrio cholerae*, and *Clostridium difficile*. Compromised or toxic patients with *Salmonella* may also be treated with antibiotics. Antibiotics that are prescribed for patients with infectious diarrhea include

*Text continued on p. 201*

**Table 21-3.** Representative pharmacologic agents used in gastroenterology

| Agent | Trade name | Indications | Adult dosage | Adverse effects |
|---|---|---|---|---|
| **Antacids** | | | | |
| aluminum hydroxide | Gaviscon | Heartburn, sour stomach, acid indigestion | 2-4 tablets 4×/day | Not to be taken with tetracycline or by patients on a sodium-restricted diet. |
| aluminum OH$^+$ magnesium OH$^+$ simethicone | Mylanta; Maalox | Temporary gastric hyperacidity and gas | 2-4 tsp or 2-4 tablets between meals and hs | CNS depression and other symptoms of hypermagnesemia in patients with renal insufficiency. |
| calcium carbonate | Tums | Hyperacidity and acid indigestion | 1 g po, 4-6 ×/day | Constipation; hypercalcemia; hypophosphatemia. |
| magnesium hydroxide | Phillips' Milk of Magnesia (suspension) | Acid indigestion; sour stomach; heartburn; constipation | Antacid dose: 1-3 tsp up to 4×/day laxative dose: 2-4 tsp | Contraindicated for patients with kidney disease. |
| magaldrate | Riopan (suspension) | Hyperacidity; heartburn; sour stomach; acid indigestion | 1-2 tsp between meals and hs | Not to be taken with tetracycline or by patients with kidney disease. |
| **Antibiotics** | | | | |
| ampicillin | Ampicillin | Antibiotic prophylaxis; *Salmonella* infections; shigellosis | Prophylaxis: 250-400 mg 4×/day; *Salmonella*: 6-8 g/day IV; shigellosis: 1 g po q 6hr for 5 days | Most frequent are nausea, vomiting, and diarrhea. Laryngeal edema and anaphylaxis may occur in sensitive patients. |
| chloramphenicol | Chloromycetin | Acute *Salmonella* infections | 50 mg/kg/day in 4 divided doses | Bone marrow depression; gastrointestinal reactions; neurotoxic reactions; hypersensivity. |
| gentamicin | Garamycin | Antibiotic prophylaxis | 3 mg/kg 3×/day | Most frequent are ototoxicity and nephrotoxicity. |
| tetracycline | Tetracycline, Achromycin | Shigellosis; cholera | Shigellosis: 2.5 g/day po or 500 mg po q 6hr for 5 days; cholera: 500 mg q 6hr for 3 days | Dental staining in children under age 10. |
| tobramycin | Nebcin | Antibiotic prophylaxis for serious infections caused by susceptible aerobic gram negative bacilli | Normal renal function: 3-5 mg/kg IV, IM in 3 equal doses q 8hr; Impaired renal function: modify, individualize dose; Duration: No more than 10 days | Irreversible ototoxicity, both cocklear and vestibular. Nephrotoxicity usually mild and reversible. Classified FDA Pregnancy Category D. |
| vancomycin | Vancocin | Antibiotic prophylaxis in patients allergic to penicillin; pseudomembranous colitis | Colitis: 125 mg po q 6hr for 1-2 weeks | Bad taste, toxicity in patients with renal failure. |
| **Anticholinergics** | | | | |
| atropine sulfate | Atropine | Premedication for endoscopic procedures; to avert vasovagal reactions, arrhythmia, and bradycardia and to reduce bowel motility and secretion | 0.4 mg IM | Use caution with patients with bladder outlet obstruction; increases intraocular pressure in patients with narrow-angle glaucoma. |

*Continued.*

**Table 21-3.** Representative pharmacologic agents used in gastroenterology—cont'd

| Agent | Trade name | Indications | Adult dosage | Adverse effects |
|---|---|---|---|---|
| dicyclomine HCl | Bentyl | Antispasmodic for treatment of irritable bowel syndrome (IBS) | 80-160 mg/day in 4 equally divided doses | Dry mouth; dizziness; blurred vision; nausea; light-headedness. |
| glycopyrrolate | Robinul | Adjunctive therapy of peptic ulcer disease; premedication for endoscopic procedures | 2-8 mg/day in 2 or 3 equally divided doses | Headache; dizziness; palpitations; constipation; urine retention. |
| methantheline Br | Banthine | Adjunctive therapy for peptic ulcer disease; pylorospasm; spastic colon; pancreatitis; gastritis | 50-100 mg po q 6hr | Palpitations; blurred vision; dry mouth; paralytic ileus; urinary hesitancy or retention. |
| propantheline Br | Pro-Banthine | Adjunctive therapy for peptic ulcer disease; IBS; reduction of gastrointestinal motility for diagnostic testing | 15 mg 30 min before each meal and 30 mg hs | Dry mouth; decreased sweating; blurred vision; tachycardia. |
| **Cholinergics** | | | | |
| bethanechol Cl | Urecholine | Cholinergic drug that relieves urinary retention, stimulates gastric motility, restores impaired peristalsis | 10-50 mg po, 3-4×/day or 5 mg SC, 3-4×/day | Dizziness; light-headedness; abdominal discomfort; urinary urgency. |
| edrophonium | Tensilon | Cholinergic used in provocative tests of esophageal motility disorders that present as chest pain | 0.08 mg/kg IV | Lacrimation; dizziness; gastrointestinal discomfort; rarely, bradycardia; pupillary constriction; laryngospasm. |
| **Antidiarrheals** | | | | |
| bismuth subsalicylate | Pepto-Bismol | Diarrhea; Heartburn; Indigestion; upset Stomach; nausea | Two 262-mg tablets or 2 Tbs (262 mg each) every 30-60 min, up to 8 doses/24 hr | Contraindicated for patients who are allergic to aspirin or salicylates. |
| difenoxin HCl$^+$ with atropine sulfate | Motofen | Acute, nonspecific diarrhea and acute exacerbations of chronic diarrhea | 2 mg, then 1 mg after each loose stool or 1 mg every 3-4hr as needed, up to 8 mg/24 hr | Nausea; vomiting; dry mouth; dizziness and light-headedness; drowsiness. |
| diphenoxylate HCl$^+$ atropine sulfate | Lomotil | Diarrhea | Up to 5 mg 4×/day | Sedation; dizziness; dry mouth; paralytic ileus. |
| kaolin + pectin | Kaopectate | Mild, nonspecific diarrhea | 60-120 ml po after each bowel movement | Absorbs nutrients, drugs, and enzymes; constipation. |
| loperamide HCl | Imodium | Acute, nonspecific diarrhea and chronic diarrhea associated with irritable bowel syndrome (IBS) | 4 mg after the first loose bowel movement + 2 mg after each subsequent loose movement, up to 16 mg/24 hr | Hypersensitivity reactions; abdominal pain; distention or discomfort, nausea and vomiting; constipation. |
| **Antiemetics** | | | | |
| chlorpromazine | Thorazine | Control of nausea and vomiting | 10-25 mg po prn; 25-50 mg IM q 3-4hr prn; one 100-mg suppository q 6-8hr prn | Tardive dyskinesia. |

**Table 21-3.** Representative pharmacologic agents used in gastroenterology—cont'd

| Agent | Trade name | Indications | Adult dosage | Adverse effects |
|---|---|---|---|---|
| dimenhydrinate | Dramamine | Prevention and treatment of motion sickness | 1-2 50 mg tablets q 4-6hr, up to 8 tablets/24 hr; 4-8 tsp q 4-6hr, up to 32 tsp/24 hr | Drowsiness, especially with alcohol, sedatives, or tranquilizers. |
| metoclopramide HCl | Reglan | Short-term therapy for esophageal reflux; enhances gastric emptying; facilitates small bowel intubation | 10-15 mg qid | Restlessness; drowsiness; fatigue; and lassitude. |
| prochlorperazine | Compazine | Control of severe nausea and vomiting | Not to exceed 40 mg/day | Dizziness; extrapyramidal symptoms; blurred vision; skin reactions; and hypotension. |
| scopolamine | Transderm-Scop | Prevention of motion sickness | 1 patch applied to the skin behind the ear delivers 0.5 mg over 72 hr | Drowsiness; dry mouth. |
| trimethobenza-mide HCl | Tigan | Control of nausea and vomiting | One 250 mg capsule, 200 mg suppository, or 200 mg (2 ml) IM injection tid or qid | Hypersensitivity reactions; Parkinson-like symptoms; drowsiness; Reye's syndrome. |

**Antiflatulents**

| | | | | |
|---|---|---|---|---|
| simethicone | Mylicon | Relief of painful symptoms of excess gas in the digestive tract | 1 40 mg tablet after meals and hs or as needed, up to 12 tablets daily | |

**Antiparasitic agents**

| | | | | |
|---|---|---|---|---|
| metronidazole | Flagyl | Giardiasis | 250 mg 3×/day for 1 week | Convulsive seizures; peripheral neuropathy. |

**Antiulcer agents**

| | | | | |
|---|---|---|---|---|
| cimetidine | Tagamet | Short-term treatment of duodenal ulcers | 300 mg po qid with meals and hs | Agranulocytosis; neutropenia; thrombocytopenia; mild and transient diarrhea. |
| famotidine | Pepcid | Duodenal ulcer; pathologic hypersecretory conditions | Acute therapy: 40 mg po once daily hs; maintenance: 20 mg po once daily hs | Headache; diarrhea; constipation. |
| misoprostol | Cytotec | Prevention of NSAID-induced ulcers | 200 mcg po qid with food | Diarrhea; abdominal pain; menstrual disorders. |
| nizatidine | Axid | Duodenal ulcers | Acute therapy: 300 mg hs or 150 mg bid; maintenance therapy: 150 mg hs | Thrombocytopenia; somnolence; sweating; exfoliative dermatitis. |
| omeprazole | Prilosec | Short-term treatment of esophageal reflux; long-term treatment of pathologic hypersecretory conditions | esophageal reflux: 20 mg/day for 4-8 weeks; Hypersecretory states: lowest effective dose | Headache; diarrhea; abdominal pain; nausea; dizziness; vomiting; rash; constipation. |
| ranitidine HCl | Zantac | Duodenal and gastric ulcers; hypersecretory conditions; esophageal reflux | 150 mg bid or 300 mg once daily hs; 150 mg once daily for maintenance therapy | Headache. |
| sucrulfate | Carafate | Short-term treatment of duodenal ulcer | 1 g po qid 1 hr before meals and hs | Constipation; dizziness; sleepiness. |

*Continued.*

**Table 21-3.** Representative pharmacologic agents used in gastroenterology—cont'd

| Agent | Trade name | Indications | Adult dosage | Adverse effects |
|---|---|---|---|---|
| **Corticosteroids** | | | | |
| hydrocortisone | Hydrocortone | Ulcerative colitis; Crohn's disease | Approx. 120-240 mg/day, depending on the severity of the disease and the patient's response | Acne; Cushingoid changes; fluid and electrolyte disturbances; osteoporosis; pancreatitis; gastric ulcer. |
| methylprednisolone | Medrol | Ulcerative colitis; Crohn's disease | 4-48 mg/day, depending on the severity of the disease and the patient's response | Acne; Cushingoid changes; fluid and electrolyte disturbances; osteoporosis; gastric ulcer. |
| prednisolone sodium phosphate | Hydeltrasol injection | Ulcerative colitis; Crohn's disease | 4-60 mg/day, depending on the severity of the disease and the patient's response | Fluid and electrolyte disturbances; peptic ulcer; menstrual irregularities; Cushingoid changes; osteoporosis. |
| triamcinolone acetonide | Kenalog | Relief of dysphagia in patients with benign esophageal strictures | 5 mg injections in each quadrant of the narrowest region of the stricture. Adult Dosage: 2.5-15 mg | Myopathy; anorexia with weight loss, sedation and depression. |
| **Agents used in diagnostic tests** | | | | |
| bentiromide | Chymex | Screening for pancreatic exocrine insufficiency | 500 mg po, followed by 250 ml water | Diarrhea; headache; flatulence; nausea. |
| glucagon | Glucagon | Inhibition of gastrointestinal motility, especially in conjunction with ERCP | Increments of 0.2-0.4 mg IV | Nausea, vomiting. |
| pentagastrin | Peptavlon | Stimulates gastric acid secretion | 6 mcg/kg SC | Abdominal discomfort; nausea; flushing; lightheadedness. |
| secretin | Secretin | Stimulates pancreatic exocrine secretion; diagnosis of gastrinoma | 2 units/kg IV over a 1 min period | Clinically significant side effects are unusual. |
| **Gallbladder therapeutic agents** | | | | |
| chenodiol (chenodeoxycholic acid) | Chenix | Dissolution of radilucent cholesterol stones | 250 mg po bid for the first 2 weeks, followed by weekly increases of 250 mg/day, up to 13-16 mg/kg/day for up to 24 months | Diarrhea; cramps; heartburn; reversible elevated hepatic enzymes. |
| monooctanoin | Moctanin | Dissolution of cholesterol stones retained in the biliary tract after cholecystectomy | Continuous infusion (3-5 ml/hr) directly into the common bile duct for 7-21 days | Gastrointestinal pain and discomfort; nausea; vomiting. |
| ursodiol (ursodeoxycholic acid) | Actigall | Dissolution of radiolucent cholesterol stones less than 20 mm in diameter | 8-10 mg/kg po daily in 2 or 3 divided doses for up to 12 months | Rarely, diarrhea; pruritus; cough; headache; nausea. |
| **Laxatives, cathartics, and bulk agents** | | | | |
| bisacodyl | Dulcolax | Acute or chronic constipation; preoperative preparation or postoperative care | 2-3 5 mg tablets or 1 10 mg suppository | Abdominal cramping. |

**Table 21-3.** Representative pharmacologic agents used in gastroenterology—cont'd

| Agent | Trade name | Indications | Adult dosage | Adverse effects |
|---|---|---|---|---|
| docusate sodium | Modane Soft | Constipation, especially to lessen the strain of defecation | 1-3 100 mg capsules daily | Diarrhea; nausea; cramping pains; and rash (all uncommon). |
| lactulose | Chronulac; Cephulac; Duphulac | Constipation (Duphulac, Chronulac); portal-systemic encephalopathy (Cephulac) | Constipation: 15-30 ml po daily; portal-systemic encephalopathy: 20-30 g po (30-45 ml) tid or qid, or as a retention enema to reverse hepatic coma | Abdominal cramps; belching; diarrhea; hypernatremia. |
| methylcellulose | Citrucel | Chronic constipation | 5-20 ml liquid po tid with a glass of water or 15 ml syrup po morning and evening | Nausea; abdominal cramps. |
| phenolphthalein | Correctol; Ex-Lax | Constipation | 30-270 mg po, preferably hs | Colic in large doses; abdominal cramps; hypersensitivity. |
| polyethylene glycol | CoLyte; GoLYTELY | Bowel preparation before gastrointestinal examination | 240 ml po q 10 min until 4 L are consumed | Nausea; bloating; cramps; vomiting. |
| psyllium | Metamucil | Constipation, bowel management | 1-2 rounded tsp po in full glass liquid daily, bid or tid, followed by a second glass of liquid | Nausea; vomiting; diarrhea with excessive use; contraindicated in intestinal obstruction or fecal impaction. |
| **Narcotics and antagonists** | | | | |
| fentanyl citrate | Sublimaze | Premedication and conscious sedation for endoscopic procedures; postprocedural analgesia | 2 mcg/kg | Respiratory depression; apnea; rigidity; and bradycardia. |
| meperidine HCl | Demerol | Relief of moderate to severe pain; preoperative medication | For pain relief: 50-150 mg IM, SC, or po q 3-4hr; for preoperative medication: 50-100 mg IM or SC | Respiratory depression and, to a lesser extent, circulatory depression; nausea and vomiting. |
| morphine sulfate | Roxanol | Relief of severe acute or chronic pain | 10-30 mg q 4hr | Respiratory depression and, to a lesser extent, circulatory depression; nausea and vomiting. |
| naloxone HCl | Narcan | Reversal of narcotic depression | 0.2-0.4 mg IV every 2-3 min; may also be given IM or SC | Nausea; vomiting; sweating; tachcyardia; hypertension; tremulousness; seizures and cardiac arrest. |
| **Sclerosing agents** | | | | |
| ethanol (100%) | | Variceal bleeding | 0.1 ml/injection | |
| ethanolamine oleate | Ethamolin | Esophageal varices that have recently bled, to prevent rebleeding | 1.5-5 ml per varix; maximum total dose per treatment session not to exceed 20 ml | Pleural effusion and/or infiltration; esophageal ulcer; pyrexia; retrosternal pain; esophageal stricture; pneumonia. |
| morrhuate sodium (5% or 1%) | Scleromate | Obliteration of esophageal varices; varicose veins | 1-2 ml per varix | Esophageal ulceration; allergic reactions; stricture; chest pain. |

*Continued.*

**Table 21-3.** Representative pharmacologic agents used in gastroenterology—cont'd

| Agent | Trade name | Indications | Adult dosage | Adverse effects |
|---|---|---|---|---|
| sodium tetradecyl sulfate (1% or 3%) | Sotradecol | Obliteration of esophageal varices; varicose veins | 1-2 ml per varix; not to exceed 15 ml per session | Esophageal ulceration; allergic reactions; stricture; chest pain. |
| **Sedatives and antagonists** | | | | |
| diazepam | Valium | Relief of preprocedural anxiety and tension and reduction of recall of the procedure | 5-15 mg IV immediately before the procedure and prn during the procedure; titrate individually | Respiratory depression and arrest, especially when used for conscious sedation. |
| flumazenil | Mazicon | Reversal of sedation from use of benzodiazepines (Valium, Versed) | 0.2 mg to 1.0 mg given at 0.2 mg/min IV. No more than 1 mg should be given at once; no more than 3.0 mg per hr. | Dizziness; injection site pain; blurred vision; headache; flushing; sweating; nausea and vomiting; agitation; dry mouth; tachycardia. |
| midazolam HCl | Versed | Premedication for anxiety relief and reduced recall; conscious sedation | Conscious sedation: titrate individually, beginning with 1 mg | Respiratory depression and arrest, especially when used for conscious sedation. |
| **Smooth muscle relaxants** | | | | |
| isosorbide dinitrate | Isordil | Achalasia | 5-10 mg before meals, sublingually | Headache. |
| nifedipine | Procardia, Adalat | Achalasia | 10-20 mg, capsule broken in patient's mouth | Lightheadedness; flushing; headache. |
| **Topical anesthetics** | | | | |
| benzocaine | Hurricaine | Suppresses gag reflex and controls pain | 2 oz aerosol spray, 1 oz liquid, or 1 oz gel; liquid may be used as a gargle, gel as a lubricant | No significant adverse effects. |
| benzocaine spray | Cetacaine | Preparation for upper GI endoscopy; elimination of gag reflex | Administered as a spray before UGI endoscopy | |
| dyclonine HCl | Dyclone | Topical anesthetic for mucous membranes; blocks gag reflex | Lowest dose needed to provide effective anesthesia, up to 30 ml of 1% solution | Excitatory and/or depressant CNS effects; drowsiness; cardiovascular depression; allergic reactions. |
| lidocaine HCl | Xylocaine | Topical anesthesia in spray or gel form for use in the oral cavity | 10% oral spray: up to 2 metered doses per quadrant; 2% viscous solution: 4.5 mg/kg | Excitatory and/or depressant CNS effects; drowsiness; cardiovascular depression; allergic reactions. |
| **Other agents** | | | | |
| Mesalamine (5-ASA) | Rowasa | Suspension retention enema for distal ulcerative colitis, proctosigmoiditis, or proctitis | 1 enema daily hs, retained for approximately 8 hr; course of therapy, 3-6 wks | Cramping; acute abdominal pain; bloody diarrhea; sometimes fever, headache, and rash. |
| cholestyramine | Questran powder | Relief of pruritus in patients with partial biliary obstruction | 9 g powder (4 g cholestyramine) mixed with 2-6 oz fluid po 1-6 times daily | Constipation; nausea. |
| interferon alfa | Intron A | Hepatitis C | 3 million units SC, 3×/week for at least 6 months | Mild to moderate flulike symptoms; reactions at the injection site. |

**Table 21-3.** Representative pharmacologic agents used in gastroenterology—cont'd

| Agent | Trade name | Indications | Adult dosage | Adverse effects |
|---|---|---|---|---|
| olsalazine sodium | Dipentum | Remission maintenance in sulfasalazine-intolerant patients with ulcerative colitis | 1.0 g/day in 2 divided doses, preferably with food | Transient diarrhea; abdominal pain; rash and/or itching. |
| pancreatin | Entozyme | Steatorrhea; pyrosis; flatulence; belching | 2 tablets with each meal and 1 or 2 tablets with each snack; swallowed whole | Skin rash; laxative effect at excessively high doses. |
| pancrelipase | Cotazym | Pancreatic exocrine insufficiency; cystic fibrosis; steatorrhea | 1-3 capsules or tablets po before or with meals and 1 capsule or tablet with snacks | Nausea; diarrhea with high doses. |
| neomycin sulfate | Mycifradin sulfate | hepatic encephalopathy | 4-6 g/day in divided doses | Diarrhea; malabsorption; ototoxicity; nephrotoxicity. |
| penicillamine | Cuprimine | Wilson's disease | 1-2 g/day po, in divided doses, on an empty stomach | Fever; rash; leukopenia; thrombocytopenia. |
| sulfasalazine | Azulfidine | Ulcerative colitis; Crohn's disease | Adjust to patient's tolerance; administer in evenly divided doses after meals | Hypersensitivity; abdominal discomfort; nausea; vomiting; headache. |
| vasopressin | Pitressin | Variceal bleeding | IV | Bradycardia; coronary vasoconstriction; bowel ischemia; water retention. |

ampicillin, chloramphenicol (Chloromycetin), tetracycline (Achromycin), and vancomycin (Vancocin). The specific drug prescribed depends on the agent involved.

Prophylactic antibiotics may be prescribed before endoscopic procedures for selected patients. The frequency of bacteremia during endoscopic procedures varies with the type of procedure. In most individuals, bacteremia is transient and resolves without complications. Bacterial endocarditis is a concern in patients with valvular heart disease, internal prosthetic devices, or a previous episode of endocarditis. Antibiotics ordered for prophylaxis against endocarditis include ampicillin, gentamicin (Garamycin), vancomycin (Vancocin), and tobramycin (Nebcin). It is important to recognize that the criteria for the use of prophylactic antibiotics continue to be controversial.

**Anticholinergics and cholinergics**

**Anticholinergic** medications, such as atropine and dicyclomine hydrochloride (Bentyl) inhibit gastric acid secretion at its source by blocking the acetylcholine receptor on gastric parietal cells. These medications decrease the output of hydrochloric acid and pepsin and block vagal stimulation of smooth muscle, thus decreasing gastrointestinal tone and motility. They also decrease

gastric emptying time, presumably through their inhibition of vagal and cholinergic-mediated motility.

Anticholinergics may be used in the treatment of diffuse esophageal spasm, peptic ulcer disease, ileitis, irritable bowel syndrome (IBS), pancreatitis, gastritis, and ulcerative colitis. They can help to relieve the gastric distress caused by gastric spasms, hyperperistalsis, and rapid emptying of the stomach. Anticholinergic medications are contraindicated in patients who experience bleeding or who have tachycardia, glaucoma, achalasia, obstruction, or suspected toxic megacolon.

Anticholinergics are best given about 1 hour after meals, when food-stimulated acid is at its peak. Their effects persist for 4 to 5 hours.

Adverse effects of anticholinergics include dryness of the lips, nose, and throat; hoarseness; tachycardia; blurred vision; urinary hesitancy or retention; headache and dizziness; flushing of the skin; and constipation. Because of their side effects, they are used primarily as an adjunctive therapy for peptic ulcer disease, in combination with antacids or histamine-2 (H2) blockers.

In contrast to anticholinergics, **cholinergic** agents increase gastrointestinal tone and motility. They produce the same effects as stimulation of the parasympathetic nervous system, thereby stimulating gastrointestinal secretion and motility, diaphoresis, and bladder contractions. Bethanechol (Urecholine) may be used to increase lower esophageal sphincter (LES) pressure in patients suffering from gastroesophageal reflux. It is also used in children with gastroesophageal reflux who are unresponsive to metoclopramide (Reglan). Cholinergics are contraindicated in the presence of peptic ulcer or possible gastrointestinal obstruction.

## Antidiarrheals

**Antidiarrheal** agents are used for symptomatic relief of diarrhea. They include drugs that decrease intestinal motility (opium alkaloids and synthetic opium alkaloids), and drugs that decrease the fluid content of the stool or inhibit intestinal secretions. Antidiarrheal agents may also be used judiciously to decrease the frequency of bowel movements in patients with ulcerative colitis or Crohn's disease.

- Opium alkaloids, such as morphine, methylmorphine, and camphorated tincture of opium, and synthetic opium alkaloids, such as loperamide (Imodium) and diphenoxylate hydrochloride (Lomotil), may be used as antidiarrheal agents. These agents act primarily by inhibiting intestinal motility. Because these drugs may be habit-forming, patients must be cautioned not to exceed the recommended dosage. Opium alkaloids are contraindicated in patients with toxic causes of diarrhea and should be used cautiously by patients with asthma, liver disease, prostatic hypertrophy, and narcotic dependence.
- Some antidiarrheal preparations are inert powders that act by decreasing the fluid content of the stool. They are most effective for acute short-term treatment of diarrhea. Kaolin and pectin (Kaopectate) fall in this category.
- Bismuth subsalicylate (Pepto-Bismol) is useful for mild diarrhea and upset stomach. It acts by inhibiting intestinal secretions. In addition, it may absorb toxins and provide a protective coating for the mucosa. Bismuth may also be used in combination with antibiotics for the treatment of *H. pylori* infection.

In general, antidiarrheal agents delay the intestinal clearance of pathogens. They are not recommended for patients with fever or bloody diarrhea or in patients younger than 2 years old. Agents that inhibit intestinal motility are associated with toxic megacolon in patients suffering from pseudomembranous enterocolitis, acute dysentery, and acute ulcerative colitis.

Even in suitable patients, continued use of antidiarrheal agents over an extended period is not recommended. If it is not possible to control diarrhea promptly, diagnostic tests should be ordered. In seriously ill patients the etiologic agent should be isolated, and specific antimicrobial therapy should be started.

## Antiemetics

**Antiemetics** produce symptomatic relief of nausea and vomiting. They include both phenothiazines and antihistamines, as well as trimethobenzamide hydrochloride (Tigan).

Phenothiazines are the most common type of antiemetic drugs. They appear to exert their effects on the cells of the chemoreceptor trigger zone (CTZ) and prevent the vomiting center from being activated. Phenothiazines such as prochlorperazine (Compazine) and chlorpromazine (Thorazine) are effective in relieving vomiting associated with gastroenteritis, radiation sickness, and drug therapy, but they do not relieve motion sickness. Adverse effects of phenothiazines include sedation, hypotension, restlessness, dry mouth, blurred vision, constipation, and muscle twitching. They should be used only when nondrug antiemetic measures or other drugs fail.

Certain antihistamines, such as dimenhydrinate (Dramamine), act on the CTZ to suppress centrally mediated nausea and vomiting associated with motion sickness or drug or radiation therapy, or following surgery. The primary side effect of antihistamines is drowsiness.

The mechanism of action of trimethobenzamide hydrochloride is unknown, but it may act on the CTZ.

Metoclopramide (Reglan) may also be considered an antiemetic drug, although its principle function is to increase LES pressure and the rate of gastric emptying. Metoclopramide appears to produce its antiemetic effects as a result of its antagonism of central and peripheral dopamine receptors.

## Antiflatulents

**Antiflatulent** agents, such as simethicone (Mylicon), are used to relieve painful symptoms of excess gas in the GI tract that may be caused by air swallowing, postoperative gaseous distention, peptic ulcers, spastic or irritable colon, or diverticulosis. The agents act by dispersing and preventing the formation of mucussurrounded air or gas pockets in the GI tract. Simethicone is also added to some antacid preparations.

## Antiparasitic/Antifungal agents

There are a number of agents available to combat the effects of intestinal parasites and fungi. One important agent is metronidazole (Flagyl), which is the drug of choice in the treatment of adults with giardiasis.

## Antiulcer agents

The various drugs prescribed for peptic ulcer disease promote healing by reducing gastric acid secretion, buffering secreted gastric acid, and/or enhancing intrinsic mucosal defenses. The classes of drugs used for these purposes include antacids, anticholinergic agents, H2 blockers, and sucralfate (Carafate). Antacids and anticholinergics have been discussed previously.

**Histamine-2 (H2) blockers** include cimetidine (Tagamet), famotidine (Pepcid), nizatidine (Axid), and ranitidine (Zantac). They reduce the secretion of gastric acid by blocking histamine's action on the H2 receptors in the parietal cells. H2 blockers may also be used to reduce gastric acidity in patients with upper GI bleeding that stems from a peptic ulcer.

The most common side effects of H2 blockers are diarrhea, headaches, dizziness, fatigue, muscle pain, rash, impotence and mild gynecomastia, leukopenia, and thrombocytopenia.

Sucralfate (Carafate) is a basic aluminum salt of sucrose octasulfate that forms a viscous adhesive gel that adheres to the ulcer crater, thereby preventing further digestive action by both acid and pepsin. It has been approved for the treatment of duodenal ulcers but not for gastric ulcers. The main side effect of sucralfate is constipation, which occurs in approximately 10% of patients who take this drug. Other rarely occurring side effects include dizziness, vertigo, sleepiness, dry mouth, skin rashes, pruritus, back pain, diarrhea, nausea, gastric discomfort, and indigestion.

Synthetic **prostaglandins,** such as misoprostol (Cytotec), have both antisecretory and cytoprotective effects. They may be used to prevent the gastric ulcers and mucosal injury that have been associated with the use of nonsteroidal antiinflammatory drugs (NSAIDs). The most common side effect is diarrhea, followed by abdominal pain as the second most common. Because of its abortifacient properties, misoprostol is contraindicated in pregnant women and generally is not recommended for women of childbearing age.

Omeprazole (Prilosec) is another relatively new antiulcer agent. It is a substituted benzimidazole that blocks acid production by all three direct acid secretagogues: gastrin, **histamine,** and acetylcholine. Use of these delayed-release capsules is indicated for the short-term treatment of patients with severe erosive esophagitis of grade 2 or above who have responded poorly to customary treatment. Omeprazole also inhibits gastric acid secretion and controls symptoms of diarrhea, anorexia, and pain in patients with pathologic hypersecretory conditions, such as Zollinger-Ellison syndrome. Adverse reactions may include abdominal pain, asthenia, constipation, diarrhea, nausea, vomiting, and headache.

## Corticosteroids

**Corticosteroids** are used in gastroenterology practice primarily for their antiinflammatory properties in the management of inflammatory bowel disease. They in-

clude hydrocortisone (Hydrocortone), prednisone, and synthetic analogues, such as prednisolone (Hydeltrasol) and methylprednisolone (Medrol). In addition, injection of the synthetic corticosteroid triamcinolone acetonide (Kenalog) may relieve dysphagia in patients with benign esophageal strictures.

In patients with proctitis or distal colitis, corticosteroids may be administered topically (by rectal suppository, foam, or retention enema). Oral administration is effective for patients with more extensive disease and more prominent symptoms. For patients with severe and fulminant forms of the disease, intravenous hydrocortisone, methylprednisolone, or prednisolone may alter the course of the disease and avert colectomy. Corticosteroids are also routinely used for patients with Crohn's disease; in patients with Crohn's colitis, corticosteroids may be used in combination with sulfasalazine (Azulfidine).

Patients on prolonged corticosteroid therapy should be monitored for signs of Cushing's syndrome, which is characterized by rapidly developing adiposity of the face, neck, and trunk; kyphosis; hypertension; diabetes mellitus; amenorrhea; hypertrichosis; impotence; and muscular wasting and weakness.

## Agents used in diagnostic tests

A number of different pharmacologic agents may be used in the diagnosis of gastrointestinal disorders, including pentagastrin (Peptavlon), which stimulates gastric acid secretion, and bentiromide (Chymex) and secretin, which are used in tests of pancreatic exocrine secretion. The cholinergic agent edrophonium chloride (Tensilon) is used for provocative testing in patients with noncardiac chest pain. Glucagon is also used in diagnostic and therapeutic procedures, primarily to reduce gastrointestinal motility. Exogenous administration of the gastrointestinal hormone, cholecystokinin (Kinevac), may be used in diagnostic procedures in which an increase in gastric or colonic motility is desired.

## Gallstone therapeutic agents

A number of chemical agents are available that may be used to dissolve gallstones, including monooctanoin (Moctanin) and the bile salts chenodeoxycholic acid (CDCA, Chenix) and ursodeoxycholic acid (UDCA, Actigall).

Both CDCA and UDCA are used to dissolve cholesterol gallstones. They decrease the rate of secretion of cholesterol into bile thus causing the bile to become desaturated with cholesterol. This unsaturated bile dissolves cholesterol molecules from gallstones and holds them in micellar or vesicular solution until gallbladder contraction discharges them into the duodenum. Therapy must be continued until the stones dissolve completely, typically 6 to 24 months.

Medical dissolution therapy dissolves gallstones completely in up to 50% of selected patients with cholesterol stones. It is contraindicated for patients without patent cystic ducts, patients with radiopaque (pigment) stones, women who are or may be pregnant, and patients with stones that are larger than 15 mm in diameter. Contraindications to CDCA, but not UDCA, include severe obesity, liver disease, and inflammatory bowel disease. Potential adverse effects of CDCA include hepatic toxicity, diarrhea, and increases in serum LDL cholesterol. These adverse effects are not associated with UDCA.

Monooctanoin is used to dissolve cholesterol stones that are retained in the biliary tract after cholecystectomy. It is administered as a continuous infusion through a catheter inserted directly into the common bile duct via a T-tube or through a nasobiliary catheter. Administration of monooctanoin is contraindicated in patients with clinical jaundice, significant biliary tract infection, or a history of recent duodenal ulcer or jejunitis. Adverse reactions, including gastrointestinal pain and discomfort, nausea, and vomiting, may be relieved by slowing the infusion rate or discontinuing infusion between meals.

### Laxatives, cathartics, and bulk agents

**Laxatives** and **cathartics** are used to induce defecation. They are most commonly classified by their mechanisms of action.

- Hyperosmotic colonic lavage solutions act by increasing intraluminal pressure, which stimulates peristalsis. These solutions are used primarily to cleanse the bowel in preparation for gastrointestinal examination. Polyethylene glycol (Colyte) is an example of a colon electrolyte lavage preparation. It can be administered orally or by nasogastric intubation.
- Stimulant cathartics act by producing local irritation or by stimulating Auerbach's plexus, thus resulting in increased intestinal motility. They are contraindicated in the presence of obstruction or peritonitis or immediately after bowel surgery. Bisacodyl (Dulcolax) and phenolphthalein (Correctol, Ex-Lax) are examples of stimulant cathartics.
- Bulk-forming cathartics are composed of natural or synthetic polysaccharides or cellulose derivatives that expand in the intestine without being absorbed and thus facilitate normal elimination. They are used to relieve chronic constipation and to ease passage of stool in patients with anorectal disorders. Psyllium (Metamucil) is an example of a bulk-forming laxative. The addition of fruits and natural fiber to the diet has the same effect.
- Lubricant cathartics soften the stool by acting as wetting agents. The most common drug in this category is mineral oil.
- Emollient laxatives act as surfactants that soften the fecal mass by facilitating the mixture of aqueous and fatty substances. They increase the secretion of water in both the small bowel and the colon. Docusate sodium (Modane) is an emollient laxative.

Laxatives may be used to cleanse the bowel before radiographic examination, colonoscopy, flexible or rigid sigmoidoscopy, or surgery; to eliminate a substance or organism from the GI tract; or to prevent hardened stools in patients with a colostomy or hemorrhoids. They may also be used to prevent straining, to obtain a stool specimen, or simply to treat constipation.

### Narcotics and antagonists

Narcotic analgesics, particularly meperidine (Demerol), may be used for premedication of patients undergoing endoscopic procedures. They may also be used for postoperative pain relief.

**Narcotics** should be used sparingly because they tend to mask symptoms and complications and may cause physical and psychologic dependence. Abrupt discontinuance of the drug may precipitate withdrawal symptoms, including convulsions and a decrease in bowel motility.

Morphine should not be given to patients with biliary or pancreatic problems, either preoperatively or postoperatively, because it may increase smooth muscle spasm. Meperidine is usually the drug of choice for these patients. Morphine must also be restricted in patients with severe liver disease.

Fentanyl citrate (Sublimaze) appears to have less emetic activity than either morphine or meperidine. In addition, clinically significant histamine release rarely occurs with fentanyl.

The most dangerous side effect of narcotic medications is respiratory depression. Respiratory depression and sedation and hypotension can be reversed by administration of naloxone (Narcan), which is thought to antagonize the opioid effects by competing for the same receptor sites.

### Sclerosing agents

Sclerosing agents, such as morrhuate sodium (Scleromate), sodium tetradecyl sulfate (Sotradecol), ethanolamine oleate (Ethamolin), and 100% ethanol are injected intravariceally or paravariceally to promote intima inflammation and thrombus formation in patients with esophageal varices. The subsequent formation of fibrous tissue results in partial or complete vein obliteration.

### Sedatives and antagonists

**Sedatives** and antianxiety agents, such as diazepam (Valium) and midazolam (Versed) are used in the practice of gastroenterology primarily to medicate patients before and during endoscopic or invasive procedures. They may be used to relieve preprocedural anxiety and tension and to decrease recall of the procedure.

The most serious side effect of conscious sedation with diazepam or midazolam is a centrally mediated respiratory depression, which seems to occur in at least 1% of patients. Apnea is associated with rapid IV injection of either drug. The extent of respiratory depression is dependent on dosage, rate of administration, and individual susceptibility. Sedative effects are accentuated by the concomitant administration of other central nervous system depressants, such as opiates, barbiturates, or alcohol. Compared with diazepam, midazolam is more potent and faster acting and has a greater amnesic effect. Diazepam is associated with more injection site complications, such as thrombophlebitis.

Respiratory depression from benzodiazepine sedatives (i.e., diazepam, midazolam) may be reversed with flumazenil (Mazicon). Flumazenil is given intravenously in individualized doses (0.2 mg/min.), not to exceed 1 mg at a time and not more than 3 mg per hour. The drug acts in minutes but may wear off, and patients must be watched for resedation and subsequent respiratory depression. Patients physically dependent on benzodiazepines may develop withdrawal symptoms, including convulsions, upon receiving this drug.

The ability to reverse the action of narcotics or sedatives does not replace the need for judicious induction of conscious sedation or careful monitoring during and after procedures, or the need for assistance with transportation or other activities requiring alertness.

### Smooth muscle relaxants

Agents that have a direct relaxant effect on the smooth muscle fibers of the LES can alleviate symptoms of achalasia and improve esophageal emptying in some patients. Sublingual isosorbide dinitrate (Isordil) can improve symptoms as well as radionuclide transit time. Calcium channel blockers, such as nifedipine (Procardia), also have recognized relaxant effects on LES muscle.

### Topical anesthetics

Topical **anesthetics,** such as benzocaine (Cetacaine), lidocaine (Xylocaine), and dyclonine (Dyclone), are used in gastroenterology to suppress the gag reflex and to control pain for upper GI endoscopic procedures.

### Other agents

Other drugs used in the treatment of gastrointestinal disorders include 5-aminosalicylic acid (Rowasa), sulfasalazine (Azulfidine), pancrelipase (Cotazym), cholestyramine (Questran), penicillamine (Cuprimine), vasopressin (Pitressin), neomycin (Mycifradin), lactulose (Cephulac), and interferon alfa (Intron A).

Mesalamine, or 5-ASA, (5-Aminosalicylic acid) may be administered in the form of a suspension retention enema for patients with distal ulcerative colitis; proctosigmoiditis, or proctitis; and radiation enteritis and colitis. The suspension enema also contains potassium metabisulfite, which may cause life-threatening allergic reactions in patients with sulfite sensitivity. Epinephrine is the preferred treatment for serious allergic or emergency situations.

Sulfasalazine, which is a complex of sulfapyridine and 5-ASA, has been proven effective in the maintenance of clinical remission and in the treatment of mildly to moderately severe attacks of ulcerative colitis. It is also effective in active Crohn's colitis and ileocolitis, although it does not appear to be as effective in ileitis alone. Side effects are common, and include nausea, vomiting, and headache.

5-ASA may also be administered orally as olsalazine sodium (Dipentum). Olsalazine sodium consists of two molecules of 5-ASA that are split and released by colonic bacteria. It has been proved as effective as sulfasalazine in preventing relapse of ulcerative colitis, but without the side effects associated with the sulfapyridine moiety.

Pancrelipase is a combination of digestive enzymes, including lipase, protease, and amylase. It is used to decrease the number of bowel movements and improve stool consistency in patients with pancreatic exocrine insufficiency, cystic fibrosis, steatorrhea, and other disorders of fat metabolism. Pancreatin (Entozyme) is also prescribed to relieve steatorrhea, pyrosis, flatulence, and belching associated with incomplete digestion of food caused by a deficiency of digestive enzymes.

Cholestyramine is an anion exchange resin that is used to lower plasma cholesterol levels. It adsorbs and combines with bile acids in the intestine to form an insoluble complex that is excreted in the feces. This increased fecal loss of bile acids leads to an increased oxidation of cholesterol to bile acids, a decrease in plasma LDLs, and a decrease in serum cholesterol. In patients with partial biliary obstruction, the reduction of serum bile acid levels reduces excess bile acids deposited in the skin, resulting in a decrease in pruritus. Cholestyramine is contraindicated in patients with complete biliary obstruction. The most common adverse reactions are constipation, abdominal discomfort, and nausea.

Penicillamine is the drug of choice for patients with Wilson's disease, which is a hereditary disorder of copper metabolism. Patients with Wilson's disease must be committed to lifelong administration of a daily dose of penicillamine, which chelates to copper and then is excreted in the urine. Complete reversal or improvement of hepatic, neurologic, and psychiatric abnormalities can be expected in most patients, although a small proportion develop serious toxic reactions and may require administration of an alternative chelating agent.

Intravenous vasopressin is used to stop variceal bleeding. Studies have shown that approximately 52% of patients stop bleeding when treated with vasopressin. The preferred method of administration is by constant IV infusion. Side effects include an increase in peripheral vascular resistance, bradycardia, coronary vasoconstriction (which may precipitate myocardial infarction in patients with coronary artery disease), and bowel ischemia. Vasopressin should be used only in intensive care settings with close cardiac monitoring.

Neomycin and lactulose are both used in the treatment of hepatic encephalopathy. Neomycin acts by reducing the production of the nitrogenous breakdown products that cause encephalopathy. Bacterial breakdown of lactulose acidifies the colonic contents, resulting in the retention of ammonia in the colon and a concomitant reduction in blood ammonia levels.

Recent research has shown that interferon alfa (Intron A) is effective in controlling disease activity in many patients with hepatitis C (non-A, non-B hepatitis). Interferon's mechanism of action is not known, but it may act through an antiviral effect or by modulating the effects of the patient's immune system in handling hepatitis C.

---

**CASE SITUATION**

---

Davy Simms is admitted to the endoscopy unit with a persistent reflux problem manifested by vomiting or "spitting up." Regurgitation occurs within 1½ to 2 hours following ingestion of food or fluids. Davy is 6 months old and was diagnosed as having a patent ductus arteriosus at the age of 4 weeks. He is a poor feeder, highly irritable and fussy, and is on the low borderline developmental scale for his age. He weighs 13½ pounds (6.1 kg), is 24½ inches in length, and has a body surface area of 0.33 meters (based upon a precalculated approximation). Because he lives in a high streptococcus incident area of the country and has two siblings, ages 5 and 7, he is on a daily dose of prophylactic ampicillin (20 mg). He is to have general anesthesia for the endoscopic procedure. His pediatrician orders 65 mg of ampicillin and 12 mg of gentamycin to be given by intravenous drip over a 1-hour period. Sedation will be by diazepam (Valium), given orally 1 hour before the procedure.

*Points to think about*

1. What might be the rationale for not using the drug Versed (midazolam) to sedate this patient?
2. What are the benefits of using diazepam as an adjunct to an anesthetic agent?

3. Why would diazepam be given orally in this patient rather than intravenously or intramuscularly?
4. What are the responsibilities of the gastroenterology nurse when conscious sedation is used on an adult patient?

*Suggested response*

1. The most important reason for not using midazolam is that the manufacturer of the drug cannot recommend its use in children at this time. Although it has been used in several series of cases, the manufacturer has not conducted clinical trials in children and no dosage range has been established.

   Conscious sedation in a 6-month-old is risky because of the inherent danger associated with esophagoscopy in an infant who cannot be sedated enough or cannot understand the need to remain still during the procedure. General anesthesia, while it has its own associated difficulties, precludes movement during the procedure.

2. The benefits of diazepam as a premedication include the following:
   • Reduction of fear and anxiety resulting from the unknown and, in this case, parental separation
   • Sedation and amnesia
   • Probable better acceptance of face mask
   • Few nightmares
   • Not likely to cause hypotension, tachycardia, dizziness, excitement and/or postoperative nausea and vomiting

3. Diazepam probably would be given orally to this patient for the following reasons:
   • It absorbs rapidly from the gastrointestinal tract.
   • The rate of absorption from the IM route is erratic and absorption depends upon the muscle into which the drug is injected (deltoid and upper thigh preferred rather than buttock). These muscles are relatively small in an infant.
   • The drug cannot be mixed with other drugs for intravenous use.
   • The drug may cause persistent pain at the injection site if given intramuscularly and may cause superficial, painless venous thrombosis when given intravenously in small veins.

4. The responsibilities of the registered nurse in the gastroenterology lab when conscious sedation is used for an adult are as follows:
   Preoperative phase
   • Perform a nursing assessment
   • Verify presence of signed, informed consent
   • Establish venous access
   • Explain procedure, medications, what patient can expect before, during, and after procedure, and review post endoscopy instructions
   Intraoperative phase
   • Monitor the patient's physical parameters

- Document all events occurring during the procedure and patient's status upon completion
- Reassure patient verbally and by touch

Postoperative phase
- Monitor patient's condition and level of consciousness
- Document all findings and events
- Provide verbal and written instructions regarding diet, medications, activities, and signs and symptoms of complications with action to take if complications develop
- Ensure that the patient meets institutional discharge criteria

**REVIEW TERMS**

anesthetic, antacid, antibiotics, anticholinergic, antidiarrheal, antifungal, antiemetics, antiflatulent, cathartics, cholinergic, corticosteroids, histamine, histamine-2 (H2) blockers, laxatives, narcotics, narcotic antagonist, oral, parenteral, prostaglandins, sedatives, topical

**REVIEW QUESTIONS**

1. When used in a medication order, the abbreviation "hs" indicates that the drug is to be administered:
   a. At mealtime.
   b. At bedtime.
   c. Every hour.
   d. As needed.
2. One kilogram is equivalent to approximately:
   a. 2.2 pounds.
   b. 22 ounces.
   c. 20 pounds.
   d. 1,000 ounces.
3. Probably the most accurate methods of calculating a pediatric dose from a known adult dose are based on the child's:
   a. Height.
   b. Weight.
   c. Surface area.d. Age.
4. For optimal effect, antacids should be given:
   a. Before meals.
   b. Immediately after meals.
   c. 1 hour after meals.
   d. At bedtime.
5. Which of the following classes of drugs inhibits gastric secretion and motility?
   a. Anticholinergics.
   b. Cholinergics.
   c. Laxatives.
   d. Antiemetics.
6. By what mechanism do the opium alkaloids exert their antidiarrheal effect?
   a. Adsorption of liquids.
   b. Inhibition of intestinal motility.
   c. Inhibition of intestinal secretions.
   d. Stimulation of the parasympathetic nervous system.
7. Corticosteroids are used most often in gastroenterology patients who have:
   a. Inflammatory bowel disease.
   b. Peptic ulcers.
   c. Pancreatic exocrine exocrin insufficiency.
   d. Cholelithiasis.
8. The purpose of glucagon in gastrointestinal diagnostic testing is to:
   a. Reduce gastrointestinal motility.
   b. Stimulate gastric acid secretion.
   c. Stimulate production of bile.
   d. Increase gastrointestinal motility.
9. The most dangerous side effect of narcotic medications is:
   a. Constipation.
   b. Respiratory depression.
   c. Physical dependence.
   d. Hypotension.
10. When vasopressin (Pitressin) is administered for the control of variceal bleeding, the preferred route of administration is:
    a. Intravenous.
    b. Oral.
    c. Intramuscular.
    d. Subcutaneous.

**BIBLIOGRAPHY**

Albanese, J. *Nurses' Drug Reference*. 2nd ed. New York: McGraw–Hill, 1982.

Barnhart, E, publisher. *Physicians' Desk Reference*. 44th ed. Oradell, NJ: Medical Economics Company, 1990.

Blume, D. *Dosages and Solution*. 3rd ed. Philadelphia: F.A. Davis, 1980.

Bongiovanni, G, ed. *Essentials of Clinical Gastroenterology*. 2nd ed. New York: McGraw–Hill, 1988.

Chopra, S, and May, R, eds. *Pathophysiology of Gastrointestinal Diseases*. Boston: Little, Brown & Co., 1989.

Damsgard, C. *G.I.A. Certification Review Manual*. Rochester, N.Y.: Society of Gastrointestinal Assistants, 1985.

Davis, G, et al. "Treatment of Chronic Hepatitis C with Recombinant Interferon Alfa: A Multicenter Randomized Controlled Trial." *New England Journal of Medicine* 321(November 30, 1989): 1501-06.

Given, B, and Simmons, S. *Gastroenterology in Clinical Nursing*. 4th ed. St. Louis: Mosby–Year Book, 1984.

Gruber, M, and Camara, D. "Injection Sclerotherapy: Seven Years' Experience." In *SGA Journal Reprints*, ed. Trivits, S, 127-29. Rochester, N.Y.: Society of Gastrointestinal Assistants, 1988.

Hamilton, H, editorial director. *Procedures*. Nurse's Reference Library. Springhouse, PA: Intermed Communications, 1983.

Kirby, D. "Management of Esophageal Varices: A Review of Treatment Options and the Role of the Gastroenterology Nurse and Associate." *Gastroenterology Nursing* 12(Summer 1989): 10-14.

Kirsch, M, Blue, M, Desai, R, and Sivak, M, Jr. "Intralesional Steroid Injections for Peptic Esophageal Strictures." *Gastrointestinal Endoscopy* 37(1991): 180-82.

*Nursing90 Drug Handbook.* Nursing90 Books. Springhouse, PA: Springhouse Corporation, 1990.

Schroeder, S, Krupp, M, and Tierney, L, Jr., Editors. *Current Medical Diagnosis and Treatment.* Norwalk, CT: Appleton and Lange, 1988.

Swartz, M. "Cytotec (Misoprostol)." *Gastroenterology Nursing* 13(Summer 1990): 37-39.

Swartz, M. "Losec (Omeprazole/MSD)." *Gastroenterology Nursing* 12(Spring 1990): 274-76.

Van Ness, M, and Gurney, M, eds. *Handbook of Gastrointestinal Drug Therapy.* Boston: Little, Brown & Co., 1989.

Williams, S, and DiPalma, J. "Constipation in the Long-Term Care Facility." *Gastroenterology Nursing* 12(Winter 1990): 179-82.

# Chapter 22

# INTRAVENOUS THERAPY

This chapter will acquaint the gastroenterology clinician with the principles of intravenous (IV) therapy. In addition to parenteral hyperalimentation, which is discussed in Chapter 23, IV lines are used in gastroenterology practice to administer **crystalloids** for the maintenance of fluid and electrolyte balance; to administer certain drugs; and to transfuse **colloids,** such as whole blood, packed red blood cells, fresh frozen plasma, platelets, and albumin.

To maximize continuity and quality of care, many institutions have designated trained IV teams, including registered nurses and pharmacists, who manage specific aspects of IV therapy. However, gastroenterology clinicians are often responsible for patient observation and for routine IV care, such as tubing changes, site care, and dressing changes.

## Learning objectives

After reviewing the content of this chapter, the gastroenterology nurse should be able to:
1. Discuss the maintenance in gastroenterology patients of fluid and electrolyte balance through the use of IV solutions.
2. Explain techniques for the administration of IV drug therapy in gastroenterology patients.
3. Describe techniques for transfusing blood and blood products in gastroenterology patients, along with signs, symptoms, and treatment of adverse reactions.

## FLUIDS AND ELECTROLYTES

One important nursing goal for gastroenterology nurses is to maintain the patient's fluid and electrolyte balance.

### Basic principles

A solution is a liquid that contains dissolved substances. The liquid portion of a solution is the solvent; the substance that is dissolved in the solvent is called the solute. **Osmosis** is the passage of a solvent, usually water, through a selectively permeable membrane that separates solutions of different concentrations. The solvent passes through the membrane from the region of lower concentration of solute to that of higher concentration of solute, thus tending to equalize the concentration of the two solutions.

**Electrolytes** are salts that dissociate in solution into electrically charged particles (ions), including anions (negative ions), such as chloride, sulfate, bicarbonate, phosphate, organic acids, and proteins; and cations (positive ions), such as sodium, potassium, calcium, and magnesium. Electrolytes help to maintain osmotic pressure within cells. The concentration of particles is expressed as milliequivalents per milliliter (mEq/ml). One mEq of any cation is able to react with one mEq of any anion. Ordinarily, electrolyte solutes are balanced so there is an equal distribution of cations and anions.

Nonelectrolytes, such as glucose, urea, bile salts, creatinine, and cholesterol, do not dissociate in water into anions and cations, but they do affect the acid-base balance and osmotic pressure gradients.

The osmolality of a solution is determined by the concentration of solute in that solution. Osmotic pressure develops because of the differing concentrations of solute on either side of a membrane, expressed in units called osmols (Osm). One osmol is the number of particles in 1 g molecular weight of undissociated solute. One thousandth of an osmol is a milliosmol (mOsm).

Body fluid makes up about 60% of the average adult's body weight. It consists largely of water (45% to 70%) and dissolved minerals, proteins, and other nutrients and gases that are necessary for normal cell function. Body fluid exists in two main compartments: the intracellular compartment (within the cells) and the extracellular compartment (outside the cells). The extracellular compartment includes the plasma, the interstitial fluid (the fluid around the cells), and the fluid and electrolytes from certain secreting and excreting organs and tissues. Usually, two thirds of body fluid are in the intracellular compartment and one third is in the extracellular compartment.

Water moves freely between the intracellular and extracellular compartments, maintaining an osmotic equilibrium. Thus, if the extracellular electrolyte concentration increases, water diffuses from the intracellular compartment to the extracellular compartment, thereby increasing cellular tonicity and diluting the extracellular compartment and vice versa.

### Fluid and electrolyte imbalances

The body receives water through the oral intake of fluids and solid foods. Water is also produced by the chemical oxidation of nutrients. In addition, approximately 8 L of water are secreted daily by the gastrointestinal organs.

Under normal conditions, the body loses water daily in the urine and feces, by perspiration, and via insensible (immeasurable) losses through the skin and the lungs. Patients may also lose fluids and electrolytes during surgery or through vomiting, diarrhea, suction, draining wounds, intestinal obstructions, draining fistulas, hemorrhage, infections, or prolonged use of enemas and laxatives. Infants are especially vulnerable to fluid loss because of their high proportion of body fluid, immature kidneys, increased heat production, and rapid growth.

Excessive loss of body water can result in dehydration. The goal of nursing in dehydrated patients is to restore the circulating volume of fluid without causing an overload. Careful observation, recording, and reporting of the patient's signs and symptoms and fluid intake and output are essential in such patients.

In addition to fluid imbalances, patients should be monitored for possible electrolyte disturbances. The most common imbalances of electrolytes in the GI tract are excesses or deficits of chloride, magnesium, sodium, potassium, bicarbonate, calcium, or hydrogen ions.

Systematic observations to detect fluid and electrolyte imbalances include changes in temperature, pulse rate, respirations, and blood pressure. Fatigue and changes in skin and in mucous membranes and/or in speech, behavior, facial appearance, skeletal muscle, sensations, and body weight are also significant. Desire for food and water, anorexia, or thirst are important signs in detecting imbalances. Observations of importance relative to urine output include the specific gravity, pH, volume, and character. Significant observations should be relayed to the physician to facilitate early diagnosis and treatment before serious imbalances occur.

### Administration of fluids and electrolytes

One way of correcting fluid and electrolyte disturbances is by IV administration of solutions containing the necessary electrolytes and nutrients. All IV solutions are considered medications and their infusion requires a physician's order. The order should include the name of the solution/medication, volume/dose, rate, frequency, and route of administration. Consent of the patient or a legally authorized representative and the patient's identity must be confirmed before initiation of IV therapy.

### Equipment

The equipment needed for IV therapy generally includes needles and/or catheters, containers, tubing, filters, tourniquets, tape, antimicrobial agents, stands, clamps, and sometimes electronic pumps and controllers.

• Most **needles** are made of stainless steel that is coated with silicone. Because needles tend to dislodge and infiltrate more frequently than catheters, the use of stainless-steel needles should be limited to single-dose or short-term therapy. Needles carry less risk of site infection than plastic catheters. Winged infusion sets are used for short-term therapy in cooperative adult patients and for therapy of any duration in infants, children, or elderly patients with veins that are fragile or sclerotic (hardened and thickened).

• **Catheters** are made of plastic, such as polyvinyl chloride, Teflon, or Silastic. They are generally considered better than needles alone for long-term therapy. Over-the-needle catheters that are radiopaque (that is, appear light or white on x-ray films) should be used for routine IV therapy. In-the-needle catheters are used for central venous pressure monitoring and for administration of total parenteral nutrition and other highly concentrated dextrose solutions. They are inserted into large veins and secured in place with skin sutures. Because of the risk of puncture or shearing, through-the-needle catheters are not recommended for routine peripheral venous access.

• The word *cannula* may be used to refer either to a stainless-steel needle or to a catheter. The cannula selected for peripheral insertion should be of the smallest diameter and shortest length that will accommodate the prescribed therapy.

• Before use, IV fluid containers should be checked for cracks or tears, foreign matter, cloudiness, precipitation (that is, settling out of solid particles), any other signs of contamination, and the expiration date.

• Intravenous tubing may be a regular (macrodrip) solution administration set that delivers 10 to 20 drops per ml, or a microdrip set that delivers 60 drops per ml. Tubing with a secondary injection port permits separate or simultaneous infusion of two solutions; tubing with a piggyback port and a back-check valve permits intermittent infusion of a secondary solution. Vented tubing is used for solutions contained in a nonvented bottle, and nonvented tubing is used for solutions in vented bottles or containers.

- Intermittent infusion sets (heparin locks) consist of a winged-tip needle with tubing ending in a resealable rubber injection port. The device is filled with dilute heparin to prevent blood clot formation. Heparin locks are used both to provide immediate access in case IV therapy is needed during a procedure and to maintain venous access in patients who are receiving IV medication regularly or intermittently but do not require continuous infusion of fluids.
- Several different types of filters are utilized in IV therapy, including 0.2-micron bacteria-retentive, air-eliminating filters, which are recommended for routine use to decrease the complications of infection and air embolism; particulate-matter filters of 1 or 5 microns, which are used to remove particulate matter in situations where bacteria-retentive filters are contraindicated; and blood filters, which range from microaggregate filters that are 20 to 40 microns in size to standard 170-micron filters.
- Tourniquets are applied above the intended insertion site to distend a vein with a larger-than-average amount of blood. Vein distention may also be enhanced by application of warm, moist heat, light slapping of the skin over the veins, having the patient open and close a fist several times, or manually stroking the part. The tourniquet should impede venous, but not arterial, flow. Tourniquets should be routinely discarded or disinfected after every procedure. To avoid circulatory impairment, they should be applied only for the short time needed to perform the venipuncture.
- Half-inch tape or a transparent semipermeable membrane dressing may be used to anchor the needle or catheter on the skin. One-inch tape is used to secure the armboard or handboard, to secure a loop of tubing, and to secure the site dressing. When tape is used, it must not be applied directly to the skin-cannula junction site. Instead, an adhesive bandage with a gauze pad may be used. Hypoallergenic tape is available for patients who have tape allergies.
- Antimicrobial agents, such as alcohol or povidone-iodine (Betadine), are used to cleanse the IV site before venipuncture.
- Intravenous stands may be portable or may be attached to the bed or wall. To achieve the maximum flow rate, the infusion tubing drip chamber should be suspended approximately 3 feet above the injection site.
- Mechanical flow-control clamps, including roller, screw, and slide clamps, are suitable for the regulation of most infusions, but electronic infusion pumps or controllers should be used when warranted by the patient's age and condition, the setting in which the therapy is delivered, and the prescribed therapy. Controllers regulate gravity flow either by counting drops or by measuring volume. Infusion pumps generate flow under positive pressure; they operate independently of gravity flow.
- Patient-controlled analgesia (PCA) devices may be used to deliver IV analgesic agents. When these devices are used, patients must be educated as to the purpose of the PCA therapy, operating instructions, expected outcomes, precautions, and potential side effects. Because the medications administered through PCA devices are controlled substances, they must be obtained, delivered, administered, documented, and discarded in accordance with state and federal regulations.

**Intravenous solutions**

The **tonicity** of body fluids refers to the effective osmotic pressure equivalent. Intravenous fluids may be categorized as **isotonic** (having the same tonicity as the extracellular fluid), **hypotonic** (having a tonicity lower than the extracellular fluid), or **hypertonic** (having a tonicity greater than the extracellular fluid).

- The tonicity of plasma is approximately 290 mOsm; this is considered isotonic. Isotonic solutions are considered to be compatible with body fluids when introduced into the vascular system.
- Solutions less than 240 mOsm are considered hypotonic. Hypotonic solutions, unless they are balanced with sufficient numbers of electrolytes, can flood the red blood cells, causing them to burst, a condition known as **hemolysis.** NaCl in water (0.45%).
- Solutions with a tonicity greater than 340 mOsm are considered hypertonic. Improperly balanced hypertonic solutions can cause red blood cells to shrink, a condition known as **plasmolysis.** 10% dextrose in water.

Intravenous fluids may be administered for maintenance or replacement purposes. Maintenance therapy meets the patient's ordinary needs by providing approximately 3,000 ml of fluid per 24 hr, along with added electrolytes, nutrients, and vitamins. Replacement therapy restores lost fluids on a volume-to-volume basis, often in excess of 3,000 ml/24 hr. The electrolyte concentration of replacement therapy is generally equal to the concentration of electrolytes in the extracellular fluid.

For maintenance therapy, a balanced hypotonic electrolyte solution with the addition of 5% dextrose for calories is ideal. This balanced electrolyte solution typically contains sodium, potassium, magnesium, chloride, and acetate.

Ideally, replacement therapy solutions should contain ions in the same composition as that of the plasma and interstitial fluid. Five percent dextrose may or may not be included, depending on the caloric needs of the patient. A balanced isotonic multiple-electrolyte solution would include sodium, potassium, magnesium, chloride, acetate, and gluconate, with an average pH of 6.2. Most IV solutions have an acid pH, thus making them more stable and better able to withstand the effects of bacterial overgrowth.

The IV fluids administered most often are 5% dextrose in water (D5W), normal saline solution, and lactated Ringer's solution. Other IV solutions include carbohydrate in water, carbohydrate in sodium chloride, isotonic sodium chloride, potassium, vitamins, protein hydrolysates, and alcohol solutions. Fructose may be added instead of dextrose because fructose is more rapidly metabolized and converted to glycogen.

### Insertion sites

Selection of an insertion site for IV therapy depends on the type of solution; the type, frequency, and duration of therapy; the patient's age, size, diagnosis, and condition; and the patency, size, and location of available veins. The vessel chosen must accommodate the size of the catheter. When a heparin lock is used to administer conscious sedation during endoscopic procedures, it is usually placed in a large vessel in the right arm. A large vessel is more appropriate because the medications used to produce sedation can irritate the vessel wall.

When choosing an insertion site it is important to distinguish between veins and arteries. If a vessel pulsates, it is an artery. Puncture and the inadvertent injection of certain medications into arteries can lead to complications such as inflammation, necrosis, sloughing, and even gangrene and loss of function of the affected part.

Peripheral IV infusions are typically inserted in a superficial vein on the nondominant arm, including but not limited to the metacarpal, cephalic, basilic, and median veins. Jointed areas, thrombosed veins, varicosed veins, shunted areas, veins over joints, and traumatized or heavily scarred areas should be avoided. It is best to begin with distal veins and then work up. If an infiltration occurs, cannulation must always be performed proximal to the previously cannulated site.

Generally, cannulation of the lower extremities should be avoided in adults because it increases the risk of thrombophlebitis and embolism. If an IV cannula must be placed in a lower extremity, it should be changed as soon as an alternative site can be established.

### Insertion technique

Before insertion the selected site should be cleansed with soap and water, if necessary. Then the site should be swabbed with an antimicrobial agent, most often povidone-iodine (Betadine), and permitted to air dry. A tourniquet should be applied above the intended insertion site. The use of intradermal lidocaine to numb the insertion site is controversial, and it need not be used routinely for cannula insertion.

For peripheral insertion, the skin is held taut and the vein is anchored with the thumb below the injection site. The needle is inserted slowly into the vein until blood return is noted, the needle or catheter is advanced, and the tourniquet is released. Primed tubing is connected and fluid is run at a fast rate to flush blood from the tubing. Once blood is cleared, the IV drip is regulated at the prescribed rate.

The cannula should be stabilized so it does not interfere with assessment and monitoring of the IV site or impede delivery of the prescribed therapy. An antimicrobial ointment is applied to the insertion site if desired, followed by a sterile gauze or transparent semipermeable membrane dressing. All edges of the dressing should be securely taped. Roller bandages obstruct visualization of the IV site and may impair circulatory flow. They are not recommended on an extremity where an IV cannula is placed. An arm or hand board may be used if the cannula is placed close to an area of flexion.

A 3- to 6-inch portion of tubing is looped and taped at the insertion site. (The loop allows some slack to prevent dislodgement of the catheter caused by tension on the line.) Flow rate is adjusted and all pertinent information is recorded.

Frequent monitoring of patients receiving IV therapy minimizes the risk of potential complications. Monitoring should include observation of the insertion site, flow rate, clinical data, and patient response to the prescribed therapy.

Intravenous therapy can be discontinued on the order of a physician, on completion of therapy, for needle or catheter changes, or when infection or infiltration is suspected. The patient and/or a legally authorized representative also has the right to request discontinuation of treatment.

To remove a peripheral line, first the tubing is clamped, then the tape is removed from the skin, and the needle or catheter is withdrawn slowly and smoothly. Pressure should be maintained with a gauze pad at the insertion site until bleeding stops. When bleeding stops, the site should be cleansed with an antiseptic and a dry, sterile bandage should be applied.

### Complications

Intravenous therapy is an invasive procedure that is not without risks. Since the IV system provides direct access into the vascular system, stringent infection-control measures must be applied.

If an intravenous-related infection is suspected, the

cannula, any purulent drainage, and the infusate should be cultured to identify the responsible microorganism. Blood cultures may be considered to determine the extent of the infection.

Other potential local, systemic, and mechanical complications associated with IV therapy include the following:

- **Infiltration,** the inadvertent administration of a solution/medication into surrounding tissue
- Hematoma

- **Phlebitis** (inflammation of a vein), marked by infiltration of the coats of the vein and thrombus formation
- Pyrogenic reactions, including septicemia (blood poisoning) and bacteremia (presence of bacteria in the blood)
- Air embolism
- Catheter embolism, or catheter fragments in the vascular system
- Pulmonary edema

**Table 22-1.** Potential complications of intravenous therapy

| Complication | Possible cause | Signs and symptoms | Intervention |
|---|---|---|---|
| Infiltration | Puncture of the vein wall or needle or cannula slipping out of the vein | Edema, pain and burning at the venipuncture site | Discontinue infusion; remove cannula; restart at a different, more proximal location; elevate the affected part; apply cold compresses for the first 24 hrs, followed by warm, moist compresses |
| Hematoma | Unsuccessful attempt at venipuncture or infiltration of a blood transfusion | Painful, raised area, with blue or purplish patches | Remove needle or cannula; apply pressure and cold compresses |
| Phlebitis with or without clot formation | Vein irritation and inflammation; may occur postinfusion | Edema along the affected vein; sore, hard, cordlike, and warm vein | Discontinue infusion; remove cannula; apply warm, moist compresses; notify physician |
| Pyrogenic reactions | Contaminated equipment or solutions | Fever, chills, nausea and vomiting, backache, malaise | Discontinue infusion; culture cannula and solution and record lot number of solution; notify physician |
| Air embolism | Air in tubing; loose connections allowing air to enter tubing | Hypotension; cyanosis; heart murmur; tachycardia; syncope; vascular collapse; and loss of consciousness | Turn the patient on his or her left side with the head down; notify physician; check the system for leaks |
| Catheter embolism | Portion of a plastic cannula breaks off and flows into the vascular system; attempting to rethread the catheter with a needle; unsecured catheter | Vein discomfort; cyanosis; decreased blood pressure; weak, rapid pulse; loss of consciousness | Discontinue infusion; apply tourniquet above insertion site; notify physician; x-ray film taken to locate fragment |
| Pulmonary edema | Circulatory overload; excessive infusion flow rate | Headache; venous dilatation; hypertension; coughing; dyspnea; tachycardia | Slow infusion to a keep-open rate; elevate the head of the bed and raise the patient's knees; notify physician |
| Speed shock | Too-rapid administration of solutions and medications | Shock; syncope; and cardiac arrest | Slow infusion to keep-open rate; resuscitate; notify physician |

Modified from Hamilton, H, ed. *Procedures.* Nurse's Reference Library. Springhouse, PA: Internal Communications, 1983.

- Speed shock, a systemic reaction that occurs when a foreign substance is introduced too rapidly into the circulation

These complications are listed in Table 22-1, with respective causes, signs and symptoms, and appropriate interventions.

### Dosage calculations

The rate of flow of IV fluids can be affected by many factors, such as height of the fluid container, bent or kinked tubing, use of filters, medication additions, needle or catheter size, needle or catheter position, needle or catheter occlusion, or infiltration of IV fluid to the surrounding tissue. Patient movement or manipulation of the clamp may also be a factor. Flow rate can be easily monitored by using a time tape, which indicates the prescribed solution level at hourly intervals.

The rules of ratio and proportion can be used to calculate the rate of flow of IV fluids. It is important to check the rate of flow at least every 15 minutes for infants and children and at least every 30 minutes for adults. Every time the rate is checked, it is necessary to determine how much fluid is left in order to refigure the rate of flow needed and in what period of time it is to be administered.

Calculated infusion flow rates are only guidelines. Maintaining the calculated rate of flow does not relieve nurses of the responsibility to observe the patient for signs that the infusion is too rapid or too slow. Observation of pediatric patients for indications of too-rapid infusion is imperative. Pumps and controllers that automatically regulate the flow at a set rate should be used for infants and small children and occasionally for older children and adults. Smaller volume administration containers are also recommended for these groups.

### Patient education

The establishment of rapport and an effective system of communication between the nurse and the patient is of utmost concern. It is important to explain the procedure to ensure cooperation and reduce anxiety, which can cause a vasomotor response resulting in venous constriction. Intravenous therapy should be initiated only after the patient has exhibited signs of understanding and acceptance.

Before starting a continuous infusion, patient education should cover patient mobility, the importance of avoiding pressure to the IV site, keeping the site dry, and the need to keep the fluid container at an appropriate height. Patients should be given an estimate of the approximate duration of therapy and should be warned not to adjust the flow rate. They should be advised to notify the nurse if they experience pain or other complications.

Patient education and understanding should be documented.

### Documentation

Documentation of IV therapy should be legible and accessible to all healthcare professionals involved in the patient's care. Distinctive labeling should provide pertinent and easily identified information relative to the cannula, dressing, solution, medication, and administration set.

Documentation of any venipuncture should include the date and time of initiation, the amount and type of solution used, the type of needle or catheter and its gauge, the venipuncture site, and the rate of flow. The rate of flow should be recorded in ml/hr; rates of flow in drops per minute are misleading because drop factors vary from tubing to tubing. Any complications, anxiety, or untoward reactions on the part of the patient should be included in the record, along with nursing interventions taken.

## INTRAVENOUS MEDICATION ADMINISTRATION

Intravenous administration of medications has a number of advantages. Some drugs, including antibiotics, are frequently given intravascularly to provoke a quick, continuous therapeutic response. Other drugs may be given by the IV route because they are ineffective or dangerous by other routes. Some drugs are contraindicated for IV administration, including certain non-aqueous or suspension medications, because they obstruct blood flow.

### Techniques and routes of administration

Intravenous medications must have a physician's written order. Before medication administration, the nurse must assess the appropriateness of the prescribed therapy; the patient's age and condition; and the dose, route, and rate of the medication ordered. The nurse should be aware of the medication's indications, actions, and side effects and appropriate nursing interventions in the event of adverse reactions. Before administering any medication it is important to verify the patient's identity and to check the label on the medication against the order on the patient's medication record and against the physician's order.

Before adding any drug to an IV solution it is also necessary to establish that the drug is compatible with the solution. Mixing of drugs in a continuous infusion should be done only after consultation with incompatibility lists and with the pharmacist. Aseptic technique should be used for admixing. The expiration date of solutions/medications must be ascertained. In addition, the physical and chemical compatibility of the delivery systems used must be confirmed. Incompatibilities can cause leakage, air embolism, occlusion, infection, and other undesirable effects. The addition of a drug to blood transfusions complicates identification of the source of adverse reactions, if any, and therefore should not be done.

Various methods can be used for IV drug administration, including the addition of drugs to the IV solution (continuous infusion); infusion through a secondary line (piggyback or add-a-line method); use of an intermittent infusion injection device (heparin lock); and IV push injections.

- Continuous infusions are diluted in a large quantity of fluid, from 250 to 1,000 ml, and delivered over a 2- to 24-hour period. The medication is typically added to the infusion container by using a needle and syringe. After injecting the drug it is important to rotate the bottle or squeeze the bag to mix the solution thoroughly, observing the solution after the addition for any precipitation, discoloration, or cloudiness. After adding the medication, a label noting that medication has been added must be placed on the IV container.
- Implementing the piggyback method, a moderate quantity of fluid (usually 50 to 100 ml) is administered over a 5-minute to 2-hour period, using a separate small volume IV fluid container that is attached either through the top of the drip chamber for the primary container or through a Y-connector on the tubing of the main line. This secondary container must be elevated above the level of the main-line IV container. If the drug to be added through the piggyback set is incompatible with the primary IV solution, the line must be flushed with 0.9% sodium chloride before starting the drug infusion.
- Intermittent infusion sets (heparin locks) may be used for patients who are receiving IV medications regularly, either by the push method or intermittently, but who do not require continuous infusion of fluids. After insertion, heparinized saline is injected every 6 to 12 hours to maintain the patency of the infusion set. If the medication to be administered is compatible with heparin, the medication is injected in the time recommended, followed by an injection of heparinized saline to flush the medication and refill the catheter. If heparin is incompatible with the administered medications/solutions, the SASH (saline, administration, saline, heparin) procedure should be used. In this procedure, saline is used before and after administration of the medication, and is followed by a final flush of heparinized saline.
- Intravenous push (bolus) medications may or may not be diluted in 0.25 to 50 ml of fluid. They are administered over a 5-second to 5-minute period, either by direct venipuncture or using in-progress

infusion setups. If administered through an in-progress setup, the IV tubing above the injection site should be pinched during injection so the medication does not flow up to the bottle. The IV fluid should be permitted to flow rapidly for 30 to 60 seconds after injection to move the medication through the tubing.
- The IV push method is often used in endoscopic procedures. It may be used to give conscious sedation, to provide an immediate drug effect in an emergency, to achieve peak drug levels in the bloodstream, or to deliver drugs that cannot be diluted or administered intramuscularly. A winged-tip needle is often used for this purpose because it can be quickly and easily inserted, thereby making it ideal for the repeated administration of drugs, such as in weekly or monthly chemotherapy.

## Indications for intravenous medication in gastroenterology

Intravenous medications may be administered to gastroenterology patients for the following purposes:
- Conscious sedation and/or analgesia; for example, use of diazepam (Valium), meperidine (Demerol), midazolam (Versed), or fentanyl (Sublimaze)
- Control of variceal hemorrhage; for example, use of vasopressin (Pitressin)
- Treatment of narcotic-induced respiratory depression with naloxone (Narcan)
- Treatment of bradycardia; for example, use of atropine
- Reducing peristalsis; for example, use of glucagon

In addition, IV antibiotics are given for prophylaxis in gastroenterology patients who are at risk for bacterial endocarditis or for patients with abdominal abscess, cholangitis, diverticulitis, or ulcerative colitis. Whenever prophylactic antibiotics are given, it is important to weigh the risks of infection against potential side effects of the drugs.

## Adverse reactions

After administering any drug it is important to observe the patient for signs of drug sensitivity or intolerance. If adverse effects occur, the medication should be discontinued and the physician should be notified.

Appropriate steps should be taken to reduce the risk of infection, as detailed above. To reduce vein irritation, the following steps may be taken:
- Use the smallest gauge needle possible for IV push medications.
- Use heparinized saline following a 50 to 100 ml dose of antibiotic to prevent thrombus formation and vein irritation at the injection site.
- Use intermittent, rather than continuous, infusions.

- When possible, use normal saline as the IV fluid or diluent.
- Use at least 50 to 100 ml of diluent with all antibiotics.
- For IV therapy extending beyond 72 hours, rotate injection sites.

Medications should be timed as they are administered; too-fast administration can produce speed shock.

Certain complications of IV drug administration are specific to the method of administration.

- Excessively high drug concentrations in the IV solution can cause complications, such as sclerosis, thrombosis (clot formation), hemolysis, or phlebitis.
- With piggyback infusions, side effects and reactions to the infused drug can occur. Repeated punctures of the secondary injection port can cause an imperfect seal, with possible leakage or contamination.
- Infiltration and a specific reaction to the infused drug are the most common complications of intermittent infusion devices.
- With IV push injections, effects are often immediate, and signs of an acute allergic reaction or anaphylaxis can develop rapidly. If signs of anaphylaxis occur (i.e., dyspnea, cyanosis, convulsions, or increasing respiratory distress), the physician should be notified immediately and emergency measures should be instituted as necessary.

Infiltration is the leakage of infused solution from a vein into surrounding tissue, resulting from a needle puncturing a vascular wall or leakage around the venipuncture site. It causes local pain and itching, edema, blanching, and decreased skin temperature in the affected extremity. Infiltration of some drugs can severely damage tissue through irritative, sclerotic, vesicant, corrosive, or vasoconstrictive actions. Treatment of infiltrations of IV solutions and nonirritating drugs involves routine comfort measures, such as application of warm soaks. Infiltrations of corrosive drugs require emergency treatment to prevent tissue necrosis. If signs of infiltration occur, such as swelling, the absence of blood back-flow, and/or a sluggish flow rate, the injection should be stopped, the amount of infiltration estimated, and the physician notified.

### Documentation

Documentation requirements are similar to those that apply when administering fluids and electrolytes. In addition, it is important to document any medications added, the drip rate, and by whom they were added. For patients who arrive in an endoscopy unit with a line in place, the condition of the IV should be documented. The patient's response to IV medications should also be recorded. All unusual occurrences should be reported to the physician immediately. Written reports of adverse effects should include all signs, symptoms, treatment, and outcome. Encourage the physician to examine the patient and to draw a diagram on the chart indicating the location of pain or complications.

In the case of infiltration, record the site of the infiltration, the patient's symptoms, the estimated amount of infiltrated solution, the nursing treatment, the time, and the name of the physician notified. Continue to document the appearance of the infiltrated site and any associated symptoms.

## BLOOD AND BLOOD COMPONENTS

Each year, more than 6 million patients in the United States receive blood therapy. Of those, 3,000 (approximately 1 in 5,000) die annually as a result of complications of blood therapy. This is approximately the same number who die from the untoward effects of general anesthesia.

Many states require that registered nurses be specially trained before administering blood therapy. Blood therapy includes ordering blood, checking blood, hanging blood, observing the patient for expected actions and adverse reactions, regulating blood, discontinuing blood, obtaining blood samples for type and cross-matching, and documenting the therapy provided.

### Techniques of blood administration

The trend in blood therapy is to administer fractionated blood components, as opposed to **whole blood,** to avoid circulatory overload. Whole blood can be fractionated into red blood cells (**erythrocytes),** platelet suspensions and concentrates, white blood cells (**leukocytes,** fresh plasma, frozen and stored plasma, cryoprecipitates or factor VIII concentrates, fibrinogen, factors II, VII, IX, and X concentrates (prothrombin complex), albumin, and gammaglobulin.

- Whole blood contains red and white blood cells, serum, platelets, proteins (albumin, globulin, and fibrinogen), and other intravascular nutrients and substances. It is the best substance to transfuse in massive gastrointestinal bleeding because it replaces both blood volume and oxygen-carrying capacity.
- Packed red blood cells (RBCs) raise the hemoglobin and hematocrit faster than whole blood, with less risk of circulatory overload. Packed RBCs are used in severe anemia, in patients whose bleeding has ceased and whose vascular volume has been replenished with saline or lactated Ringer's solution, and cautiously in patients with underlying cardiac disease or renal failure. Red blood cells may be frozen and then thawed for autotransfusions.
- Leukocyte-poor blood is produced by removing

leukocytes and platelets from whole blood. It is administered to patients who are candidates for transplants because it prevents sensitization to tissue antigens.

- **Platelets** are administered to patients with thrombocytopenia (a decreased number of platelets), marked splenomegaly (enlargement of the spleen), or chronic depletion of platelets. In septic and/or febrile patients, platelet infusion should be doubled to effect an increase in platelet count. Most patients require four or more units of platelets to prevent or control bleeding.

- **Plasma** is the fluid portion of blood that remains after centrifuging whole blood to remove the red blood cells. It contains most clotting factors, but no platelets. The plasma may be prepared as a liquid or it may be frozen or dried. It is used to treat clotting factor deficiencies when specific concentrates are not available or when the precise factor deficiency has not been determined.

- Fresh frozen plasma is used when there is little or no actual blood loss, such as in burns and in crush injuries. In emergencies, fresh frozen plasma may be used as a volume expander in hypovolemic bleeding until fresh whole blood is available. It is not required in most patients unless there is a clinically important disturbance in coagulation. Because a deficiency of coagulation factors is a preexisting phenomenon in many patients with cirrhosis, consideration should be given to providing these patients with fresh frozen plasma after every second or third unit of packed RBCs.

- **Cryoprecipitates** are **serum** proteins, including factors VIII, XIII, and fibrinogen, that settle out of solution at temperatures below 20° C. Cryoprecipitates are administered to patients with hemophilia A and von Willebrand's disease.

- **Prothrombin** complex, which comprises Factors II, VII, IX, and X, may be administered to treat hemophilia B, severe liver disease, and deficiencies of these specific factors. It carries a relatively high risk of transmitting hepatitis.

- Volume expanders include 25% normal serum albumin; Plasmanate (a commercially prepared hypertonic solution of alpha and beta globulins, human albumin, sodium, and chloride), which is used in burn cases, hypovolemic shock, or hypoproteinemia; and the plasma substitutes dextran-40 or dextran-70, which have a molecular weight higher than that of blood, and therefore cause osmotic diuresis and a resulting increase in blood volume when introduced into the vascular system.

- Gammaglobulin is transfused to prevent infectious hepatitis, rubeola, mumps, pertussis, tetanus, and hypogammaglobulinemia and agammaglobulinemia.

The equipment required for transfusing blood and blood products includes whole blood or components, a straight or Y-type blood administration set with a regular or microaggregate filter, infusion equipment, including a 19- or 21-gauge needle or catheter, and a portable infusion standard. Both whole blood and packed cells contain cellular debris, thereby necessitating in-line filtration during administration.

Nursing responsibilities in the administration of blood and blood components include but are not limited to the following:

- Blood product inspection
- Verification of product expiration date
- Confirmation of compatibility between recipient and donor
- Confirmation of informed patient consent
- Patient education
- Monitoring the patient at least 5 minutes postadministration
- Identification of immediate and delayed reactions
- Intervention in the case of adverse reactions
- Written documentation
- Communication with other healthcare providers
- Adherence to aseptic technique

All blood to be used for transfusion must be cross-matched with a sample of the patient's blood. Institutional protocols should be followed to ensure that the blood to be transfused is identified and double-checked with the patient's name, assigned hospital number, the number on the unit of blood, and the date of collection and cross-matching. It is vital that this identifying information be absolutely accurate; *transfusing the wrong blood to the wrong patient can be fatal!* It is advisable that two parties, registered nurses or physicians, check the blood before transfusion and report any discrepancies to the blood bank before administration.

After verifying the identifying information, the blood bag should be gently rotated to distribute the blood cells. The tubing, drip chamber, and filter(s) should be primed and flushed with 30 to 60 ml of sterile normal saline, which is accomplished by connecting an infusion container of saline to the tubing and filter. After flushing at a keep-open rate (about 10 drops per minute), the saline container is disconnected and the blood bag is connected to the tubing.

The blood is administered at a keep-open rate (25 to 30 drops per minute) for the first 30 minutes, while observing the patient for adverse reactions. After that, the flow should be adjusted to the prescribed rate, checking every 30 to 60 minutes for rate of flow, infiltration, and side effects. When the transfusion is complete, the blood bag, used tubing, and tag should be disconnected and returned to the blood bank.

To preserve blood and prevent contamination, it should be refrigerated at 4° C. If hanging of blood is delayed more than 30 minutes from the time it is received from the blood bank, it should be returned to the bank for refrigeration. Rapid transfusion of cold blood can lead to hypothermia. When multiple units of blood are required, portable or stationary blood warmers may be used to keep the blood at a constant temperature of 98.6° F.

If an infusion is to be administered following the transfusion, the tubing should be changed, the filter removed, and the needle or cannula flushed with 10 to 20 ml normal saline before reconnecting the infusion.

Whole blood and red blood cells should not be used after 21 days. Frozen blood should be used within 24 hours after thawing and cannot be refrozen. Fresh frozen plasma should be used within 4 hours of thawing because it does not contain preservatives. Blood may be heparinized to prevent clotting. Citrate is added to stored whole blood to prevent coagulation. If the blood is administered slowly, the patient's liver can remove citrate.

In autotransfusion, the patient's own blood may be salvaged after a traumatic injury or during an operative procedure and reinfused into a vein after it is filtered and treated with an anticlotting agent. Or, the patient may donate his or her own blood before elective surgery. Potential complications of autotransfusion include blood clotting, hemolysis, coagulopathies, thrombocytopenia, particulate and air emboli, sepsis, and citrate toxicity.

### Indications and contraindications

The primary purpose of blood transfusions is to improve tissue oxygenation (with red blood cells) and/or to improve coagulation (with plasma and platelets). Other indications may include improving hemoglobin/hematocrit levels, increasing intravascular volume, or replacing certain substances, such as protein, platelets, or clotting factors.

Transfusions may be indicated for treatment of massive gastrointestinal bleeding if the patient continues to bleed despite therapy, is in shock, has a very low hematocrit, or has symptoms related to poor tissue oxygenation. Treatment for massive bleeding is aimed at preventing hypovolemic shock, preventing dehydration and electrolyte imbalance, stopping the bleeding, and providing rest. Transfusions may also be given to increase the blood volume and help correct anoxia resulting from decreased RBCs. Infusion of crystalloids may dilute the red cell count. Stabilization of blood values may take 6 to 8 hours after volume replacement.

Exchange blood transfusions may be used in the treatment of hepatic coma. Fresh blood is used to replace the blood volume. This may be repeated in 12, 24, and 48 hours. Cross-circulation of blood between a donor and the patient may be done without the need for a large volume of typed and cross-matched blood. Either procedure gives the patient's liver cells time to regenerate, and provides fresh blood or enables the donor to correct some of the patient's metabolic and electrolyte disturbances. In advanced cirrhosis when there is irreversible damage, these methods are of little benefit.

Patients should receive blood until their vital signs are stable, bleeding ceases, and enough RBCs are circulating to provide adequate oxygenation. A hematocrit of 30% is a reasonable goal in most patients.

### Adverse reactions

Any nurse who administers blood must be able to recognize the signs and symptoms of adverse reactions. Potential adverse reactions to blood and blood component therapy include the following:

- Circulatory overload, which occurs when too much fluid or too rapid an infusion is administered to patients with underlying cardiac, renal, liver, pulmonary, or hematologic disease. Signs and symptoms include cough, chest pain, dyspnea, tachycardia, and cyanosis.
- Bacterial reaction to the transfusion, which is characterized by the development of a fever, chills, abdominal and extremity pain, vomiting, hypotension, and bloody diarrhea. Bacteremic shock and death may follow the administration of as little as 25 ml of contaminated blood.
- Allergic reactions, which may occur when the donor has ingested substances to which the recipient is allergic. They may be manifested in mild cases by a mild urticaria, pruritus, and nasal congestion, or in severe cases, by bronchospasm, severe dyspnea, laryngeal edema, and circulatory collapse. Allergic reactions are usually treated with antihistamines.
- Hemolytic reactions, which usually occur within the first 30 minutes of the transfusion and are caused by incompatibility between the transfusing blood and the patient's blood. Signs and symptoms in the initial phase include anxiety, headache, flushing, chest pain, shortness of breath, tachycardia, and low back pain or pains of the long bones. The reaction may progress to fever, nausea, vomiting, cyanosis, oliguria, anuria, uremia with shock, jaundice, and vascular collapse.
- Hepatitis B, which may develop as long as 6 months after the use of contaminated blood, needles, catheters, tubing, or other equipment. Signs and symptoms include anorexia, jaundice, dyspepsia, abdominal pain, malaise, and weakness, often with hepatomegaly and splenomegaly.
- Massive transfusions of 8 to 10 or more units of blood may result in overtransfusion reactions (uncontrollable hemorrhage), citrate intoxication (con-

vulsions, impaired clotting, hyperkalemia, and ammonia intoxication), acid-base imbalances, or rapid pressure reactions.

If an adverse reaction occurs, the nurse should immediately stop the transfusion, save the substance being transfused, and keep the vein open with normal saline. The patient's vital signs should be assessed, and a urine specimen should be collected and sent to the laboratory immediately. The physician and the blood bank should be notified of a possible transfusion reaction. The labels of all blood containers should be compared to corresponding patient identification forms. Blood samples, all transfusion containers, and the administration set should be sent immediately to the blood bank.

The patient should be treated symptomatically and supportively. If ordered, oxygen, epinephrine, or other drugs should be administered. An alcohol bath or a hypothermia blanket may be used to reduce fever. The patient should be made as comfortable as possible, and reassurance should be provided as necessary. In the case of an anaphylactic reaction, emergency resuscitative measures must be instituted immediately.

## Patient education

Blood transfusions always require a signed consent form from the patient.

To prevent recurrence of a transfusion reaction, patients who experience hypersensitivity reactions should be educated as to the cause and encouraged to carry this information in their wallets.

## Documentation

After the transfusion is complete, it is important to record the time, date, and duration of transfusion, the type and amount of transfused blood or blood components, baseline vital signs, and the check of all identifying data.

In the case of a transfusion reaction, the nurse should record the time and date of the reaction, the type and amount of transfused blood or blood products, the clinical signs of the transfusion reaction in order of occurrence, the patient's vital signs, any specimens that were sent to the laboratory, any treatment, and the patient's response to treatment. Some institutions require completion of a transfusion reaction form.

In autotransfusion, the nurse should record the duration of collection, suction pressure, type and amount of anticoagulant, the duration of transfusion, the use of a blood filter or washed cells, the amount and characteristics of drainage, and any complications.

---

**CASE SITUATION**

---

Davy Simms, the 6-month-old infant with a patent ductus described in the previous chapter, is sched-

uled for an esophagoscopy under general anesthesia. He is to receive ampicillin and gentamycin intravenously during the procedure.

*Points to think about*

1. Using the surface-area formulas provided in chapter 21, the nurse should calculate the amount of ampicillin Davy should be given when the therapeutic dose of ampicillin for an adult is 1000 mg over a 24-hour period.
2. The nurse should calculate the dose of ampicillin using Fried's and Clark's rules and compare them with calculations using body surface area.
3. The nurse should convert the dosage to minims of medication needed when there are 250 mg of ampicillin in 5 cc of diluent.
4. With what solution should the ampicillin be diluted?
5. How might the potential adverse reactions to ampicillin be described?
6. What is the reason for giving Davy prophylactic ampicillin?

*Suggested responses*

1. Surface-area formulas used in chapter 21 to calculate the pediatric dose of ampicillin are as follows:
   - $0.33 \times 0.33 \times 1000$ mg $\div 1.7 = 64$ mg in a 24-hour period
   - $0.33 \times 0.33 \times 60 = 6.5\%$ of 1000 mg $= 65.4$ mg in 24 hours
2. Fried's and Clark's rules for pediatric doses are as follows:
   - Fried's rule: $6 \div 150 \times 1000$ mg $= 40$ mg in 24 hours
   - Clark's rule: $13.5 \div 150 \times 1000$ mg $= 90$ mg in 24 hours

   Comparison of the figures obtained here and in the previous question indicates that the two surface-area calculations yield very similar dosages. The results of applying Fried's and Clark's rules, however, seem to be too divergent for infants of this size.
3. The conversion of calculations to minims when 250 mg of a drug are contained in 5 ml of diluent is as follows:
   If 5 ml = 250 mg, then 1 ml = 50 mg
   According to the conversion chart, 1 ml = 16 minims
   Therefore, 50 mg = 16 minims
   If the prescribed dosage (x) = 65 mg, then:

   $$\frac{50\ mg}{16\ minims} = \frac{65\ mg}{x\ minims}$$

   (50 mg) (x minims) = (65 mg) (16 minims)
   50x = 1040
   x = 20.8 minims
4. Ampicillin sodium can be diluted with either sterile distilled water or sterile normal saline. In this

instance, the diluent used depends on the fluid used to keep the vein open. That will probably be D5W, so the ampicillin would be diluted with sterile distilled water.

5. Potential adverse reactions to ampicillin include the following:
   • Gastrointestinal reactions, such as nausea, vomiting, or diarrhea
   • Hypersensitivity reactions, such as urticaria, fever, laryngeal edema, and anaphylaxis. Skin rashes occur more frequently with ampicillin than with other penicillins.
   With a patient this age, it is imperative that precise intake and output records be kept.

6. Davy is on prophylactic ampicillin to prevent bacterial endocarditis or great vessel arteritis while the physician evaluates the possibility of surgically closing the patent ductus. Ampicillin is the drug of choice in nonpenicillin-allergic persons to prevent throat and ear infections caused by beta-hemolytic *Streptococcus*, which is the organism most commonly implicated in these problems in endemic areas of the country.

## REVIEW TERMS

cannula, catheters, colloids, cryoprecipitates, crystalloids, D5W, electrolytes, erythrocytes, hemolysis, hypertonic, hypotonic, infiltration, isotonic, leukocytes, needles, normal saline, osmosis, phlebitis, plasma, plasmolysis, platelets, prothrombin, Ringer's solution, serum, tonicity, whole blood

## REVIEW QUESTIONS

1. Salts that dissociate in solution into positive and negative ions are called:
   a. Anions.
   b. Cations.
   c. Electrolytes.
   d. Colloids.

2. The preferred instrument for delivering long-term, routine IV therapy is a(n):
   a. Stainless-steel needle.
   b. Over-the-needle catheter.
   c. In-the-needle catheter.
   d. Cannula.

3. A peripheral IV cannula would most likely be inserted in the:
   a. Cephalic vein.
   b. Femoral vein.
   c. Superior vena cava.
   d. Radial artery.

4. Elevation of the affected part and application of cold compresses for the first 24 hours, followed by warm,

moist compresses, is the appropriate treatment for what complication of IV therapy?
   a. Hematoma.
   b. Infiltration.
   c. Air embolism.
   d. Catheter embolism.

5. Drugs should never be added to blood transfusions because:
   a. they are incompatible.
   b. It complicates determination of the source of any adverse reaction.
   c. Drugs can cause clotting.
   d. The rate of infusion is too slow.

6. If heparin is incompatible with the solution/medication to be administered through a heparin lock, then saline, solution/medication, and heparin must be administered in the following order:
   a. Saline, administration, saline, heparin.
   b. Heparin, administration, saline, heparin.
   c. Saline, administration, heparin, saline.
   d. Administration, saline, heparin, saline.

7. When administering IV medications, vein irritation can be minimized by:
   a. Using continuous, rather than intermittent, infusions.
   b. Using the same injection site continuously.
   c. Using 50 to 100 ml of diluent with antibiotics.
   d. Avoiding the use of normal saline as the diluent.

8. What is the best substance to transfuse in patients with massive gastrointestinal bleeding?
   a. Whole blood.
   b. Packed red blood cells.
   c. Platelets.
   d. Plasma.

9. If the patient experiences an adverse reaction to a blood transfusion, the first thing the nurse should do is:
   a. Assess the patient's vital signs.
   b. Stop the transfusion.
   c. Compare labels on blood containers with the patient's identification forms.
   d. Return the blood to the blood bank.

10. Hemolytic reactions to blood transfusions usually occur:
   a. Immediately.
   b. Within the first 30 minutes of the transfusion.
   c. Within 24 hours.
   d. As long as 6 months after the transfusion.

## BIBLIOGRAPHY

American Medical Association, Department of Drugs, Division of Drugs and Toxicology. *Drug Evaluations Annual 1991*. Chicago: American Medical Association, 1991.

Blume, D. *Dosages and Solutions*. 3rd ed. Philadelphia: F.A. Davis, 1980.

Coco, C. *Intravenous Therapy: A Handbook for Practice.* St. Louis: Mosby–Year Book, 1980.

Crass, R, and Vanderveen, T. "IV Pumps & Controllers: New Technology Stimulates Increased Sophistication." *Journal of Healthcare Material Management* 6(January 1988): 52-61.

Damsgard, C, *G.I.A. Certification Review Manual.* Rochester, N.Y.: Society of Gastrointestinal Assistants, 1985.

Given, B, and Simmons, S. *Gastroenterology in Clinical Nursing.* 4th ed. St. Louis: Mosby–Year Book, 1984.

Hamilton, H, editorial director. *Procedures.* Nurse's Reference Library. Springhouse, PA: Intermed Communications, 1983.

Intravenous Nurses Society. "Intravenous Nursing Standards of Practice." *Journal of Intravenous Nursing* Supplement(1990): S1-S98.

Kneedler, J, and Dodge, G. *Perioperative Patient Care: The Nursing Perspective.* 2nd ed. Boston: Blackwell Scientific Publications, Inc., 1987.

Langfitt, D. *Critical Care: Certification Preparation and Review.* Bowie, MD: Brady Communications, 1984.

Sleisenger, M, and Fordtran, J. *Gastrointestinal Disease: Pathophysiology, Diagnosis, Management.* 4th ed. Philadelphia: W.B. Saunders, 1989.

Society of Gastroenterology Nurses and Associates, Inc., Practice and Education Committees. *Nursing Care of the Patient Receiving Conscious Sedation in the Gastrointestinal Endoscopy Setting.* Rochester, N.Y.: Society of Gastroenterology Nurses and Associates, 1991.

Wiggins, M, and Sesin, P. "Guidelines for Administering I.V. Drugs." *Nursing 90* 20(April 1990): 145-52.

# Chapter 23

# NUTRITIONAL THERAPY

This chapter will acquaint the gastroenterology nurse with the basic principles of nutrition and nutritional therapy. These principles are followed by detailed discussions of special diets in the practice of gastroenterology and the care of patients who are receiving enteral or parenteral nutrition. The insertion and removal of percutaneous endoscopic gastrostomy/ jejunostomy (PEG/PEJ) devices are also discussed.

## Learning objectives

After reviewing the content of this chapter, the gastroenterology nurse should be able to:
1. Outline the basic principles of good nutrition and nutritional assessment, and nutritional therapy.
2. Describe a number of special diets that may be prescribed for patients with gastrointestinal disorders.
3. Discuss the techniques used in the administration of enteral and parenteral nutrition, and factors to be considered in the care of patients receiving this type of therapy.
4. Explain indications and techniques for the insertion and removal of PEG/PEJ devices.

## BASIC PRINCIPLES

A patient's nutritional status depends on the balance between the nutrient intake and energy expenditures. This balance may be affected by internal factors, such as age and physical condition, or by external factors, such as the quantity and quality of food available.

In patients with gastrointestinal disorders, nutritional status may also be affected by the following:
- Factors that interfere with food consumption, such as impaired appetite, disease, or a special diet
- Factors that increase tissue destruction, such as cancer, ulceration, or necrosis
- Factors that interfere with the patient's ability to absorb nutrients, including absence of normal digestive secretions, intestinal hypermotility, or decreased absorptive surface
- Factors that interfere with nutrient utilization or storage, such as impaired liver function, neoplasms, or pancreatitis
- Factors that increase nutrient excretion or loss, including hemorrhage, abscess or fistula formation, nausea and vomiting, surgery, or diarrhea
- Factors that increase nutritional requirements, including fever, chronic infection, and malignancy

For any patient, **nutrition** is an integral part of the total plan of care. A poor nutritional state can affect recovery, contribute to complications, and cause increased morbidity and mortality.

There are six general classes of essential nutrients, including carbohydrates, lipids, proteins, vitamins, minerals, and water.

## Carbohydrates

**Carbohydrates,** which comprise starches and/or sugars, are found in grains, vegetables, fruits, syrups, and sugars. They are all sources of glucose, which is needed for energy metabolism.

Ptyalin, an α-amylase secreted by acinar cells of the salivary glands, hydrolyzes about 40% of ingested starches into **disaccharides** in the mouth and stomach. In the duodenum, pancreatic amylase hydrolyzes the remaining 60% of ingested starch. In the jejunum, these newly formed disaccharides and ingested disaccharides are split into **monosaccharides** and are then absorbed with ingested monosaccharides. Any condition that compromises the duodenum or jejunum inhibits carbohydrate absorption.

The end product of carbohydrate **catabolism** is **glucose,** a monosaccharide that is the chief source of energy for all living organisms. Glucose is taken up by all of the cells of the body and burned for immediate energy. Excess glucose can be converted to **glycogen,** which is a long-chain polymer that is stored mainly in the liver and muscles. When necessary, liver glycogen can be converted to glucose for systemic distribution, but muscle glycogen is used primarily by the muscle itself. Excess dietary carbohydrates are also converted to triglycerides for storage in adipose tissue.

### Lipids

**Lipids** consist of fats, oils, waxes, and related compounds. They provide a concentrated stored energy source, cushion vital organs, and insulate the body to help maintain a constant body temperature. The primary sources of lipids are dairy products, egg yolks, meats, and nuts and seeds.

Ingested lipids are hydrolyzed and passed into the small bowel, where they form **triglycerides.** Short-chain triglycerides are broken down by gastric lipase and pancreatic lipase. Long-chain triglycerides, on the other hand, are emulsified by bile, which allows pancreatic lipase to cleave them into **monoglycerides,** end-stage **fatty acids,** and **glycerol.** In the jejunum, these products form micelles, which allow fat to be absorbed. Both bile and lipase disorders and jejunal or ileal disease can cause fat malabsorption.

### Proteins

**Proteins** are made up of various combinations of **amino acids.** Nine of the 22 recognized amino acids are considered essential for adequate nutrition. The chief dietary sources of protein are meats, dairy products, and vegetables. Ingested proteins may either be used to synthesize the proteins needed to build new tissue or may be catabolized for energy. There is no storage form of protein; ingested protein must supply all of the amino acids needed for internal protein synthesis.

**Nitrogen balance** is an indication of the effect of diet on the body's protein supply. Depending on the patient's condition, nitrogen balance may be neutral, positive, or negative.

- In a healthy adult, protein synthesis is equal to protein degradation, and the individual is said to be in neutral nitrogen balance.
- Positive nitrogen balance occurs when protein synthesis exceeds protein degradation. This state is normal and to be expected in children, who are building new tissue. In adults it may signify a rebuilding of wasted tissue.
- Negative nitrogen balance occurs when carbohydrate and lipid intake are less than body requirements, thus necessitating the use of the body's protein for fuel and resulting in protein breakdown in excess of protein synthesis.

Metabolism of ingested protein begins in the stomach, where pepsin, in the presence of hydrochloric acid, hydrolyzes proteins into amino acids and polypeptides of varying lengths. Then, in the duodenum and jejunum, pancreatic enzymes reduce these products to their basic peptides and amino acids. In the lower jejunum and ileum, the remaining peptides are hydrolyzed into amino acids and are absorbed. Protein absorption may be reduced by disorders that reduce gastric hydrochloric acid secretion, by duodenal or jejunal inflammation or infection, or by gastric or intestinal resection.

### Vitamins

**Vitamins** are organic compounds that are essential in minute quantities for specific cellular metabolic reactions and for normal growth and health. They are classified as either fat-soluble or water-soluble.

- Vitamins A, D, E, and K are soluble in fat solvents. They are absorbed with dietary fats and tend to be stored in the body in moderate amounts.
- All other vitamins are soluble in water. They are excreted in urine and are not stored in the body in appreciable amounts.

The general functions of vitamins are to regulate metabolism, convert fats and carbohydrates to energy, and aid bone and tissue formation.

### Minerals

**Minerals** are inorganic nutrients. They include major minerals, trace minerals, and trace elements. Major minerals include calcium, chloride, sodium, magnesium, potassium, sulfur, and phosphorus. These essential mineral nutrients are found in the human body in amounts in excess of 5 grams. Trace minerals include chromium, cobalt, copper, fluorine, iodine, iron, manganese, and zinc. These essential mineral nutrients are found in the human body in amounts less than 5 grams.

Among other things, minerals serve to regulate enzyme metabolism, maintain nerve and muscle integrity, and facilitate membrane transfer of essential compounds.

### Water

Water acts as an intracellular and extracellular solvent and provides a medium for transportation of nutrients and metabolic waste products. It also lubricates the tissues and helps maintain body temperature.

## NUTRITIONAL ASSESSMENT

A thorough assessment of a patient's nutritional status includes the following:
- A complete health and dietary history, including reports of any recent gain or loss of weight; recurrent nausea, vomiting, or diarrhea; any chronic illness; and dietary habits
- A physical examination to obtain data, such as height, weight, weight-to-height ratio, body frame size, mid-arm circumference, and skin fold thick-

ness, and to note signs of nutritional deficiency, such as edema, loss of subcutaneous fat, and muscle wasting

- Diagnostic studies, including laboratory tests for serum proteins, total lymphocyte count, nitrogen balance calculations, hemoglobin and hematocrit, serum iron, and serum albumin

For patients with recognized nutritional deficits, the physician may order oral, enteral, or parenteral nutritional therapy. Oral intake is the preferred means of administering a special diet but it requires that the patient have a functioning GI tract and be able to ingest foods. Enteral (tube) feedings are used when patients are unable or unwilling to use the normal oral route, such as when a patient is unable to swallow, has altered central nervous system function, or has severe anorexia secondary to the primary underlying illness. Parenteral feeding (intravenous hyperalimentation) is provided through an IV line for patients without a functional GI tract or for whom a period of bowel rest is indicated.

## SPECIAL ORAL DIETS

Many diets used in the treatment of gastrointestinal illnesses involve restriction of a particular dietary component, such as fats or protein. Others alter the consistency of the diet or the amount of dietary fiber. When prescribing a special diet it is important to remember that dietary habits or customs are difficult to change. As much as possible, the patient's cultural, socioeconomic, and religious patterns should be taken into account.

### High-fiber diets

Dietary fiber is made up of the complex polysaccharides and other polymers that are not digested in the small bowel, including cellulose, hemicelluloses, gums, mucilages, pectins, and lignins. Fiber acts to increase stool bulk and weight and also affects bowel transit time. The object of a high-fiber diet is the production of a regular pattern of defecation, with formed stools. High-fiber diets should not be used routinely for the treatment of chronic constipation because there is a distinct subset of patients with irritable colons, which can be exacerbated by the gas produced by the digestion of a high-fiber diet.

High-fiber diets may be indicated for patients with irritable bowel syndrome (IBS), ulcerative colitis, Crohn's disease, or diverticulitis. Approximately 10 g of additional crude fiber is recommended. This additional fiber can either be supplied in the diet, with emphasis on whole-grain breads and cereals, fresh fruits, and fresh vegetables, or can be consumed in the form of psyllium seed, which is a rich source of hemicellulose, or bran, which provides both cellulose and hemicellulose. Bran has the highest fiber content of any food. If the additional fiber is to be supplied by diet alone, it is important to recognize that the fiber content in unprocessed foods may be altered significantly by processes that remove the fiber, such as eating fruits without the peels.

### Low-fiber diets

The primary indication for a low-fiber diet is acute diarrhea. A low-fiber diet is also recommended in children who have active inflammatory bowel disease. Preparation for certain gastrointestinal procedures, including air-contrast barium enema, colonoscopy, and intestinal surgery, also requires adherence to a very low-fiber diet, or even enteral nutrition, for a few days. Partial low-fiber diets may be necessary to avoid recurrence of gastric phytobezoars or for patients with a very narrow ileal segment as a result of Crohn's disease.

Typically, a low-fiber diet used for chronic problems involves a reduction in the quantity of grains, fruits, and vegetables and limiting the intake of fats and proteins. The major drawback of low-fiber diets is that they may provide an inadequate amount of calories. If the patient's nutrition is marginal, the diet can be supplemented by enteral feedings.

### Gluten-free diets

Gluten is a protein found in wheat, oats, rye, and barley. A lifelong gluten-free diet is used in the treatment of celiac sprue, which is a disease characterized by malabsorption of nutrients, absence of normal intestinal villi on the small bowel mucosa, and prompt clinical improvement following withdrawal from the diet of all glutens to which the patient is sensitive.

Only the gliadin fraction of gluten protein is implicated in mucosal damage. To remove all cereal grains containing gliadin (i.e., wheat, barley, rye, and, in a few patients, oats), it is necessary for patients with celiac sprue to avoid the following:

- Obvious sources of such nutrients, including baked goods, dry cereals containing wheat and/or oats, and pastas
- Less obvious sources of gluten, including wheat that has been used as an extender in processed foods and beverages, such as ice cream, salad dressings, canned foods, catsup, mustard, candy bars, and instant coffee
- Foods with ingredients such as modified food starch, hydrolyzed vegetable protein, and malt

Because many sources of gliadin are not readily apparent to the consumer, it is very important that patients on gluten-free diets read all labels and carefully study the ingredients of all processed foods. Rice, soybean, corn, buckwheat, potato, and tapioca flours are appropriate substitutes or alternatives for gluten-sensitive patients.

Healthcare providers must remember that lifelong adherence to a gluten-free diet is a big commitment and may represent a significant social liability, especially for children and teenagers. Studies show that only 30% to 70% of celiac patients comply with their gluten-free diet. Patient education regarding the importance of compliance for continued good health is essential. Patients should be informed that failure to comply with a gluten-free diet results in lower stature and weight in young adults. Closely monitored follow-up and continued counseling are recommended.

Within a week of removal of gluten from the diet, patients may experience a decrease in diarrhea, improved appetite, and an overall improvement in attitude and behavior. In other patients, clinical improvement may take several months.

The most common cause of failure to respond to a gluten-free diet is incomplete removal of gluten. Sometimes it may be necessary to hospitalize the patient for supervision by a knowledgeable dietician to be certain that no glutens are consumed.

Some patients with celiac sprue may develop other nutritional deficiencies secondary to their gluten intolerance. If a secondary lactase deficiency develops, milk and milk products should be limited initially. In young children, initial dietary management also may require adequate calories and protein to sustain catch-up growth, multivitamin supplements, and iron and folic acid supplementation if the child is anemic. Most patients develop an increased tolerance to lactose and decrease their need for supplementation after gluten withdrawal as their intestinal structure and function begin to return to normal.

### Lactose-free diets

A low-lactose diet is indicated for patients with symptoms of lactose intolerance, which is evidenced by a history of diarrhea, bloating, and gas following ingestion of lactose and/or a positive lactose tolerance or hydrogen breath test.

Lactose intolerance may be the result of either a lactase deficiency or a decreased time of exposure to the intestinal mucosa, such as in short bowel syndrome or dumping syndrome. A low-lactose diet may be used in the treatment of patients with IBS or during the acute phase of a diarrheal illness in which intestinal transit is rapid or lactase deficiency is transient, as in acute gastroenteritis, ulcerative colitis, or Crohn's disease. A low-lactose diet may also be helpful in the initial phase of therapy for celiac sprue.

Patients with lactose intolerance should avoid milk and milk products, including ice cream, cheeses, and butter. Lactose-intolerant patients should also be alert to processed foods containing milk solids, whey, lactose, milk sugar, galactose, or skim milk powder. Yogurt may be well tolerated by lactose-intolerant individuals because fermentation continues in the intestinal lumen.

Most lactose-intolerant patients can tolerate up to 3 g of lactose per day. More severe restrictions may be necessary in certain patients, such as patients with galactosemia. Because dairy products typically provide a significant percentage of dietary calcium, calcium supplements may be necessary for patients on low-lactose diets, particularly for postmenopausal women.

Cow's milk substitutes containing corn syrup solids and sodium caseinate may be used by patients on low-lactose diets. Nondairy creamers and fruit and vegetable juices may be used as substitutes for milk products. Also available are yeast preparations that may be added to milk to hydrolyze the lactose, and prehydrolyzed milk. Patients with a limited tolerance of lactose can use this milk in cooking or on cereal. In addition, tablets that contain lactose can be swallowed with meals to improve lactose tolerance.

The object of a low-lactose diet is relief of symptoms. After a period of time, small amounts of lactose can be carefully reintroduced into the diet, as long as the patient remains asymptomatic.

### Low-protein diets

Restriction of dietary protein is indicated both in patients who have symptoms of chronic renal insufficiency and in patients with severe liver disease who are at risk for portosystemic encephalopathy. Severe dietary restriction of protein requires restricting intake of milk, cheese, meat, fish, poultry, and eggs, and limiting amounts of breads, cereals, and some vegetables.

To avoid a negative nitrogen balance and further deterioration of liver function, special mixtures of orally or intravenously administered amino acids may be prescribed. Supplementation with iron, calcium, B-complex vitamins, and calories may be required.

Some infants are intolerant to the protein constituents of cow's milk. A variety of substitute formulas that are prepared from hydrolyzed casein, vegetable proteins, or a meat base are available. Food labels must be checked for ingredients such as butter, cream cheese, any form of milk, casein, curds, whey, beef, and veal. After the infant has been symptom-free for 3 to 4 months, small amounts of milk may be reintroduced carefully and, if tolerated, may be slowly increased.

### Low-fat diets

Low-fat diets are used to control symptoms of gastrointestinal disease, particularly steatorrhea or diarrhea. They are indicated in all acute and chronic diseases in which the functions of lipolysis, micellar solubilization, mucosal absorption, transport out of the absorptive cell, or transport in the lymphatic system is impaired. A short-term low-fat diet may also be helpful in patients with acute gastroenteritis.

Because small amounts of cooking fats provide a large percentage of dietary fat, all foods prepared on a low-fat diet must be broiled, boiled, or baked. Chicken and turkey with the skin removed are the staples of a low-fat diet. If red meat is eaten, all fat must be trimmed. Fish should be served without sauces. Consumption of breads, cereals, vegetables, and fruits should be emphasized. Dairy products made with whole or 2% milk should be avoided, as well as most desserts, cheeses, nuts, olives, bacon, mayonnaise, salad dressings, and cream sauces or gravies.

If table foods must be severely restricted to control fat intake, low-fat dietary supplements may be required to deliver adequate calories. Supplements containing preparations of vitamins E, K, D, and A may be necessary. Medium-chain triglycerides are available in oil and dry powder preparations that supply minerals, carbohydrates, and fat-soluble vitamins.

### Low-sodium diets

The restriction of dietary sodium is indicated for gastroenterology patients with ascites and edema caused by severe liver disease. A combination of sodium restriction and diuretic administration is the mainstay of treatment for ascites. Sodium restriction prevents further expansion of the extracellular fluid volume and may be used alone for outpatients with minimal ascites. Once diuretic therapy has mobilized the ascites, patients may be maintained on a low-sodium diet without diuretics.

Patients on low-sodium diets should not add salt to their food, nor should they use salt in food preparation. Water that has been treated with sodium-containing water-softening compounds should be avoided, along with over-the-counter medications that contain sodium. Foods that are particularly high in sodium should be eliminated, including tomato juice, organ meats, smoked meats, shellfish, cheese, dry cereals, commercial mixes, commercially prepared desserts, spices, and commercially prepared soups. Supplementation with iron and B-vitamin preparations that do not contain sodium may be necessary.

## ENTERAL NUTRITION

**Enteral nutrition** refers to the administration of a prescribed diet by means of a flexible tube that may be inserted into the stomach or small bowel either transnasally, surgically, or endoscopically.

### Indications and contraindications

Enteral nutrition is indicated for maintenance of nutritional status in patients who have a functioning GI tract, but cannot ingest sufficient food and nutrients to meet energy requirements. Examples of conditions for which enteral nutrition may be indicated are **anorexia,** malabsorption syndromes, chronic malnutrition, infants with failure to thrive, major burns, severe trauma, hepatic or renal failure, and dysphagia resulting from cerebrovascular accident or esophageal tumor. It is contraindicated in patients with bowel obstruction, ileus, or severe diarrhea and should not be used immediately following a massive small bowel resection.

For patients in whom the gastrointestinal tract is functional but oral feeding is not possible, enteral nutritional support is preferred over **total parenteral nutrition (TPN).** Compared to TPN, enteral nutrition is safer, less expensive, and makes reintroduction of table foods easier. The use of a transnasal tube is one-tenth to one-twentieth the cost of comparable support with parenteral nutrition, and significant complications are less frequent. At the same time, enteral nutrition is just as effective as TPN in reversing malnutrition and restoring positive nitrogen balance.

### Administration of enteral nutrition

Enteral nutrition is administered through a tube that may be inserted transnasally, surgically, or endoscopically.

Transnasal insertion of a feeding tube involves the use of a nasogastric, nasoduodenal, or nasojejunal tube. Nasogastric tubes are indicated when pharyngeal reflexes are intact and there is little risk of aspiration. Nasojejunal or nasoduodenal intubation is indicated when the potential for aspiration is high or when a simple formula is required to assist nutrient breakdown in an impaired gut. However, it may be difficult to place a tube in the duodenum and maintain it there for any length of time. In addition, duodenal and jejunal tubes tend to be smaller in diameter and clog easily. Discomfort and esophagitis may occur with any transnasal tube.

Tubes made of silicone or polyurethane plastics are thinner and more flexible than older tubes made of polyvinyl plastic. In addition, they do not stiffen or become brittle in the GI tract. Nasoenteral tubes come in a variety of lengths and diameters. Tubes for gastric feeding measure approximately 76 cm, while the longer tubes used for intestinal feeding are up to 120 cm. Some tubes are weighted at the distal end with tungsten; mercury is no longer used to weight these tubes because of complicated disposal problems. Nasoduodenal tube feedings are currently preferred for enteral nutrition because they offer less potential for aspiration than nasogastric tubes. Other disadvantages of nasogastric tubes include discomfort, which is a result of lumen size, and reflux esophagitis.

For patients who require long-term enteral nutrition, the feeding tube may be inserted by gastrostomy or jejunostomy. Intermittent bolus feeding through a gastrostomy tube (G-tube) is most suitable for the ambulatory patient who does not wish to be confined by a continuous infusion. G-tubes do not have most of the problems associated with nasogastric intubation but can be complicated by aspiration.

Jejunostomy tubes (J-tubes) are most useful for patients who will undergo surgery for esophageal, gastric, pancreatic, or biliary disease. Experience with jejunostomy is limited in infants and children. It seems to be indicated primarily in older children with severe neurologic or esophagogastric disorders who have a functioning lower tract.

Feeding tubes may also be inserted transnasally, orally, or endoscopically, such as in a percutaneous endoscopic gastrostomy or jejunostomy (PEG/PEJ), which are described in detail at the end of this chapter.

Once the tube is in place, enteral feedings may be administered in the form of intermittent gravity drips or continuous drip infusion. With continuous drip infusion, a defined amount is given continuously every hour with the use of an infusion pump. This method minimizes the risk of aspiration, abdominal distention, and diarrhea. Intermittent drip infusion may be used once a patient has been stabilized on maintenance therapy.

It is important to check for proper tube placement before each intermittent feeding and at least once a shift during continuous feedings. The most promising bedside method for verification of tube placement may be pH testing of aspirates. Radiographic verification of tube placement may be needed before tube feedings are begun and after any event that may predispose a patient to tube dislocation.

The patient's head and thorax should be elevated at least 30 degrees. To minimize diarrhea, the solution should be diluted as ordered by the physician.

To allow the patient to adjust to tube feeding, the rate of administration of the solution should be increased gradually. For most patients, a lactose-free, 1 kcal/ml formula is used, beginning with 50 ml/hr and increasing the rate each day by 25 ml/hr intervals until a rate of 100 to 125 ml/hr is reached. Once the prescribed rate is reached, the strength of the formula may be increased. Antidiarrheal agents and/or water supplements should be given as ordered.

The tube should be irrigated before and after each feeding and every 3 to 4 hours when the patient is not receiving a continuous drip. It should be irrigated every 6 hours when the patient is receiving a continuous drip. To maintain optimum patency, the tube should be considered for replacement every 4 weeks.

## Enteral diets

There are three basic types of enteral diets. The type of diet used depends on the status of the patient's GI tract and on his or her caloric and nutrient requirements.

- Elemental diets are predigested, nutritionally complete powdered mixtures of basic nutrients that are reconstituted with water. Such diets are low-residue and lactose-free. They require little lipolytic or proteolytic activity and are relatively nonstimulating to pancreatic, biliary, and gastrointestinal secretions. Elemental diets are used for patients with definite evidence of maldigestion and malabsorption. Disease-specific elemental diets are available for patients with renal failure, respiratory insufficiency, or hepatic encephalopathy.
- Formulas with intact nutrients include blenderized meat-based meals; lactose-free feedings containing polymeric mixtures of proteins, fats, and carbohydrates in high-molecular weight forms; and nutrient-dense feedings that provide 1.5 to 2.0 kcal/ml compared with the 1.0 kcal/ml in blenderized or lactose-free feedings. Polymeric formulas are used when lipolytic and proteolytic gastrointestinal function are almost normal.
- Modular preparations contain only one nutrient group (fats, proteins, or carbohydrates). Modular preparations may be added to formula diets to increase specific components or to increase calories for patients on fluid restrictions.

Enteral calorie requirements may be calculated by using the Harris-Benedict equation for basal energy expenditures (BEE), where W is the patient's actual or usual weight in kilograms; H is the height in centimeters; and A is the age in years.

Women:
$$BEE = 655 + (9.6 \times W) + (1.8 \times H) - (4.7 \times A)$$
Men:
$$BEE = 66 + (13.7 \times W) + (5 \times H) - (6.8 \times A)$$

The enteral maintenance requirement is $1.2 \times BEE$; the enteral anabolic requirement is $1.5 \times BEE$.

## Potential complications

Less than 1% of patients receiving enteral nutrition experience serious complications. The most common complication is aspiration. Aspiration may be minimized by placing nasojejunal or jejunostomy tubes well beyond the ligament of Treitz, by keeping gastric volumes less than 100 ml, and by elevating the patient's head and shoulders.

Other potential complications of enteral feedings include the following:

- Tube obstruction
- Pharyngeal discomfort
- Nausea, vomiting, or cramping
- Diarrhea
- Dumping syndrome
- Hyperglycemia
- Excessive carbon dioxide production

- Hyponatremia and/or hypokalemia
- Constipation
- Nasal or pharyngeal irritation or necrosis

To avoid nausea, vomiting, or abdominal cramping, a slow rate of administration through a tube placed well into the stomach is best, with the patient in a sitting or low Fowler's position. Diarrhea can result from too-rapid infusion, infusion of hyperosmolar solutions, or use of concomitant antibiotic or fat malabsorption.

### Nursing care

To avoid complications, patients on tube feedings should be monitored continuously to assess patient position, tube position and patency, and gastric residuals. For intermittent feedings, the position of the tube should be checked before each feeding. Adult patients should be given at least 50 ml of water before and after each intermittent feeding. In addition, fluid intake and output and weight gain or loss should be checked daily. The effectiveness of enteral support should be assessed periodically by testing for metabolic imbalances and repeating nutritional assessments.

Patients who are receiving enteral feedings will also need psychologic support. Ambulation should be encouraged if possible, and both patient and family should be reassured that these feedings are necessary and that normal eating will be resumed as soon as possible.

Patients who are receiving enteral nutrition at home must be instructed in techniques of administration, record keeping of intake and output, and what physical symptoms to note.

## PARENTERAL NUTRITION

Parenteral nutrition refers to the administration of a carefully controlled diet through an IV line that has been inserted in a central vein, or occasionally in a peripheral vein.

### Indications and contraindications

Parenteral nutrition is indicated for patients who are moderately to severely malnourished or for those who are in negative nitrogen balance at presentation and are not expected to meet their nutritional requirements orally within a short period of time.

Parenteral nutrition may be ordered for patients with gastrointestinal disease, such as inflammatory bowel disease, radiation enteritis, acute pancreatitis, and short-bowel syndrome; for preoperative preparation of malnourished patients; for patients with postoperative surgical complications, particularly fistulas; for postoperative care of neonates; for infants with intractable diarrhea; and for patients with extensive burns or trauma, anorexia nervosa, liver disease, and renal failure.

Parenteral nutrition should not be used if oral or enteral nutrition is possible.

### Administration of parenteral nutrition

To be practiced safely and successfully, parenteral nutrition should be administered by a trained TPN team consisting of a physician, nutritionist, pharmacist, and nurse. Parenteral nutrition is administered through an IV line. Most often, parenteral feedings are administered through an indwelling subclavian vein catheter via the superior vena cava. A Broviac or Hickman catheter may be used to permit capping of the catheter between infusions. For pediatric patients, a Broviac catheter with an inner diameter of 0.12 mm is available, compared to the regular size of 0.20 mm. In some cases the catheter is inserted via the femoral vein or tunneled under the skin to the subclavian vein.

For some patients, **peripheral parenteral nutrition (PPN)** may be administered through a peripheral, rather than central, vein. PPN may be ordered for a patient who cannot ingest food orally for 2 or 3 days but who has adequate fat stores; for patients in whom a central line is precluded; and for patients who are eating but are not getting sufficient calories. PPN also is appropriate for low–birth-weight infants and for infants and children who need parenteral supplementation. PPN solutions contain a mixture of **dextrose** and amino acids. The concentration of dextrose should not be greater than 10%, however, because more concentrated solutions may be associated with vein sclerosing and thrombosis. Lipids may be given with peripheral alimentation to further dilute the dextrose concentration. Because of the limitations on dextrose content, the number of calories that can be given with PPN may be inadequate for long-term **anabolism**.

The initial infusion should be administered gradually, beginning with a rate of approximately 1 L in the first 24 hours. The concentration of the solution is increased slowly until the desired number of calories is delivered.

### Parenteral diets

Parenteral formulas are concentrated liquids that usually provide 1 kcal/ml and about 42 G/L protein. Typically, parenteral formulas contain protein, carbohydrates, electrolytes, vitamins, trace minerals, and water.

In addition, lipid emulsions are often administered to meet essential fatty acid requirements. Fat should provide 30% or more of total calories.

In most hospitals, TPN solutions are ordered by the physician on a daily solution order form. Formulation of a parenteral solution must be carefully calculated so that it meets the complete needs of the patient in terms of calories, nitrogen, fatty acids, vitamins, trace elements, and water. Dextrose solutions and lipid emulsions are the main sources of energy in patients who are fed by central catheter.

The minimal amount of energy (calories) required to prevent weight loss or autocannibalism is $1.5 \times$ BEE (the parenteral maintenance requirement). To achieve anabolism and positive nitrogen balance, the parenteral anabolic requirement is $1.8 \times$ BEE.

Protein requirements are usually supplied by crystalline amino acids. The amount of protein needed is calculated according to the following formula:

Protein (g) $= 6.25 \times$ Energy requirements/day $\div$ 150

Daily fluid requirements are calculated according to the following formula:

1000 ml for the first 10 kg body weight
500 ml for the next kg
$+$ 20 ml for each kg of body weight thereafter
_____
Daily fluid requirements

The maximum daily fat allowance is 2.5 g/kg. Not more than 60% to 70% of the total calories per day should be from fat. Usually, a lipid solution is added to the carbohydrate and protein solutions, and the combined mixture is administered to the patient. Some patients receive lipid solution only 1 or 2 times per week.

Vitamins and trace minerals are provided in parenteral alimentation solutions in amounts designed to meet daily requirements of patients with disease.

### Potential complications of total parenteral nutrition

Serious complications occur in 5% to 10% of patients receiving TPN. The most common complication is catheter-related sepsis, which occurs in less than 5% of TPN patients. TPN-related infection may result from contamination of the catheter by skin flora, contamination of the TPN solution or tubing, or bacteremia originating from another source in the body. To avoid catheter infections, specific aseptic techniques must be followed in the care of the catheter and dressing. If the patient has a positive blood culture, the catheter should be removed for 24 to 48 hours and 10% dextrose should be administered peripherally during this time. After removal, the catheter should be cultured and intravenous antimicrobials should be administered to cover the causative organism.

Potential mechanical complications of parenteral nutrition include thoracic injury during catheter insertion, such as subclavian artery puncture or myocardial perforation; air embolism from air entering the catheter during a line change; or venous thrombosis and thrombophlebitis. Metabolic imbalances may include hyperglycemia or hypoglycemia, electrolyte or mineral imbalances, and ketoacidosis. Hepatic complications may include hepatomegaly, fatty liver, enzyme elevations, and cholestasis.

### Nursing care for patients receiving parenteral nutrition

Nursing goals in the administration of parenteral nutrition include prevention of infection, maintenance of the prescribed rate of flow, ongoing patient assessment, and the provision of patient/family education and support.

All aseptic precautions must be observed when preparing parenteral solutions and when caring for patients who are receiving parenteral nutrition. Careful aseptic insertion of the central venous catheter is the first step. Over the long term, care of the catheter dressing, tubing, and the catheter itself must be meticulous. Hands should be washed with an antimicrobial solution before any contact with the TPN system or dressing. Most TPN teams have a nurse who changes dressings, or else a protocol is established for the floor nurses. Dressings are usually changed 3 times per week and more often if they become soiled, wet, or nonocclusive. Institutional policies and procedures for insertion-site care should be consulted, because they may vary.

Parenteral feeding solutions should be kept refrigerated until needed, then allowed to reach room temperature before infusion to prevent irritation to the GI tract. The solution should be administered at a steady rate. To prevent air embolism, the patient should bear down or perform Valsalva's maneuver when the tubing is being changed.

The patient on TPN should be monitored daily for fluid intake and output and weight gain or loss. Vital signs should be checked every 4 to 8 hours and the urine should be checked for glucose every 4 to 6 hours. Regular laboratory tests should include creatinine and urea nitrogen, serum chemistries, electrolytes, magnesium, transferrin, triglycerides, complete blood count with differential, and platelet count. When parenteral nutrition is to be stopped, the glucose concentration should be decreased gradually.

For patients who continue to need parenteral nutrition but no longer require skilled nursing care, home parenteral nutrition can be safe and cost-effective. Home TPN with infusion done overnight permits the patient to return to a reasonably normal daytime routine and aids in social adjustment. Both the patient and his or her family members need to be trained before discharge regarding dressing changes, addition of fluids, record keeping of fluid intake and output, what symptoms to note, and how to contact a healthcare provider.

## PERCUTANEOUS ENDOSCOPIC GASTROSTOMY/JEJUNOSTOMY

Percutaneous endoscopic gastrostomy and jejunostomy* are techniques for endoscopic placement of gastrostomy/jejunostomy feeding tubes, without the need for laparotomy or general anesthesia. It has been used with low morbidity in infants, children, and adults.

PEG placement is indicated to provide enteral nutrition:

_____
* Also discussed in the SGNA *Manual of Gastrointestinal Procedures.*

- In patients for whom swallowing is difficult or impossible, such as those with neurologic impairments or anatomic or physiologic abnormalities that prevent normal alimentation
- In patients who cannot tolerate an indwelling nasogastric tube
- In patients who need long-term nutritional support, but are at high risk for surgical placement of a feeding tube

In patients with biliary obstructions who require placement of an external biliary drainage catheter for decompression, loss of bile may be excessive. To avoid distasteful oral administration of bile, the external biliary catheter may be connected to a PEG tube, thus creating an external biliary-gastric fistula for refeeding of bile.

PEJ is indicated for patients with an incompetent gag reflex or incompetent lower esophageal sphincter, which leave the patient at risk for aspiration, or to provide jejunal feeding and gastric decompression. If continued gastroesophageal reflux is a risk to aspiration and its attendant complications, jejunal enteral feedings are preferred to PEG feedings.

PEG/PEJ placement may be contraindicated in patients with the following:

- Uncorrected coagulopathy
- Prior gastric or duodenal surgery (relative)
- Compromised gastric wall
- Inadequate gastric emptying (PEG only)
- Upper small bowel or gastroduodenal obstruction
- Sepsis
- Ascites (relative)
- Morbid obesity
- Hiatal hernia with the stomach located in the chest
- Recent myocardial infarction

In patients in whom it is not possible to visualize the light through the anterior abdominal wall at the time of endoscopy, the physician may locate the proper site by ballottement.

### Percutaneous endoscopic gastrostomy (PEG)

Several manufacturers provide **Percutaneous endoscopic gastrostomy (PEG)** kits. All of the necessary materials should be assembled or the contents of preassembled kits should be checked before diagnostic endoscopy is completed.

Before beginning the procedure it is important to obtain baseline vital signs and laboratory results, remove dentures, and establish a patent IV line. The patient should be NPO for at least 8 hours, including tube feedings. If the patient has a nasogastric tube, it should not be removed until the endoscopist passes the scope. If there is edema or stricture, the nasogastric tube may serve as a guide for the endoscopist. A single parenteral dose of a prophylactic antibiotic may be administered if ordered by the physician.

The patient's mouth may be swabbed several times to reduce flora and the incidence of infection. Intravenous sedation is administered, and the patient's throat may be anesthetized with a topical anesthetic. The patient is placed in a fully supine position with the limbs restrained as necessary. The head of the bed may be elevated to a semi-Fowler's position. The abdomen is prepped and draped as for a surgical procedure. During the procedure the patient's mouth is suctioned as necessary.

The esophagus, stomach, and duodenal bulb are examined endoscopically for any pathologic conditions. The stomach is distended with air, causing it to come in close contact with the abdominal wall. The room lights are dimmed and the abdomen is transilluminated with the endoscope. The endoscopist marks the skin at the site of maximum transillumination, which is usually about one third the distance from the midpoint of the left costal margin to the umbilicus. The assistant applies finger pressure to the selected area as the endoscopist observes the indentation on the interior of the stomach. The selected site should be more than 2 cm from the lower margin of the left rib cage. The skin is anesthetized and a small (approximately 5 mm) incision is made with a pointed blade and extended into the subcutaneous fat.

Commercially available PEG tubes may be inserted by using either push or pull techniques. In the pull method, a polypectomy snare is passed through the biopsy channel of the endoscope. The snare loop is positioned over the place where the puncture will occur. The physician inserts an IV needle and sheath through the abdominal incision and into the gastric lumen, passing it through the center of the open snare loop. The snare is then closed around the sheath, and the trocar of the needle is removed. A long suture is passed through the sheath into the stomach. The snare is loosened from around the sheath and tightened around the suture. The snare and suture are then retracted into the biopsy channel of the endoscope, and the scope, snare, and suture are removed through the patient's mouth. Ultimately, the suture can be seen to enter the patient's abdominal wall and exit the mouth.

The gastrostomy tube is a feeding catheter that is tapered on one end and has a bolster on the other end. A suture extending from the tapered end is tied to the orally extruded suture, and the G-tube is introduced by pulling on the abdominal end of the first suture, thereby causing the PEG device to progress down through the mouth, esophagus, and stomach. The tapered end of the catheter exits the abdominal wall. The gastroscope is then reinserted, and under direct vision, the bolster is snugged up against the gastric wall and an external bolster is applied. Care must be taken to ensure that the bolster is not so snug as to apply undue pressure on the skin or gastric mucosa.

When a "push" method is to be used to insert the PEG tube, a Seldinger needle is introduced into the stomach through a 5- to 6-mm incision. The needle's inner stylet is withdrawn, thus leaving the outer cannula in place. A snare wire is passed through the endoscope and looped over the outer cannula. A specialized, flexible-tip guidewire is threaded through the cannula and grasped by the snare loop. The endoscope, snare, and guidewire are then withdrawn through the patient's mouth, leaving the guidewire extending from the abdominal wall and out through the patient's mouth.

Next, the G-tube is threaded continuously over the guidewire, ultimately pushing the cannula out through the abdominal wall. The external portion of the G-tube is pulled into place outside the abdominal wall and the guidewire is removed. A radiopaque bolster secures the tube inside the stomach and a retention disk secures it outside the abdomen. The endoscope is reinserted to check the position of the inner bolster against the stomach wall. Patency of the device is tested with injection of air and/or water. An adapter is placed on the external end of the G-tube for attaching an irrigation syringe or feeding pump.

During the procedure, one nurse is responsible for assisting the endoscopist, while a second nurse monitors the patient, maintains an open airway, and provides mouth suction as necessary. After the procedure a topical antibiotic ointment is applied at the insertion site. The site should be checked daily for signs of infection. The tube should be marked with indelible ink at the point where it exits the abdomen, thereby allowing the nurse to recognize if the tube moves after insertion.

### Percutaneous endoscopic jejunostomy (PEJ)

**Percutaneous endoscopic jejunostomy (PEJ)** is a modification of PEG. It permits continuous jejunal feedings in combination with gastric decompression. A J-tube with a weighted distal tip is usually passed through an existing PEG tube, under endoscopic and possibly fluoroscopic guidance. A biopsy forceps, snare, or grasper is passed through the instrument channel of the endoscope. The end of the PEJ tube is grasped and the scope pulls the PEJ tube into the duodenum. The jejunal tube is then released and the forceps and scope are removed from the patient, thus leaving the J-tube in the duodenum. A universal adapter is placed in the common end of the two tubes. Immediate feeding may be started via the jejunal tube.

After either PEG or PEJ, the skin should be cleansed gently and topical antibiotics applied around the insertion site. After 24 hours the site can be left open to air. Prophylactic antibiotics may be administered if ordered by the physician.

Usually, for the first 24 hours the G-tube is clamped. After the initial 24 hours the patient can receive tube feedings and/or medications. The PEG site should be inspected daily for signs of swelling, redness, drainage, or leakage around the tube and any signs should be reported to the physician. Following any instillation, the G-tube and/or J-tube must be flushed thoroughly with water to prevent blockage and maintain patency. All medications instilled should be in liquid form; crushed tablets frequently will obstruct the tube. It may be helpful to permanently mark the G-tube at the exit site to monitor for continued proper placement.

Patients and caregivers should receive instruction on the feeding tube and its care. Signs and symptoms of infection should be reviewed, and information should be provided on replacement tubes and supplies. Caregivers should be instructed to notify the physician immediately if the tube is removed at any time. A replacement tube must be placed quickly, because the tract will begin to heal over rapidly. Patients with long-term PEG or PEJ tubes and their families need to be taught how to wash the skin surrounding the catheter and to keep the catheter patent by flushing it after feedings.

Most patients are able to tolerate full-strength bolus feedings, rather than a continuous drip infusion. Some blenderized foods may be placed through the G-tube if they are liquid in consistency.

Potential major complications of PEG/PEJ insertion include sepsis or inadvertent puncture of another viscus (usually the colon). The most frequent minor complication is wound infection, which may respond to local treatment, antibiotics, or a small incision at the tube site to allow drainage of purulent material. Rarely, wound infection may result in discontinuation of the gastrostomy. To avoid superficial wound infections, a prophylactic antibiotic may be given.

Other possible complications include leakage into the peritoneal cavity because of tube dislodgement, transient fever, respiratory depression secondary to administration of medication, aspiration, bleeding, and/or perforation. Gastrocolic fistula may occur as a result of pinching of the colon between the gastric and abdominal walls; it is rare and can be managed effectively by removing the tube. Fistulas close spontaneously within several hours to several days.

### PEG replacement

If the patient's condition improves or the tube deteriorates, the PEG device can be removed and replaced if necessary.* Typically, the tube is cut off at the abdominal site and the internal portion is snared and removed endoscopically. During removal, care must be taken to keep the internal portion from hanging up at the

---

* Also discussed in the SGNA *Manual of Gastrointestinal Procedures.*

lower esophageal sphincter or from dropping into the bronchus as it comes through the hypopharynx. In some cases the catheter may be cut close to the skin and allowed to pass spontaneously into the stool.

If the tube is not replaced, the opening in the abdominal wall will close rapidly. The replacement tube must be inserted into the fistula within hours to maintain easy passage and avoid the need to establish a new fistula PEG.

When replacement with a new catheter is desired, PEG reinsertion may be accomplished with a replacement device designed for that purpose. The tract must be well-established (at least 10 to 14 days after insertion). PEG tubes should be changed when necessary if used for long-term nutritional support. PEG replacement may also be indicated to replace a blocked feeding tube or to enhance patient comfort and aesthetics.

To prevent leakage of gastric acid onto the abdominal skin, the replacement device should be fitted to the stoma carefully. It is therefore necessary to have tubes in graduated sizes on hand and ready for use.* Various types of PEG replacement devices are available, including the PEG *button* and prepackaged gastrostomy replacement tubes.

- The PEG *button* is inserted flush with the skin. It is especially good for ambulatory patients because it has an antireflux valve and a cap to close it completely between feedings.
- Prepackaged gastrostomy replacement tube kits include all of the necessary parts needed to insert and stabilize the tube. The tubes are manufactured from materials designed to enhance the passage of feedings and to reduce the risk of blockage.
- In an emergency, if a regular replacement tube cannot be placed immediately, Foley catheters are readily available and inexpensive and can be inserted into a mature tract without special equipment by any physician. However, their thick, rubber tubing causes the inner diameter to be substantially smaller than the outer diameter. Foley catheters block more easily and may require repeated replacement. Latex Foley catheters deteriorate when exposed to gastric acid for long periods of time.

After insertion of a replacement device, it is important to gently clean the skin and apply a topical antibiotic ointment around the insertion site. Potential complications of inserting a PEG replacement device are bleeding, infection, and perforation.

---

**CASE SITUATION**

Mrs. Ellen Marshall is a 60-year-old woman who is 5'6" and weighs 179 pounds. She has been diag-

---

* Also discussed in the SGNA *Manual of Gastrointestinal Procedures.*

nosed by endoscopy as suffering from reflux esophagitis. The gastroenterology nurse's initial assessment notes that Mrs. Marshall is overweight. Excessive weight gain can increase intraabdominal pressure and exacerbate reflux. Furthermore, eating the wrong foods can add calories, decrease LES tone, exacerbate pain, and increase the gastric acid secretion rate. One appropriate nursing diagnosis in Mrs. Marshall's case is "altered nutrition: more than body requirements, related to caloric intake exceeding metabolic need."

*Points to think about*

1. How might the gastroenterology nurse differentiate between the meanings of overweight and obesity?
2. What are the critical indicators (NANDA) in making a nursing diagnosis of "altered nutrition: more than body requirements, related to caloric intake exceeding metabolic need?"
3. How might the gastroenterology nurse describe the approach to obtaining these indicator data to confirm or refute such a nursing diagnosis?
4. What additional data are needed to complete a basic dietary assessment on Mrs. Marshall?
5. What nutritional advice might the nurse give Mrs. Marshall that might alleviate symptoms of esophageal reflux?

*Suggested responses*

1. The generally accepted definitions of overweight and obesity are as follows:
   - Overweight is any weight in excess of the ideal/desirable body weight for age, height, and body size. A person may be overweight but not obese because of muscle mass.
   - Obesity is an excess of body fat; that is, 120% or more above the ideal/desirable body weight.
2. The critical indicators for the nursing diagnosis "altered nutrition: more than body requirements related to caloric intake exceeding metabolic need are as follows:
   - Body weight 10% to 30% over ideal weight for height and frame
   - In women, triceps skin fold greater than 25 mm (measures body fat)
3. To confirm or refute such a nursing diagnosis, it would be appropriate to do the following:
   - Obtain accurate weight, height, triceps skin fold, and wrist measurements.
   - Calculate body frame size as small, medium, or large (height in cm divided by wrist circumference in cm). For a woman: small = >11.0, medium = 10.1 to 11.0, large = <10.1.

- Using derived frame size, use weight/height norms for age to arrive at ideal weight. (U.S. Public Health Service probability statistical norms are probably more accurate than insurance actuarial tables.)
- Calculate actual weight percentage over ideal weight.
  NOTE: There are other methods for calculating amount of body fat.
4. In addition to weight, height, and body frame, data needed to complete a dietary assessment on Mrs. Marshall might include the following:
  - Usual food and fluid intake including frequency of meals, snacks, method of food preparation, portion size, types of foods normally consumed
  - Elimination patterns
  - Activity and energy levels
  - Ethnic or cultural background
  - Conditions surrounding food consumption
5. Nutritional advice that the nurse could give Mrs. Marshall to alleviate symptoms of esophageal reflux might include the following:
  - Avoiding large meals and refraining from snacking before going to bed to keep gastric volume at a minimum
  - Keeping dietary fat to a minimum because fat slows gastric emptying and also decreases LES pressure
  - Minimizing dietary intake of chocolate, alcohol, and coffee, which also reduce basal LES pressure
  - Avoiding carminative substances, such as spearmint and peppermint, because they impair LES function
  - Avoiding citrus juices, tomato products, and coffee, which are direct esophageal irritants
  - Encouraging other dietary modifications to promote weight loss

---

**REVIEW TERMS**

**amino acids, anabolism, anorexia, carbohydrates, catabolism, dextrose, disaccharides, enteral nutrition, fatty acids, glucose, glycerol, glycogen, lipids, minerals, monoglycerides, monosaccharides, nitrogen balance, nutrition, percutaneous endoscopic gastrostomy (PEG), percutaneous endoscopic jejunostomy (PEJ), peripheral parenteral nutrition (PPN), proteins, total parenteral nutrition (TPN), triglycerides, vitamins**

---

**REVIEW QUESTIONS**

1. Excess glucose is stored in the liver and in the muscles in the form of:
   a. Adipose tissue.
   b. Glycogen.
   c. Disaccharides.
   d. Triglycerides.
2. If a patient is in negative nitrogen balance, that means he or she is:
   a. Building new tissue.
   b. Ingesting the proper amount of protein.
   c. Eating too much protein.
   d. Not getting enough carbohydrates and lipids to meet energy requirements.
3. Patients with celiac sprue must avoid eating:
   a. Gluten.
   b. Fiber.
   c. Sodium.
   d. Protein.
4. Low-fat diets are usually used to control:
   a. Steatorrhea and diarrhea.
   b. Intestinal gas and bloating.
   c. Ascites.
   d. Constipation.
5. The primary disadvantage of using a nasogastric feeding tube is:
   a. Risk of aspiration.
   b. Patient discomfort.
   c. Risk of infection.
   d. High cost.
6. Diarrhea may be avoided in patients receiving enteral nutritional support by:
   a. Placing the patient in a sitting or low Fowler's position.
   b. Slowing the rate of infusion.
   c. Increasing the strength of the formula.
   d. Using aseptic technique.
7. Peripheral parenteral nutrition is most appropriate for:
   a. Patients who need long-term hyperalimentation.
   b. Patients with inadequate fat stores.
   c. Patients who require concentrated feeding solutions.
   d. Infants with low birthweights.
8. To prevent an air embolism when central lines are being changed, the nurse should:
   a. Place the patient in an upright position.
   b. Use sterile technique.
   c. Have the patient perform Valsalva's maneuver.
   d. Flush the tubing with water.
9. The most common complication in patients receiving TPN is:
   a. Thoracic injury.
   b. Air embolism.
   c. Metabolic imbalance.
   d. Catheter-related sepsis.
10. How long does it take for a well-formed tract to develop around a PEG tube?
    a. 6 weeks.
    b. 10 to 14 days.

c.  3 to 4 days.
d.  24 hours.

## BIBLIOGRAPHY

Beck, M. "Percutaneous Endoscopic Gastrostomy." *Nursing89* 19(April 1989): 76-77.

Beck, M. "Reflux Esophagitis." *SGA Journal* 9(Fall 1986): 77-78.

Chobanian, S, and Van Ness, M, eds. *Manual of Clinical Problems in Gastroenterology.* Boston: Little, Brown & Co., 1988.

Eastwood, G, and Avunduk, C. *Manual of Gastroenterology: Diagnosis and Therapy.* Boston: Little, Brown & Co., 1988.

Fullenkamp, P. "Gluten-Sensitive Enteropathy. Part II. Dietary Treatment of Celiac Disease." In *Journal Reprints II,* ed. Trivits, S, 203-05. Rochester, N.Y.: Society of Gastroenterology Nurses and Associates, 1990.

Given, B, and Simmons, S. *Gastroenterology in Clinical Nursing.* 4th ed. St. Louis: Mosby–Year Book, 1984.

Goldberg, K, ed. *Gastrointestinal Problems.* Nurse Review Series. Springhouse, Pa.: Springhouse Corporation, 1986.

Hardick, M, and Beck, M, eds. *Manual of Gastrointestinal Procedures.* 2nd ed. Rochester, N.Y.: Society of Gastroenterology Nurses and Associates, 1989.

Jackson, B. "Care of Patients After Percutaneous Endoscopic Gastrostomy (PEG) Tube Placement." *Gastroenterology Nursing* 12(Fall 1989): 131.

Kundtz, J. "PEG/PEJ: Implications for Nursing Care." *SGA Journal Reprints,* ed. Trivits, S, 173-76. Rochester, N.Y.: Society of Gastrointestinal Assistants, 1988.

Messner, R. "Infection Control in Total Parenteral Nutrition." In *SGA Journal Reprints,* ed. Trivits, S, 265-67. Rochester, N.Y.: Society of Gastrointestinal Assistants, 1988.

Short, N. "Gastrointestinal Intubations: Nursing Considerations." In *Journal Reprints II,* ed. Trivits, S, 105-11. Rochester, N.Y.: Society of Gastroenterology Nurses and Associates, 1990.

Silverman, A, and Roy, C. *Pediatric Clinical Gastroenterology.* 3rd ed. St. Louis: Mosby–Year Book, 1983.

Sleisenger, M, and Fordtran, J, eds. *Gastrointestinal Disease: Pathophysiology, Diagnosis, Management.* 4th ed. Philadelphia: W.B. Saunders, 1989.

Waye, J, Geenen, J, Fleischer, D, and Venu, R. *Techniques in Therapeutic Endoscopy.* Philadelphia: W.B. Saunders, 1987.

# DIAGNOSTIC PROCEDURES AND TESTS

# Chapter 24

# ENDOSCOPY

This chapter will acquaint the gastroenterology nurse with endoscopic techniques that are used to diagnose disorders of both the upper and lower GI tract.* Therapeutic endoscopy is discussed in subsequent chapters.

**Learning objectives**

After reviewing the content of this chapter, the gastroenterology nurse should be able to:

1. Describe the different types of endoscopes used in gastrointestinal procedures and their main components.
2. Discuss the responsibilities of the gastroenterology nurse with respect to IV conscious sedation of gastroenterology patients.
3. Explain the indications, contraindications, techniques for, and potential complications of endoscopic investigations of the upper and lower GI tract, including esophagogastroduodenoscopy (EGD), endoscopic retrograde cholangiopancreatography (ERCP), colonoscopy, and flexible and rigid sigmoidoscopy.
4. Discuss nursing considerations involved in each of these procedures.
5. Describe several recent advances in endoscopic diagnosis, including small bowel enteroscopy, endoscopic ultrasonography, and videoendoscopy.

## TYPES OF ENDOSCOPES

Gastrointestinal **endoscopy** is the direct visual examination of the lumen of the GI tract. It is a safe, effective way of evaluating the appearance and integrity of the gastrointestinal mucosa, detecting lesions, and providing access for therapeutic procedures.

---

* All techniques in this chapter, except anoscopy and small bowel enteroscopy, are also discussed in the SGNA *Manual of Gastrointestinal Procedures.* 2nd ed. Rochester, N.Y.: Society of Gastroenterology Nurses and Associates, 1989.

The first endoscopes were rigid, metal instruments. Most have now been replaced by flexible fiberoptic or video scopes, which increase visibility and promote patient safety and comfort. Depending upon the section of the GI tract that is to be explored, the endoscopist may use one of the following:

- Flexible end-viewing or side-viewing (oblique) endoscopes, which are used to visualize the esophagus, stomach, and proximal duodenum, or to cannulate the biliary tract in ERCP.
- An anoscope, which is a rigid plastic or metal speculum that is used to inspect the anal canal.
- A proctosigmoidoscope or rectosigmoidoscope, which is a 15- or 25-cm rigid endoscope that is used to examine the rectum and the sigmoid colon.
- A flexible sigmoidoscope, which may be up to 65 cm in length and is used for examining the rectum and the sigmoid and descending colon.
- A colonoscope, which is a 120- to 180-cm flexible endoscope that is used to visualize the entire lower GI tract, from the rectum to the ileocecal valve.

Although they are designed for specific uses, all endoscopes have certain common parts, which include the following:

- A flexible insertion tube that is usually 8 to 12 mm in diameter. The insertion tube contains air/water and biopsy channels, fiber bundles, and cables. It extends from the distal end to the control head.
- An umbilical cord that extends from the control head and inserts into the light source.
- An optic system, which consists of **fiberoptic bundles** that conduct light through the shaft and transmit the image to the eye, used with a lens system that focuses the image at the eyepiece. In a video endoscope, the optic system consists of a one-piece, solid-state video camera (including the camera head, coupler, and focusable optics), which

transmits the image to a television screen without the need for fiber optics.

- A control head that houses the lenses, controls for maneuvering the tip up and down and left and right, and valves that regulate irrigation, air or carbon dioxide insufflation, and suction.
- Cables that extend the length of the insertion tube and serve to control the movement of the flexible tip.
- Channels for air and water flow.
- A suction/biopsy channel that also allows the passage of accessories, such as biopsy forceps, cytology brushes, polypectomy snares, laser fibers, electrocautery devices, or prostheses (stents). The suction channel also allows for suctioning fluid that obstructs the endoscopist's vision.
- Optional cameras that can be attached to the endoscope to allow the taking of still 35-mm or instant photographs or video recordings.

Taken together, the various types of endoscopes and their accessories provide a powerful armamentarium for the diagnosis and treatment of gastrointestinal disease.

## CONSCIOUS SEDATION

Many diagnostic and therapeutic procedures in the endoscopy unit, including esophagogastroduodenoscopy (EGD), endoscopic retrograde cholangiopancreatography (ERCP), and colonoscopy, are performed under conscious sedation. By definition, conscious sedation provides a minimally reduced level of consciousness in which the patient retains the ability to maintain an airway independently and to respond appropriately to physical stimulation and/or verbal command. The objectives of conscious sedation are to do the following:

- Allay anxiety and fear
- Maintain the patient's ability to respond to commands
- Maintain the patient's protective reflexes
- Ensure patient cooperation
- Elevate the pain threshold
- Minimize changes in vital signs
- Provide some degree of retrograde amnesia

In endoscopy settings, conscious sedation is most often induced by the intravenous administration of the benzodiazepines diazepam (Valium) or midazolam (Versed). These agents may be administered in combination with atropine and narcotic analgesics, such as meperidine (Demerol).

It is the responsibility of the registered nurse to administer and maintain conscious sedation during endoscopic procedures, in the presence of and by the order of a physician. In procedures that are complicated by the severity of the patient's illness and/or the complex technical requirements of the procedure, a second nurse may be needed to assist the physician while the first nurse monitors the patient. It may be necessary to have the anesthesia department monitor pediatric patients.

Before the administration of conscious sedation, it is important that the gastroenterology nurse assess the patient's vital signs, drug allergies, medication history, and relevant medical-surgical history; verify signed informed consent; establish venous access; and explain the procedure clearly.

Both diazepam and midazolam must be titrated slowly until the desired effect is reached. Individual response varies with age, physical status, and present medications. Particular care must be taken with elderly or debilitated patients.

During any procedure that is conducted under conscious sedation, it is the nurse's responsibility to monitor the patient's vital signs. Minimal monitoring should include blood pressure, pulse, respirations, level of consciousness, warmth and dryness of skin, and pain tolerance. Continuous ECG, intermittent mechanical blood pressure monitoring, and pulse oximetry are also useful but not required. Although automatic monitoring devices may enhance the nurse's ability to assess the patient accurately, they are no substitute for watchful, educated assessment.

It is important to document the diagnostic or therapeutic technique(s) used, any unusual events, and the status of the patient upon completion of the procedure. The nurse must also document the dose/amount and route of all drugs, fluids, and blood products administered. In the event of an adverse reaction, the nurse must document any subsequent intervention(s) and the patient's response. Potential adverse reactions to IV conscious sedation include anaphylaxis, respiratory distress, tachycardia, bradycardia, and seizures. Pediatric patients may have a paradoxical reaction to IV conscious sedation, becoming incoherent, uncontrollable, and inconsolable.

After the procedure is complete, it is important that the nurse monitor the patient's vital signs and level of consciousness; observe and document any unusual events or postprocedural complications, along with any interventions and patient responses; provide verbal and written postprocedural instructions to the patient and/or a responsible person; and ensure that institutional discharge criteria are met.

## ESOPHAGOGASTRODUODENOSCOPY

In **esophagogastroduodenoscopy (EGD),** a flexible endoscope less than 10 mm in diameter is passed into the upper GI tract. The entire esophagus and stomach and the proximal duodenum are easily visualized. Smaller pediatric endoscopes may be used for younger patients or for patients with strictures. Larger-diameter gastroscopes with a larger suction channel or two suction channels may be used for therapeutic procedures.

EGD allows the physician to diagnose and document gastrointestinal abnormalities through the use of direct vision and still and video photography. Diagnostic EGD may be indicated for patients with any of the following:

- Dysphagia or odynophagia
- Dyspepsia (selected patients)
- Esophageal reflux that persists despite appropriate therapy
- Persistent, unexplained vomiting
- Upper GI x-ray films showing lesions that require biopsy
- Acute or chronic upper GI bleeding (hematemesis or melena)
- Suspected esophageal or gastric varices
- Suspected esophageal stenosis, esophagitis, hiatal hernia, gastritis, obstructive lesions, and gastric or peptic ulcers
- Chronic abdominal pain
- Suspected polyps or cancer
- Follow-up of patients with Barrett's esophagus; large, indeterminate ulcers; or previous gastric or duodenal surgery

Diagnostic EGD may be contraindicated in uncooperative patients and in patients with any of the following:

- Suspected perforated viscus
- Shock
- Seizures
- Recent myocardial infarction
- Severe cardiac decompensation
- Large aortic aneurysm
- Respiratory compromise
- Severe cervical arthritis
- Acute oral or oropharyngeal inflammation
- Acute abdomen

To decrease the risk of aspiration, the patient should be NPO for 6 hours or more before EGD. A thorough medical and drug history and physical examination are important, with special attention given to any history of drug reactions, bleeding disorders, or associated cardiac, pulmonary, renal, hepatic, or central nervous system (CNS) disease. If ordered, a topical anesthetic should be applied to the oral pharynx to suppress the gag reflex.

IV sedation is usually ordered. If a sedative is used, it is titrated slowly until the appropriate level of consciousness is achieved. Reversal agents can be given intravenously to reverse severe respiratory depression caused by overdose or oversensitivity. One precaution to consider, however, is that naloxone can induce drug withdrawal if the patient is on narcotics for pain control or if the patient is a drug user. General anesthesia with endotracheal intubation is usually recommended for neonates, infants, and young children.

Before insertion, the endoscope should be lubricated with a water-soluble lubricant. The patient should be placed in the left lateral position. The chin should be tilted toward the chest, keeping the head in the midline. The endoscope is passed in stages, examining each structure as the scope advances. To obtain the best possible view, mucus or other secretions are aspirated and air is instilled to distend structures.

As the endoscope passes the pylorus, the patient may experience some abdominal discomfort or may retch. At this time, it may help to have the patient breathe deeply and slowly to help relax the abdominal muscles. The patient may also experience a feeling of fullness or an urge to defecate as air passes into the stomach and duodenum. It is important to reassure the patient and hold his or her head and shoulders to help maintain the proper position, keeping the chin tilted toward the table to allow secretions to drain.

Occasionally, duodenal spasm makes visualization of this structure difficult. Administration of a smooth-muscle relaxant, such as glucagon, decreases contractions so the mucosa and contour of the duodenum can be examined thoroughly.

During EGD it is important to maintain the patient's oral airway, suctioning secretions and regurgitated material when necessary from the pharynx. Nasal oxygen should be used to treat hypoxia, and resuscitation equipment should be immediately available in the event of adverse cardiopulmonary reactions.

After the procedure the patient should remain NPO until the gag reflex returns, which may take 1 to 2 hours. After the gag reflex returns, any residual sore throat or hoarseness may be relieved by drinking liquids, using a normal saline gargle, or using anesthetic throat lozenges.

The nurse should monitor the patient's vital signs regularly and observe the patient for signs of bleeding, vomiting, change in vital signs, pain, and abdominal distention. The patient should be instructed to report any hematemesis, pain, or difficulty breathing, because these are symptoms of complications.

EGD is generally regarded as safe, but adverse events can occur, including the following:

- Respiratory depression or arrest
- Perforation of the esophagus, stomach, or duodenum
- Hemorrhage related to trauma or perforation
- Pulmonary aspiration of blood, secretions, or regurgitated gastric contents
- Infection
- Cardiac arrhythmia or arrest
- Localized phlebitis related to IV diazepam (Valium). This reaction is seen less often now that midazolam (Versed) is in widespread use.
- Vasovagal response
- Allergic reaction to the topical anesthetic or IV medications

The rate of complications increases when therapeutic maneuvers are performed. Patients at the highest risk are the elderly and those with advanced cardiac, pulmonary, hepatic, or CNS disease.

## ENDOSCOPIC RETROGRADE CHOLANGIOPANCREATOGRAPHY

**Endoscopic retrograde cholangiopancreatography (ERCP)** uses a combination of endoscopic and radiologic techniques to visualize the biliary and pancreatic ducts.

ERCP is indicated for the following:

- Evaluation of signs or symptoms suggesting pancreatic malignancy when results of ultrasonography and/or CT scan are normal or equivocal
- Evaluation of acute, recurrent, or chronic pancreatitis of unknown etiology
- Before therapeutic endoscopy of the biliary tree; for example, removal of retained common bile duct stones, endoscopic sphincterotomy, balloon dilatation of strictures, or placement of a stent or biliary drain
- Unexplained chronic abdominal pain of suspected biliary or pancreatic origin
- Evaluation of jaundiced patients suspected of having treatable biliary obstruction
- Evaluation of patients without jaundice whose clinical presentation suggests bile duct disease
- Preoperative or postoperative evaluation to detect common duct stones in patients who undergo laparoscopic cholecystectomy
- Manometric evaluation of the ampulla and common bile duct

The use of ERCP in pediatric patients is limited to rare cases of obstructive jaundice without dilated biliary ducts (such as in sclerosing cholangitis or congenital stricture of common hepatic duct), relapsing pancreatitis of unknown cause, and preparation of patients for pancreatic surgery when knowledge of the ductal anatomy is important.

ERCP is contraindicated in uncooperative patients and in patients who are physically unable to tolerate the procedure. It is also contraindicated in patients with recent myocardial infarction, severe pulmonary disease, coagulopathy, or pregnancy. The physician should be notified if the patient has a known allergy to contrast media and any necessary precautions should be taken. ERCP may be contraindicated in patients with acute pancreatitis, unless the clinical situation necessitates the procedure.

Before ERCP, patients should fast for 6 hours. Barium studies should not be conducted within 72 hours preceding ERCP because the residual barium can obstruct the view of the contrast medium in the ducts. ERCP usually takes longer than routine EGD and therefore IV sedation is likely to be heavier.

Before the procedure, all equipment should be set up and tested in a radiographic examination room. The patient should be in either the prone or left lateral position. A side-viewing duodenoscope is passed into the second part of the duodenum. Glucagon may be injected intravenously to suppress duodenal peristalsis and enhance visualization.

When the endoscope is in the proper position to view the ampulla of Vater, the patient is moved to the prone position. The endoscopist then passes a plastic cannula through the endoscope and maneuvers it into the orifice of the ampulla. Further adjustment of the cannula using the endoscope's elevator control allows it to enter the pancreatic duct or the common bile duct.

Radiocontrast material is injected through the cannula. To be certain that the contrast medium is free of air bubbles, the cannula must be primed with contrast before being inserted into the endoscope. When the contrast medium is injected, the amount injected should be stated verbally. Contrast should be injected slowly to avoid overfilling the duct. X-ray films are then taken to identify the configuration of the appropriate ductal system. The patient should be observed for any allergic reactions to the radiocontrast dye. Before the scope is withdrawn, a biopsy exam or cytologic brushing may also be done.

After the procedure is completed, delayed x-ray films may be ordered to determine the time and amount of drainage of the ducts. It is the responsibility of the nurse to perform the following procedures:

- Monitor and document vital signs
- Observe the patient for abdominal distention and signs of pancreatitis, including chills, low-grade fever, pain, vomiting, and tachycardia
- Maintain NPO status until the patient's gag reflex returns or further orders are written
- Administer antibiotics as ordered

The patient's temperature should be checked every 4 hours for 48 hours. In 2 to 4 hours a light meal may be served; the day following the procedure, a full diet may be resumed.

The most significant complications associated with ERCP are pancreatitis and sepsis. Injury to the pancreas can be the result of mechanical, chemical, enzymatic, microbiologic, thermal, or hydrostatic factors. If pancreatitis does result, it usually occurs within 2 to 4 hours after the procedure.

Another frequent complication of ERCP is biliary sepsis, especially in patients with partial obstruction of either the pancreatic or common bile ducts. The introduction of infection into a stagnant duct system can result in cholangitis and septicemia. If a pseudocyst is present, ERCP should be used only as an immediate preoperative procedure under antibiotic prophylaxis.

Parenteral antibiotics, usually gentamicin (Garamycin) and/or ampicillin, should be given immediately to anyone diagnosed by ERCP as having biliary or pancreatic stasis.

In many patients an asymptomatic rise in serum amylase is noted following ERCP. Unless accompanied by abdominal pain, this rise in amylase is usually insignificant and subsides shortly. Additional potential complications include aspiration, bleeding, perforation, respiratory depression or arrest, and cardiac arrhythmias or arrest. Patients may experience a rise in temperature, chills, nausea, vomiting, abdominal pain, or ascending cholangitis.

## ANOSCOPY

An anoscope is a clear plastic or metal speculum designed for examining the anus and lower rectum. One type is cylindrical, with one side that is incomplete or slotted. The mucosa to be evaluated protrudes through this slot. By withdrawing and reinserting the anoscope in multiple orientations, excellent visualization of the entire circumference of the anal canal is possible.

The most common causes of bright red rectal bleeding are hemorrhoids and fissures. **Anoscopy** is indicated for identification of these disorders. It may also be used before sigmoidoscopy or colonoscopy.

For anoscopy, the patient is positioned in Sims' left lateral position or the knee-chest position, which allows the sigmoid colon to straighten, thus promoting better visualization. Special proctologic tilt tables (breakaway tables) are available that permit the patient to be placed in an inverted position with the head down, against a headrest. To minimize embarrassment, the patient is draped, exposing only the lower buttocks area.

A thorough visual and digital rectal examination is performed first, using a gloved, well-lubricated index finger (the little finger is used for infants under 2 years of age). At this time the examiner looks for anal anomalies, sphincter tone, polyps or adenomas, rectal prolapse, extracolonic masses, and hemorrhoids. Any stool remaining on the examining finger may be checked for blood.

Severe spasm induced by digital examination usually signifies low-lying inflammatory bowel disease, such as proctitis or ulcerative colitis (UC).

A warm, well-lubricated anoscope is inserted slowly, with the beveled surface of the tip facing laterally. The general appearance of the mucosa is noted, and the area is examined for fissures, abscesses, or signs of anal papillitis or cryptitis.

## PROCTOSIGMOIDOSCOPY

**Proctosigmoidoscopy,** also known as **rectosigmoidoscopy,** is an examination of the rectum and the sigmoid colon using a rigid proctosigmoidoscope. The proctosig-

moidoscope is a small, hollow, stainless steel or plastic disposable tube that is 25 to 30 cm long and approximately 1.5 cm in diameter. A smaller **proctoscope** may be used with newborns or infants or for patients with strictures. A light source is attached to the end of the scope.

Indications for proctosigmoidoscopy may include the following:

- Melena or bleeding from the anorectal area
- Persistent diarrhea
- A change in bowel habits
- Passage of pus and mucus
- Suspected chronic inflammatory bowel disease
- Bacteriology and histologic studies
- Surveillance of known rectal disease
- Rectal pain
- Screening for suspected polyps or tumors
- Foreign body removal
- As an adjunct to a barium enema
- Surveillance following rectal surgery

Contraindications include severe necrotizing enterocolitis, toxic megacolon, painful anal lesions, severe cardiac arrhythmias, and uncooperative patients.

Most patients should be given a hypertonic phosphate or saline enema the morning of the examination. Patients who have UC or acute diarrhea can be examined without the use of cleansing enemas or laxatives. Medication is rarely needed for adult or adolescent patients, but infants and young children should be sedated.

With the patient in either a knee-chest or Sims' left lateral position, a thorough visual and digital rectal examination is conducted. The scope is warmed under running water and then gently pressed against the anal opening. While the patient is asked to bear down, the instrument is easily passed into the rectum, the obturator is removed, and the instrument is passed slowly into the colon. If spasm or difficulty is encountered, the scope should be withdrawn until the full lumen is seen and a second attempt should be made.

During insertion, the patient should breathe deeply with the mouth open, to keep the abdominal muscles relaxed. Cramping or a desire to defecate can be relieved by having the patient relax and take deep breaths or pant. If air is insufflated into the lumen to enhance visualization, the patient will normally experience some flatulence as the air moves down the bowel and escapes.

Once the desired depth is reached, the sigmoidoscope is gradually withdrawn, thus allowing examination of all sides of the bowel. A large cotton swab or suction may be used to remove any fecal matter, blood, or mucus that is obscuring vision. The examiner will note the color and friability of the mucosa, bleeding sites, petechiae, and ulcers. (Mucosal friability is established if pinpoint bleeding is noted immediately after application of mechanical pressure with a cotton swab or cytology brush.) If a biopsy exam is indicated, the site of the lesion or specimen and its distance from the anus should be recorded.

Throughout the procedure, the nurse should monitor the patient for vital signs, abdominal distention, pain tolerance, and warmth, color, and dryness of the skin. Sudden changes in position during the procedure should be prevented.

After the procedure is finished, the table should be returned to a low position and the patient should be brought slowly to a seated position before standing. The patient should be observed for signs of bleeding or perforation. Diet, fluids, and activity can return to normal following the procedure, unless complications occur.

Potential complications of rigid proctosigmoidoscopy include perforation, minimal bleeding from lacerations, transient abdominal discomfort, and cardiac arrhythmias. If perforation is suspected and confirmed by clinical symptoms and roentgenographic examination, prompt surgical intervention is indicated. If there is excessive bleeding from a biopsy site, the patient's bleeding status should be checked and the biopsy site reexamined. Either silver nitrate or electrocautery of the bleeding area will usually stop the bleeding.

## FLEXIBLE SIGMOIDOSCOPY

**Sigmoidoscopy** is the examination of the rectum and the sigmoid and descending colon using a flexible sigmoidoscope or colonoscope. In recent years, the flexible fiberoptic sigmoidoscope has largely replaced the standard 25-cm rigid sigmoidoscope for routine examination. The newer, flexible fiberoptic sigmoidoscopes, which measure up to 65 cm in length, have a much greater range than the older, rigid scopes. Flexible instruments are capable of reaching the descending colon in over 80% of patients, and it is possible to reach the splenic flexure. In addition, patients seem to tolerate flexible sigmoidoscopy better than rigid proctosigmoidoscopy.

Flexible sigmoidoscopy is indicated for the following:
- Routine screening of adults over age 50
- Screening of asymptomatic patients at risk for colon neoplasia or polyps
- Evaluation of suspected distal colonic disease when there is no indication for colonoscopy
- Inflammatory bowel disease
- Chronic diarrhea
- Pseudomembranous colitis
- Radiation colitis
- Sigmoid volvulus
- Foreign body removal
- Lower gastrointestinal bleeding
- Evaluation of the colon in conjunction with a barium enema

Sigmoidoscopy is contraindicated in patients with fulminant colitis; toxic megacolon; severe, acute diverticulitis; peritonitis; or uncooperative patients.

Except in patients with watery diarrhea or suspected colitis, preparation for flexible sigmoidoscopy includes 2 warm tap-water or sodium biphosphate (Fleet) enemas 1 to 2 hours before the examination. Compliance with the bowel preparation ordered by the physician should be verified. A medical history should be obtained, including medications, allergies, and any information pertaining to the current complaint. Antibiotic prophylaxis should be administered if ordered. Patients usually do not require sedation.

After a thorough digital rectal exam, the patient is instructed to breathe slowly and deeply to relax the anal sphincters and the well-lubricated endoscope is inserted. While the endoscope is being advanced to the rectosigmoid junction, air is insufflated to facilitate passage into the sigmoid and descending colon. While the instrument is slowly withdrawn, the physician examines the sigmoid colon and then the rectal and anal mucosa. Suction may be used to remove residual matter, blood, or mucus that obscures vision.

During the procedure it is important for the nurse to monitor the patient's vital signs; color, warmth, and dryness of skin; abdominal distention; level of consciousness; pain tolerance; and vagal response. The physician should be notified if the abdomen is becoming excessively distended secondary to air insufflation. To help the patient cooperate, it may be helpful to offer back rubbing or instructions in breathing technique.

After the procedure is completed the patient may resume normal activity if no sedation has been administered. The patient should be observed for postbiopsy bleeding and persistent abdominal pain or distention.

Potential complications of flexible sigmoidoscopy include bleeding and perforation.

## COLONOSCOPY

**Colonoscopy** involves direct visualization of the lower GI tract from the rectum to the ileocecal valve and even the distal ileum, using a long, flexible endoscope. Modern fiberoptic and video colonoscopes are similar in design to upper GI endoscopes, but are longer, ranging in length from 120 to 180 cm. Suction removes liquid secretions that obscure vision, thereby permitting safe advancement of the instrument. Air and water controls help keep the lumen distended and the optics of the tip of the instrument clean.

An experienced endoscopist may view the entire colon and often the distal ileum, reaching the cecum in most patients.

Diagnostic colonoscopy is indicated for the following:

- Evaluation of active or occult lower GI bleeding, such as hematochezia, melena with a negative upper GI investigation, unexplained fecal occult blood, and unexplained iron deficiency anemia
- Evaluation of abnormalities found on radiographic examination
- Suspected cecal or ascending colonic disease
- Surveillance for colon neoplasia in patients who have had a previous colon cancer or previous colon polyps; in patients with a family history of colon cancer; and in patients with chronic UC of several years' duration
- Diagnosis or management of chronic inflammatory bowel disease
- Chronic, unexplained abdominal pain
- Confirmation of suspected polyps, rectal or colonic strictures, or cancer

Colonoscopy is contraindicated in patients with fulminant UC; acute ischemic colitis; acute radiation colitis; suspected toxic megacolon; suspected perforation; acute, severe diverticulitis; the presence of barium; infectious bowel disease; imperforate anus; massive colonic bleeding; shock; acute surgical abdomen or a fresh surgical anastomosis; or patients who are physically unable to tolerate the procedure. Relative contraindications include massive hematochezia, pregnancy, coagulation abnormalities, unstable cardiovascular status, and uncooperative patients.

Standard bowel preparation for colonoscopy is to administer about 1 gallon of an iso-osmolar electrolyte lavage solution. The solution may be consumed either orally or through a nasogastric tube over a 4-hour period, beginning 6 to 12 hours before the procedure. The only problem with this type of preparation is that some patients have difficulty consuming such a large quantity of fluid over a short period. If rectal bleeding or severe abdominal pain occurs during bowel preparation, the physician should be notified immediately.

The patient should be given an opportunity to urinate before the procedure. Because colonoscopy takes longer and is more uncomfortable than flexible sigmoidoscopy, it is customary to administer IV sedation to promote relaxation and diminish discomfort. General anesthesia is used routinely in pediatric patients.

Colonoscopy is usually begun with the patient in the left lateral decubitus position. After a digital examination, the lubricated colonoscope is inserted into the rectum while the patient breathes slowly and deeply. Then the physician insufflates a small amount of air to help dilate the bowel lumen. When appropriate, the nurse should assist the physician in repositioning the patient smoothly to facilitate passage through the splenic flexure, the transverse colon, the hepatic flexure, the ascending colon, and the cecum. In addition, the nurse may apply pressure to areas of the abdomen as requested by the physician to assist with passage of the instrument.

Throughout the procedure it is important that the nurse monitor the patient for vital signs; color, warmth, and dryness of the skin; abdominal distention; level of consciousness; vagal response; and pain tolerance. The physician should be notified if the abdomen becomes excessively distended secondary to air insufflation. To help the patient cooperate more readily, instructions in breathing technique may be offered.

During the procedure the physician may order the administration of atropine or glucagon in an attempt to decrease bowel spasms and/or motility. If either drug is used, the nurse should closely monitor the patient for hypotension and irregular or rapid pulse.

During insertion of the colonoscope, the objective is to reach the cecum as quickly and as safely as possible. During withdrawal, the objective is meticulous inspection. The mucosa is scanned by changing the position of the flexible tip while the instrument is slowly withdrawn. The bowel wall is examined for abnormalities, such as bleeding sites, polyps, inflammation, or tumors. Direct visualization allows for therapeutic procedures, such as polypectomy, dilatation, decompression, and fulguration of bleeding sites.

Following colonoscopy it is important for the nurse to monitor and document vital signs every 15 to 30 minutes until the patient is stable. The patient should be observed for signs of complications, such as bleeding, vomiting, a change in vital signs, severe or persistent abdominal pain and/or distention, and abdominal rigidity.

Major complications occur in less than 1% of patients undergoing colonoscopy. The two major complications, perforation and hemorrhage, are most likely to occur during or after polypectomy, which is discussed in Chapter 32. Other potential complications of colonoscopy include medication reactions, such as cardiac arrhythmias or arrest and respiratory depression or arrest; explosion of colonic gases; vasovagal reactions; and cardiac failure or hypotension, related to overhydration or underhydration of a susceptible patient during bowel preparation. Excessive bleeding from biopsy sites is rare unless the patient has a coagulation disorder or has been on products that contain aspirin. Unsuspected serosal tears and retroperitoneal emphysema have occasionally been found at laparotomy. Excessive use of air and advancement of the scope without a clear view of the lumen are most likely to cause these difficulties.

Colonoscopic complications may be minimized by advancing the colonoscope or sigmoidoscope with care and avoiding overdistention of the colon. Fluid and electrolyte status of elderly patients and those with renal and cardiac disease should be considered during bowel preparation. If soreness occurs at the IV injection site, it can be relieved with warm compresses.

## ADDITIONAL TECHNIQUES

The technology available for endoscopic visualization of the gastrointestinal tract continues to advance. Additional diagnostic techniques that are available to the endoscopist include small bowel enteroscopy, endoscopy through an ostomy, videoendoscopy, and endoscopic ultrasonography.

### Small bowel enteroscopy

**Small bowel enteroscopy** permits visualization of all 20 feet of the small bowel, using a long, thin, and extremely flexible endoscope. This enteroscope has two internal channels, one for intraluminal air insufflation, and one to distend a balloon located at the tip of the instrument.

The complete procedure lasts 8 to 10 hours and can be performed on an outpatient basis. It has been most useful in patients with continued or intermittent blood loss, in whom a bleeding site has not been found despite exhaustive testing.

The lubricated tip of the enteroscope is passed through the nose and into the patient's stomach. A pediatric colonoscope acting as a push-enteroscope is passed orally into the duodenum, while the esophagus, stomach, and duodenum are examined for possible causes of bleeding. The push-enteroscope is then withdrawn to the stomach, where the biopsy forceps grasp a suture on the tip of the small bowel enteroscope. The two instruments are advanced into the small bowel, and a balloon on the tip of the small bowel enteroscope is inflated, thereby holding it in place as the push-enteroscope is removed. IV metoclopramide (Reglan) is administered and the patient is sent to a recovery area for several hours while peristalsis advances the enteroscope through the small bowel. After the enteroscope is positioned in the distal ileum, the small bowel is examined thoroughly while the enteroscope is slowly withdrawn.

Sources of bleeding may be documented by photography, but no therapeutic procedures are possible through the long, narrow, internal channel of the enteroscope. The chance of finding a lesion with this procedure is approximately one in three.

### Endoscopy through an ostomy

Occasionally it may be necessary to directly visualize a segment of small or large intestine using a flexible endoscope that has been inserted through a stoma.

This procedure is indicated for evaluation of an anastomotic site, identification of recurrent disease (e.g., Crohn's disease or cancer), or visualization and/or treatment of gastrointestinal bleeding. It is contraindicated in patients with recent ostomy/bowel surgery, poor bowel preparation, suspected bowel perforation, presence of a large peristomal hernia, or massive lower gastrointestinal bleeding.

Before the procedure it is necessary to examine the ostomy site to determine the size of the stoma, the type of effluent that can be expected during the procedure, and what ostomy appliance will be needed following the procedure. Compliance with bowel preparation orders should be confirmed and their effectiveness ascertained. The old ostomy appliance should be removed gently, working from the top downward, taking care to push the skin away from the appliance.

The patient should be in the supine position, with fluid-impervious towels draping the stoma. A large supply of sponges should be provided, especially for an ileostomy. The endoscope should be held at a right angle to the abdominal wall to facilitate entry through the ostomy. The patient's vital signs should be monitored throughout the procedure, as should the color, warmth, and dryness of the skin; abdominal distention; level of consciousness; and pain tolerance. The nurse should also provide emotional support to the patient while also maintaining a tight seal around the endoscope as it enters the stoma so the physician is able to accomplish adequate insufflation.

After the procedure is completed it is important that the nurse monitor and document vital signs. The peristomal area should be cleaned carefully with a mild soap and water, and the skin should be thoroughly dried. An appropriate skin barrier and collecting pouch should be applied immediately. The patient should be observed for stomal bleeding, vomiting, a change in vital signs, severe or persistent abdominal pain, and abdominal rigidity.

### Videoendoscopy

Videoendoscopes have no coherent fiberoptic image bundle. Instead, a distal sensing device in the tip of the instrument electronically transmits an image to a video processor for display in color or black and white on a television monitor. Endoscopy is performed by reference to the monitor. An advantage of this technology is that all members of the endoscopy team are able to view the procedure, thus enhancing collaboration among team members.

A videotape deck may be added to the system for recording the procedure on videotape. The video processor has a freeze-frame function, and a character-generator keyboard is provided to make marginal notes on the video screen next to the endoscopic image. Individual photographs may be generated by adding a mavigraph to the system. New computer programs are continually being developed to enhance the capabilities of **videoendoscopy.** Now, patient data can be accessed for statistical purposes and reports of procedures can be generated by computer.

Controls for tip deflection are similar to those of conventional fiberoptic scopes, with two coaxial knobs, for left and right and up and down deflections. Valves are provided for air and water insufflation and for suction. An accessory/suction channel is also provided. Because of its high photosensitivity, the videoendoscope requires less light and provides greater depth of visual field than fiberoptic endoscopes. However, because of the decreased light output, it is more difficult to transilluminate the right lower quadrant of the abdomen when the tip of the colonoscope is in the cecum.

The use of videoendoscopy or any form of photography is secondary to patient needs. It should be postponed if the safety of the patient is compromised in any way.

## Endoscopic ultrasonography

New technology has combined the endoscope with ultrasonography to enhance visualization of the GI tract, which is obscured in conventional ultrasonographic examinations by intraabdominal gas and bony structures. With an oblique-viewing endoscope that has an ultrasonic transducer built into the tip, high-frequency, ultrasonic beams can be targeted in close proximity to existing lesions.

This procedure results in better-quality resolution, which enhances evaluation of the histologic structure of targeted lesions. In addition, esophageal wall thickness may be evaluated and assessed. The walls of the esophagus, stomach, duodenum, and colon may be visualized, as well as the structure of several contiguous organs.

The act of scanning through the gastric wall, combined with changes in the patient's position, is sufficient for the study of the gastric wall itself, the gallbladder, pancreas, kidneys, left lobe of the liver, spleen, aorta, inferior vena cava, and various tributaries of the extrahepatic portal vein system.

An inflatable balloon covers the ultrasonic transducer and can be filled with water to compress the esophageal wall, eliminate the air space, and improve the quality of resolution, which enhances the evaluation of the targeted lesion. Endoscopic ultrasonography, as compared with radiographic and endoscopic examinations, has many advantages for detecting lesions in the wall of the GI tract.

---

**CASE SITUATION**

The nurse manager of a busy hospital endoscopy unit is adding a new nurse. Susie Jones has finished her hospital orientation and started in the unit. She is vaguely familiar with gastroenterology procedures, but has no gastroenterology experience. The nurse manager needs to set up a training program for Susie.

*Points to think about*

1. The nurse manager begins by showing Susie the orientation manual. What should be included in this manual?
2. What other manuals and books should the manager make available to Susie to help her do her job?
3. It is Susie's third week and she is beginning to learn how to assist with a colonoscopy. What has she probably learned so far?
4. The manager is now showing Susie how to assist with a colonoscopy. What types of things must she be taught?

*Suggested responses*

1. The orientation manual should include the following:
   - Hospital and department philosophy statements and standards
   - Job descriptions and lists of essential duties
   - An overview of the training period
   - An outline of expected learning experiences with time frames for completion
   - A tool for evaluating learning experience
   - Copies of policies specific to employee conduct (e.g., reporting on-the-job accidents, or infection-control policies)
   - Policy and statements on patient rights
2. Other manuals and books that the nurse manager might make available to Susie include the following:
   - Hospital and department policy manuals
   - The hospital's fire and disaster manual
   - The hospital's manual on hazardous materials
   - The SGNA procedure manual
   - The SGNA core curriculum
   - A good GI anatomy and physiology book
   - A drug reference book
   - Other GI endoscopy books (see bibliography)
   - Recent volumes of *Gastroenterology Nursing*
3. After her first 3 weeks, Susie has probably read the pertinent policy and procedure manuals and at least part of the core curriculum. In addition, she has probably learned the following:
   - How to handle the various forms and paperwork required in the department
   - How to admit a patient to the unit and how to perform the nursing assessment and plan of care
   - The necessary infection-control techniques
   - The different types of scopes and how to set up equipment for EGD and colon examination procedures

- How to assist with a simple EGD with minimal supervision
- How to process biopsy and cytology specimens

4. Before Susie assists with a colonoscopy, it is important that she know the following:
   - Basic colon anatomy and physiology
   - Indications for colonoscopy
   - Techniques of preparing the colon for colonoscopy
   - How to relate possible diagnosis with the equipment setup
   - How the nurse can facilitate the passage of the scope by using gentle external hand pressure to prevent the scope from bowing in the sigmoid; how different patient positions can facilitate passage of the scope in difficult cases
   - How to comfort the patient by talking gently and providing encouragement and praise, and that gently stroking the patient's back or forehead can be comforting and reduce the need for medication
   - Pertinent information that should be provided to the patient before discharge

Patients are usually receptive and supportive of a teaching situation if they feel that they will not be left alone in the care of a novice. The nurse manager should let the patient know that he or she will be teaching a new nurse, but will be present throughout the procedure. The manager should leave technical discussions of any pathologic conditions encountered and the treatment that will be used for them until after the procedure to avoid causing the patient any additional stress. When teaching, the nurse manager should always remember to support statements with a rationale.

---

### REVIEW TERMS

**anoscopy, colonoscopy, endoscopic retrograde cholangiopancreatography (ERCP), endoscopy, esophagogastroduodenoscopy (EGD), fiberoptic bundles, proctoscopy, proctosigmoidoscopy, rectosigmoidoscopy, sigmoidoscopy, small bowel enteroscopy, videoendoscopy**

---

### REVIEW QUESTIONS

1. The endoscopes used in EGD can visualize the upper GI tract as far as the:
   a. Pylorus.
   b. Ampulla of Vater.
   c. Proximal duodenum.
   d. Ileocecal valve.
2. Before EGD, the patient should be NPO for at least:
   a. 2 hours.
   b. 6 hours.
   c. 12 hours.
   d. 24 hours.
3. The major complication(s) associated with ERCP is (are):
   a. Perforation.
   b. Adverse effects of medication.
   c. Hemorrhage.
   d. Pancreatitis and sepsis.
4. The most common cause(s) of bright red rectal bleeding is (are):
   a. Inflammatory bowel disease.
   b. Perforation.
   c. Hemorrhoids and fissures.
   d. Bleeding ulcers and varices.
5. One contraindication for rigid proctosigmoidoscopy is:
   a. Severe cardiac arrhythmias.
   b. Previous rectal surgery.
   c. Rectal bleeding.
   d. Rectal pain.
6. The usual bowel preparation for flexible sigmoidoscopy is:
   a. A single warm tap-water enema.
   b. Two warm tap-water or Fleet enemas.
   c. A 2-day liquid diet, followed by a strong laxative.
   d. Electrolyte lavage.
7. For flexible sigmoidoscopy, the patient should be in the knee-chest or:
   a. Prone position.
   b. Supine position.
   c. Right lateral position.
   d. Left lateral position.
8. Patients who will undergo colonoscopy usually receive:
   a. Local anesthesia only.
   b. IV sedation.
   c. General anesthesia.
   d. No sedation or anesthesia.
9. Distention of the abdomen during colonoscopy is most likely caused by:
   a. Excessive insufflation of air.
   b. Excessive amounts of water used for irrigation.
   c. Perforation.
   d. Colonic obstruction.
10. Small bowel enteroscopy is indicated for patients with:
    a. Peptic ulcers.
    b. Inflammatory bowel disease.
    c. Persistent blood loss with no identifiable source.
    d. Intestinal polyps.

### BIBLIOGRAPHY

Bertagnolli, M, Loebenberg, M, Benjamin, S, Fleischer, D, Collen, M, Lewis, J, Cattau, E, Jr., and Jaffe, M. "Use of Endoscopic Ultrasound in Patients with Esophageal Motility Disorders." In

*Journal Reprints II,* ed. Trivits, S, 74-75. Rochester, N.Y.: Society of Gastroenterology Nurses and Associates, 1990.

Eastwood, G, and Avunduk, C. *Manual of Gastroenterology: Diagnosis and Therapy.* Boston: Little, Brown & Co., 1988.

Given, B, and Simmons, S. *Gastroenterology in Clinical Nursing.* 4th ed. St. Louis: Mosby–Year Book, 1984.

Hamilton, H, editorial director. *Procedures.* Nurse's Reference Library. Springhouse, Pa.: Intermed Communications, 1983.

Hardick, M, and Beck, M, eds. *Manual of Gastrointestinal Procedures.* 2nd ed. Rochester, N.Y.: Society of Gastroenterology Nurses and Associates, 1989.

Lewis, B, and Czachor, K. "Small Bowel Enteroscopy: The GIA's Role." In *Journal Reprints II,* ed. Trivits, S, 168-71. Rochester, N.Y.: Society of Gastroenterology Nurses and Associates, 1990.

Mathews, J, Maher, K, and Cattau, E, Jr. "The Role of Endoscopic Retrograde Cholangiopancreatography Injection Training Sessions for the Gastroenterology Nurse and Associate." In *Journal Reprints II,* ed. Trivits, S, 120-22. Rochester, N.Y.: Society of Gastroenterology Nurses and Associates, 1990.

Ravenscroft, M, and Swan, C. *Gastrointestinal Endoscopy and Related Procedures: A Handbook for Nurses and Assistants.* Baltimore: Williams & Wilkins, 1984.

Rayhorn, N, ed. *Manual of Gastrointestinal Procedures: Pediatric Supplement.* Rochester, N.Y.: Society of Gastroenterology Nurses and Associates, 1991.

Silverman, A, and Roy, C. *Pediatric Clinical Gastroenterology.* 3rd ed. St. Louis: Mosby–Year Book, 1983.

Sivak, M, Jr., and Petrini, J, eds. *Gastrointestinal Endoscopy: Old Problems, New Techniques.* Gastrointestinal Series, Vol. 4. New York: Praeger, 1986.

Society of Gastroenterology Nurses and Associates, Practice and Education Committees. *Nursing Care of the Patient Receiving Conscious Sedation in the Gastrointestinal Endoscopy Setting.* SGNA Monograph Series. Rochester, N.Y.: Society of Gastroenterology Nurses and Associates, 1991.

Watson, D. *Monitoring the Patient Receiving Local Anesthesia.* Denver: Association of Operating Room Nurses, 1990.

Waye, J. "Diagnostic and Therapeutic Endoscopy." In *Gastroenterology for the House Officer,* eds. Sachar, D, Waye, J, and Lewis, B, 309-16. Baltimore: Williams & Wilkins, 1989.

Waye, J, Atchison, M, Talbott, M, and Lewis, B. "Light in the Right Lower Quadrant During Colonoscopy: A Comparison of Fiberoptic Versus Video Colonoscopes." *SGA Journal* 11(Winter 1988): 157-58.

Zfass, A, and Brennan, P. "Endoscopy of the Bowel." In *Principles and Practice of Gastroenterology and Hepatology,* ed. Gitnick, G, and Hollander, D, 669-77. New York: Elsevier, 1988.

# Chapter 25

# MANOMETRY

This chapter will acquaint the gastroenterology nurse with manometric procedures that are used in the diagnosis of gastrointestinal disorders, focusing on esophageal manometry.*

**Learning objectives**

After reviewing the content of this chapter, the gastroenterology nurse should be able to:
1. Describe the equipment and techniques typically used in manometric studies.
2. List the indications and contraindications for manometric procedures involving the esophagus, stomach, sphincter of Oddi, and anorectum.
3. Discuss the types of manometric tracings that are observed in normal subjects and in patients with selected gastrointestinal disorders.

## BASIC PRINCIPLES

Gastrointestinal **manometry** is a diagnostic test that measures changes in intraluminal pressure and coordination of activity in the muscles of the GI tract. Although it is primarily used to measure esophageal motility, manometric techniques may also be used in the stomach, the sphincter of Oddi, and the anorectum. The instrumentation used may vary, but virtually all manometric techniques involve a series of catheters and pressure transducers that measure gastrointestinal motor activity and transform this activity into electrical signals that, in turn, produce graphic images on a physiograph or a computer.

## ESOPHAGEAL MANOMETRY

Esophageal manometry is the standard process whereby most motility disorders of the esophageal body

---

* All techniques in this chapter, except gastroduodenal manometry, are also discussed in the SGNA *Manual of Gastrointestinal Procedures,* 2nd ed. Rochester, N.Y.: Society of Gastroenterology Nurses and Associates, 1989.

and lower esophageal sphincter (LES) are diagnosed. Disorders of the upper esophageal sphincter (UES) and the oropharyngeal region may be better diagnosed with radiography.

**Indications and contraindications**

Esophageal manometry is indicated for patients with primary esophageal motility disorders, such as achalasia, diffuse esophageal spasm, nutcracker esophagus, hypertensive LES, and nonspecific esophageal motility disorders. Secondary esophageal motility disorders for which esophageal manometry may be indicated include diabetes mellitus, scleroderma, and chronic idiopathic intestinal pseudoobstruction.

With the addition of provocative tests, esophageal manometry may also be used to evaluate patients with symptoms that are suspected to be esophageal in origin, such as dysphagia, odynophagia, or noncardiac chest pain.

Esophageal manometry is contraindicated in uncooperative patients; in patients with cardiac instability, recent gastric surgery, or severe esophageal ulcers; or in patients that have ingested, within the previous 24 hours, any medications that affect esophageal motor function. Complications of this procedure are rare.

**Equipment**

In esophageal manometry, the only piece of equipment that enters the patient's esophagus is a long, flexible catheter; either a water-infusion catheter, in which the transducers are external, or a solid-state catheter, in which the transducers are small and part of the catheter itself.

The **water-infusion catheter** is a multilumen catheter that is typically 5 mm or less in diameter. Each of the three to eight lumens has a side opening or port in a set location, usually 1 to 5 cm apart. Each recording port is connected to a separate, external **pressure transducer.**

The transducers, in turn, are connected to a **physiograph** or to a computer with light-sensitive paper, either of which records contractions in millimeters of mercury (mm Hg). An infusion pump powered by compressed nitrogen continuously perfuses the catheter with water. As contractions of the GI tract occlude one or more of the recording orifices on the catheter, the flow of water is stopped. The resulting change in water pressure is translated by the transducer into an electrical signal and recorded as a contraction on the physiograph.

The water-infusion system is reliable and easy to use and maintain. Unlike solid-state systems, external transducers can easily be replaced, and malfunction of one transducer does not render the entire system inoperable.

**Solid-state catheters** contain miniature pressure transducers that directly record contractions exerted by the esophageal wall or sphincters. No water or infusion pump is used. Compared with water-infusion systems, solid-state catheters are more expensive and less reliable. They are also more difficult to repair or replace because malfunction of a single transducer requires that the entire system be sent for repair.

## Procedures

Before conducting an esophageal manometric study, it is important to verify the patient's NPO status; obtain the patient's medical history; remove eyeglasses, plates or dentures, if any; obtain and document vital signs; and reassure the patient. In adult patients the procedure is performed while the patient is awake and without sedation, because premedication may interfere with swallowing and may have direct effects on motor events. In children, however, sedation is required. Nitrates, calcium channel blockers, anticholinergics, promotility agents, and sedatives should be discontinued 24 to 48 hours before the study because they can interfere with normal esophageal function. However, it is important to consult with the attending physician before discontinuing any medication.

The recording equipment and the manometry catheter are calibrated and connected. Then the manometry catheter is inserted nasally or orally with the patient in a sitting position. For comfort, the patient's nasal passage may be anesthetized with a topical anesthetic that may be applied with a cotton-tipped applicator, an atomizer, or a syringe. When the tip of the tube is in the back of the throat, the patient is instructed to tuck his or her chin down to the chest and swallow. It may be helpful to give the patient some water to drink to facilitate movement of the catheter through the esophagus and, finally, past the LES and into the stomach. Once the tube has been inserted into the stomach, the patient may be helped into a supine position.

Before beginning to withdraw the catheter, it is important to check that everything is working properly.

- If all of the recording ports are in the patient's stomach, the physiograph should initially show a relatively flat, smooth tracing with a small pressure increase on inspiration or abdominal pressure. This pattern confirms placement in the stomach and is called the gastric baseline.
- If one or more of the channels shows a straight line, the equipment may be malfunctioning or one of the catheter orifices may be blocked. To avoid this problem, patency of the catheter lumens should be checked before tube placement.
- If one of the channels shows very rapid activity, this may be a result of cardiac interference. This type of pattern is most often seen during study of the esophageal body, when the recording orifice lies adjacent to the aortic arch.

Once it has been established that the recording equipment is working properly, the next step is to attach the equipment necessary to monitor the patient's swallows and respirations.

### Lower esophageal sphincter

The first step in a manometric study is to measure LES pressure. The catheter may be moved steadily through the LES into the esophagus while the patient is not breathing or swallowing (rapid pull-through method) or may be withdrawn in a step-wise fashion while the patient breathes regularly and evenly (station pull-through). Under normal conditions, a **rapid pull-through** should show a rise in LES pressure, followed by a drop in pressure to below the gastric baseline as the recording ports enter the esophagus.

The **station pull-through** gives a more complete assessment of LES function. Using this method, the catheter is moved through the LES 1.0 cm at a time, with a pause at each point or station to observe LES pressure and relaxation. Relaxation of the sphincter is assessed by having the patient perform a series of controlled swallows, beginning with dry swallows and adding wet swallows. The swallow and accompanying relaxation of the LES should be reflected by a drop in pressure to about the level of the gastric baseline.

The point where the tracing goes down, rather than up, with an inspiration is called the *pressure inversion point* and represents the point where the recording port moves from the abdominal cavity into the thoracic cavity. If LES pressure is very weak, this inversion point may be the only way to locate the LES.

### Esophageal body

The motility of the esophageal body is usually evaluated after anchoring the catheter at a point where the recording ports span the esophagus, usually at 3, 8, 13, and 18 cm above the LES. Motility can be assessed by giving the patient about ten 3- to 5-ml swallows of water at 20- to 30-second intervals. The mean values for the last 10 swallows are analyzed, either manually or by computer. The precise steps to be followed in this procedure may vary according to the physician's preference. In some cases, food swallows may be given.

A normal tracing of a wet swallow should show an orderly progression of contractions from top to bottom, which is representative of normal esophageal peristalsis. Abnormal responses may include the following:

- Simultaneous contractions, which occur at the same time throughout the esophageal body
- Retrograde contractions, which progress from the distal to the proximal esophagus
- Repetitive triple-peaked contractions; double contractions are considered a variant of normal contractions, whereas triple-peaked contractions are considered abnormal
- Nontransmitted contractions
- Very strong or very weak contractions

**Upper esophageal sphincter**

If assessment of the UES is desired, it is the final step in an esophageal motility study. For this process, each pressure port is pulled through the UES and relaxation of the sphincter with a swallow is assessed. Normally, a swallow causes a rapid decrease (or relaxation) in UES pressure, coordinated with pharyngeal activity and a resumption of resting UES pressure.

After the entire manometric study is completed, the water-infusion catheter lumens are flushed with detergent, followed by thorough rinsing and drying, and ethylene oxide gas sterilization. Solid-state manometry catheters undergo high-level disinfection only.

Before discharge, it is important to obtain and document the patient's vital signs and to assess and document patient status.

## PROVOCATIVE TESTING

Provocative testing is an optional technique that is designed to reproduce chest pain that may be esophageal in origin. It is imperative initially to exclude coronary disease, because of its more serious prognosis, as the cause of the patient's pain. In addition, an upper GI series and gallbladder evaluation are usually performed to exclude other GI tract abnormalities.

Provocative testing is accomplished while the recording ports of the manometry catheter are located in the esophageal body. Interpretation is based on the patient's subjective pain and on manometric tracings.

### Bernstein test

Noncardiac chest pain associated with acid reflux may be simulated by performing the **Bernstein test;** that is, alternating infusions of a placebo (normal saline) and 0.1N hydrochloric acid through one of the recording ports of a manometry catheter. The test is indicated in patients with atypical chest pain and is contraindicated in patients with an inability to tolerate intubation, with

active or recent gastrointestinal bleeding, or with known active ulcer disease (relative).

Before this test the patient should avoid ingesting antacids or coating agents, anesthetic gargle, or pain medication and should be NPO.

Because the patient's subjective pain is the diagnostic endpoint, the patient should be informed only that the test will attempt to determine the source of his or her chest pain. The two irrigating fluids should be out of the patient's visual field. With the patient in a sitting position, a nasogastric (NG) or motility tube is placed at midesophagus, and alternating solutions of normal saline and 0.1N hydrochloric acid are dripped through the tube in an attempt to reproduce the patient's symptoms. If the Bernstein test is performed following a manometric study, the manometry catheter may be used to instill saline and acid.

If discomfort occurs at any time, the patient should be instructed to point to the area and to describe the pain verbally, comparing it to previous symptoms (Fig. 25-1). A true positive response to the Bernstein test requires that the symptoms be stimulated by acid infusion, lessened with saline infusion, and worsened with a subsequent acid infusion. If pain is related to gastric or duodenal lesions, it will not be relieved by the infusion of normal saline. Normal saline should be infused at the end of the test to flush hydrochloric acid from the esophagus.

Potential complications of the Bernstein test include aspiration and misplacement of the NG tube.

### Edrophonium testing

The purpose of this test is to confirm the esophageal origin of noncardiac chest pain. It is indicated in patients with noncardiac chest pain and contraindicated in patients with an unstable cardiac history, atrial fibrillation, arrhythmias (or bundle branch block), severe asthma, bradycardia, or bronchial constrictive disease.

Before the test, any pain medications or any medications that could affect esophageal contractions should be withheld for 48 hours, as ordered by the patient's physician. Baseline esophageal manometry is conducted first. A motility catheter with at least four lumens should be positioned with the distal opening 3, 8, 13, and 18 cm above the LES. During continuous recording of esophageal pressures, a saline placebo is administered intravenously, after which the patient performs 10 wet swallows 30 seconds apart, is administered a rapid IV bolus of the cholinesterase inhibitor **edrophonium chloride** (Tensilon), and performs 10 wet swallows. The amplitude and duration of esophageal contractions should increase following edrophonium provocation. The test is complete after 5 minutes of manometry tracings or 10 wet swallows. It is considered positive if typical chest pain is reproduced by edrophonium injec-

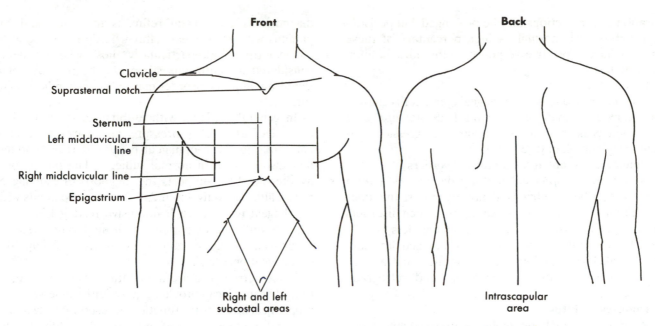

**Fig. 25-1.** Anatomic landmarks for differentiating discomfort evoked during intraesophageal acid drip test.

tion, and if abnormal motility is noted on motility tracings.

Adverse reactions to edrophonium may occur and are usually transient. They include tearing, dizziness, gastrointestinal discomfort and, less often, bradycardia, pupillary constriction, and laryngospasm. Atropine should be available as an antidote to bradycardia.

### Disorders diagnosed using esophageal manometry

Esophageal manometry may be used in the diagnosis of both primary and secondary esophageal motility disorders.

#### Achalasia

Achalasia is characterized by long-standing, progressive dysphagia for both solids and liquids, often with weight loss, nocturnal regurgitation, and pulmonary symptoms. Definitive manometric findings include aperistalsis, usually with incomplete LES relaxation (with or without an increase in resting sphincter pressure). Patients with early achalasia may show complete LES relaxation, but of unusually short duration. In addition, LES pressure may be elevated, the length of the high-pressure zone may be increased, and intraesophageal pressures may be elevated relative to gastric pressure, a condition that is opposite to the normal relationship.

When assessing patients with suspected achalasia, it is important to advance the manometry catheter through the LES even though it may be difficult, because LES characteristics are important for manometric diagnosis. Fluoroscopy is occasionally needed to confirm the location of the catheter and to aid in passage into the stomach. LES relaxation should be assessed with wet swallows, using a station pull-through technique. Demonstration of incomplete sphincter relaxation following a swallow is needed to distinguish achalasia from other disorders with aperistalsis. In most cases, sphincter pressure drops by only approximately 30% of its elevation over gastric baseline.

Patients with so-called *vigorous* achalasia demonstrate high-amplitude (greater than 60 mm Hg), simultaneous, often repetitive contractions of the esophageal body in response to swallows, along with elevated LES pressure.

#### Diffuse esophageal spasm

Diffuse esophageal spasm (DES) may also be diagnosed manometrically. The primary symptoms of DES are chest pain and dysphagia. Manometrically, patients with DES must demonstrate simultaneous contractions in more than 10% of wet swallows, along with intermittent normal peristalsis. Such patients may also show repetitive contractions.

Manometric findings in patients with esophageal spasm are generally restricted to the smooth muscle portion of the esophagus and are most pronounced in the 5- to 10-cm segment proximal to the LES. They do not seem to affect the skeletal muscle portion of the esophagus.

#### Nutcracker esophagus

Nutcracker esophagus is an abnormality of contraction wave amplitude, typified by a mean contraction amplitude greater than 2 standard deviations above a well-documented normal range. Patients with this disorder complain of chest pain and/or dysphagia. The duration of contractions may be prolonged, but peristaltic progression is normal. A high percentage of these patients have a positive response to the edrophonium chloride test.

### Hypertensive LES

A hypertensive lower esophageal sphincter is characterized by abnormally high resting LES pressure. LES relaxation is normal, as is peristaltic progression. Patients may complain of chest pain.

### Nonspecific esophageal motility disorders

Nonspecific esophageal motility disorder is a term used to describe any abnormal motility pattern that does not fall into one of the other categories. Such disorders include weak (low-amplitude) contractions (less than 30 mm Hg), peristaltic contractions of prolonged duration, triple-peaked contractions, nontransmitted contractions (more than 20% of wet swallows), and retrograde contractions.

### Diabetes mellitus

Patients with diabetes mellitus often exhibit manometric abnormalities, possibly as a result of the degenerative effects of diabetes on the autonomic nervous system. Esophageal motility is abnormal in approximately 80% of patients with diabetic neuropathy. These abnormalities may include occasional nontransmitted swallows and spontaneous contractions or may resemble diffuse esophageal spasm. In the majority of cases, esophageal dysfunction is asymptomatic. In symptomatic patients, complaints are mild, consisting of heartburn and, rarely, dysphagia.

### Scleroderma

Scleroderma, which is a form of progressive systemic sclerosis, is a connective tissue disorder characterized by a progressive thickening and induration of the dermis. A majority of patients with typical skin manifestations have evidence of esophageal involvement at autopsy, characterized by muscle atrophy and fibrosis that affect predominantly the smooth muscle region of the esophagus. The end results are failure of muscle contraction in the distal esophagus and incompetency in the LES. Manometry in these patients shows reduced contraction, aperistalsis in the distal esophageal body, and low to absent LES pressure.

### Primary chronic intestinal pseudo-obstruction

Chronic intestinal pseudoobstruction is a syndrome that is characterized by intermittent signs and symptoms of bowel obstruction, in the absence of a demonstrable obstructing lesion. It most commonly affects the small bowel. Esophageal manometry is abnormal in more than 80% of cases. Typical findings include incomplete LES relaxation, abnormal esophageal contractions (simultaneous and repetitive), and absent peristalsis.

### Esophageal reflux

Esophageal manometry has limited usefulness in the diagnosis of esophageal reflux. It is indicated when the diagnosis of esophageal reflux is in doubt, and for patients with esophageal reflux who do not respond to medical treatment, particularly those who are being considered for antireflux surgery. (The presence of a significant motility disorder may be a contraindication to surgery.)

In general, patients with esophageal reflux tend to have decreased LES pressure and lower peristaltic amplitude in the esophageal body, but these findings may also be seen in normal subjects. The finding of a hypotensive LES supports the diagnosis of esophageal reflux, although only about 25% to 50% of patients with esophageal reflux have hypotensive resting LES pressure. About 50% of patients with moderate or severe esophageal reflux exhibit some degree of impaired esophageal peristalsis.

Manometry is also useful in patients with esophageal reflux because it can provide a quantitative assessment of esophageal body motor function in response to swallowing and esophageal acid infusion. In addition, the intraesophageal pH measurements used to assess the competence of the antireflux barrier typically require placement of a pH probe 5 cm above the LES, and manometric measurements are the best method for defining correct placement of such probes.

### Anorexia nervosa

A recent study found abnormal esophageal motility in up to 50% of patients with primary anorexia nervosa. Many of these patients had previously undiagnosed achalasia. Following the manometric diagnosis, pneumatic dilatation resulted in weight gain. The authors of this study conclude that esophageal motility studies should be performed in every patient diagnosed with primary anorexia nervosa.

## GASTRODUODENAL MANOMETRY

Gastric manometry may be indicated in patients with symptoms of delayed gastric emptying or clinically evident gastric motility disorders. Clinical conditions that have been associated with gastric dysrhythmias include idiopathic gastroparesis; gastroparesis secondary to diabetes mellitus or anorexia nervosa; gastric ulcer disease; or gastric adenocarcinoma. Gastric dysrhythmias have also been associated with the effects of certain drugs and hormones, including anticholinergics, metenkephalin, β-endorphin, epinephrine, glucagon, prostaglandin E2, secretin, and insulin. Transient abnormal rhythms have also been observed postoperatively in otherwise normal individuals. Clinical signs of these disorders include severe gastric retention, nausea, vomiting, and weight loss.

Impaired gastric motor activity in patients with diabetic neuropathy may cause symptoms ranging from vague postprandial abdominal discomfort to invariable postprandial nausea and vomiting. Gastric stasis may

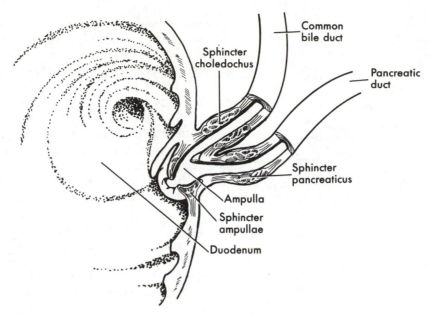

**Fig. 25-2.** Sphincter of Oddi anatomy.

also cause more serious problems, such as weight loss, poor diabetic control, and bezoars. The most commonly seen gastric motor abnormality in these patients is absence of the antral component of the interdigestive motor complex, which is normally responsible for clearance of indigestible solids. These patients may be helped by prescriptions of metoclopramide (Reglan) before meals and at bedtime.

Gastroduodenal motility studies include recording both fasting and fed patterns of phasic pressure activity in the antrum and upper small bowel, and responses to provocative testing. Both catheter perfusion techniques and transducer-containing probes are available. Perfusion catheters are inexpensive and easy to build or buy, but they are thicker than most transducer tubes.

The transducer tube is passed over a guidewire, and its location is confirmed fluoroscopically. Transducers are arranged spatially to sense the antrum, duodenum, and small bowel and are encased in a flexible polyurethane sheath that can be tolerated for long periods of time. Measurements can be made for up to 24 hours to sample a number of interdigestive, migrating motor complexes and to provide more opportunity to observe a disturbed or disrupted complex.

## SPHINCTER OF ODDI MANOMETRY

The sphincter of Oddi is a circular smooth muscle that surrounds the ampulla of Vater, the distal common bile duct, and the pancreatic duct (Fig. 25-2). During fasting, it exhibits peristaltic-like contractions that propel bile into the duodenum and prevent reflux of duodenal contents. Food causes the release of cholecystokinin from the duodenum, which inhibits contraction of the sphincter of Oddi and lowers the basal pressure.

Sphincter of Oddi manometry is indicated for diagnosis of papillary stenosis and for motility disorders of the sphincter of Oddi, which may be associated with choledocholithiasis, biliary pain, abdominal pain, or pancreatitis. Possible factors causing obstruction of bile flow include spasm of the sphincter of Oddi or retrograde contractions.

Sphincter of Oddi manometry is usually obtained during endoscopic retrograde cholangiopancreatography (ERCP) (Fig. 25-3). Like ERCP, sphincter of Oddi manometry is contraindicated in the following:

- Uncooperative patients
- Recent myocardial infarction
- Acute pancreatitis
- Coagulopathy
- Barium in the GI tract
- Pregnancy
- Severe pulmonary disease

Before beginning sphincter of Oddi manometry, it is important to verify informed consent and NPO status, obtain the patient's medical history and laboratory results, establish a patent IV line, remove dentures, administer antibiotic prophylaxis as ordered, and record baseline vital signs.

The patient should be mildly sedated. (Anticholinergic drugs and opiates are not used before manometry because they can alter sphincter pressures.) A triple-lumen catheter is inserted through the biopsy channel of a side-viewing duodenoscope.

The duodenoscope is inserted orally. The ampulla of Vater is identified and cannulated with the triple-lumen manometry catheter, which is passed through the sphincter of Oddi into the common bile duct. This catheter is attached to a capillary infusion system, and

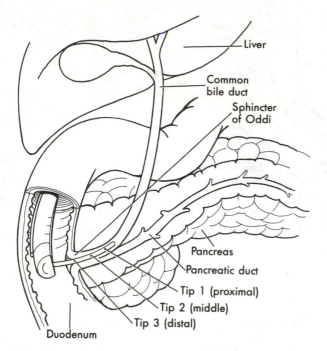

**Fig. 25-3.** Placement of pressure catheter in sphincter of Oddi.

three external transducers transmit the pressures to a physiograph. As the catheter is withdrawn slowly at 1-mm increments, a normal tracing shows basal pressures of less than 30 mm Hg, with peristaltic-like phasic waves. If a motility disorder is confirmed, the physician may choose to perform an endoscopic sphincterotomy.

After the procedure is completed, it is important to monitor and document the patient's vital signs, observe for abdominal distention and signs of pancreatitis, maintain NPO status until the gag reflex returns, administer antibiotics as ordered, remove the IV line, provide written discharge instructions, and ensure that outpatients have someone to drive them home.

The most common complication of sphincter of Oddi manometry is pancreatitis, which may present as mild to incapacitating pain, beginning in the midepigastrium and radiating to the patient's back; nausea and vomiting; fever; distended abdomen; and decreased bowel sounds. Less likely complications are perforation, which may present with abdominal rigidity, rebound tenderness, an increase in pulse rate, and shallow and rapid respirations; or bleeding, which may present as a decrease in blood pressure and increased pulse rate.

## ANORECTAL MANOMETRY

Anorectal manometry is indicated in patients with chronic constipation and/or fecal incontinence, after construction of a rectal pouch, before and after rectal surgery, in suspected scleroderma and dermatomyositis, and to rule out Hirschsprung's or Chagas' disease. It may be useful as a screening procedure in newborns with the meconium plug syndrome or with difficulty in passing stools. Anorectal manometry is also used as an operant conditioning technique to improve bowel control in patients with incontinence secondary to previous anorectal surgery, obstetrical trauma, spinal injury, irritable bowel syndrome, diabetic neuropathy, rectal prolapse, multiple sclerosis, scleroderma, or stroke.

Anorectal manometry is contraindicated in patients suffering from any severe or unstable medical or psychologic condition, infectious diarrhea, or anal or rectal disease.

Before the procedure, it is important to verify informed consent and to review the patient's medical and surgical history and results of the physician's physical examination. The patient should be encouraged to have a bowel movement before the procedure; a Fleet's enema may be administered if necessary. Baseline vital signs should be obtained and documented.

The equipment used for anorectal manometry consists of two pressure transducers, two balloons that are attached to a hollow metal cylinder, and a third balloon connected to a small catheter.

- An inner, doughnut-shaped balloon is positioned at the internal anal sphincter.
- An outer, pear-shaped balloon is placed at the external sphincter.
- The third balloon is passed through the hollow cylinder and positioned in the rectum, proximal to the inner balloon.

Alternatively, a perfused catheter system similar to the equipment used in esophageal manometry may be employed.

The test procedure consists of recording the reflex response of the two anorectal sphincters to transient distention of the rectal balloon. In most individuals, distention of the rectal balloon causes the internal sphincter to relax, while the external sphincter contracts to prevent defecation.

Anorectal manometry may also be used for biofeedback therapy in patients with fecal incontinence.* Such patients should be shown their baseline manometric tracings of external sphincter pressure and then should be instructed in the maneuver necessary to produce a rise in pressure on the tracing. Following this instruction, the patient should be asked to contract the external sphincter briefly whenever he or she perceives an increase in the distending volume in the rectal balloon. As appropriate responses are made, the distending volume in the rectal balloon should be decreased progressively, out of sight of the patient, until the patient responds appropriately to smaller volumes. After the initial instruction period the patient should be asked to apply the learned techniques consciously for 2 weeks whenever the sensation of fecal distention is felt. In addition, the patient should practice sphincter contrac-

---

* Also discussed in the SGNA *Manual of Gastrointestinal Procedures.*

tions 30 to 50 times a day for the first few weeks.

After anorectal manometry is completed, it is important to obtain and document vital signs and to check for rectal bleeding and abdominal distention. Potential complications of anorectal manometry include hemorrhage, perforation, and sepsis.

## PATIENT EDUCATION

Before any manometric procedure, it is important that the patient be fully informed. Patients should be advised of the following:

- The purpose of the test
- The positioning that will be used
- Effective relaxation methods
- The techniques to be used
- The approximate length of the procedure
- Sensations the patient is likely to experience
- The risks of the procedure
- The importance of patient cooperation

Patient education and comprehension should be documented. After the procedure, the physician may want to discuss the results of the test with the patient. The nurse should discuss and document postprocedural instructions and recommendations for follow-up care.

### CASE SITUATION

We met Doris Johnson in Chapter 14. She has suffered significantly with chest discomfort. She has heartburn, reflux of sour, bitter-tasting liquid up into her mouth, and she has even had several chest colds that her physician said were caused by the acid getting into her lungs at night. On upper endoscopy, she was found to have esophagitis. Mrs. Johnson says she has had trouble adhering to her antireflux regimen. She does not have the head of her bed up on blocks yet, but she has been sleeping on several pillows. She thought the pillows would be sufficient, but she admits that when she wakes up in the morning she has invariably rolled off the pillows. She is in the endoscopy department now for esophageal manometry.

### Points to think about

1. The gastroenterology nurse has set Mrs. Johnson up for her motility study. The equipment is all ready and the nurse is prepared to place the tube into her esophagus. Mrs. Johnson jumps up in alarm and says, "You mean you aren't going to put me to sleep like the last time?" How should the nurse respond?
2. What techniques might help the nurse pass the manometry tube successfully?
3. The nurse would expect that Mrs. Johnson has a hypotensive LES, which allows reflux of gastric

material into the esophagus. What else might be seen on the tracing?
4. There are two types of esophageal motility disorders: primary and secondary. What does that mean?

### Suggested responses

1. When Mrs. Johnson expresses surprise that she will not be sedated, the nurse might respond as follows:
   - Explain that this is not the same procedure she had before.
   - Explain that this test will determine how the muscles in her esophagus contract and that the sedating medication could affect the test by artificially relaxing those muscles.
   - Reassure Mrs. Johnson that the tube to be inserted through her nose is much smaller than an ordinary NG tube and that everything possible will be done to make her comfortable.
2. To help pass the manometry tube successfully, the nurse might:
   - Measure the tube to know how far to insert it. The manometry tube must pass through the esophagogastric junction into the stomach, with all of the lower side openings positioned below the diaphragm.
   - Have the patient remove her dentures, if any.
   - If the physician allows, anesthetize the inner nares with lidocaine (Xylocaine) jelly.
   - Ask Mrs. Johnson if she breathes better through one side of the nose. If so, that side should be tried first.
   - Listen to Mrs. Johnson if she says she has had problems in the past with NG tube insertion. Even if the nurse is an expert at passing tubes, listening and being compassionate fosters trust and confidence.
   - Advance the tube slowly and carefully around the back of the nose and into the back of the throat. The nurse must never push against an obstruction, and if one naris is obstructed, the other side should be tried. After some experience the nurse will know how to maneuver the tube from one side to the other, or up or down, or curl the tip to get around the back of the nose and throat.
   - When ready to enter the esophagus, the nurse should have the patient bend her head forward and swallow. This causes the epiglottis to open the esophagus and close the trachea. Unless there is suspicion of achalasia or other obstruction, it is usually permissible for the patient to take a few sips of water.
   - Once the patient is able to swallow, the tube usually passes easily into the stomach. If any obstructions are met, the nurse should stop and check tube placement on the manometry machine. If the tube is pushed against a lower esophageal obstruction, it will curl back on itself.

- If the patient gags inordinately, it may be a good idea to have another nurse sit by the patient to calm her and coach her while the tube goes down.

3. In addition to a hypotensive LES, the nurse might expect to see a secondary spasm of the esophagus. Reflux of gastric contents into the esophagus is usually caustic to the esophageal mucosa, causing esophagitis. In turn, esophagitis can cause secondary spasm of the esophagus, which can be painful. On manometry, DES may show normal peristalsis interspersed with simultaneous contractions, often of high amplitude and prolonged duration. These contractions may be repetitive and there is usually an incomplete relaxation of the LES.

4. Primary motility disorders are those that involve only the esophagus, such as achalasia, DES, nutcracker esophagus, hypertensive LES, and nonspecific esophageal motility disorders. Secondary motility disorders occur when the esophagus is affected as part of a more generalized disease process, such as diabetes mellitus, scleroderma, or chronic idiopathic pseudo-obstruction.

---

## REVIEW TERMS

**Bernstein test, edrophonium chloride, manometry, physiograph, pressure transducer, rapid pull-through, solid-state catheters, station pull-through, water-infusion catheter**

---

## REVIEW QUESTIONS

1. The function of a pressure transducer is to:
   a. Convert electrical signals to pressure readings.
   b. Convert pressure changes to electrical signals.
   c. Record ink tracings that represent gastrointestinal motility.
   d. Apply pressure to the GI tract.
2. Esophageal manometry is contraindicated in patients with:
   a. Dysphagia.
   b. Recent gastric or esophageal surgery.
   c. Diabetes mellitus.
   d. Noncardiac chest pain.
3. Compared to water-infusion systems, the transducers used in solid-state manometry catheters are:
   a. Larger.
   b. Less expensive.
   c. More difficult to repair.
   d. More reliable.
4. If one of the recording channels shows unusually rapid activity during an esophageal motility study, this is most likely a result of:
   a. Esophageal spasm.
   b. Pull-through is too rapid.
   c. A malfunctioning transducer.
   d. Cardiac interference.
5. Motility of the esophageal body is best assessed while the patient:
   a. Performs a series of wet swallows.
   b. Performs a series of dry swallows.
   c. Takes a series of deep breaths.
   d. Holds his or her breath and does not swallow.
6. The Bernstein test is used to:
   a. Stimulate esophageal peristalsis.
   b. Calibrate the pressure transducers.
   c. Reproduce chest pain that may be a result of acid reflux in the esophagus.
   d. Reproduce chest pain that may be a result of esophageal spasm.
7. Aperistalsis of the esophageal body and incomplete relaxation of the LES are manometric symptoms associated with:
   a. Achalasia.
   b. Diffuse esophageal spasm.
   c. Nutcracker esophagus.
   d. Nonspecific esophageal motility disorders.
8. Manometric manifestations of advanced scleroderma include:
   a. Simultaneous and repetitive esophageal contractions.
   b. Aperistalsis in the distal esophageal body and low to absent LES pressure.
   c. Abnormally high resting LES pressure.
   d. A mean contraction amplitude at least two standard deviations above normal.
9. Anticholinergic drugs and opiates are not used before manometric procedures primarily because they can:
   a. Make the patient nauseous.
   b. Sedate the patient.
   c. Change the patient's breathing pattern.
   d. Alter gastrointestinal motility.
10. In anorectal manometric studies of normal subjects, distention of the rectal balloon causes the external anal sphincter to:
    a. Spasm.
    b. Relax.
    c. Contract.
    d. No change in sphincter pressure.

## BIBLIOGRAPHY

Arndorfer, R. "Techniques of Esophageal Manometry." In *SGA Journal Reprints,* ed. Trivits, S, 47-48. Rochester, N.Y.: Society of Gastrointestinal Assistants, 1988.

Carlson, L, and Anderson, B. "Sphincter of Oddi Dysfunction: A Cause of Biliary Obstruction." In *SGA Journal Reprints,* ed. Trivits, S, 101-04. Rochester, N.Y.: Society of Gastrointestinal Assistants, 1988.

Castell, D, Richter, J, and Dalton, C, eds. *Esophageal Motility Testing.* New York: Elsevier, 1987.

Chobanian, S, and Van Ness, M, eds. *Manual of Clinical Problems in Gastroenterology.* Boston: Little, Brown & Co., 1988.

Chopra, S, and May, R, eds. *Pathophysiology of Gastrointestinal Diseases.* Boston: Little, Brown, & Co., 1989.

Dalton, C, Richter, J, and Castell, D. "Esophageal Manometry." In *Journal Reprints II,* ed. Trivits, S, 52-55. Rochester, N.Y.: Society of Gastroenterology Nurses and Associates, 1990.

Hardick, M, and Beck, M, eds. *Manual of Gastrointestinal Procedures.* 2nd ed. Rochester, N.Y.: Society of Gastroenterology Nurses and Associates, 1989.

Sachar, D, Waye, J, and Lewis, B, eds. *Gastroenterology for the House Officer.* Baltimore: Williams & Wilkins, 1989.

Silverman, A, and Roy, C. *Pediatric Clinical Gastroenterology.* 3rd ed. St. Louis: Mosby–Year Book, 1983.

Sleisenger, M, and Fordtran, J, eds. *Gastrointestinal Disease: Pathophysiology, Diagnosis, Management.* 4th ed. Philadelphia: W.B. Saunders, 1989.

Stachner, G, Kiss, A, and Wiesnagrotzki, S. "Oesophageal and Gastric Motility Disorders in Patients Categorized as Having Primary Anorexia Nervosa." *Gut* 27(1986): 1120-26.

# Chapter 26

# LAPAROSCOPY

This chapter will acquaint the gastroenterology nurse with the use of laparoscopy (peritoneoscopy) in the diagnosis of gastrointestinal disease.* General indications and contraindications for laparoscopy are outlined, followed by descriptions of the equipment used and methods employed in the care and cleaning of this equipment. The general procedure followed in laparoscopic visualization of gastrointestinal structures is also outlined, and patient care considerations before, during, and after the procedure are discussed.

## Learning objectives

After reviewing the content of this chapter, the gastroenterology nurse should be able to:
1. List indications and contraindications for laparoscopy in gastroenterology patients.
2. Describe the basic equipment and techniques used in laparoscopy.
3. Discuss patient care and patient education considerations that are applicable to gastroenterology patients who are undergoing laparoscopy.

## BASIC PRINCIPLES

**Laparoscopy,** also known as **peritoneoscopy,** makes use of specialized equipment for direct visualization of the structures and organs within the abdominal cavity, and for biopsy of suspicious intraabdominal tissue. The procedure involves the introduction of a fiberoptic **laparoscope** through the anterior abdominal wall under local or general anesthesia. Laparoscopic procedures often permit the physician to make a specific diagnosis

without incurring the risks associated with general anesthesia or exploratory laparotomy.

## INDICATIONS

Laparoscopy provides a view of the anterior and superior surfaces of the liver and the gallbladder, the spleen and omental surfaces, and the mesentery. It is estimated that 80% of the surface of the liver can be inspected laparoscopically; the left hepatic lobe and the left portion of the right lobe are most easily seen. Areas that cannot be readily visualized include the dome and the most lateral segment of the right lobe of the liver, and retroperitoneal structures and the porta hepatis.

The major indication for laparoscopy is usually evaluation of hepatic disease to help exclude malignancy, assess benign disease, or follow up on abnormal hepatic imaging studies. It may also be used to evaluate suspected peritoneal disease or to stage lymphomas, including Hodgkin's disease or non-Hodgkin's lymphoma. Less common indications include chronic abdominal pain, intraabdominal masses, pancreatic disease, and assessment of the operability of patients with neoplasms. A definitive diagnosis is possible in more than 90% of patients with ascites, focal liver disease, and abdominal masses, but the success rate is much lower in patients with chronic abdominal disease.

### Liver disease

Laparoscopy should be considered when abnormal laboratory data or hepatomegaly suggest the possibility of liver metastases, or when results of screening with ultrasonography (US) or computed tomography (CT scan) are inconclusive. Among the applications of laparoscopy in the evaluation of liver disease are the following:
- Detection of visible metastases as small as a few millimeters in diameter, both on the liver surface

* Laparoscopy is also discussed in the SGNA *Manual of Gastrointestinal Procedures,* 2nd ed, Rochester, N.Y. Society of Gastroenterology Nurses and Associates, 1989.

and on the **peritoneum.** Once identified, these lesions may undergo biopsy examination under direct vision.

- Identification of subcapsular tumor masses through location of a visible bulge on the liver surface.
- Selection of a biopsy site that is away from large surface vessels in the case of hypervascular tumors.
- Determination of the extent of the tumor in the hepatocellular carcinoma and the condition of the uninvolved portion of the liver, thus aiding in an assessment of its resectability.

### Hodgkin's disease and non-Hodgkin's lymphomas

Laparoscopy may eliminate the need for **laparotomy** in patients being staged for Hodgkin's disease. In staging Hodgkin's disease, visible tumor implants on the liver surface should be examined by biopsy under direct vision. If no such lesions exist, multiple biopsy specimens should be obtained from various sites in both hepatic lobes. Fewer than 10% of patients with negative laparoscopic biopsies are found to have hepatic Hodgkin's disease on wedge biopsy obtained at subsequent laparotomy. In staging non-Hodgkin's lymphoma, on the other hand, about half of the patients with negative laparoscopic biopsies have positive surgical wedge biopsies, which show only rare, focal lymphomatous involvement of portal areas.

Laparoscopy is also useful for repeated abdominal examinations to evaluate the effects of treatment on liver metastases in patients with previously documented Hodgkin's disease and non-Hodgkin's lymphoma.

### CONTRAINDICATIONS

Laparoscopy is contraindicated in each of the following:

- Uncooperative patients
- Severe hemostatic abnormalities
- Advanced cardiac or respiratory disease
- Acute bacterial peritonitis or a history of peritonitis
- Intestinal obstruction
- Infections of the abdominal wall
- Tense ascites (relative)
- Previous surgery that may have caused abdominal adhesions

### EQUIPMENT

The equipment used for laparoscopic procedures includes the laparoscope, a cannula with a trumpet valve, a **Verres needle,** and a **trocar** (Fig. 26-1). If a biopsy will be performed, biopsy forceps and/or a liver biopsy needle, such as a Tru-Cut needle, will be required. Additional equipment needed for the procedure includes an insufflator with tubing, a light source, carbon dioxide or nitrous oxide for **insufflation,** and a preheater for the laparoscope and insertion cannula.

During set-up of the sterile equipment before the procedure, each piece should be inspected as the

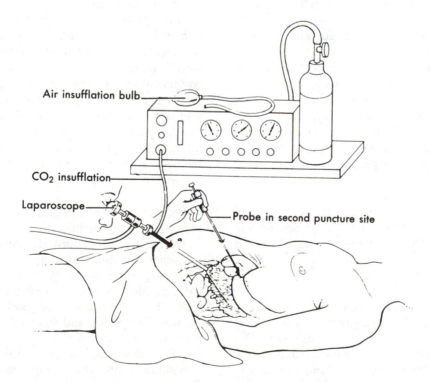

**Fig. 26-1.** Entrance site, field of view, and instrument setup for laparoscopy.

equipment is assembled. A defogger should be put on the lens and eyepiece. The laparoscope lens must be clear and the lens seal must fit well. There should be no perforations in the light carrier. Seals on the trocar and cannula must fit well and should be replaced when worn. The trumpet valve should be disassembled, lubricated with silicone, and then reassembled. The teaching attachment should be checked, if one is used.

After use, all of the parts should be washed meticulously with a detergent solution according to the manufacturer's instructions, rinsed well, dried, and sent for ethylene oxide gas sterilization and aeration.

## PREPROCEDURAL ASSESSMENT AND CARE

Laparoscopy is usually performed as an inpatient procedure, and coagulation studies and cross-matching have usually been performed ahead of time. The patient should have fasted overnight. Before beginning the procedure, it is important to verify the following:

- The patient's signed informed consent
- The length of his or her NPO status
- The patient's medical history, including past surgery, allergies, current medications, and information pertaining to the current complaint
- Laboratory results, informing the physician if the patient is on anticoagulation therapy or nonsteroidal antiinflammatory drugs (NSAIDs), or if the laboratory results are abnormal in any way
- Completion of a bowel preparation

It is also important that the nurse obtain baseline vital signs, establish a patent IV line, have the patient empty his or her bladder, and shave the abdomen if there is excessive hair growth.

Also before the procedure, the patient should be informed of the purpose of the procedure; type of positioning to be used; the use of restraints, if any; anticipated effects of anesthesia; techniques to be used; and any sensations the patient may experience during and after the procedure. The nurse should also document patient teaching and the patient's comprehension.

The sterile laparoscope and sometimes the sterile insertion tube should be placed in the preheater. All valves, needles, and gauges on the insufflator unit should be checked. It is important that all pieces of the insufflation set fit snugly to prevent leakage of the gas during the procedure.

## PROCEDURE

For the procedure itself, the patient is positioned on the table in a supine position, using restraints as needed. The patient is sedated by slow IV injection. The abdomen is exposed and cleansed with a skin preparation fluid and sterile drapes are placed in position. The insertion site on the anterior abdominal wall is anesthetized.

Once the anterior abdominal wall is suitably anesthetized, a Verres needle is inserted at the insertion site through a 1-cm incision made from the skin through the subcutaneous tissue. Aspiration is performed to rule out the possibility of intestinal or large vessel perforation. To separate the anterior abdominal wall from the organs, either nitrous oxide or carbon dioxide is instilled into the abdominal cavity. An insufflation apparatus and sterile attachments deliver the gas intraabdominally, using a sterile Verres needle connected to polyethylene tubing that is attached to the insufflator. Usually, 2 to 3 L of gas produce adequate distention. The insufflation unit can then be set to "automatic" to maintain the desired pressure throughout the examination. Gauges on the insufflator that indicate the amount of gas injected into the cavity are carefully monitored by the endoscopist and the circulating nurse.

**Pneumoperitoneum,** or the presence of gas in the peritoneal cavity, causes the abdomen to become distended and tympanitic, providing free space for safe insertion of the examining cannula and its trocar. At this time, the incision is enlarged, the Verres needle is removed, and the laparoscopic trocar and cannula are inserted through the incision. The trocar is removed, and the preheated laparoscope is inserted through the cannula. The fiber-optic light guide and insufflation tube are attached. A full examination of the liver, gallbladder, pancreas, omentum, and pelvis may now be made for diagnostic purposes. Fogging of the lens may occur during the procedure.

If malignant disease is suspected, a biopsy examination of the liver or peritoneum is required. A second site is anesthetized and a trocar and sleeve are inserted. The trocar is withdrawn and a biopsy needle or other equipment may be inserted through the sleeve. A long biopsy needle may be inserted through the abdominal wall at a point near the proposed biopsy site. The needle can be guided under direct vision into the area of interest. The specimen thus obtained is expelled from the needle into a specimen container for transfer to the histopathology department. It is important that all specimens be properly handled, preserved, and labeled. The site of internal biopsy may be inspected for evidence of secondary hemorrhage.

During the procedure the scrub nurse assists the physician and maintains aseptic technique, and the circulating nurse monitors the patient's condition, provides emotional support, gives additional medications as ordered, and observes the patient for hypotension, vasovagal response, and signs or symptoms of perforation or hemorrhage.

After the examination is completed, the laparoscope is withdrawn and the pneumoperitoneum is reduced. The incision sites are closed in two layers, both insertion sites are cleaned, and simple dressings are applied. If ascites is present, additional pressure dressings are required.

## POSTPROCEDURAL ASSESSMENT AND CARE

After the procedure is completed, the patient should be reassured and made comfortable. It is important to monitor and document the patient's vital signs, observe for shoulder or subcostal discomfort, bleeding, signs and symptoms of peritonitis, and abdominal pain. Intravenous fluids should be continued as ordered. A verbal report must be provided to the nurse who is responsible for further patient care. The patient should be evaluated 6 to 24 hours before discharge as per the physician's orders.

## POTENTIAL COMPLICATIONS

Laparoscopy is completed safely and successfully in more than 90% of cases. According to retrospective studies reported in the literature, the minor complication rate is approximately 1%, the major complication rate is 0.3%, and the mortality rate is approximately 0.03%. Even though a recent prospective study suggested that these rates may be higher, the complication rates for laparoscopy still compare favorably with other methods of direct visualization, especially exploratory laparotomy.

The most important major complications experienced by patients undergoing laparoscopic procedures are bleeding and perforation. Minor complications include ascites leakage, abdominal pain and discomfort, dehiscence, hematoma, subcutaneous emphysema, cellulitis, ileus, and hypotension.

Abdominal discomfort is common after laparoscopy and is usually caused by residual gaseous distention. Manipulation of adhesions during the procedure can also be painful. More persistent pain and symptoms of shock suggest bleeding from a biopsy site or the development of a hematoma within the peritoneal ligaments or mesentery. Hypotension and shock suggest that more severe hemorrhage has occurred. In such cases, the physician must be informed.

---

**CASE SITUATION**

---

Mr. Robert Allen, age 66, had cardiac bypass surgery 10 years ago and unfortunately contracted hepatitis C (non-A, non-B hepatitis) from blood transfusions. Since then, he has bled from esophageal varices and has undergone sclerotherapy. Recently he has had upper right epigastric pain and tenderness. He has had a negative US and CT scan. His physician performs a laparoscopy and biopsy of a suspicious lesion on the liver. Mr. Allen is diagnosed as having hepatocellular carcinoma.

*Points to think about*

1. A percutaneous liver biopsy is an easier, less expensive method of obtaining a liver biopsy sample. Why would the physician perform a laparoscopy?
2. What atypical symptoms of cirrhosis would lead the nurse to suspect further pathologic process, which laparoscopy might help to diagnose?
3. The gastroenterology nurse is accustomed to seeing laparoscopy done in the operating room. Can this procedure be done in the endoscopy suite?
4. One nursing diagnosis for patients undergoing laparoscopy would certainly be "anxiety related to a knowledge deficit of the procedure." What can the nurse tell Mr. Allen to help relieve his anxiety?

*Suggested responses*

1. Reasons that the physician might perform laparoscopy instead of a percutaneous liver biopsy examination include the following:
   - Percutaneous liver biopsies may only be accurate in 49% of patients. Ultrasonography can be diagnostic, but results are often based on the skill of the operator. Newer CT scanners can detect lesions in the 1- to 2-cm range.
   - The accuracy of laparoscopy in malignant liver disease ranges from 70% to 90%. Because the liver is actually visualized, the specificity is very high.
   - A directed or targeted biopsy sample is much easier to obtain during laparoscopy.
   - Laparoscopy can differentiate a hepatocellular carcinoma from regenerative nodules of cirrhosis.
2. Atypical symptoms of cirrhosis that might lead the nurse to suspect further pathology might include any of the following:
   - Abdominal pain and/or tenderness. This is an unusual finding in uncomplicated cirrhosis and may indicate a hepatic neoplasm.
   - Prolonged fever. In a patient with cirrhosis, prolonged fever may be associated with an inflammation of the gallbladder, peritoneal inflammation, or hepatic tumor.
   - Deep, prolonged jaundice. Mild jaundice may vary in intensity in cirrhosis, but deep, prolonged jaundice may indicate cholestasis or a primary or metastatic tumor.
   - Hepatomegaly. Even though it is seen in cirrhosis, a markedly enlarged liver may mean a hepatocarcinoma in conjunction with the cirrhosis.
3. Laparoscopy can be safely done in the endoscopy suite. There are no published statistics indicating an increase in infection rate for laparoscopy performed in an endoscopy room. The gastroenterology nurse must have a thorough knowledge of aseptic technique, and all equipment must be sterile. The

patient's abdomen must be given a thorough surgical preparation, but shaving is not usually necessary. All participants must don surgical attire, including gown, sterile gloves, masks, and hair covers.

Laparoscopy can be done with local anesthesia and mild conscious sedation or with general anesthesia. However, the risk of general anesthesia equals the risk of laparoscopy, and the patient may need to be awake to cooperate with the physician in performing some maneuvers.

4. To relieve Mr. Allen's anxiety, the nurse might:
- Tell him that the procedure takes about an hour, and that he may be in the hospital overnight. (Some laparoscopies are done on an outpatient basis.)
- Explain the preprocedural tests that may be done and why they are necessary. Routine blood work may be ordered, along with a chest radiograph and electrocardiogram (ECG). It is also important to know the bleeding time and ascertain any problem with clotting. The nurse's assessment should include questions about any bleeding tendency in the patient and/or his family.
- Assure the patient that he will receive some sedation and explain whether it will be local or general.
- Tell the patient that he may experience some pain at the puncture site. Patients may also experience shoulder pain, which can result from elevation of the diaphragm during carbon dioxide or air insufflation. This pain is usually mild and is treated with analgesics; it subsides in a few days.
- Explain the preparatory stages and assure the patient that he will be informed of each step in the procedure and what sensations he may expect. Routine enemas are not necessary unless the patient has been constipated, but he should empty his bladder before the procedure.
- Teach the patient any maneuvers he will be asked to perform during the procedure, such as a Valsalva maneuver with the spine pressed flat against the table.
- Inform the patient of what to expect after the procedure. Most patients are encouraged to ambulate once the sedation has worn off enough to make it safe. Patients who have had a liver biopsy during the procedure are kept on bed rest for 24 hours and vital signs are closely monitored. Activity may be restricted for 2 to 7 days. Patients can usually shower with the puncture site covered. Stitches are removed in 5 to 7 days.

## REVIEW TERMS

insufflation, laparoscope, laparoscopy, laparotomy, peritoneoscopy, peritoneum, pneumoperitoneum, trocar, Verres needle

## REVIEW QUESTIONS

1. Laparoscopy is generally performed under:
   a. Epidural anesthesia.
   b. No anesthesia.
   c. General anesthesia.
   d. Local anesthesia and conscious sedation.
2. The abdominal organ that is least visible during laparoscopy is the:
   a. Left lobe of the liver.
   b. Right lobe of the liver.
   c. Pancreas.
   d. Gall bladder.
3. The major indication for laparoscopy in gastroenterology patients is:
   a. Chronic abdominal pain.
   b. Pancreatic disease.
   c. Hepatic disease.
   d. Peritonitis.
4. Laparoscopy is contraindicated in patients with:
   a. Hodgkin's disease.
   b. Pancreatitis.
   c. Abdominal adhesions from previous surgery.
   d. Liver metastases.
5. The laparoscope is sterilized by using:
   a. Ethylene oxide.
   b. Glutaraldehyde.
   c. Steam.
   d. Hydrogen peroxide.
6. The surgical position used for laparoscopy is the:
   a. Supine position.
   b. Prone position.
   c. Lithotomy position.
   d. Trendelenburg position.
7. In patients undergoing a laparoscopic procedure, the purpose of the first incision is insertion of the:
   a. Trocar and cannula.
   b. Laparoscope.
   c. Menghini needle.
   d. Verres needle.
8. Distention of the abdomen before laparoscopy usually requires intraabdominal infusion of how much gas?
   a. 1 L.
   b. 2 to 3 L.
   c. 5 L.
   d. 500 ml.
9. The lens of the laparoscope may become fogged during the procedure. This may be avoided by:
   a. Cleaning the lens with lens wax.
   b. Sterilizing the lens with glutaraldehyde.
   c. Using a defogger.
   d. Wiping the lens with 70% alcohol.
10. One of the rare major complications of laparoscopy is:
    a. Perforation.

b. Abdominal discomfort.
c. Residual gaseous distention.
d. Hypotension.

## BIBLIOGRAPHY

Hardick, M, and Beck, M, eds. *Manual of Gastrointestinal Procedures.* 2nd ed. Rochester, N.Y.: Society of Gastroenterology Nurses and Associates, 1989.

Kneedler, J, and Dodge, G. *Perioperative Patient Care: The Nursing Perspective.* 2nd ed. Boston: Blackwell Scientific Publications, Inc., 1987.

Langfitt, D. *Critical Care: Certification Preparation and Review.* Bowie, Md.: Brady Communications, 1984.

Ravenscroft, M, and Swan, C. *Gastrointestinal Endoscopy and Related Procedures: A Handbook for Nurses and Assistants.* Baltimore: Williams & Wilkins, 1984.

Sivak, M. *Gastroenterologic Endoscopy.* Philadelphia: W.B. Saunders, 1987.

Sleisenger, M, and Fordtran, J, eds. *Gastrointestinal Disease: Pathophysiology, Diagnosis, Management.* 4th ed. Philadelphia: W.B. Saunders, 1989.

# Chapter 27

# BIOPSY AND CYTOLOGY

This chapter will acquaint the gastroenterology nurse with the techniques used to obtain biopsy samples, cell cultures, and cytology specimens for the diagnosis of gastrointestinal disease.* Endoscopic methods used to obtain biopsy specimens from the esophagus, stomach, small bowel, and colorectum are detailed. Procedures for percutaneous liver biopsy and pancreatic fine-needle aspiration are outlined, in addition to techniques for suction biopsies of the small bowel and rectum. Methods employed in the collection of tissue specimens for cell culture and cytologic analysis are also explored.

**Learning objectives**

After reviewing the content of this chapter, the gastroenterology nurse should be able to:

1. Describe the techniques used for endoscopic biopsy of the esophagus, stomach, small bowel, and colorectum, including indications, contraindications, potential complications, and patient care and patient education considerations.
2. Explain the techniques that are used for percutaneous liver biopsy, fine-needle aspiration of the pancreas, and suction biopsy of the small bowel and rectum.
3. Discuss the methods used in gastroenterology for the collection of specimens for cell culture and cytology.

**BASIC PRINCIPLES**

**Biopsy** and **cytology** both allow direct sampling of gastrointestinal tissue for diagnostic purposes. Biopsy involves excision of pieces of living tissue from a suspected pathologic site, with subsequent **histopathologic analysis** in the laboratory. Specimens may be obtained either by using biopsy forceps that are passed through the biopsy channel of an endoscope or by using a suction method (e.g., small bowel or rectal suction biopsy) or a needle that is inserted percutaneously (e.g., percutaneous liver or pancreatic fine-needle aspiration). Liver biopsy specimens may also be obtained surgically or laparoscopically, as described in Chapter 26.

Specimens for cell culture or cytologic analysis may be obtained either endoscopically, by using brushings, or by using **washing** and/or **aspiration** techniques.

**ENDOSCOPIC BIOPSY**

Endoscopic biopsy is indicated when there is a suspicion of abnormal mucosal tissue or for confirmation of normal tissue in any portion of the GI tract. It is contraindicated in patients with severe coagulopathy or active bleeding. A current bleeding profile should be obtained, if clinically indicated. Caution must be exercised in patients who are currently using anticoagulants, or who have recently ingested nonsteroidal antiinflammatory drugs (NSAIDs) or medications containing acetylsalicylic acid (aspirin), unless bleeding time is verified as normal. Ideally, patients should discontinue ingestion of aspirin and NSAIDs for one week before endoscopic biopsy.

To obtain an endoscopic biopsy specimen, an endoscope is inserted into the esophagus, stomach, small bowel, or colon, as described in Chapter 24. Once the endoscope is in place, biopsy forceps are passed down the biopsy channel.

A whole range of **biopsy forceps** are available, with different-shaped jaws and sometimes a central spike or bayonet. The most common biopsy forceps are simple

---

* All techniques in this chapter, except fine-needle aspiration of the pancreas, are also discussed in the SGNA *Manual of Gastrointestinal Procedures.* 2nd ed. Rochester, N.Y.: Society of Gastroenterology Nurses and Associates, 1989.

cupped forceps, but elongated or even fenestrated types, with smooth or dentate edges, are available. Forceps with a central spike can be especially helpful to hold the tissue in place and prevent the forceps from slipping so an accurate biopsy specimen can be taken. Jumbo forceps can be used with large-channel scopes to obtain larger pieces of tissue.

Electrocoagulating, or **"hot," biopsy forceps** are used to coagulate tissue when the patient is at an increased risk of bleeding. Hot forceps are insulated by a nonconducting sheath. An active cord connects the handle of the forceps to the cautery unit. The sheath on these forceps also decreases friction in the biopsy channel, thereby allowing the forceps to pass more readily. Because of the thin wall of the right colon and the greater risk of perforation, care should be taken when using hot biopsy forceps in this location.

Once the forceps are in place, the nurse opens and closes the forceps, in response to the physician's request. The act of closing the forceps and pulling on the tissue tears off a specimen of the target tissue. The specimen is then retrieved by bringing the biopsy forceps out through the channel of the endoscope. As the forceps are withdrawn, the shaft should be wiped with a gauze sponge to remove secretions.

In most cases the accuracy of histopathologic interpretation of endoscopic biopsy specimens can be improved by obtaining multiple specimens of the suspicious area. Specimens should be prepared according to institutional policy, and the container should be labeled with patient information and the site of the biopsy.

If immediate denial or confirmation of malignancy is required, the endoscopic biopsy specimen, in the form of a **frozen section,** may be sent to the laboratory for immediate microscopic examination by a pathologist. No fixative of any kind is used for frozen sections. Instead, the specimen is placed on mounting material, labeled, and immediately taken to the laboratory.

After use, reusable forceps should be cleaned and steam-sterilized, in accordance with SGNA infection control guidelines. Disposable biopsy forceps are also available.

Excessive bleeding or perforation are the most likely complications of endoscopic biopsy. After the procedure is completed, the patient should be instructed to notify the physician of signs and symptoms of bleeding.

### Endoscopic esophageal biopsy

Endoscopic biopsy of the esophagus is indicated for the diagnosis of mucosal abnormalities in the esophagus, such as a radiologically demonstrated stricture or suspected carcinoma. It may be used to look for evidence of Barrett's esophagus in patients with esophageal reflux or, in children, to verify esophagitis.

When radiologic interpretation identifies a stricture as benign, endoscopy with multiple biopsies and brush cytology are also recommended to rule out any possibility of malignancy.

To correctly diagnose esophageal cancer, it is important to dilate any strictured lesion sufficiently to allow passage of the endoscope down to its distal margin. Numerous biopsy specimens should be obtained from tissue that is clearly abnormal but not necrotic. Specimens for cytology may be obtained by using a sheathed disposable brush that is inserted through the endoscope. Brush cytology can also be helpful in some cases.

Esophageal biopsy specimens from patients with chronic esophageal reflux often show thickening of the esophageal squamous epithelium. Findings of polymorphonuclear leukocytes and ulceration in esophageal biopsy specimens also provide strong support for a diagnosis of acute esophagitis.

### Endoscopic gastric biopsy

Endoscopic biopsy is indicated in the diagnosis of gastric mucosal abnormalities associated with chronic gastritis, gastric polyps, carcinoma, or gastric ulcers. In addition, biopsy specimens may be used for the diagnosis of *Helicobacter pylori* infections.

All polyps of the stomach should be examined by endoscopic biopsy. The biopsy technique used depends on the type and size of the protruding lesion. If possible, polyps should be removed endoscopically. If polyps cannot be removed, biopsies should be performed. Adenomatous polyps, large hyperplastic polyps, and any polyp with a stalk should be removed by using an endoscopic snare technique, as described in Chapter 32.

Endoscopic visualization is not sufficient for a definitive diagnosis of gastric cancer; a biopsy should be performed in all suspect cases. Most neoplasms of the stomach are adenocarcinomas. For patients with suspected gastric adenocarcinoma, the appearance of the lesion can be assessed, a biopsy of the lesion can be performed, and the lesion brushed for cytology. Biopsies of the ulcer edges are necessary to be certain whether or not the lesion is cancerous. It is possible to detect lesions as small as 2 to 3 mm in diameter, and to obtain a histologic diagnosis.

For submucosal tumors, the mucosa overlying the tumor can be lifted off with biopsy forceps, but this will not always provide a positive diagnosis for the tumor itself. To obtain submucosal tissue, a large-particle biopsy, hot biopsy, or a lift-and-cut biopsy employing a snare may be used. Needle biopsy may also be used to aspirate tissue from submucosal nodules.

The benign appearance of a gastric ulcer should always be confirmed by multiple biopsies and **exfoliative brush cytology** (Fig. 27-1). When endoscopy is performed, six to ten biopsy specimens should be obtained in a circumferential pattern from the ulcer margin.

In patients with suspected *H. pylori* infections, the specimen may be obtained by using standard biopsy forceps from the dependent portion of the antrum, along the greater curvature. The sample can then be inserted into an agar gel test kit that contains urea, a pH indicator, buffers, and a bacteriostatic agent. A rapid color change indicates the presence of the urease enzyme typically produced by *H. pylori.* Tissue may also be sent to the pathology lab and stained for *Helicobacter;* the gastroenterology nurse should request either a silver stain (Warthin) or a hematoxylin and eosin (H & E) stain.

After an endoscopic gastric biopsy, the patient should be observed for signs and symptoms of complications such as bleeding and perforation, including abdominal pain, tenderness, distention, nausea, vomiting, chills, hypotension, or temperature elevation.

**Endoscopic small bowel biopsy**

Small bowel biopsy is a simple technique that provides important diagnostic information. Small bowel biopsies can be obtained in two ways, either endoscopically, using biopsy forceps, or by suction biopsy, using a capsule or a multipurpose biopsy tube (**Rubin tube** or **Quinton tube**) that is passed orally under fluoroscopic guidance. The direct visualization that is permitted by endoscopic biopsy is advantageous in patients with focal disease.

Small bowel biopsy is indicated for the differential diagnosis of malabsorption syndromes and other entities that are responsible for chronic diarrhea or weight loss. A diagnosis of celiac sprue, for instance, should never be made without a biopsy. Diseases such as intestinal lymphangiectasia, agammaglobulinemia, and Whipple's disease also give rise to highly specific lesions. Small

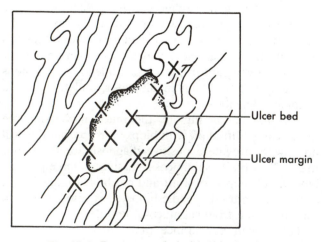

**Fig. 27-1**. Recommended ulcer biopsy sites.

bowel biopsy is also useful for obtaining tissue to check for *Giardia.*

Requirements for small bowel biopsies to be of maximum diagnostic value include the following:
- Precise localization of the biopsy site
- Proper orientation and prompt fixation of biopsy specimens
- Careful study of serial sections of the central half or two thirds of each biopsy specimen
- Obtaining the specimen from the region of the duodenal-jejunal junction, in the area of the ligament of Treitz

**Endoscopic colorectal biopsy**

Although colonoscopy permits visualization of the entire inner surface of the colon, mucosal biopsy is often necessary to arrive at a specific diagnosis. Colonic biopsies of the mucosa and colonic lesions are obtained routinely for diagnostic purposes. The main advantages of taking biopsy specimens through an endoscope are the ability to sample the entire colon and to precisely target the area of interest. In addition, multiple specimens are easily obtained endoscopically.

It is important to note that significant and potentially diagnostic abnormalities may be present in tissue obtained by colorectal biopsy, despite a normal endoscopic appearance of the mucosa. Colorectal biopsies are indicated in the following situations:
- Suspected collagenous or microscopic colitis in middle-age women with unexplained, chronic non-bloody diarrhea and grossly normal colonic mucosa.
- Suspected neoplastic lesions of the rectum and sigmoid colon.
- Suspected Crohn's disease, in which the typical mucosal biopsy shows a focal ulcerative and inflammatory process, rather than the diffuse abnormality seen with ulcerative colitis. Histologic documentation of granulomatous inflammation of bowel mucosa argues strongly for a diagnosis of Crohn's disease, particularly when discrete noncaseating granulomas are found and other causes of granulomatous disease have been excluded.
- Suspected ulcerative colitis, which is characterized by inflammation of the colonic mucosa, with changes ranging from mild degrees of inflammation to microscopic erosions of the epithelium and crypt abscesses. A complete colonoscopy with biopsy is especially useful when prior sigmoidoscopic findings are equivocal.
- As an adjunct to cultures and smears of rectal mucosa for detecting an infectious process in men and women who engage in anal intercourse and may be at risk for AIDS. Mucosal biopsy in such patients may demonstrate focal crypt epithelial cell degen-

eration, which has been described as a characteristic pathologic feature in AIDS. When doing a culture for AIDS-related diseases, the tissue should be examined for cytomegalovirus (CMV), herpes, cryptosporidium, *Micrococcus,* and amoeba.

- Suspected Hirschsprung's disease. The deeper specimens provided by rectal suction biopsy are particularly useful for a definitive diagnosis of Hirschsprung's disease, which requires demonstration of an absence of ganglia in Meissner's plexus.
- Diagnosis of a suspected neural lipidoses and patients with unexplained signs of a degenerative nervous system disorder. Morphologic and histochemical staining characteristics of the biopsy specimen can help diagnose certain neural diseases, including Niemann-Pick disease, amaurotic idiocies like Tay-Sachs disease, and Hurler's syndrome.
- Schistosomiasis, in which the eggs of the parasite can be identified in a squash preparation of the mucosal specimen.
- Amebiasis, in which volcano-like lesions are seen; the center of the volcano may have organisms.
- Assessment of progress in patients who are undergoing therapy.

To provide useful diagnostic information from a colorectal biopsy specimen, the following activities should be performed:

- The intestinal location of the biopsy specimens must be clearly defined by anatomic area (e.g., rectum, descending colon, splenic flexure). Centimeter designation is not usually accurate, especially if that number is used to find that location a second time.
- Labeled, separate containers must be used for tissue specimens from different biopsy sites.
- Multiple sections should be made of all specimens and thoroughly examined.

## SMALL BOWEL SUCTION BIOPSY

**Suction biopsy** has been proved safe, provided there is no tendency to bleed. In addition, the tube can be positioned rapidly and is easily visualized fluoroscopically. Compared to endoscopic biopsies, suction biopsies of the small bowel can be larger, easier to orient, and less traumatized. In addition, suction biopsies can avoid the more proximal duodenum, where Brunner's glands and lymphoid follicles are abundant and potentially complicate histologic interpretation. The procedure can be performed on an outpatient basis and is particularly valuable in the evaluation of patients with malabsorption syndromes.

Small bowel biopsy is diagnostic in Whipple's disease, agammaglobulinemia and severe hypogammaglobulinemia, and abetalipoproteinemia.

It *may* be diagnostic in any of the following:
- Intestinal lymphoma
- Intestinal lymphangiectasia
- Eosinophilic enteritis
- Mastocytosis
- Amyloidosis
- Crohn's disease
- Giardiasis
- Coccidiosis

Small bowel biopsy is abnormal, but not diagnostic, in the following:
- Celiac sprue, unclassified sprue, and tropical sprue
- Viral gastroenteritis
- Intraluminal bacterial overgrowth
- Folate and/or B12 deficiency
- Acute radiation enteritis

Small bowel biopsy is contraindicated in patients with coagulopathy, in uncooperative patients, and in patients who are not NPO.

Platelet count or platelet smear, prothrombin time, partial thromboplastin time, and bleeding times should be obtained before suction biopsy if clinically indicated. Aspirin-containing products, anticoagulants, and NSAIDs should be avoided for 2 weeks before biopsy. The patient should fast for 4 to 8 hours, depending on age. The posterior part of the pharynx may be anesthetized with a topical anesthetic; infants and uncooperative younger children may be sedated.

Before beginning the procedure, it is important to complete the following activities:
- Verify a written informed consent and the length of the patient's NPO status
- Obtain lab results, medical history, and baseline vital signs
- Notify the physician if the patient is currently on anticoagulant therapy, ASA, or NSAIDs; if laboratory results are abnormal; or if the patient's history indicates a need for prophylactic antibiotics (e.g., prosthetic heart valve)
- Inform the patient of the purpose of the test, the techniques to be used, and the sensations he or she is likely to experience

A number of instruments of various designs can be used for small bowel biopsy, including a **Carey capsule, Crosby capsule,** or a Quinton or Rubin tube.

A dissection microscope or a hand lens permits a reasonably good assessment of villous morphology and often leads to an immediate diagnosis of the atrophy that is typical of celiac disease. In addition to histologic examination, biopsy samples may be useful for enzymatic, metabolic, immunologic, and microscopic studies. Tissue for morphology is placed in formalin, while the portion for intestinal enzymology is immediately quick-frozen at $-40°$ C on a piece of aluminum foil lying on dry ice. Enzymatic studies include the determination of enzyme activity in tissue homogenates from patients with isolated lactase deficiency, congenital sucrase-isomaltase deficiency, or a general decrease of disaccharidase activity associated with various mucosal disorders.

In addition, a small portion of the tissue sample can be placed in glutaraldehyde for electron microscopy. Another portion can be quick-frozen in isopentane, to be evaluated later by immunofluorescent studies designed to confirm the presence of immunity defects or to identify bacteria, viruses, or parasites.

Intestinal mucosa specimens may also be incubated with a radioactive substrate placed in an incubation medium to help characterize inborn errors of intestinal transport, such as cystinuria and glucose-galactose malabsorption.

Complications of small bowel biopsy are rare, but may include perforation, hemorrhage, or entrapment of the capsule in the duodenum. The patient's hematocrit should be checked 4 to 6 hours after completion of the biopsy. Risk of perforation is greatest in severely hypoproteinemic, edematous patients.

## FINE-NEEDLE ASPIRATION OF THE PANCREAS

Pancreatic abnormalities may be diagnosed by direct percutaneous **fine-needle aspiration** of the pancreas using ultrasonography or computed tomography (CT) guidance. Pancreatic aspiration appears to be a highly successful method of obtaining a cytohistologic diagnosis of pancreatic cancer, with reported diagnostic accuracy rates of 80% to 90%. False positive biopsy results are unlikely, but the absence of malignant cells in an aspirated biopsy does not definitively exclude pancreatic cancer.

Fine-needle aspiration is indicated in patients with large pancreatic masses that have been identified by noninvasive imaging studies. Cytologic examination of biopsy specimens can provide tissue diagnosis and differentiation of lymphoma or endocrine tumors from adenocarcinoma without surgery, which is especially useful in elderly patients in whom the morbidity and mortality from laparotomy is high. For patients with small focal mass lesions, diffuse enlargement of the pancreas with calcification, or equivocal findings on ultrasonogram or CT scan, endoscopic retrograde cholangiopancreatography (ERCP) should be performed first, as described in Chapter 24.

In performing a fine-needle aspiration, either ultrasonography or CT guidance is used to pass a needle directly into the mass lesion. The aspirated material is then used for cytologic examination. Several attempts at aspiration may be needed to obtain an adequate number of cells for cytologic examination. Accuracy may be improved by the presence of a cytologist in the examining room to immediately prepare the cytology slides and quickly fix them in alcohol.

Complications of fine-needle aspiration are infrequent, but there has been at least one report of seeding of malignant cells along the needle tract after aspiration. Accuracy depends greatly on the skill of the operator and the experience of the cytologist.

## PERCUTANEOUS LIVER BIOPSY

In most cases, liver biopsy is done percutaneously, but it can also be done under direct vision via laparoscopy or surgery. **Percutaneous liver biopsy** is a relatively low-cost bedside procedure. Traditionally it was performed only on inpatients, but recently it has been used for selected outpatients, providing they do not have severe liver disease, a clotting disorder, or some other serious illness, and providing facilities are available to observe the patient for 6 to 8 hours after the procedure.

Percutaneous liver biopsy is indicated for the evaluation of the following:
- Acute and chronic cholestatic jaundice, after extrahepatic bile duct obstruction has been ruled out.
- Acute viral hepatitis, pathologic features of which include diffuse spotty parenchymal infiltration of hepatic lobules by lymphocytes and occasional plasma cells; ballooning degeneration of hepatocytes; acidophilic body formation; swollen Kupffer cells; cholestasis; and inflammation of the portal tracts.
- Alcoholic hepatitis, histologic features of which include Mallory bodies, scattered fat, hepatocyte swelling, neutrophilic inflammation, and varying degrees of fibrosis, progressing to cirrhosis.
- Documentation of cirrhosis and provision of information about the etiologic agent. In alcoholic cirrhosis, liver biopsy is used to establish the stage of hepatic injury and to exclude the presence of non–alcohol-related liver disease. In primary biliary cirrhosis, liver biopsy shows four progressive histologic stages: florid duct lesions, followed by bile ductule proliferation, scarring, and micronodular cirrhosis. Percutaneous liver biopsy is complicated in cirrhotic patients, because penetration into the liver is made more difficult by subcapsular fibrosis and bile duct proliferation. In some patients, diagnostic laparotomy may be more productive because it helps to eliminate sampling errors.
- $\alpha$1-Antitrypsin deficiency. In cirrhotic patients with $\alpha$1-antitrypsin deficiency, liver biopsy shows globules in the cytoplasm of liver cells that stain positively with periodic acid-Schiff stain and resist digestion with diastase.
- Unexplained hepatomegaly or liver abnormalities, as identified by ultrasonography, CT, or radionuclide scanning.

- Space-occupying lesions or infiltrative neoplastic disease. Biopsy will indicate malignancy in patients with hepatocarcinoma only if the specimen is obtained from the site of the malignant lesion. Blind percutaneous needle biopsy with cytology is positive in 75% of patients with metastatic liver disease. CT-guided and peritoneoscopic needle biopsies may have higher diagnostic yields.
- Assessment of a patient's response to therapy.
- Lipid or glycogen storage diseases.
- Wilson's disease. In the absence of Kayser-Fleischer rings, a liver biopsy for quantitative copper determination is essential in patients with suspected Wilson's disease. It is important in these patients that the biopsy needle and container be free from copper contamination.
- Hemochromatosis, a genetic disorder of iron absorption. Liver biopsy permits estimation of tissue iron stores by histochemical staining, measurement of hepatic iron concentration by dry weight by chemical analysis, and histologic assessment of liver damage.
- Screening of relatives of patients with familial liver disease.
- Staging of malignant lymphoma.

Percutaneous liver biopsy is contraindicated in uncooperative or confused patients and in patients with any of the following:
- Significant coagulopathy (although, if necessary, such patients may be prepared with infusions of fresh-frozen plasma and platelets)
- Severe anemia
- Extrahepatic obstructive jaundice
- Inadequate movement of the right diaphragm secondary to right pleural effusion, right lower lung pneumonia, or fibrosis
- Moderate to large amounts of ascites
- Severe uremia, unless bleeding time is normal
- Excessive obesity
- Local skin infections involving the planned biopsy site
- Peritonitis
- Suspected hemangioma or hepatoma
- Suspected hepatic vein thrombosis
- Amyloidosis (relative), because of the possible risk of liver rupture

Before performing percutaneous liver biopsy, it is important that laboratory studies (hemoglobin, hematocrit, white blood cell count, platelet count, prothrombin time, and partial thromboplastin time) be done to establish proper clotting factors and adequate blood volumes, absence of infection, and absence of high-grade obstruction. Other preliminary procedures may include obtaining baseline vital signs, blood typing and cross-matching, prophylactic vitamin K, chest and abdominal radiographs and scans, and a history of drug allergies. Foods and fluids should be withheld for at least 6 hours and NPO status verified.

Written informed consent must be obtained and the patient's medical history verified, including nonuse of anticoagulants, aspirin, or NSAIDs. The patient should be reassured, and the risks of the procedure and possible alternatives should be explained. An IV line may be started, if ordered. Because the patient will have to remain in bed for several hours after the biopsy, he or she should be encouraged to void before the procedure. The purpose of the test, techniques to be used, and sensations the patient is likely to experience should be explained. Breathing techniques that will be needed during the procedure should be explained and reinforced.

To minimize discomfort, the patient may be premedicated with sedatives, analgesics, mild narcotics, and/or barbiturates. The patient is placed in a supine position near the right edge of the bed with a pillow under the right side; the right arm is placed under the head and the head is turned toward the left. Because pediatric patients cannot be expected to cooperate, they must be adequately sedated. Infants may be restrained on a circumcision board or held by assistants.

The biopsy site is chosen, and the surrounding skin is cleansed with acetone-alcohol and iodine solutions. Sterile drapes are arranged around the biopsy site (Fig. 27-2). The skin, subcutaneous tissues, and the deeper intercostal muscles at the insertion site are infiltrated with a local anesthetic, such as procaine (Novocain) or

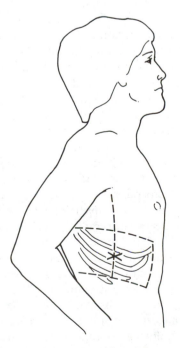

**Fig. 27-2.** Liver biopsy site.

lidocaine (Xylocaine), assuming that the patient has no known allergy to these substances.

A 4-mm skin incision is made at the biopsy site. A biopsy needle is attached to a syringe that contains a small amount of nonbacteriostatic sterile saline. The type of needle used depends on the probable nature of the lesion. For example, a standard biopsy needle (Klatskin, Menghini, or similar) has the potential for causing a serious hemorrhage, but a fine needle may not obtain enough tissue for diagnosis. Tru-Cut disposable needles are commonly used, even for children.

After the needle is attached to the syringe, it is pushed through the skin incision and advanced into the intercostal muscles. The saline is injected to expel any tissue fragments from the needle. To prevent pleural cavity or diaphragm puncture, the patient holds his or her breath at full expiration while the biopsy needle is pushed into the liver. For pediatric patients, the biopsy should be timed to the respiratory cycle.

While constant aspiration is maintained, the needle is advanced 4 to 5 cm and then quickly withdrawn. Throughout the procedure, the needle is actually in the liver for only a fraction of a second. The patient resumes breathing 5 to 10 seconds after the specimen is obtained. A second biopsy through the same incision at a slightly different angle may be necessary.

The biopsy sample may be expelled from the needle temporarily into saline or directly into 10% formalin and then sent to the laboratory for analysis. If lymphoma is suspected, accurate diagnosis requires that a portion of the biopsy specimen be placed in saline, not formalin. The minimal amount of tissue necessary for evaluation by the pathologist is usually a core sample longer than 1 cm.

If the apparent tumor is of a size or in a location unlikely to be reached with the standard blind-needle technique, sonography-guided or CT-guided biopsy may be more appropriate. Lesions that are more than 3 cm in diameter and peripherally located may be biopsied with sonographic guidance. CT guidance makes it easier to perform a biopsy of smaller, deeper lesions or those in relatively inaccessible locations. Angiographic techniques may be used to obtain liver tissue in patients with abnormal clotting parameters or massive ascites.

After the procedure is completed, an adhesive bandage is applied to the insertion site, and the patient is turned onto his or her right side against a firm support (e.g., a bath blanket, sandbag, or pillow). The patient maintains that position for the first 2 hours, with strict bed rest for the next 6 to 8 hours. If bleeding from the site persists, a pressure dressing may be needed. The insertion site must be observed closely for intraperitoneal hemorrhage or peritonitis. Vital signs should be taken regularly during this time. Patients may be allowed

clear liquids shortly after biopsy. Solid food may be reintroduced after several hours if no serious complications have developed. If vital signs do not change, and hemoglobin and hematocrit are normal, outpatients may be discharged after 4 to 6 hours of observation, but they must remain on bed rest for 8 to 12 hours.

The physician should be notified immediately if:
- The patient's pulse increases and systolic blood pressure decreases
- The patient experiences prolonged pain that radiates to the back, abdomen, or shoulder
- There is abdominal distention or obvious bleeding from the insertion site
- The patient's temperature increases
- The patient's respiration changes

Major complications have been reported in about 3 out of every 1,000 biopsies and deaths have been reported in about 1 out of every 1,000. Potential complications of percutaneous liver biopsy are listed in the box below.

Complications can be minimized by using a needle that is 1.2 mm in diameter or less, avoiding biopsy in high-risk patients, and adhering strictly to protocol for obtaining the biopsy.

---

**Potential complications: percutaneous liver biopsy**

| | |
|---|---|
| Local pain and infection | Needle breakage |
| Hemorrhage into the peritoneum | Hemobilia |
| Bile peritonitis | Liver laceration |
| Perforated gallbladder | Pleurisy and perihepatitis |
| Subcapsular or intrahepatic hematoma | Shock |
| Pleural pain and pneumothorax | Hemothorax |
| Penetration of abdominal viscera | Anesthetic reactions |
| Capsular bleeding | Endotoxic shock |
| Bacteremia | Septicemia |
| Arteriovenous fistulae | Tumor seeding |

---

## CELL CULTURE AND CYTOLOGY

When the presence of an infection is suspected, tissue specimens may be needed for the **culture** of bacteria, fungi, or other organisms. Specimens for culture may be obtained by using a cytology brush, by washing, or by aspiration. When whole cells are needed for microscopic examination, cytology specimens are collected, using either a cytology brush or a washing technique.

**Brush cytology**

Information about the nature of some lesions can be obtained by **brush cytology,** using a tiny brush that is passed through the endoscope in much the same way as the biopsy forceps.

Inexpensive, sheathed disposable brushes are available in various sizes and lengths. Once it is in line with the suspicious mucosal area, the brush can be extended beyond its plastic sheath and rubbed across the mucosa. After harvesting cells from the suspect lesion, the head of the brush is withdrawn into the outer sheath before it is removed from the endoscope. Use of a sheathed brush minimizes the shedding of cells into the suction/biopsy channel.

After the brush is removed from the endoscope, thin smears of cells are made on clean microscope slides. The brush is gently rotated over the slide, brushing in one direction only. The slide is placed in a slide holder or an alcohol solution, labeled, and sent to the laboratory. The tips of disposable brushes may be cut off after the sample has been taken and sent intact to the laboratory, after moistening with 1 or 2 drops of sterile nonbacteriostatic saline for culture, or in a container of 3 to 6 drops of nonbacteriostatic saline for cytologic examination. If cell smears are used, they should be fixed according to hospital protocol.

For brush cytology of the pancreatic ducts, a commercially available sleeved brush may be used. The brush is passed through the papillary opening and pushed through the duct and into the ductal lesion, or as near to it as possible. Smears are made, fixed, and stained.

**Obtaining specimens by washing**

If a washing technique will be used to obtain specimens for culture or cytology, a specimen trap is attached to the endoscope suction port and the specimen is aspirated through the endoscope into the trap, injecting 20 to 30 ml of nonbacteriostatic saline through the biopsy channel to obtain the specimen. The trap is disconnected from the endoscope and sealed, and the endoscopic cytology specimen is labeled and sent immediately to the laboratory.

**Indications for cytology**

There are a number of different indications for obtaining endoscopic cytology specimens, including the following:
- Suspected malignancy
- Suspected candidiasis
- Examination of duodenal aspirate for *Giardia,* secretory immunoglobulins, bile acid patterns, pan-

creatic amylase and trypsin levels, or evidence of strongyloidiasis
- Pancreatic ductal lesions

Esophageal secretions may be obtained during esophagoscopy or by aspiration of iced saline that is injected through a nasogastric tube positioned at progressively higher positions in the esophagus.

For gastric cytology, vigorous gastric lavage is performed with a large volume of normal saline. This solution is aspirated and placed in an ice-water bath for later analysis. Then, a buffered solution of sodium acetate with chymotrypsin is instilled to promote exfoliation of malignant cells. Lavage is performed with the patient in different positions and the solution is then aspirated, placed on ice, and taken to the laboratory for analysis.

For aspiration or lavage cytology of the pancreatic duct, pancreatic juice is collected into tubes containing a fixative. The tubes are centrifuged, and smears are made and fixed. For lavage cytology, small amounts of saline are injected into the main pancreatic duct and then aspirated with a syringe.

For colon cytology, the patient is prepared with a cathartic and with cleansing enemas. Warm saline, with or without chymotrypsin added, is instilled. After several minutes the solution is collected, placed on ice, and taken to the laboratory.

---

**CASE SITUATION**

This is the second hospital admission for Gary H., age 28, who is HIV-positive with AIDS. Initially, Gary was admitted for severe dysphagia (difficulty swallowing) and odynophagia (pain on swallowing). His upper endoscopy at that time revealed severe esophageal inflammation with whitish patches. Specimens taken at that time revealed candidiasis. Gary now has diarrhea and weight loss in addition to some continuing odynophagia. He is scheduled for both upper and lower endoscopy, with biopsy and cytology.

***Points to think about***

1. Immunocompromised patients, especially those with AIDS, are susceptible to a host of gastrointestinal problems. What are some of the normal defenses the gut has to prevent invasion by pathologic organisms and how are these defenses affected by AIDS?
2. On upper endoscopy, Gary is found to have dense patches of creamy, waxy exudate, esophagitis, and two very large, deep ulcerations. His duodenum is normal, but there are two raised, dark red, 10-mm lesions in

his stomach. What types of specimens will help diagnose the cause of these problems?

3. The gastroenterology nurse is now involved in much more specimen collection than in the past. Why is it important to develop a good working relationship with lab personnel?

4. Diarrhea can have many causes in the patient with AIDS, including amebiasis, shigellosis, gonorrhea, CMV, herpes simplex, syphilis, lymphogranuloma venereum, cryptosporidiosis, and *Chlamydia*. What tests would help determine the cause of Gary's diarrhea?

5. In dealing with infectious specimens, what special practices should be employed?

### Suggested responses

1. The normal defenses the GI tract has against pathologic organisms include the bactericidal effect of gastric acid, intestinal motility, normal bowel flora, intact mucosa, humoral immunity, and lymphocytes, macrophages, and neutrophils. In patients with AIDS, deficiencies in the immune system (neutropenia and alterations in hormonal and cell-mediated immunity) affect the normal defense mechanisms of the GI tract. In addition, infections can disrupt intact mucosa, decrease motility, and overrun normal flora. Because of this, the gut is susceptible to local and systemic infections.

2. In AIDS patients, the esophagus is often involved with opportunistic infections such as *Candida,* herpes simplex, and CMV. Comprehensive testing is recommended because having the scope in place allows for easy specimen acquisition. Specimens that will help diagnose the cause of Gary's symptoms include the following:

   • Brush cytology to test for *Candida.* Disposable brushes are packaged sterile and are inexpensive enough that nondisposable brushes should no longer be used for specimen acquisition. It is important to know the institution's routine for preparing specimens. Often, the brush may be delivered to the lab in its package with orders for fungal culture and stains, and the lab will prepare it. Although symptoms of *Candida* infections may improve or disappear with therapy, this does not always indicate disappearance of mucosal lesions. Follow-up endoscopies are often necessary.

   • Biopsy of the deep esophageal ulcerations. If the pathologist knows the suspected diagnosis, special stains can be applied to identify fungal, viral, or parasitic invasion.

   • Viral cultures. Special media are usually obtainable from the lab for viral cultures. They are kept refrigerated and have a relatively short outdate. A forceps biopsy specimen is placed in the viral culture and labeled.

   • Biopsy of the dark red lesions in the stomach. These lesions are most likely Kaposi's sarcoma. They can appear anywhere in the gut and vary in color from red to deep purple. Fifty percent of AIDS patients who present with Kaposi's skin lesions will also have GI tract lesions, which present a much poorer prognosis. In the gut, these lesions lie submucosally; standard forceps biopsy, which only penetrates mucosal tissue, may be negative. It would be helpful to use the largest forceps that will fit through the channel of your scope. This may be a time for the snare lift-and-cut technique. Care should be taken in case there is excessive bleeding from these lesions at biopsy.

3. Laboratory personnel can be very helpful. Specimens must often be taken to different departments within the lab (e.g., pathology for biopsy and cytology, or bacteriology for cultures and staining). There are many different ways to order tests, and many specimens need special collection methods and media. Having this knowledge before the procedure can save time and can help avoid making mistakes and losing specimens.

4. Tests that can help specify the cause of Gary's diarrhea include:

   • A colonoscopy, to examine the whole large bowel and ascertain the extent of disease

   • A flexible sigmoidoscopy for specimen collection

   • Stool cultures and microscopic examinations. In the colon, it may be difficult to determine what agent is causing a suspicious colitis. The list of possible agents is long. Many of these organisms may be present simultaneously, or they may not appear in every specimen. This means that stool cultures and microscopic examinations may need to be done on a serial basis and must often be repeated.

   • Specimens for Gram stain, bacterial culture, ova and parasites, viral cultures, and special staining techniques. Again, each institution uses different methods and media. It is important to be familiar with institutional procedures and to give the pathologist and lab personnel as much information as possible regarding the potential diagnosis.

   • Biopsy to help differentiate colitis from Crohn's disease or ulcerative colitis

   • Biopsy of the characteristic red lesions of Kaposi's sarcoma

5. It is unlikely that handling infectious specimens would cause infection in healthcare personnel unless they are immunocompromised. However, the contaminated hands or clothing of healthcare personnel may spread infections to other patients who might be

immunocompromised. It is important to remember that AIDS patients are immunocompromised and therefore more susceptible to infection than most patients. Special practices to think about when dealing with infectious specimens include the following:

- Wearing gloves, protective gowns, masks, and protective eyewear when collecting specimens
- Washing hands thoroughly when gloves are removed and leaving protective clothing in the procedure room hamper
- Not handling patient care equipment when exudative lesions or weeping dermatitis are present
- Putting all specimens in well-constructed containers with secure lids to prevent leaking during transport
- Collecting each specimen carefully to avoid contaminating the outside of the container and the laboratory form accompanying the specimen
- Implementing universal blood and body fluids precautions for *all* patients. This eliminates the need for warning labels on specimens because all specimens should be considered infective.
- Subjecting endoscopes used on HIV-positive patients to the same scrupulous cleaning and disinfecting regimen given to all endoscopes
- Using biopsy forceps that are sterile because they are designed to break the mucosal barrier. They may be disposable and packaged sterile or they may be reusable and sterilized after use by ultrasonic cleaning and steam under pressure.
- Using disposable cytology brushes

---

### REVIEW TERMS

**aspiration, biopsy, biopsy forceps, brush cytology, Carey capsule, Crosby capsule, culture, cytology, exfoliative brush cytology, fine-needle aspiration, frozen section, histopathologic analysis, hot biopsy forceps, percutaneous liver biopsy, Quinton tube, Rubin tube, suction biopsy, washing**

---

### REVIEW QUESTIONS

1. Endoscopic biopsy is contraindicated in patients with:
   a. Carcinoma.
   b. Severe coagulopathy.
   c. Inflammatory bowel disease.
   d. Gastrointestinal polyps.
2. Frozen sections are used when:
   a. The biopsy specimen will be preserved for a long period of time.
   b. A fixative is needed to preserve the specimen.
   c. Immediate denial/confirmation of malignancy is required.
   d. A pathologist is not immediately available.
3. The most likely complication of endoscopic biopsy is:
   a. Excessive bleeding.
   b. Infection.
   c. Tumor seeding.
   d. Nausea and vomiting.
4. Suspect esophageal tissue is most often sampled using what technique?
   a. Suction.
   b. Needle aspiration.
   c. Endoscopic biopsy.
   d. Polypectomy.
5. Specimens for small bowel biopsy are usually taken from what general area?
   a. The duodenum.
   b. The jejunum.
   c. The ileum.
   d. The ligament of Treitz.
6. A Carey capsule is used for:
   a. Esophageal biopsy.
   b. Liver biopsy.
   c. Gastric biopsy.
   d. Small bowel biopsy.
7. During small bowel suction biopsy, the purpose of flushing the suction tubing with saline is to:
   a. Sterilize the tubing.
   b. Remove any accumulated liquids or debris.
   c. Close the capsule.
   d. Remove the specimen.
8. To prevent pleural cavity or diaphragm puncture during the procedure, insertion of the needle for percutaneous liver biopsy in pediatric patients should be:
   a. Timed to the patient's respiratory cycle.
   b. Done while the patient holds his or her breath on expiration.
   c. Done slowly.
   d. Done under ultrasonography or CT guidance.
9. If disposable cytology brushes are sent intact to the laboratory, they should be moistened with:
   a. Nonbacteriostatic saline.
   b. Glutaraldehyde.
   c. Isopentane.
   d. Cellular fixative.
10. An abrasive solution that may be instilled in the GI tract to promote exfoliation of malignant cells is:
    a. Normal saline.
    b. Secretin-cholecystokinin.
    c. Chymotrypsin.
    d. Formalin.

## BIBLIOGRAPHY

Bongiovanni, G, ed. *Essentials of Clinical Gastroenterology.* 2nd ed. New York: McGraw–Hill, 1988.

Chobanian, S, and Van Ness, M, eds. *Manual of Clinical Problems in Gastroenterology.* Boston: Little, Brown & Co., 1988.

Chopra, S, and May, R, eds. *Pathophysiology of Gastrointestinal Diseases.* Boston: Little, Brown & Co., 1989.

Eastwood, G, and Ayunduk, C. *Manual of Gastroenterology: Diagnosis and Therapy.* Boston: Little, Brown & Co., 1988.

Given, B, and Simmons, S. *Gastroenterology in Clinical Nursing.* 4th ed. St. Louis: Mosby–Year Book, 1984.

Hardick, M, and Beck, M. *Manual of Gastrointestinal Procedures.* 2nd ed. Rochester, N.Y.: Society of Gastroenterology Nurses and Associates, 1989.

Hoffman, S, Marshall, B, Dye, K, and Caldwell, S. "Gastric Urease, *Campylobacter Pylori* and the Interpretation of CLOtest®." *Gastroenterology Nursing* 11(Spring 1989): 217-20.

Hugg, D. "Liver Biopsy: The Role of The Gastrointestinal Assistant." In *SGA Journal Reprints,* ed. Trivits, S, 125-26. Rochester, N.Y.: Society of Gastrointestinal Assistants, 1988.

Katsugai, T, ed. *Endoscopic Diagnosis in Gastroenterology.* New York: Igaku-Shoin, 1982.

Misiewicz, J, Bartram, C, Cotton, P, Mee, A, Price, A, and Thompson, R. *Atlas of Clinical Gastroenterology.* Volume 1. London: Gower Medical Publishing, 1985.

Ravenscroft, M, and Swan, C. *Gastrointestinal Endoscopy and Related Procedures: A Handbook for Nurses and Assistants.* Baltimore: Williams & Wilkins, 1984.

Silverman, A, and Roy, C. *Pediatric Clinical Gastroenterology.* 3rd ed. St. Louis: Mosby–Year Book, 1983.

Sivak, M, Jr., and Petrini, J, eds. *Gastrointestinal Endoscopy: Old Problems, New Techniques.* Gastroenterology Series, Volume 4. New York: Praeger, 1986.

Sleisenger, M, and Fordtran, J, eds. *Gastrointestinal Disease: Pathophysiology, Diagnosis, Management.* 4th ed. Philadelphia: W.B. Saunders, 1989.

Waye, J, Geenen, J, Fleischer, D, and Venu, R. *Techniques in Therapeutic Endoscopy.* Philadelphia: W.B. Saunders, 1987.

# Chapter 28

# OTHER PROCEDURES AND TESTS

This chapter will acquaint the gastroenterology nurse with nonendoscopic diagnostic tests and procedures that are used in the practice of gastroenterology. Radiographic and nonradiographic imaging techniques are discussed, including plain and contrast radiography, ultrasonography, and computed tomography. Studies involving the analysis of gastrointestinal secretions are described and laboratory tests involving the analysis of blood, urine, and fecal samples are reviewed.

## Learning objectives

After reviewing the content of this chapter, the gastroenterology nurse should be able to:

1. Describe several types of radiographic and nonradiographic imaging studies that are performed on gastroenterology patients, including indications, contraindications, and patient care instructions.
2. Discuss a variety of diagnostic tests and procedures that are used to analyze gastrointestinal secretions.
3. Briefly explain the diagnostic tests that are used most frequently to analyze the blood, urine, or feces of gastroenterology patients.

## BASIC PRINCIPLES

In addition to the diagnostic techniques discussed in the preceding chapters, gastroenterology patients are often required to undergo a variety of other laboratory tests and procedures.

The importance of discussing these tests with the patient cannot be overemphasized. To educate and prepare patients for such tests, it is important that the nurse understand the role of these tests in the diagnostic process and communicate this information to the patient. Complete instructions and explanations help ensure the patient's compliance and also allay any feelings of anxiety. Most patients do better during a test

when they have received information about the procedure they will undergo and the sensations they are likely to experience. It may be helpful to provide patient instruction when a member of the patient's family is there to offer support and to reinforce the teaching. Upon completion, patient education and comprehension should be documented.

It is also important to review the patient's history before any diagnostic testing is conducted and to verify compliance with any necessary preparations, such as length of NPO status, withholding of certain medications, or preliminary blood work. During the procedure the nurse may be responsible for patient positioning, handling specimens or test samples, gathering instruments and supplies, and calibrating any recording devices.

After the procedure is completed, the patient should be monitored for adverse effects, provided with discharge instructions, and told how to obtain test results.

## RADIOGRAPHIC AND NONRADIOGRAPHIC IMAGING

**Radiographic studies** of the GI tract help detect abnormalities such as obstructions, strictures, ulcers, or structural changes. Flat and upright plain x-ray films of the abdomen and upright chest x-ray films are often the first tests performed on patients with acute abdominal symptoms. In most cases, other tests are also required.

Generally speaking, radiology is easier for the patient than endoscopy and has fewer direct complications; however, endoscopy has greater diagnostic potential. The local availability of radiologic and endoscopic expertise may also influence the physician's choice of diagnostic method.

Administration of a contrast medium before or during radiographic studies accentuates differences in the densities of abdominal regions and structures, thus facilitating interpretation of the radiographs. Most radiographic tests for gastrointestinal disorders use **barium sulfate** as the contrast medium. Barium is a chalky, radiopaque, inert, nonallergenic substance that enables **fluoroscopic** and **x-ray (roentgenographic) examination** of the esophagus, stomach, and small and large intestines. It may be administered orally, rectally, or via intestinal stoma. Any routine x-ray examinations, lower GI studies, or oral cholecystograms should be done *before* barium studies because the ingested barium may obscure other films. Barium studies are contraindicated in patients with digestive tract obstruction or perforation.

Patients who undergo barium studies must be cautioned to report failure to pass the barium within 2 to 3 days so cathartics or enemas may be prescribed to avoid constipation or obstruction. In some institutions, an enema or a laxative is given routinely after barium studies. Patients may also be advised to increase their intake of fluids. They should be told to expect stools to be chalky and light-colored for 24 to 72 hours after the barium.

Iodine-based contrast media are administered intravenously for radiographs of the gallbladder, pancreas, spleen, and the various ducts. Radiographic studies with iodine-based contrast media require careful review of the patient's history of allergies to iodine, seafood, or iodine-based contrast agents. They also require careful patient preparation before the test and close observation afterward for delayed hypersensitivity reactions.

### Barium swallow

A **barium swallow** permits radiographic examination of the esophagus after ingestion of a thick barium solution. This test can reveal the presence or absence of peptic strictures, foreign bodies, diverticula, ulcerations, varices, polyps, tumors, a hiatus hernia, or motility disorders. It may discover, but is not sensitive for, esophagitis or Barrett's esophagus. A barium swallow is contraindicated in patients with intestinal obstructions. For patients with suspected perforations, Gastrografin is the preferred contrast medium.

Patients scheduled for a barium swallow should not ingest any food, fluids, or oral medications after midnight. On the day of the test, the patient swallows a barium mixture while in a supine position. The Trendelenburg position may be used to detect gastric reflux or a sliding hiatus hernia. For patients with dysphagia, a barium tablet or food/marshmallow bolus should be used in addition to the liquid barium, so that strictures can be better identified.

### Upper gastrointestinal series

In an **upper gastrointestinal (UGI) series** with small bowel follow-through, the esophagus, stomach, and small intestine are all examined following ingestion of a barium solution. A UGI series can be used for diagnosis of hiatal hernia, diverticula, varices, strictures, ulcers, tumors, regional enteritis, malabsorption syndromes, or motility disorders. Gastric x-ray films may show benign or malignant tumors or ulcers, while films of the small intestine may indicate obstruction, regional ileitis, or diverticula.

Before this procedure, patients must be instructed to remain NPO after midnight. In addition, some institutions may instruct their patients to do the following:

- Follow a low-residue diet for 2 to 3 days
- Avoid anticholinergic or narcotic medications for 24 hours
- Refrain from smoking after midnight
- Avoid antacids for several hours before the test

After swallowing the barium, the patient assumes various positions on the x-ray examination table so the barium will outline all parts of the gastric wall. In addition, the abdomen may be palpated or compressed. Air may be introduced into the abdomen to improve visualization of the rugae.

Occasionally the entire small bowel is examined using **enteroclysis**, which is a **double-contrast technique** that involves infusing barium and later methylcellulose through a catheter that is passed into the small bowel under fluoroscopic guidance. Usually, a film is taken every 30 to 60 minutes; the entire series, including the small bowel, can take up to 6 hours. Enteroclysis may be helpful in diagnosing patients with suspected partial small bowel obstruction, Meckel's diverticulum, or lymphoma.

### Barium enema

The **barium enema** is a common and valuable diagnostic test for patients with colon disorders. Both single-contrast and double-contrast barium enemas are safe and well-tolerated without premedication, although double-contrast enemas are generally the method of choice.

A barium enema is indicated for the diagnosis of colorectal cancer and inflammatory disease and to detect polyps, diverticula, and structural changes. The procedure is contraindicated in patients with fulminant ulcerative colitis associated with systemic toxicity, toxic megacolon, or suspected perforation or obstruction.

Before a barium enema, the patient must follow a clear liquid diet for 1 to 2 days. This is followed by evacuation of the colon with a conventional cathartic and an enema prepartion or a balanced electrolyte lavage solution. The barium is administered like any other enema, but the patient must be encouraged to retain the barium, despite any cramping or urge to defecate. In some cases the barium is administered through a Foley type of catheter, and the balloon is inflated slightly to prevent the patient from expelling the solution, although use of a catheter may increase the urge to defecate and exacerbate patient discomfort. The patient is instructed to move about to allow the barium to spread throughout the colon. In some cases a tilt table may be used to achieve a semierect or Trendelenburg position that will allow the barium to cover all areas of the colon.

In double-contrast studies, a thicker barium solution is used. After rotation to cover the bowel wall, air is introduced into the bowel so that smaller lesions can be seen. As in any barium study, defecation of barium should be noted and corrective steps taken if it is not passed within 2 to 3 days.

## Percutaneous transhepatic cholangiography

**Percutaneous transhepatic cholangiography (PTC)** is used to visualize the biliary ductal system. It may be used to distinguish between obstructive and nonobstructive jaundice or to determine the location, extent, and cause of mechanical bile duct obstruction, which may be caused by stones, tumors, inflammation, stenosis, or stricture. PTC is contraindicated in patients with cholangitis, massive ascites, allergies to iodine, or uncorrectable coagulopathy.

Under fluoroscopic visualizaton, a thin needle (Chiba needle) is introduced into the liver, through the locally anesthetized seventh or eighth intercostal space, parallel to the plane of the table. The needle is slowly withdrawn until a green fluid is aspirated, indicating that a bile duct has been entered. A radiopaque iodine dye is then injected, and radiographs are taken to define the site, cause, and extent of bile duct obstruction. Prophylactic antibiotics may be given for 2 days before and 3 days after the procedure.

After the test is completed, the patient's vital signs should be checked regularly and the nurse should observe the patient for 24 hours. For the first 6 hours, the patient should remain in bed, lying on the right side. The nurse should be alert for signs of hemorrhage from the site, including a decrease in blood pressure, an increase in pulse rate and respirations, restlessness, pallor, or diaphoresis. Bleeding may result from PTC and can be massive. Other adverse effects of PTC may include pain, temperature elevation, chills, abdominal distention, peritonitis, bile leakage, or septicemia.

**Cholangiography** can also be performed intraoperatively and postoperatively via a T-tube or cholecystectomy tube that is placed in the cystic duct.

## Oral cholecystography

Although ultrasonography is the initial diagnostic procedure of choice for the detection of gallstones, **oral cholecystography** is an acceptable alternative when ultrasonography is unavailable or equivocal or when the cholecystogram will be performed in conjunction with a UGI series. Oral cholecystography may be superior to ultrasonography for demonstrating the patency of the cystic duct, assessing gallbladder function, or showing the apparent density of stones. It is also necessary before oral dissolution therapy of gallstones to be certain the cystic duct is open.

Oral cholecystography involves oral administration of pills containing iodinated radiocontrast material. Films are taken 10 to 14 hours later. Fat may be ingested following the inital gallbladder films to cause contraction of the gallbaldder, filling the common bile duct. Radiography takes 30 to 45 minutes. After the test, the patient resumes a normal diet and medications. Oral cholecystography is contraindicated in patients with severe renal or hepatic damage or in patients with a known allergy to iodine. Potential pitfalls include patients who have elevated bilirubin, who do not take the pills correctly, or who vomit or malabsorb them.

## Arteriography

**Arteriography**, which is also called **angiography**, involves the catheterization of selected arteries, followed by injection of an iodinated dye via the catheter. Subsequent x-ray films can help to locate the source of gastrointestinal bleeding, evaluate cirrhosis and portal hypertension, or determine the extent of vascular damage to the liver and spleen after abdominal trauma. Vascular tumors may be located by selective celiac and superior mesenteric arteriograms. Selective arteriography can also be therapeutic. Autologous clots or vasopressin (Pitressin) can be injected into appropriate vessels, or chemotherapeutic agents can be delivered directly to the tumor. Arteriography is contraindicated in patients who are allergic to iodine.

## Abdominal ultrasonography

**Ultrasonography** is indicated to show the size and configuration of organs. It identifies abnormalities of the structures and spaces within the abdomen or pelvis through the transmission of sound waves. Variances in the physical characteristics of the organs through which sound travels produce different images. The procedure is noninvasive and involves no ionizing radiation.

Ultrasonography is the initial diagnostic procedure of choice for the detection of cholelithiasis because it does not involve patient preparation or radiation and is simple to perform and interpret. It is also indicated in screening for biliary dilatation. It may be useful in detecting changes caused by appendicitis, such as a dilated appendix, thickened wall, or paraappendiceal fluid accumulation. Ultrasonography is also sensitive for acute cholecystitis.

The skin over the area to be studied is exposed. To seal out air pockets and keep the transducer from rubbing the patient's skin, the skin over the area to be studied is lubricated. While the patient lies still, a microphone transducer is slowly rubbed over the skin surface for a total of 20 to 30 minutes. Through this process, an image of the structures within the target area is produced on a screen.

### Computed tomography

**Computed tomography (CT)** is a noninvasive, radiologic scanning technique that relies on differences in tissue density to reflect organ configurations. Because it gathers information in all three dimensions, CT provides a more detailed and more precise view of the area being scanned than does abdominal ultrasonography. However, CT scanning also requires more personnel and expensive equipment to operate than does ultrasonography, and it does use ionizing radiation. The diagnostic accuracy of CT scanning can be enhanced by IV injection of contrast material to visualize the biliary system or by oral ingestion of a contrast agent to delineate the gastrointestinal system.

CT scanning is indicated for evaluation of gallbladder carcinoma, common bile duct stones, liver masses, pancreatic adenocarcinoma, intraabdominal abscess, and complications of acute pancreatitis.

### Scintigraphy

**Scintigraphy** relies on the use of radioactive isotopes, such as technetium ($^{99m}$Tc), iodine ($^{131}$I), or indium ($^{111}$In), to reveal displaced anatomic structures, changes in organ size, and the presence of neoplasms or other focal lesions, such as cysts or subphrenic and subhepatic abscesses.

#### Hepatic scintigraphy

Hepatic scintigraphy with $^{99m}$Tc-labeled sulfur colloid is widely used for noninvasive evaluation of the liver. The most common use of hepatic scintigraphy is in diagnosing and following the progression of metastatic disease. In addition, its sensitivity for hepatocellular dysfunction or diffuse infiltrating diseases such as alcoholic liver disease, cirrhosis, lymphoma, amyloidosis, or infiltrating metastatic disease, may be higher than other imaging methods.

The radiolabeled chemical is absorbed by the Kupffer cells and other phagocytic littoral cells in the liver and spleen. Because most intrahepatic masses do not contain these phagocytes, such masses appear as "cold" spots on the hepatic scintigram.

#### Biliary scintigraphy

For biliary scintigraphy, the patient must be NPO after midnight. A $^{99m}$Tc-labeled iminodiacetic acid derivative is administered intravenously. In normal subjects, this labeled compound is taken up by the hepatocytes and excreted into bile. Scans obtained 5 to 60 minutes or longer after radionuclide injection should outline the bile ducts, gallbladder, and proximal small bowel.

If the ducts are visible, but the gallbladder is not, acute cholecystitis is suggested but not proved. In patients with nonacute gallstone disease, gallbladder filling may be delayed by up to 3 hours. False positive scans may occur in patients with acute pancreatitis, chronic cholecystitis, alcoholism, neoplasms of the gallbladder and liver, and patients receiving total parenteral nutrition. False negative scans may occur in patients with acute acalculous cholecystitis.

#### Radionuclide evaluation of gastric emptying

For evaluation of gastric emptying, radionuclide testing is preferred over intubation methods. Furthermore, the ability of radionuclides to tag a solid test meal offers quantitative results that are not possible with barium radiography.

The radionuclide technique is useful for evaluation of any functional cause of delayed gastric emptying, but its most common clinical use is in the diagnosis of diabetic gastroparesis. It is also of value in evaluating rapid emptying, particularly the "dumping syndrome" that may be noted after gastric surgery.

The liquid component of the meal is labeled with $^{111}$In. Either egg salad or chicken liver is labeled with $^{99m}$Tc, which serves as a marker of the solid component of the meal. Following ingestion of the radiolabeled solid and liquid meal, the patient reclines under a scintiscanner that measures the initial level of intragastric radioactivity, and the rate of passage of radioactivity out of the stomach (i.e., gastric emptying). In this manner, differential rates of solid and liquid emptying can be detected.

Gastric emptying studies may also be done without radionuclides.

## SECRETORY STUDIES

Secretory studies evaluate the secretion of bile and various gastrointestinal enzymes, with or without external stimulation.*

### Biliary drainage

For biliary drainage procedures, a duodenal tube is passed to the second portion of the duodenum, and the gallbladder is stimulated by instillation of magnesium sulfate or IV administration of sincalide (Kinevac). Specimens of bile are obtained and examined microscopically for cells, crystals, and parasites.

Although biliary drainage is no longer a major diagnostic aid, it may be helpful in special cases. It may be indicated in the following situations:

- For patients with absent or poor gallbladder function and a clinical picture of cholelithiasis
- For patients with deep jaundice or sensitivity to the iodine in the contrast medium

---

*All techniques in this section, except pancreatic stimulation, are also discussed in the SGNA *Manual of Gastrointestinal Procedures* 2nd ed. Rochester, N.Y.: Society of Gastroenterology Nurses and Associates, 1989.

- When there is a probability of common duct stones in a postcholecystectomy patient
- In patients with suspected cholesterolosis, where cholesterol crystals are imbedded in the submucosa of the gallbladder
- In diagnosing giardiasis or bacterial overgrowth

It is contraindicated in uncooperative patients, including patients who gag or retch uncontrollably or pull out the tube, and in patients with vomiting and/or pyloric obstruction.

Successful intubation depends on the nurse's ability to achieve good rapport with the patient and inspire a positive attitude. Thorough teaching techniques may include use of an anatomy chart or diagram. The patient is instructed to fast for at least 6 hours before the test, avoiding even oral medications. Pertinent allergies should be ruled out. Dentures should be removed, unless they are tight-fitting upper dentures, which may help the patient swallow more normally. Spray anesthesia may be administered to the posterior pharynx if the patient retches or gags excessively; however, pharyngeal anesthesia increases the risk of aspiration and should be avoided if possible.

A lubricated double-lumen nasogastric or intestinal tube is inserted into the duodenum, with the patient sitting upright. A triple-lumen tube, which allows isolation of the second and third portions of the duodenum between two inflatable balloons, may be used for pediatric patients. Oral passage of the duodenal tube to the stomach can be facilitated if the patient uses mind control and relaxation techniques. To prevent gagging after the initial insertion, it is best to keep the tube on the side of the mouth between the cheek and teeth.

To avoid contamination of the duodenal drainage by stomach contents, gastric contents should be aspirated as the tube passes through the stomach. The gastric aspirate is placed in a container marked "gastric residual."

With the patient in the right lateral position, the tube is then passed slowly (about 1 inch every 4 or 5 minutes) into the duodenum, until the tip of the tube is near the ampulla of Vater. To increase gastric activity and help the tube to be carried more rapidly through the pylorus, it may be helpful to suggest relaxation techniques or to ask the patient to pretend to eat a favorite meal or to walk around the room.

During intubation the tube should be allowed to drain freely by gravity drainage into a specimen container. When the tip of the tube passes through the pylorus, the drainage should change from the cloudy, colorless, or bile-tinged acid secretions of the stomach to the clear, yellow, alkaline secretions of the duodenum. The drainage should be tested for pH intermittently to determine when the tube enters the duodenum. If duodenal intubation is difficult, the physician may order metoclopramide (Reglan) to increase peristalsis.

Correct positioning of the duodenal tube is of primary importance if good specimens are to be obtained. Fluoroscopic guidance may be used to confirm correct placement. The tube shold be lying along the greater curvature of the stomach and should not coil in the stomach.

Once correct placement of the tube has been confirmed fluoroscopically or by the color and alkalinity of the drainage, bile originating in the common bile duct (A bile) should be collected for 15 to 20 minutes. Then the patient may be tested for sensitivity to the stimulant drug(s). In accordance with the physician's order, sincalide (Kinevac) may be administered intravenously to contract the gallbladder, or 30 ml of 25% magnesium sulfate may be instilled through the duodenal tube to relax the sphincter of Oddi and allow bile to flow into the duodenum.

If magnesium sulfate is used for gallbladder stimulation, the tube should be clamped for 5 minutes following instillation, then reopened, and the solution permitted to run out. If Kinevac is used, the collection of A bile should be continued by gravity drainage. When the color of the bile drainage becomes dark green, the specimen collection container should be changed and this gallbladder bile (B bile) should be collected for approximately 20 to 30 minutes. Failure to collect B bile is frequently caused by gallbladder disease with loss of the concentrating function, or cholelithiasis, which causes cystic duct obstruction. If the patient has had a cholecystectomy, of course, there will be no B bile.

When the bile drainage color becomes light yellow, this liver bile (C bile) should be collected until it almost stops, approximately 20 to 30 minutes. Finally, 30 cc of air should be injected to clear the tube, and the tube should be clamped and removed. All specimens should be labeled and delivered to the laboratory, where they will be examined microscopically for cells, crystals, and parasites. Parasites are easily identified in a fresh specimen. The laboratory may also identify cells that could be indicative of an inflamed gallbladder or biliary tract, or crystals that are diagnostic for cholelithiasis, common duct stones, or cholesterolosis.

If a topical anesthetic was used, the patient should remain NPO until the gag reflex returns. The patient should be offered mouthwash to remove the bitter taste of bile from his or her mouth.

Duodenal drainage specimens may also be collected during esophagogastroduodenoscopy (EGD). Kinevac is administered intravenously and, after 5 to 10 minutes, bile is suctioned through the biopsy channel into a specimen trap. If dark green bile is not obtained, a second Kinevac stimulation may be ordered.

Another alternative is to insert a nasobiliary catheter endoscopically and leave it in the duodenum for use in collecting bile specimens following stimulation.

Potential complications of biliary drainage include entrapment of the tube in the duodenum.

### Pancreatic stimulation

Diagnosis of pancreatic disease often depends on tests that indicate alterations in pancreatic enzyme levels or pancreatic function. Pancreatic stimulation involves the determination of the volume, bicarbonate content, and pancreatic enzyme concentration in the duodenal juice before and after direct IV stimulation of the pancreas with the hormones secretin and/or cholecysto-kinin. An orally passed radiopaque duodenal tube is guided under fluoroscopic control through the duodenum to the ligament of Treitz. Secretin is administered intravenously over a 1-minute period, and samples of duodenal fluid are collected in ice-cooled flasks for a total of approximately 50 minutes. Each specimen is examined for volume, bicarbonate concentration, pH, and the enzymes trypsin, chymotrypsin, lipase, and amylase.

Results are approximate because the duodenal aspirates consist of pancreatic and duodenal juices and bile. In addition, not all of the secreted juice will be aspirated. However, a finding of less than 90 mEq/L of bicarbonate is 74% to 90% sensitive and 80% to 90% specific for chronic pancreatitis. Increases in duodenal secretion (volume and/or bicarbonate level) may occur with chronic alcoholism, hepatic or biliary cirrhosis, gastrinomas, or hemochromatosis. Decreases in secretions are associated with pancreatic carcinoma, collagen disease, diabetes mellitus, and Billroth I and II surgeries. Patients with cystic fibrosis have a substantial reduction in volume and bicarbonate and an 80% to 90% reduction in or absence of enzymes. Normal to slightly reduced volume, reduced bicarbonate concentration, and greatly reduced enzyme secretions are found in patients with pancreatic exocrine insufficiency that is not caused by cystic fibrosis.

### Gastric analysis

The purpose of gastric analysis is the objective measurement of gastric acid secretions. It is indicated in patients with intractable ulcer symptoms, suspected Zollinger-Ellison syndrome (hypersecretory disease) or achlorhydria. It may be indicated to assess the efficacy of treatment regimens in peptic ulcer disease. For patients with suspected achlorhydria or gastric hypersecretory states, it may also be helpful to obtain a serum gastrin level, as discussed in the section on blood tests.

Gastric analysis is contraindicated in patients with gastric outlet obstruction, recent upper gastrointestinal bleeding, inability to freely pass a nasogastric tube, an allergy to the stimulating agent, or when food particles or fresh blood are present in the gastric aspirate.

The patient fasts for 12 hours before gastric analsyis. H2 receptor agonists, anticholinergics, tricyclic antidepressants, sucralfate (Carafate), and antacids should be withheld for 48 hours before testing. After anesthetizing the nares, a radiopaque polyethylene nasogatric tube is passed, preferably under fluoroscopy, so the tip lies in the most dependent part of the stomach and along the greater curvature. Proper placement is confirmed by instillation of 30 ml of water with immediate recovery of at least 80%.

With the patient lying on the left side, manual suction is used to aspirate the stomach contents as completely as possible, and the aspirate is discarded. Four 15-minute basal acid output samples are then obtained separately. Pentagastrin (Peptavlon) is injected subcutaneously, and four 15-minute maximal acid output samples of gastric secretions are again collected. Each sample is analyzed for volume, pH, free acid, color, consistency, and occult blood.

Complications of gastric analysis are rare but may include nose bleeds, tube misplacement, or an adverse reaction to the gastric stimulant.

### 24-hour pH monitoring

Prolonged esophageal pH monitoring is the most sensitive method of directly detecting esophageal reflux, quantifying it, and correlating symptoms with reflux events. It is indicated for children with sleep apnea and also for patients with noncardiac chest pain. (Noncardiac chest pain may also be evaluated by using provocative testing, including the Bernstein acid test and the edrophonium chloride (Tensilon) test, both of which are discussed in Chapter 25). **Ambulatory pH monitoring** is also indicated in patients with suspected pulmonary complications of esophageal reflux; other atypical presentations of esophageal reflux, such as nonulcer dyspepsia, wheezing, and hoarseness; typical presentation of esophageal reflux with a negative workup; and follow-up for esophageal reflux patients after medical or surgical therapy. Ambulatory pH monitoring probably should also be performed in all patients before proposed antireflux surgery, to prevent unnecessary surgery in patients with atypical symptoms who do not, in fact, have esophageal reflux. It is contraindicated for patients with any esophageal condition that would prevent correct placement of the probe.

Before prolonged pH monitoring, the patient should be NPO for at least 6 hours and should discontinue H2 blockers for 36 hours. Children should fast for 2 to 4 hours. The pH probe and equipment must be calibrated for each patient. For the test, a reference electrode is placed on the chest, or out of reach on the back for pediatric patients. A pH probe is inserted through the patient's nostril to a position 5 cm above the lower esophageal sphincter (LES). The LES is located by esophageal manometry, fluoroscopic placement, endoscopic visualization, or by measuring the pH in the stomach and withdrawing the tube until it enters the esophagus, where the pH is higher. In children, the proper location is in the distal esophagus, at a distance that is 13% above the LES. Proper placement of the tube may need to be confirmed by radiographic examination.

Both probes are connected to an external recording device. The patient proceeds with his or her daily routine while wearing the device for 24 hours, either noting all symptoms and activities in a diary or pressing an event marker on the recording device. Children may need to be hospitalized overnight if the parent or guardian is unable to record events accurately. At the completion of the monitoring period, the stored data are read into a computer that analyzes the information and prints a graphic display of pH versus time, along with a summary of these values. Normal pH in the esophagus ranges between 6.5 and 7.0. Acid reflux is defined as a fall in intraesophageal pH below 4.0.

## BLOOD TESTS

Blood tests are frequently ordered for gastroenterology patients to test for coagulopathy, to reveal alterations in basic metabolic functions, and/or to indicate the severity of a disorder.

Table 28-1 shows the reference range for some of the more commonly used blood tests. It is important to note that reference ranges are determined by testing a large group of healthy individuals and then taking as the normal range the values that fall within 2 standard deviations of the mean, thus encompassing 95% of the sample studied. The range established by this method is dependent on two important factors: the method used, including reagents and instrumentation; and the geographic location of the population tested. It may be necessary to establish more than one reference interval for any given test (e.g., for different age groups or for males and females).

Not all values that fall outside the reference range are clinically significant. A clinically significant change in a test result is a numerical change that also reflects a change in the individual's condition.

### Hemoglobin and hematocrit

**Hemoglobin** is the oxygen-carrying pigment of the red blood cells. It is formed by the developing red blood cell in bone marrow. **Hematocrit** refers to the volume percentage of erythrocytes in whole blood. Both hemoglobin and hematocrit levels are decreased when the patient is anemic and increased when the patient is dehydrated, as a result of concentration of cells proportionate to fluid volume. Normal values of

**Table 28-1.** Normal Adult Values for Selected Blood Tests

| Diagnostic Test | Low Range | High Range |
|---|---|---|
| Hematocrit (%) | 38-F | 47-F |
| Hemoglobin (g/dl) | 40-M | 54-M |
|  | 12-F | 16-F |
| Prothrombin time (seconds)* | 13.5-M | 18-M |
|  | 11-14 |  |
| Activated partial thromboplastin time (seconds)* | 32.0-47.0 |  |
| Platelets (mm$^3$) | 150,000 | 450,000 |
| Albumin (g/dl) | 3.6 | 5.1 |
| Globulin (g/dl) | 2.1 | 3.8 |
| Albumin/globulin ratio | 1.0 | 2.0 |
| Total protein (g/dl) | 6.4 | 8.3 |
| Glucose (mg/dl) | 65 | 115 |
| Cholesterol (mg/dl) | 150 | 240 |
| Triglycerides (mg/dl) | 30 | 170 |
| AST/SGOT (mU/ml) | 6 | 41 |
| (IU/l) | 10 | 40 |
| ALT/SGPT (mU/ml) | 8 | 50 |
| (IU/l) | 5 | 35 |
| Alkaline phosphatase |  |  |
| 0-15 yr (IU/ml) | 50 | 300 |
| Adult (IU/ml) | 30 | 115 |
| Total bilirubin (mg/dl) | 0.10 | 1.3 |
| Indirect bilirubin (mg/dl) | 0.0 | 0.4 |

*Every laboratory establishes its own reference range for these tests, based on their instrumentation and reagents.

hemoglobin are 12 to 16 g/100 ml for women and 13.5 to 18 g/100 ml for men. Normal hematocrit levels are 38% to 47% for women and 40% to 54% for men.

### Prothrombin level

Prothrombin is a glycoprotein in the plasma that is normally converted to thrombin upon activation. A deficiency in this factor leads to hypoprothrombinemia. Decreased prothrombin levels may be associated with impaired absorption of vitamin K from the intestine. It may also be related to decreased availability of vitamin K, resulting from absence of bile salts or decreased intestinal flora caused by antibiotic suppression. Low levels of prothrombin are seen in infectious hepatitis, cirrhosis, biliary tract obstructions, and in small bowel disorders.

### Prothrombin time

**Prothrombin time (PT)** measures the rapidity of blood clotting through examination of Factors I, II, V, VII, and X. Prolonged PTs are seen in patients with poor nutrition, vitamin K deficiency from decreased absorption, liver disease leading to decreased synthesis of clotting factors, warfarin sodium (Coumadin) therapy, and inherited blood disorders.

### Activated partial thromboplastin time

**Activated partial thromboplastin time (APTT)** also measures the rapidity of blood clotting. It reflects clotting time by examining Factors I, II, V, VIII, IX, X, XI, and XII. A prolonged APTT is observed in patients who are taking heparin, in those with liver disease, and in those with inherited coagulopathies.

### Platelet count and function

A platelet count is a count of the number of platelets present in the blood. If the platelet count is extremely low, clotting mechanisms may be impaired. To assess platelet function, bleeding time is measured by making small cuts in the patient's arm and monitoring the time until bleeding stops. Aspirin products and nonsteroidal antiinflammatory drugs (NSAIDs) such as ibuprofen (Motrin) can prolong bleeding time for up to 14 days after ingestion.

### Serum albumin-globulin ratio

Serum albumin and globulin occur in inverse proportion to one another (i.e., as one increases, the other decreases proportionately). Decreased albumin is associated with cirrhosis, chronic hepatitis, temperature elevations, far-advanced carcinoma, malabsorption, fasting, and malnutrition; very low levels are often associated with edema and ascites. The highest levels of globulin occur in posthepatic cirrhosis and active chronic hepatitis.

### Protein loss

An abnormal loss of proteins into the GI tract may be associated with a variety of disorders. In patients who present with unexplained edema and hypoalbuminemia, an enteric loss of albumin should be considered, such as protein-losing enteropathy, a decreased rate of albumin synthesis, or an increased rate of albumin catabolism. Protein-losing enteropathy can be identified by examining serum and fecal α1-antitrypsin levels. [131]I-labeled albumin may be used to evaluate the albumin pool and the rate of degradation of albumin. Albumin tagged with 51-chromium ($^{51}$Cr) is used to measure enteric albumin loss. For patients in whom the cause of hypoalbuminemia is unclear, the combined use of [131]I-albumin and $^{51}$Cr may be needed.

In another test of excessive protein loss, [131]I-labeled polyvinylpyrrolidone (povidone) is injected intravenously, and blood specimens are collected after 2, 4, 6, and 24 hours.

### Galactose tolerance

In this test, IV galactose is administered, and blood is drawn at half-hour intervals for 2 hours. The presence of large amounts of galactose in the serum after this period of time is indicative of liver disease (failure of the liver to convert galactose to glycogen).

### Glucose tolerance

In this test, oral glucose is given to a fasting patient, and blood samples and urine specimens are taken at intervals of 30, 60, 120, and 180 minutes. Failure of the glucose level to return to normal in 1 to 2 hours is indicative of impairment of glucose utilization by the body tissues. In some patients it may be more appropriate to use an intravenous glucose test, which measures the ability of the liver to maintain glucose levels in the blood.

### Disaccharide tolerance

Disaccharide intolerance may be measured by administering an oral loading dose of the suspect disaccharide after an 8-hour fast. A fasting serum glucose sample is obtained, the loading dose is given, and serum glucose is measured at 30, 60, 90, and 120 minutes after the loading dose is administered. A careful record is kept of the number, character, pH, and Clinitest results (presence of reducing substances) for all stools passed during the test and for 8 hours after the test is completed. In most individuals, serum glucose rises more than 30 mg/dl over the fasting level during the test period. In patients with disaccharide intolerance, the increase in serum glucose is usually less than 20 mg/dl.

### Serum D-xylose

Disease processes that alter or compromise the mucosa of the upper small bowel result in decreased absorption and excretion of xylose. A delay in gastric emptying time is a major reason for falsely low serum and urine levels of xylose. This test is useful in evaluating the integrity of the upper intestinal mucosa in celiac disease, idiopathic steatorrhea, regional enteritis involving the upper small bowel, starvation, short bowel syndrome, blind loop syndrome, and milk-protein sensitivity. In celiac disease, with clinical improvement and restoration of the normal mucosa while the patient is on a gluten-free diet, the serum and urine values of xylose approach and ultimately reach normal levels. Renal failure will give falsely low urine xylose levels.

To measure xylose absorption, D-xylose is given orally after an overnight fast, and serum and urine xylose are measured 1 or 2 hours later.

### Total serum cholesterol

Elevated cholesterol levels may be indicative of incipient hepatitis, bile duct blockage, nephrotic syndrome, obstructive jaundice, pancreatitis, or hypothyroidism. Decreases in serum cholesterol may indicate malnutrition, cellular liver necrosis, or hyperthyroidism.

In preparation for this test, alcohol and drugs that affect cholesterol levels must be withheld for 24 hours.

### Serum triglycerides

Alterations in triglyceride levels may be indicative of early hyperlipidemia and may suggest that a change in the patient's dietary habits is in order. Triglyceride levels must be done after a 12- to 24-hour fast.

## Serum AST and ALT

The extent of liver disease may be determined by measuring aspartate aminotransferase (AST, previously known as serum glutamate oxaloacetate transaminase or SGOT) and alanine aminotransferase (ALT, previously known as serum glutamate pyruvate transaminase or SGPT). These cytoplasmic enzymes are released into the blood following disruption of cell membranes. Normal values are less than 40 international units (IU).

ALT is a cytosolic enzyme. Very high levels of this enzyme (i.e., as much as 100 times normal) indicate viral or drug-induced hepatitis with extensive cirrhosis. ALT levels in the thousands may indicate "shock liver," which is related to prolonged hypotension. Moderate to high ALT levels (i.e., less than 10 times normal) are suggestive of other forms of liver disease, such as biliary obstruction. Slight to moderate levels of ALT indicate hepatocellular injury. ALT may be used to differentiate between alcoholic and viral hepatitis, with alcoholic hepatitis having a lower elevation of ALT.

AST is a microsomal enzyme. It is not as specific to liver damage as ALT and must be used in conjunction with other liver tests. Increases in AST reflect cell permeability and cellular response to injury.

## Serum alkaline phosphatase

Increased alkaline phosphatase levels may reflect posthepatic obstructive jaundice, hepatic metastasis, or fatty infiltration. Marked elevations usually indicated cholestatic processes, such as mechanical biliary obstruction or drug-induced secretory failure. Serum alkaline phosphatase may also rise after administration of vitamin D, albumin, or drugs such as barbiturates, oral contraceptives, or phenothiazines. Levels of alkaline phosphatase are also elevated in osteoblastic diseases, Paget's disease, and hyperparathyroidism, and normally during pregnancy and growth. If there is complete obstruction of the common bile duct, both alkaline phosphatase and bilirubin are usually elevated. If a single hepatic duct is obstructed, only alkaline phosphatase is elevated.

## γ-Glutamyl transferase

If γ-glutamyl transferase (GGT) is normal in conjunction with alkaline phosphatase elevation, the source of alkaline phosphatase elevation is probably bone. If GGT is elevated, it pinpoints the liver as the source of alkaline phosphatase elevation.

## Serum amylase

The amount of amylase activity in serum may be altered in patients with penetrating or perforated peptic ulcer, peritonitis, bowel obstruction, biliary tract disease, liver disease, pelvic inflammatory disease, diabetic ketoacidosis, acute pancreatitis, parotid or other salivary gland disease, or ischemic bowel. In patients with pancreatic pseudocysts, serum amylase is elevated. Amylase levels may be elevated as early as 6 hours after the onset of acute pancreatitis, remain high for 3 to 5 days, and drop to normal in about 7 days.

## Serum lipase

Lipase is produced in the pancreas and secreted into the duodenum, where it converts triglycerides and other fats into fatty acids and glycerol. Elevation is most common in acute pancreatitis but may also occur in perforated peptic ulcer, intestinal obstruction, acute cholecystitis, infectious hepatitis, cirrhosis, or jaundice. In patients with pancreatitis, it is not uncommon for serum lipase levels to reach 100 times the normal level. Lipase increases later and remains elevated longer than amylase, usually decreasing after 7 to 10 days.

## Serum gastrin*

Gastrin is a hormone that is secreted in the pyloric-antral mucosa of the stomach. It stimulates secretion of hydrochloric acid by the parietal cells of the gastric glands. The gastrin stimulation test is indicated in patients with severe or unusual gastric or duodenal ulcerations, suspected Zollinger-Ellison syndrome, and suspected gastric hypersecretion. In this test, timed serum gastrin levels are drawn after stimulation with IV secretin. Patients must fast for 12 hours before the test, and H2 antagonists and anticholinergics should be withheld for 24 hours.

A large-bore IV needle is inserted to secure adequate blood samples. Blood specimens are drawn 10 minutes before, immediately before, and 1, 2, 5, 10, and 30 minutes after injection of secretin. For each sample, 5 ml of blood are withdrawn and discarded, followed by collection of a 10-ml specimen for testing. Serum gastrin levels are calculated for all seven samples.

Potential complications include infiltration of the IV fluid, inability to withdraw the correct amount of blood for the sample, and a local or systemic allergic reaction to administration of secretin.

## Hepatitis antigens and antibodies

Hepatitis B surface antigen (HBsAg) is a measure of hepatitis B infection. Testing is positive in carriers and in those with acute and chronic infections. Hepatitis B surface antibody (HBsAb) is seen in patients who have

---

*Also discussed in the SGNA *Manual of Gastrointestinal Procedures*. 2nd ed. Rochester, N.Y.: Society of Gastroenterology Nurses and Associates, 1989.

recovered from hepatitis B and/or have formed antibodies to the virus by other means. HBsAb titers may be valuable in confirming immunity after immunization with the hepatitis B vaccine series.

Hepatitis B core antibody (HBcAb) is present in both acute and recovered disease states; immunoglobulins must be assessed to make a differential diagnosis. If immunoglobulin M (IgM) is positive, the patient's disease is active and infectious; if immunoglobulin G (IgG) is positive, the patient has developed the antibody and is no longer infective.

Hepatitis B e antigen (HBeAg) is indicative of a highly infectious state. Patients with hepatitis B e antibody (HBeAb) are no longer infectious.

If hepatitis A antibody (HAVAb) is negative, there is no active or history of hepatitis A virus. HAVAb is positive in both acute infections and in those who have recovered from infection. Patients with acute infectious hepatitis A are IgM positive. Patients who have recovered from hepatitis A are IgG positive.

New tests are also available for hepatitis C and the delta antibody.

### Carcinoembryonic antigen

Carcinoembryonic antigen (CEA) is a glycoprotein that is associated with fetal growth. In adults, however, plasma CEA levels are elevated with endodermal tumors or neoplasia involving the lung, breast, ovary, bladder, testes, brain, or reticuloendothelial system, in addition to a wide range of benign inflammatory disorders. It has been studied as a possible prognosticator in colorectal cancer; elevated preoperative levels should be followed postoperatively and if there is a rise after an initial fall, it may be indicative of a recurrence.

### Serum antibodies

Antibodies sometimes develop to cytoplasmic constituents, including antimitochondrial antibodies and anti-smooth muscle antibodies. Indirect immunofluorescence is used to demonstrate the presence of these antibodies. They seem to have no etiologic significance, but are useful markers for a limited range of conditions of probable immune etiology, nearly all of which involve the liver. Antibody to smooth muscle occurs in 90% or more of patients with chronic active hepatitis. Antimitochondrial antibody, usually in high titers, is found in 90% or more of patients with biliary cirrhosis. Neither antibody, however, is specific for the single disease.

### Serum bilirubin

A total serum bilirubin test measures both the secretory and excretory functions of the liver. Abnormal elevations of total bilirubin indicate hepatocellular disease, biliary tract disease, or overproduction of bilirubin at a rate beyond the liver's capacity to metabolize it. It is not a sensitive indication of biliary obstruction or liver cell injury.

Unconjugated (indirect) bilirubin measures the secretory function of the liver. Conjugated (direct) bilirubin measures excretory function. Elevations in this value usually indicate hemolysis or decreased cell permeability. Elevated direct bilirubin is indicative of hepatobiliary disease, hemolysis, liver cell damage, and obstructed bile flow in the common bile duct. Direct bilirubin may also be elevated in various genetic disorders of bilirubin metabolism, such as Dubin-Johnson syndrome or Gilbert's syndrome.

## URINALYSIS

In gastroenterology patients, urine samples may be analyzed to determine levels of bilirubin or urobilinogen, vitamin B12 absorption, or the extent of biliary obstruction. Most urinalysis is semiquantitative in nature and is done on random clean-catch samples.

### Urine bilirubin

Only direct bilirubin can be measured in the urine. Significant amounts of bilirubin in the urine are indicative of hepatic disease or biliary obstruction. The urine specimen for a bilirubin test must be collected in a dark bottle and immediately taken to the laboratory, because light decreases the bilirubin level. Alternatively, the specimen may be shaken at bedside; brown urine with yellow foam is a positive result.

### Urine urobilinogen

Elevated levels of urobilinogen indicate failure of the liver cells to reabsorb the urobilinogen that is broken down in the intestine by the action of intestinal bacteria on bilirubin. Urine specimens that will be analyzed for urobilinogen levels should be put in a dark brown container and immediately taken to the laboratory.

### Schilling test (Vitamin B12 absorption)

The **Schilling test** is used to determine vitamin B12 (cyanocobalamin) malabsorption. In preparation for this test, the patient fasts from midnight the previous night until 2 hours after the oral administration of radioactive vitamin B12 capsules. The test is done in two stages: $^{58}$Co-cyanocobalamin alone and $^{57}$Co-cyanocobalamin combined with intrinsic factor. An IM injection of 1 mg of nonradioactive vitamin B12 is administered to the patient immediately or up to 2 hours after the administration of the radioactive capsules. All urine is collected for 24 hours after the administration of the radioactive capsules. The urinary excretion of each isotope is determined, and the ratio is calculated to provide information about the relative absorptions of the two isotopes and the site of the absorptive defect.

# FECAL ANALYSIS

Stool specimens should be analyzed for patients with diarrhea, steatorrhea, constipation, bleeding, or persistent abdominal discomfort. Usually only a small amount of stool needs to be collected on a tongue blade and placed in a disposable container. If an enema is needed to obtain a specimen, only tap water or normal saline should be used.

The length of time it takes for stool passage can be determined by the administration of a carmine marker or charcoal marker when a meal is ingested. The color, form, odor, consistency, content, and pH of the stool may also be important. The nurse should explain to the patient the method to be used to collect the stool specimen, whether it should be delivered fresh, and the process whereby it should be stored. The patient should also be instructed to record the times of bowel movements and to note stool color, consistency, and any associated pain.

## Fecal urobilinogen

Specimens collected for this test should be put in light-resistant containers and immediately sent to the laboratory. If possible, the specimen should be collected between noon and 4:00 PM because urobilinogen production peaks at that time. An increased amount of urobilinogen darkens the color of the stool, whereas a decreased amount causes clay-colored stools. Decreased amounts are usually the result of biliary obstruction.

## Occult blood

**Occult blood** testing is most often used for cancer screening. It is not useful in patients with frank bleeding from the GI tract, actively bleeding hemorrhoids, or in women who are menstruating.

The most common test for the detection of occult blood in the feces is **Hemoccult***, which uses guaiac-impregnated paper slides or guaiac tape and a developing solution. It is readily available, convenient, and inexpensive. However, its effectiveness depends on the degree of fecal hydration, the amount of hemoglobin degradation, and the presence of interfering substances that enhance or inhibit oxidation of the indicator dye.

Before occult blood testing, the patient must:

- Adhere to a high-fiber diet for 48 hours, with no rare red meat
- Avoid foods that are high in peroxidase, such as turnips, broccoli, or horseradish
- Avoid iron preparation, bromides, iodides, salicylates, NSAIDs, or high doses of ascorbic acid.

*Also discussed in the SGNA *Manual of Gastrointestinal Procedures.* 2nd ed. Rochester, N.Y.: Society of Gastroenterology Nurses and Associates, 1989.

Ideally, aspirin and NSAIDs should be avoided for 1 week before Hemoccult testing.

Three stools must be collected without being contaminated by urine or toilet tissue. The delay between collection and laboratory testing should not exceed 6 days, and the specimens should not be refrigerated. For analysis, a small piece of stool is placed on the slide or tape, and wetted with the appropriate developing solution. A blue color appears in 30 to 60 seconds if blood is present. Positive results indicate gastrointestinal bleeding and may be important in the early detection of colorectal cancer. False positive results may be caused by patient noncompliance with dietary and/or medication restrictions. Vitamin C (ascorbic acid) can cause false negative results.

To increase the sensitivity and specificity of fecal occult blood testing, new methods are being developed. One relatively new, commercially available test is HemoQuant, which is a sensitive quantitative assay that is based on the fluorescence of heme-derived porphyrins. Although HemoQuant appears to be a sensitive and specific assay for human fecal hemoglobin, its predictive value for disease is still under study.

## Fecal fat

Little if any dietary fat is unabsorbed when bile and pancreatic secretions are adequate. The presence of abnormal fecal fat content (steatorrhea) is significant in malabsorptive disorders such as Crohn's disease and blind loop syndrome. Typically, fatty stools are greasy, pale, frothy, floating, and foul-smelling.

For a qualitative test of fecal fat, a random sample of stool is examined for evidence of malabsorption and various fats. Neutral fat, which accounts for 20% to 30% of total stool fat in pancreatic insufficiency, stains red with Sudan and appears as globules, whereas fatty acids do not stain with Sudan and appear as fatty acid crystals.

For a more accurate, quantitative test, the patient adheres to a high-fat diet, with no alcohol, for 3 days, followed by a 72-hour collection period. A nonabsorbable marker is given at the beginning of the test period and again 72 hours later. All stools passed from the appearance of the first marker until the appearance of the second should be collected in a polyethylene bag inside a preweighed plastic container and kept in a freezer. The stool containing the first unabsorbable marker is included in the collection; the stool showing the second marker is not. Plastic wrap inside the diaper is satisfactory for collection of stool samples from young patients.

## Fecal chymotrypsin

Fecal chymotrypsin determination is a reliable, semi-quantitative test for exocrine pancreatic insufficiency. It can be applied to the same 72-hour stool collection procedure used for quantitation of fecal fat. It is more suitable than biliary drainage for routine screening of malabsorption syndromes.

Stools are collected for 72 hours between two nonabsorbable markers, such as charcoal. Specimens are frozen as soon as possible after they are passed and are pooled in a preweighed container. Enzyme activity in the stool samples is measured titrimetrically or by using an ultraviolet spectrophotometer.

### Protein loss

$\alpha$1-Antitrypsin ($\alpha$1-AT) is a natural plasma protein that resists proteolytic digestion. The purpose of measuring fecal $\alpha$1-AT is to detect protein loss. Its concentration in the stool can be measured simply and accurately by immunologic methods. In addition, measurement of $\alpha$1-AT does not require the use of radioisotopes.

Another way of detecting excessive protein loss is to inject [131]I-labeled polyvinylpyrrolidone (PVP or povidone) intravenously and collect stool samples over a 72-hour period. A patient with a disease that involves protein loss will excrete large amounts of PVP in the stool.

Alternatively, [61]Cr-albumin may be injected intravenously, and all stools collected for a 96-hour period, taking care not to contaminate the stool specimens with urine. Normal subjects excrete less than 1% of the administered dose of tagged albumin. In patients with protein-losing enteropathy, between 4% and 20% and as much as 40% of the administered dose is recovered in the stool.

### Fecal organisms

To confirm the presence of enteric pathogens, a freshly passed stool specimen may be examined. The specimen should be sent directly to the laboratory.

### HYDROGEN BREATH TEST*

Breath tests commonly involve the ingestion of a radioactive substance and the measurement of certain exhaled gases after a given time period. Usually the patient is asked to exhale through a solution containing specific chemicals that change color in the presence of certain concentrations of the gas. **Hydrogen breath tests** are used in the diagnosis of bacterial overgrowth of the intestine, short bowel syndrome, sugar intolerance, and in tests of fat absorption.

At present the hydrogen test for malabsorption of lactose and other carbohydrates is the most widely used

breath test. Hydrogen is produced in the body by bacterial fermentation of carbohydrates. Under normal circumstances, lactose is broken down into glucose and galactose and is absorbed in the small intestine, which has virtually no anaerobic bacteria. In patients who are deficient in lactase or who have delayed transit times, mucosal damage, or colonic flora in the upper GI tract, lactose will come into contact with the fermenting bacteria in the colon and hydrogen gas will evolve.

The objective of breath hydrogen testing is to measure the volume of hydrogen that is produced in the colon, absorbed from the colon into the blood, and expelled in the breath. Breath hydrogen testing is indicated in patients with suspected carbohydrate malabsorption, abnormal gastrointestinal time, or bacterial overgrowth of the small intestine. It is contraindicated in uncooperative patients. Patients must fast for 12 hours before the test and must refrain from smoking after midnight the previous night. Antibiotics and bowel cleansers should not be given within a week before the test.

End-expired tidal air is collected twice before and every 30 minutes for 3 hours after ingestion of a carbohydrate drink. Hydrogen gas concentration is determined by gas–liquid chromatography. Normal individuals expire less than 20 ppm hydrogen, while persons with malabsorption syndromes expire greater than 80 ppm.

To avoid the problem of false positive results, a positive lactose test may be followed by a glucose breath test to differentiate between true lactose intolerance and bacterial overgrowth. At least 10% of the population lacks hydrogen-producing bacteria in the colon. To avoid false negative results, a negative lactose test may be followed by a lactulose test to confirm the presence of hydrogen-producing colonic bacteria.

If the patient is found to be carbohydrate intolerant, dietary counseling should be given before discharge, as described in Chapter 23.

---

**CASE SITUATION**

Jennifer Roth, a 28-year-old female, is scheduled for a gastroscopy on Tuesday. She is being treated for alcoholism and is presenting with gastrointestinal bleeding and acute pain.

*Points to think about*

1. What tests would most commonly be ordered before a procedure for this patient?
2. What laboratory tests might be abnormal and why?
3. From the abnormal tests identified, which values would be decreased and which would be elevated?

---

*Also discussed in the SGNA *Manual of Gastrointestinal Procedures*. 2nd ed. Rochester, N.Y.: Society of Gastroenterology Nurses and Associates, 1989.

*Suggested Responses*

1. The following tests would probably be ordered for this patient:
   - Liver profile, including ALT, AST, and lactate dehydrogenase
   - Complete blood count (CBC), including hematocrit, hemoglobin, white cell count, the proportions of the different white cells, red blood cell indices and morphology, and platelet count
   - PT and APTT
   - Urinalysis, including bilirubin and urobilinogen
   - Occult blood
2. Abnormal tests might be:

| Abnormal test result | Possible cause |
|---|---|
| Alanine aminotransferase (ALT) Aspartate aminotransferase (AST) Lactate dehydrogenase (LD) | Cirrhosis or hepatitis, depending on the degree of alcoholism |
| RBC Hemoglobin Hematocrit Red cell indices/ morphology | Gastrointestinal bleeding resulting in iron deficiency |
| Platelet count | Impaired platelet production because of toxic effects of alcohol on the bone marrow Congestive splenomegaly; platelets sequestered in the spleen |
| PT APTT | Liver disease impairs production of protein synthesis |
| Urinary bilirubin Urinary urobilinogen | Normal to elevated, depending on the degree of bleeding and the stage of liver disease. (The liver converts the hemoglobin from the red cells to bilirubin) |
| Occult blood | GI bleeding |

3. The following values would be decreased:
   - RBC
   - Hemoglobin
   - Hematocrit
   - Platelet counts
   The following values would be increased:
   - ALT
   - AST
   - LD
   - Bilirubin
   - Prothrombin time
   - Urinary bilirubin or urobilinogen, depending on stage of disease.

NOTE: Red cell indices (morphology) will be abnormal, but the values will depend on the predominant pathologic process; that is, whether it is iron deficiency or liver disease.

REVIEW TERMS

**activated partial thromboplastin time (APTT), ambulatory pH monitoring, angiography, arteriography, barium enema, barium sulfate, barium swallow, cholangiography, computed tomography (CT), double-contrast technique, enteroclysis, fluoroscopic examination, hematocrit, Hemoccult, hemoglobin, hydrogen breath tests, occult blood, oral cholecystography, percutaneous transhepatic cholangiography (PTC), prothrombin time (PT), radiographic studies, Schilling test, scintigraphy, ultrasonography, upper gastrointestinal series (UGI), x-ray (roentgenographic) examination**

REVIEW QUESTIONS

1. The usual position of the patient during a barium swallow is the:
   a. Standing position
   b. Sitting position.
   c. Prone position.
   d. Supine position.
2. In a double-contrast barium enema, visualization is improved by the introduction of:
   a. Air.
   b. An inert dye.
   c. Radioactive isotopes.
   d. Methylcellulose.
3. Before abdominal ultrasonography, the patient follows a low-carbohydrate diet for 48 hours. The purpose of this regimen is to:
   a. Promote intestinal motility.
   b. Minimize residue in the GI tract.
   c. Minimize intestinal gas.
   d. Promote gastric emptying.
4. The three-dimensional image produced by computed tomography is based on:
   a. Differences in tissue density.
   b. The differential transmission of sound waves by different tissues.
   c. The differential uptake of radioactive isotopes.
   d. Visualization of radiopaque structures.
5. In biliary drainage procedure, bile samples are collected from:
   a. The common bile duct.
   b. The pancreatic duct.
   c. The duodenum, near the ampulla of Vater.
   d. The gallbladder.

6. For gastric analysis, gastric acid secretions are stimulated by the injection of:
   a. Secretin.
   b. Metoclopramide (Reglan).
   c. Glucose.
   d. Pentagastrin (Peptavlon).

7. Clinitest tablets are used with stool specimens to detect the presence of:
   a. Disaccharides.
   b. Glucose.
   c. Reducing substances.
   d. Lactose.

8. Extremely high levels of ALT are indicative of:
   a. Viral or alcohol-induced hepatitis.
   b. Biliary obstruction.
   c. Hepatocellular injury.
   d. Hepatic metastasis.

9. The Schilling test is used to evaluate:
   a. Disaccharide tolerance.
   b. Vitamin B12 absorption.
   c. Immunity to hepatitis.
   d. Bilirubin levels.

10. In patients with lactose intolerance, most of the excess hydrogen that is detected in a hydrogen breath test is produced:
    a. In the small intestine.
    b. By aerobic bacteria.
    c. In the colon.
    d. In the lungs.

## BIBLIOGRAPHY

Beck, M "Biliary Drainage: Indications and Clinical Technique." In *SGA Journal Reprints*, S. Trivits, ed. 109–11. Rochester, N.Y.: Society of Gastrointestinal Assistants, 1988.

Chobanian, S, and Van Ness, M, eds. *Manual of Clinical Problems in Gastroenterology.* Boston: Little, Brown & Co., 1988.

Chopra, S, and May, R, eds. *Pathophysiology of Gastrointestinal Diseases.* Boston: Little, Brown & Co., 1989.

Ciarleglio, C "Gastric Analysis: Old Stand-by with a New Purpose." *SGA Journal* 10(Spring 1988): 202-04.

Ciarleglo, C "Gastric Analysis: The Renaissance of an Old Technique." *SGA Journal* 11(Fall 1988): 85-92.

Cotton, P, and Williams, C. *Practical Gastrointestinal Endoscopy.* 3rd ed. Oxford: Blackwell Scientific Publications, Inc., 1990.

Dalton, C, Sinclair, J, and Castell, D. "Prolonged Ambulatory Esophageal pH Monitoring." *Gastroenterology Nursing* 11(Spring 1989): 221-26.

Fachnie, B. "Breath Hydrogen Testing: A Current Review." *SGA Journal* 11(Summer 1988): 18-21.

Given, B, and Simmons, S. *Gastroenterology in Clinical Nursing.* 4th ed. St. Louis: Mosby–Year Book, 1984.

Hamilton, H, editorial director. *Procedures.* Nurse's Reference Library. Springhouse, Pa.: Intermed Communications, 1983.

Hardick, M, and Beck, M. *Manual of Gastrointestinal Procedures.* 2nd ed. Rochester, N.Y.: Society of Gastroenterology Nurses and Associates, 1989.

Henry, J. *Clinical Diagnosis and Management by Laboratory Methods.* 18th ed. Philadelphia: WB Saunders, 1991.

Kneedler, J, and Dodge, G. *Perioperative Patient Care: The Nursing Perspective.* 2nd ed. Boston: Blackwell Scientific Publications, Inc., 1987.

Knohl, S. "Laboratory Values in GI: Implications for Procedures and Safety Issues for Patients and Staff." *SGA Journal* 12(Winter 1989): 179-83.

Rayhorn, N, ed. *Manual of Gastrointestinal Procedures: Pediatric Supplement.* Rochester, N.Y.: Society of Gastroenterology Nurses and Associates, 1991.

Sacher, R, ed. *Widmann's Clinical Interpretation of Laboratory Tests.* 10th ed. Philadelphia: FA Davis, 1991.

Schumacher, H, Garvin, D, Triplett, D. *Introduction to Laboratory Hematology and Hematopathology.* New York: Alan R. Liss, 1984.

Silverman, A, and Roy, C. *Pediatric Clinical Gastroenterology.* 3rd ed. St. Louis: Mosby–Year Book, Inc., 1983.

Wu, W. "Testing for Gastroesophageal Reflux." In *SGA Journal Reprints*, Trivits S, 43-51. Rochester, N.Y.: Society of Gastrointestinal Assistants, 1988.

# THERAPEUTIC PROCEDURES

# Chapter 29

# DILATATION

This chapter will acquaint the gastroenterology nurse with the procedures used for endoscopic dilatation of gastrointestinal strictures.

**Learning objectives**

After reviewing the content of this chapter, the gastroenterology nurse should be able to:

1. Describe the indications, contraindications, techniques, and potential complications of using sheer force to dilate gastrointestinal strictures, using rubber bougies, metal olives, stepped dilators, or tapered polyvinyl chloride dilators.
2. Explain the indications, contraindications, techniques, and potential complications of using hydrostatic or pneumatic balloons for gastrointestinal dilatation.
3. Discuss nursing considerations pertinent to each of these techniques.

## BASIC PRINCIPLES

There are two basic types of gastrointestinal dilatation; a sheer-force method, which involves forcing a dilator through a narrowed area, using axial force to enlarge the lumen; and hydrostatic or pneumatic balloon dilatation, which involves inflating a balloon within the lumen, thereby providing a radial force that accomplishes the dilatation. Obstructing tumors may also be ablated by using a bipolar tumor probe, as discussed in Chapter 30.

There are a large number of different types of sheer-force **dilators**, including the following:

*All techniques in this chapter, except the use of the Celestin dilator, are also discussed in the SGNA *Manual of Gastrointestinal Procedures*, 2nd ed. Rochester, N.Y.: Society of Gastroenterology Nurses and Associates, 1989.

- Mercury-filled rubber bougies (Hurst or Maloney type)
- Metal Eder-Puestow olives
- Stepped dilators, such as the Celestin dilator
- Tapered polyvinyl chloride Savary-Gilliard or American dilators

The sizes of esophageal dilators are expressed in terms of their diameter in millimeters (mm) or in **French units** (Fr), which are based on the circumference of the instrument (i.e., the diameter in millimeters multiplied by pi). For convenience, a factor of 3 rather than 3.14 may be used for pi when converting from millimeters to French units.

### Procedure

Dilatation procedures are contraindicated in uncooperative patients and in patients with significant coaguloapathy, esophageal impaction, recent myocardial infarction, active ulcers, recent biopsy examination, or severe cervical arthritis.

Before upper GI dilatation, the patient should be NPO for at least 6 hours. Dentures should be removed, and a topical anesthetic or gargle may be used.

The patient is positioned in a sitting, standing, or left lateral position. It is the nurse's responsibility to ensure that the correct position is maintained throughout the procedure. If the dilators deviate from the midline during the procedure, perforation of the pharynx, esophagus, or stomach could occur.

Bougienage with Hurst and Maloney dilators is usually performed without premedication. Other forms of dilatation are performed using sedation and endoscopy. Some dilatation procedures are performed with fluoroscopic guidance, particularly when carcinomas or long strictures are being dilated. The distal 5 to 6 inches of the dilator should be lubricated with a water-soluble lubricant.

The nurse should assemble the dilators, aspirate saliva, and assist the physician during the procedure. When a guidewire is used, it is the nurse's responsibility to pass the guidewire to the physician, assuring that there are no kinks or bends. The spring tip is inserted first, while the nurse controls the loose end. Then, the lubricated dilator is fed onto the correctly placed guidewire. The nurse must stabilize the guidewire to maintain the correct position during advancement and withdrawal of the dilator. Guidewire markings should be used to confirm the correct placement. The physician should be notified if there is any blood on the used dilator or in the patient's secretions. The sizes of the dilators should be documented.

It is best to begin dilatation procedures with a dilator that is one or two sizes smaller than the diameter of the stricture. Dilatation can be repeated daily, every other day, or several times per week, depending on the patient's response, the severity of the stricture, and the sense of resistance that is felt. On subsequent sessions, the physician may begin with a dilator that is one size smaller than the largest dilator passed at the previous session. As a general rule, not more than three increasing French sizes should be used in any one session.

The esophagus is the most common target of gastrointestinal dilatation. The primary goal of esophageal dilatation is to restore the patient's ability to eat and drink normally. In most cases, dysphagia in response to solid food will not be completely relieved until a minimal luminal diameter equivalent to 38 or 40 Fr (14 mm diameter) is achieved. If the esophageal lumen can be fully dilated to 52 Fr (17 mm diameter), the patient should be able to eat a normal diet. Patients with a lumen less than 39 Fr will require a modified diet.

After any upper GI dilatation procedure, the patient should remain NPO until the gag reflex returns. Vital signs and patient condition should be monitored and documented. The patient should be instructed to notify the physician immediately in the event of chest pain, fever, regurgitation of blood, pain on swallowing, back pain, shoulder pain, abdominal pain, rectal bleeding, chills, black stools, or nausea.

Potential complications of dilatation include hemorrhage, perforation, aspiration, and bacteremia. The most common site of perforation is the area immediately proximal to a stricture. With dilators that use guidewires, the risk of perforation is more likely related to the guidewire than to the dilator. Fluoroscopy is generally advised to be sure that the guidewire does not bend to form a sharp point or loop and to verify correct placement of the dilator at the stricture. Perforation may also occur if the guidewire is misplaced or damaged. In patients who have undergone previous surgery, the use of guidewires is riskier and more complicated, because the anatomy may be distorted.

It is critically important that perforation be identified as soon as possible. Cervical perforation is usually obvious. It is associated with fever, chest pain, leukocytosis, pain on swallowing, change in the quality of the voice, and air in the subcutaneous tissues of the neck (i.e., subcutaneous emphysema). Radiographic examination usually reveals air in the retroesophageal space. The most common symptom of esophageal perforation is persistent pain, even if it is mild, after dilatation.

When perforation is suspected, it is important to obtain upright and lateral x-ray films of the chest to serve as a baseline and to search for free air under the diaphragm, pneumothorax, or pleural effusion. In addition, an x-ray barium swallow examination should be performed, using a water-soluble contrast medium. Many times, perforation can be managed conservatively by administering antibiotics, providing suction, and keeping the patient NPO. At other times, surgery may be necessary.

Bleeding is a rare complication of dilatation for the management of benign lesions. When bleeding occurs, it is usually minor and transfusions are seldom needed. Bacteremia has developed after dilatation procedures, but it is a serous problem only in immunocompromised patients and in patients with prosthetic valves or a history of endocarditis. The bacteria in the blood may originate from either the dilator or the oropharynx. For this reason, it is important to clean and disinfect dilators adequately after each use. They should be soaked in a high-level disinfectant, rinsed thoroughly, air dried, and stored in a clean, dry location.

If blood and/or mucus are present on the dilator on removal from the affected site, this observation should be documented. If there is a question about the malignancy of the stricture, any blood or mucus that is present may be rinsed into a bottle with cytologic fixative and submitted for cytologic examination.

Different types of dilators are used in different situations. Indications for the use of several different types of dilators are discussed, along with techniques for insertion and specific risks associated with each technique.

## BOUGIENAGE

**Bougienage** is the dilatation of the esophagus by using mercury-filled, soft-rubber dilators (**bougies**) of graduated sizes, ranging from 18 to 60 Fr. Dilators less than 32 Fr are so flexible that little effective pressure can be applied from above without bending them.

The mercury provides the proper combination of rigidity and flexibility, so the bougies can be swallowed, and the force applied to the shaft of the dilator can be transmitted to the stricture. There are two types of bougies: tapered **Maloney dilators** and blunt or rounded **Hurst dilators**. The Maloney dilator, with its tapered end, seems to be easier for patients to swallow. The tapered tip of the Maloney dilator is more likely to enter a small-diameter stricture, but is also more likely to bend, causing the dilator to be misdirected.

Indications for bougienage include the following:

- Esophageal strictures, including peptic, postsurgical, postradiation, or malignant strictures.
- Chemically induced strictures caused by lye ingestion or a sclerosing agent. Esophageal injury associated with a gray-white exudate, ulcers, and hemorrhage can have nonforceful dilatation 3 to 7 days after injury. Esophageal injury that is associated with extensive ulceration, gray-black exudate, mucosal sloughing, and a dilated and atonic lumen without peristalsis should not be dilated until mucosal healing is noted endoscopically.
- Esophageal rings or webs. In bougienage for lower esophageal rings, it is best to use one pass of a large dilator, such as a 50 Fr. If this treatment is not successful, it may be preferable to use a pneumatic dilator similar to that used in patients with achalasia.
- Diffuse esophageal spasm, with a normal lower esophageal sphincter (LES).
- Scleroderma.

Before the procedure a topical anesthetic may be applied to the patient's throat. The patient is usually placed in an upright sitting position, but a left lateral position may be used to avoid aspiration, to facilitate endoscopic examination preceding dilatation, or if fluoroscopy is to be used.

Maloney or Hurst dilators are passed into the hypopharynx and esophagus in much the same way as a flexible endoscope. Before use, the distal end of the bougie is well lubricated. The physician introduces the bougie into the mouth and uses a forefinger to direct it into the pharynx. A swallowing motion allows gentle passage into the upper esophagus. An experienced operator can feel when the dilator engages the stricture. When it does engage a stricture, the dilator is held lightly between the thumb and fingers, and gentle force is applied to dilate the stricture.

Aspiraton of oral secretions is usually necessary during the procedure. The physician should be notified of any blood on the used dilator or in the patient's secretions. The size of the dilators used should be documented.

Care and maintenance of rubber bougies are not difficult. Before each use, the bougies should be inspected carefully. If the rubber cracks or splits when the bougie is bent, it should be replaced. Bougies should be cleaned, disinfected, and dried after each use. They should be stored horizontally, as straight as possible, in a closed, clean, and dry area.

The problem with all bougienage techniques is that they are dependent on an externally applied axial force.

If the stricture is too tight, the axial force applied may cause the pusher to bend laterally and rupture the esophagus, rather than push the dilator through the stricture. Bougies are of little benefit when the stricture is unyielding, is angulated, or causes severe luminal narrowing.

## EDER-PUESTOW DILATORS

In 1950, Puestow introduced a dilatation technique that involves a series of metal olives screwed onto a semiflexible metal wand. The entire device is passed over a guidewire, which has a flexible tip that has been inserted through the stricture. Eder-Puestow olives come in graduated sizes (21 to 53 Fr).

The use of Eder-Puestow dilators can be a very uncomfortable experience for the patient. However, this type of dilatation is indicated in patients with severe, long, complex, or rigid strictures (usually malignant tumors).

Before use, each portion of the Eder-Puestow system should be thoroughly inspected, with special attention given to the guidewire tip. Use of a guidewire with a sharp, broken end or a bent spring increases the risk of perforation.

The physician begins the procedure by inserting an end-viewing gastroscope as for a normal esophagogastroduodenoscopy (EGD) investigation. In most cases, after assessing the degree of stricture, the endoscopist passes the guidewire through the biopsy channel of the endoscope. Under either direct endoscopic view or radiologic control, the end of the wire is manipulated into a safe place in the body of the stomach, usually with the tip pointing toward the greater curvature. The endoscope is then removed.

Next, the lightly-lubricated metal wand with attached olive is passed over the guidewire. As the physician advances the dilator, the nurse puts traction on the guidewire and fluoroscopically monitors the guidewire tip in the stomach to be sure that it does not move or bend. The wire must be kept taut so the dilator can be safely advanced over the wire; the wire should remain in a constant position as the dilator is advanced. The nurse is also responsible for ensuring that the proximal end of the guidewire tip does not flail around and injure the patient or other persons participating in the procedure. Increasingly larger olives are passed over the guidewire until the desired degree of dilatation is obtained. Usually not more than three French-size dilators are used in the same session. After passing three successive olives that meet with mild to moderate resistance, pain, or slight bleeding, the guidewire is pulled snug against the tip of the last dilator, and both are removed as a unit. Guidewires may kink during use. Kinks can cause difficulty in passing the olives and can prevent effective dilatation or prolong the procedure.

Diligent oral suction is necessary throughout the procedure because secretions or regurgitated gastric contents may accumulate in the patient's mouth.

After the apparatus is removed, the physician may again pass the endoscope through the dilated stricture to check the condition of the mucosa and examine the remainder of the esophagus, stomach, and duodenum if desired. The patient receives routine postendoscopy care. A chest radiographic examination may be performed, but is not essential.

Potential complications of dilatation using the Eder-Puestow system include perforation, bleeding, aspiration, and bacteremia. The patient may also experience transient retrosternal discomfort or throat soreness.

After each use, the Eder-Puestow system should be processed and stored according to the manufacturer's instructions.

## POLYVINYL CHLORIDE DILATORS

Strictures may also be dilated by inserting a guidewire past the affected area and introducing a semiflexible, tapered, polyvinyl chloride dilator over the guidewire. Guidewires may be introduced with or without the use of an endoscope, and the dilators may be inserted with or without fluoroscopic guidance.

**Savary-Gilliard dilators** consist of a series of semiflexible, tapered, polyvinyl bougies that have a lumen for the guidewire in the center. They range in size from 5 to 18 mm (15 to 54 Fr). The dilators fit over a stainless steel guidewire that is 182 cm long and 0.8 mm in diameter. The wire has a graduated, flexible spring tip that reduces the tendency to penetrate tissue or retroflex upon itself. A radiopaque marker is incorporated into the dilator to aid in fluoroscopic monitoring.

The **American** dilator system is an adaptation of the Savary dilators. The distal tapered end of the bougie shaft is shorter, and the bougies are completely radiopaque. Dilators in the American system range in size from 5 to 18 mm (15 to 54 Fr).

Polyvinyl chloride dilators are easily passed through the mouth, and the flexible tip readily traverses the pharynx. The plastic material is less likely to injure the patient's teeth than the metal olives of the Eder-Puestow system.

Polyvinyl chloride dilators are usually used for esophageal strictures. They are indicated for the following:
- Dilatation of peptic, malignant, postsurgical, or postradiation strictures
- Dilatation of obstructing tumors to permit passage of an endoscope so endoscopic laser therapy can begin at the distal tumor margin
- Placement of a stent
- Patients with esophageal webs or rings, diffuse esophageal spasm, chemically induced strictures, or scleroderma

Potential complications of dilatation using polyvinyl chloride dilators include perforation, bleeding, aspiraton, and bacteremia.

## CELESTIN DILATORS

A **Celestin dilator** is a stepped dilator that is passed over an endoscopically placed guidewire through an esophageal stricture. Each dilator contains a series of steps that increase in size. The advantage of using a stepped dilator over an Eder-Puestow system is that only two passes through the pharynx are necessary. A slight disadvantage is that by the time the largest step of the dilator is through the stricture, the tip of the dilator is well into the body of the stomach.

The procedure for stepped dilatation is similar to that for Eder-Puestow dilatation. The guidewire is passed through the suction channel of the endoscope, and the endoscope is withdrawn. The nurse holds the guidewire taut in the patient's mouth. The dilator is passed gently over the guidewire, and the stricture is gradually dilated. The guidewire is withdrawn with the dilator, and the patient is made comfortable. Postprocedural care is the same as for all dilatations.

## HYDROSTATIC BALLOONS

The technique of luminal dilatation by using a Gruntzig-type balloon was initially performed for occlusive vascular disorders. Today, balloon dilatation has become an integral part of therapeutic endoscopy. **Hydrostatic balloons** are made of a specially treated polyethylene, which is altered to greatly increase strength and minimize stretching. A pressure gauge keeps the applied pressure within recommended limits. The balloon is filled with fluid; for example, water or dilute radiopaque dye. (Full-strength contrast material crystallizes easily and occludes the lumen of the dilator, thereby rendering it useless.)

There are two types of balloon dilators; through-the-scope (TTS) balloons and over-the-guidewire balloons.
- TTS balloons have an inflated diameter of 4 to 25 mm. They are passed through the biopsy channel of the endoscope, and dilatation is accomplished under direct vision.
- Over-the-guidewire balloons have an inflated diameter of 4 to 40 mm. A guidewire is passed, the scope is removed, and the dilators are passed under fluoroscopic control.

Hydrostatic balloons are used for the following:
- Dilatation of benign or malignant esophageal, pyloric, duodenal, rectal, or left-colon strictures.
- Temporarily opening the rectosimgoid luminal pathway when it is obstructed by a tumor, before endoscopic laser therapy. For rectal cancers, it may be easier to use a rigid proctoscope and hand-held laser fiber.

- Pyloric stenosis.
- Biliary tract strictures.
- Food impactions above an esophageal stricture.

In patients with food impactions above an esophageal stricture, the bolus is dislodged and the guidewire is passed through the stricture. The dilator is passed and inflated, and the bolus is then pushed into the stomach. This procedure avoids the potentially greater complications of aspiration secondary to removal of the foreign object.

Esophageal strictures that lend themselves to conventional bougienage should be treated in the traditional manner because it is less complicated, less time-consuming, and less expensive than balloon dilatation.

Before the procedure it is important to check the balloons filled with water for leakage and to set the pressure gauge according to the manufacturer's directions. Spraying the balloon with silicone may assist passage through the scope. Throughout the procedure the nurse should assist the physician with guidewire control.

After the balloon is in place, a syringe should be used to inflate it with the appropriate fluid as directed by the physician. The balloon is then left inflated for a short period of time, as determined by the physician. After the appropriate time has elapsed, the balloon is deflated. Once it is removed it should be checked for signs of bleeding. Patient discomfort may serve as a guide to the number of dilatations attempted during a single session. With the use of three progressively larger inflatable balloons, esophageal peptic strictures can be dilated dramatically in one session. The schedule for subsequent dilatation sessions is based on the type of stricture, its response to initial and subsequent dilatation, and the patient's tolerance of the procedure. Each stricture requires an individually tailored approach.

After use, balloon dilators should be washed, disinfected or sterilized, dried inside and out, and stored in protective packages. If contrast material was used to inflate the balloon, it must be rinsed out completely before processing. If it is not removed the balloon walls may adhere and destroy the balloon. Hydrostatic balloons can withstand temperatures up to 65 C, which allows for sterilization with ethylene oxide. Manufacturers' directions should be followed for cleaning and disinfection and/or sterilization, and for reuse.

Potential complications of dilatation by using a hydrostatic dilator are similar to those for other dilatation procedures.

### Hydrostatic dilatation in pyloric stenosis

In patients with pyloric stenosis, a through-the-scope or over-the-guidewire technique may be used to insert a hydrostatic balloon. In the TTS technique, a well-lubricated balloon is passed through the biopsy channel of an endoscope and into the stricture. The balloon is inflated to maximum pressure with water or dilute contrast medium, using a pressure gauge. Dilatation is repeated 3 or 4 times, maintaining maximum inflation for at least 1 minute during each dilatation. After dilatation is complete, the balloon is withdrawn, and the endoscope is passed through the pyloric ring for inspection of the duodenum.

For over-the-wire balloon dilatation of the pylorus, a heavy-gauge guidewire with a spring tip is passed through the stricture and advanced far enough to serve as an anchor. Dilatation is carried out with fluoroscopic guidance, filling the balloon with dilute radiographic contrast material. Following dilatation, endoscopy is used to evaluate the pyloric ring and duodenal bulb.

### Balloon dilatation of biliary tract strictures

Bile duct strictures may be dilated with balloon catheters during endoscopic retrograde cholangiopancreatography (ERCP) or percutaneous transhepatic cholangiography (PTC). After dilatation, a biliary stent may be placed through the stricture either endoscopically or via a guidewire placed percutaneously during PTC. Indications for balloon dilatation of the biliary tract include the following:

- Inflammatory strictures
- Postoperative strictures
- Benign or malignant strictures
- Stenoses at a choledochoenterostomy site
- Sclerosing cholangitis
- Sphincter of Oddi dysfunction and biliary dyskinesia
- Before stent placement

For dilatation of the biliary tract, a Gruntzig dilating balloon is typically attached to a 180-cm double-lumen catheter with a 1.5-cm tapered tip. The distended balloon measures 2 to 4 cm in length, with a diameter of 4 to 8 mm. The guidewire that is used in conjunction with a nasobiliary catheter or stent can also be used to achieve correct placement of balloon catheters.

Before dilatation, diagnostic ERCP is performed by using a regular cannula to confirm the size, location, and anatomy of the stricture. The regular cannula is cleared of contrast medium, and a guidewire that is well lubricated with silicone is threaded into the cannula and advanced into the appropriate duct so its tip is proximal to the stricture.

With the guidewire in position, the cannula is withdrawn. The external surface of the balloon is well lubricated and the folded balloon is carefully threaded through the instrument channel of the lateral-viewing endoscope. The endoscopist slowly advances the balloon catheter over the guidewire while the nurse keeps tension on the guidewire. The balloon is stationed through the stricture, and its position is confirmed by fluoroscopically observing the radiopaque markers on the balloon.

An inflation pressure of 4 to 6 atmospheres is applied for a brief period on three successive occasions, using a syringe filled with dilute contrast medium. When fully inflated, the balloon assumes a dumbbell shape because of the circumferential pressure exerted at the stricture zone. Following dilatation, the contrast medium is removed, and the balloon is withdrawn through the endoscope.

Repeat dilatation is performed if the initial response is inadequate. In patients with common bile duct strictures, a stent can be positioned across the stricture for 1 to 3 months to promote reepithelialization of the traumatized duct lumen without restricturing.

Following balloon dilatation, a clinical improvement in jaundice and a drop in serum bilirubin should be observed, in addition to a decrease in the incidence of cholangitis. Intermediate and long-term results, however, are discouraging. The major use of dilating balloons may be in the temporary dilatation of a stricture, which will then allow the long-term placement of a biliary stent.

Complications occur in approximately 10% of patients, and notably include pancreatitis and injury to the bile duct. Most cases of pancreatitis respond to conservative management. Laceration of the bile duct often resolves spontaneously if the lacerated area is bridged by a stent.

## PNEUMATIC BALLOONS

**Pneumatic balloons** are used for forceful stretching of the LES in patients with achalasia. Forceful dilatation to a diameter of approximately 3 cm is necessary to tear the circular muscle and effect a lasting reduction in LES pressure. The success rate in treatment of achalasia with pneumatic dilators is 80% to 85% with a 0.2% mortality rate and 2.6% perforation rate.

Pneumatic dilatation may also be used in cases of diffuse esophageal spasm with a hypertensive LES. The object of this procedure is to decrease the resistance at the LES to allow the esophagus to empty. It may also be used for dilatation of lower esophageal rings, if bougienage is unsuccessful. One successful dilatation should cure this condition permanently. Although the ring may still be visible on radiographic examination, the patient's dysphagia should not recur.

Many types of balloon dilators have been used for pneumatic dilatation. Balloons are available in various lengths and diameters. Although manufacturers recommend inflation to a fixed pressure, many experts dilate by feeling the esophagus.

The patient may be hospitalized, and a liquid diet should be instituted the day before dilatation. Before the procedure the patient should be warned that moderate to severe discomfort will be experienced. The patient should be assured that additional pain medication will be administered if necessary. The procedure is done under local anesthesia, with meperidine (Demerol) given preoperatively to reduce discomfort. Atropine may be given intravenously to reduce oral secretions, and diazepam (Valium) may be administered for sedation, but it is preferred that the patient remain alert and cooperative. It is important to lavage and empty the esophagus of retained material, if present, and to set the pressure gauge according to the manufacturer's specifications.

The collapsed pneumatic balloon should always be introduced over a guidewire, and the procedure should be performed under fluoroscopic control. When the center of the balloon is positioned at the level of the LES, the bag is inflated rapidly with air, fluid, or dilute contrast medium to a preset pressure (at least 6 lbs/sq in) for 15 to 60 seconds. After the length of time determined by the physician, the balloon should be deflated and removed.

During the procedure the patient should be observed for severe chest pain and additional medication administered as ordered.

After the procedure the head of the patient's bed should be elevated. The dilator should be checked for evidence of blood. The physician should be notified if the patient experiences chest pain, fever, regurgitation of blood, pain on swallowing, back pain, shortness of breath, shoulder pain, or chills. The patient should be instructed to notify the physician of continuing chest pain, back pain, or other pain.

Some endoscopists immediately follow dilatation with a radiographic contrast study to identify any distal esophageal leaks near the region of the esophagogastric junction. If no leak is seen, the patient is observed over the subsequent 6 hours, and the diet is gradually resumed.

Because of the importance of monitoring the patient for severity and character of chest pain, the physician may prefer inpatient observation for 24 hours. In addition, the physician may want the patient to remain on a clear liquid diet for 24 hours after the procedure.

Potential complications of pneumatic dilatation include perforation, bleeding, and aspiration. Risk of perforation is somewhat higher than in standard dilatation, occurring in 2% to 4% of patients. Patients with small perforations and contrast material extending beyond the normal esophageal lumen can be managed conservatively, with antibiotics and close observation for signs of worsening pain and fever. Clinical deterioration or the presence of free-flowing contrast material into the mediastinum mandates immediate thoracotomy and repair. If the tear is small, the repair and a Heller myotomy can be performed in the same operation.

Mrs. Doris Johnson, whose case was presented in Chapters 14 and 25, suffers from esophageal reflux, which was diagnosed 2 years ago. Her husband died 18 months ago and she was unable to force herself to comply with her treatment regimen during the grieving period. Emotional recovery has been slow, and she has not returned to the prescribed therapy. Now she is experiencing dysphagia in reaction to solid food but not to liquids. She is to have an esophageal endoscopy and possible dilatation.

### Points to think about

1. Given Mrs. Johnson's history and symptoms, what might the nurse expect to find upon endoscopic examination?
2. Based upon these expectations, what equipment should the nurse have ready?
3. The nurse discovers that Mrs. Johnson has a knowledge deficit in relation to her current diagnosis and treatment. What should the nurse review with her?
4. Mrs. Johnson might be considered noncompliant in relation to her esophageal reflux medical regimen. What are the ethical issues to be considered in labeling a patient noncompliant?
5. In the nursing diagnosis, "noncompliance in relation to esophageal reflux medical recommendations," what one factor is inherent in the definition and must be known before an individual can be so labeled?
6. What areas must be assessed before a nurse can assist Mrs. Johnson in overcoming noncompliance?
7. What might the nurse tell Mrs. Johnson regarding postdilatation follow-up?

### Suggested responses

1. The endoscopic findings demonstrate a stricture of the distal esophagus. This type of stricture may or may not permit passage of the endoscope.
2. The equipment that the nurse should have available for the procedure to be performed on Mrs. Johnson would include:
   - Biopsy forceps and cytology brush. All strictures should be diagnosed histologically to rule out a malignancy or Barrett's esophagus (the presence of gastric mucosa above the squamocolumnar junction).
   - Dilators. Depending on the type of stricture and/or physician preference, the nurse may need balloon (TTS) dilators, polyvinyl (Savary) dilators, mercury-weighted bougies (Maloney dilators), and/or metal olives (Eder-Puestow dilators)

3. Information the nurse should discuss with Mrs. Johnson would include the following:
   - The current diagnosis and ways the problem can be alleviated, so that the nurse can ascertain Mrs. Johnson's recall of what her physician has told her. In addition, the nurse should answer questions or refer them to the physician.
   - The physiologic process of reflux and ways to manage it, such as not eating late at night, not lying down after meals, not wearing constricting clothing, and elevating the head of the bed on 6-inch blocks.
   - The need to reduce weight, which will help with managing reflux and hypertension. The nurse should refer Mrs. Johnson for counseling in this area.
   - Dietary and medication restrictions, such as eliminating caffeine, alcohol, ASA, and nonsteroidal antiinflammatory drugs.
4. The label *noncompliant* can carry a judgmental connotation and place blame on the patient for failing to comply with a therapeutic recommendation. Healthcare providers must be able to identify all of the variables or factors that contribute to or interfere with a person's ability to comply with recommendations before so labeling a patient. Some nursing authorities believe that such a label inflicts unnecessary discomfort or pain on patients by professionals presumably dedicated to "do no harm."
5. The definition of noncompliance involves the expressed desire and intent not to adhere to therapeutic recommendations. Without this expression, a nurse cannot apply this type of label. It is important to identify not only the variables for nonadherence but also the degree to which compliant behavior has occurred.
6. Before attempting to assist Mrs. Johnson in overcoming noncompliance, the nurse should assess the following:
   - Defining characteristics of noncompliance, such as observation of noncompliant behavior or results of objective measures that reveal noncompliant behavior (e.g., physiologic measures, development of complications, or increase in symptoms)
   - Personal factors, which include values and beliefs about health, illness, threat, and the prescribed therapy
   - Interpersonal factors, such as support from others and satisfaction gained from it
   - Environmental factors, including barriers to compliance in the environment in which the patient must exist (e.g., economic difficulties)
7. Instructions for follow-up after esophageal dilatation might include:

- Symptoms of complications, such as increased chest pain, vomiting of blood, difficulty breathing, scapular pain, and fever
- Dietary modifications needed (e.g., eat slowly and chew food well)
- Prescribed medications
- Required follow-up visits

## REVIEW TERMS

**American dilator, bougies, bougienage, Celestin dilators, dilators, Eder-Puestow dilators, French units, Hurst dilators, hydrostatic balloons, Maloney dilators, pneumatic balloons, Savary-Gilliard dilators**

## REEVIEW QUESTIONS

1. The primary goal of most esophageal dilatation procedures is to:
   a. Permit passage of the endoscope.
   b. Allow the patient to eat and drink normally.
   c. Treat achalasia.
   d. Cure esophageal cancer.
2. Before the patient can resume a normal diet, the esophageal lumen must be dilated to a diameter equivalent to at least:
   a. 20 French.
   b. 30 French.
   c. 40 French.
   d. 50 French.
3. A mercury-filled, rubber bougie with a tapered tip is called a:
   a. Maloney dilator.
   b. Hurst dilator.
   c. Eder-Puestow dilator.
   d. Savary dilator.
4. After bougienage with local anesthesia, the patient should remain NPO:
   a. For 2 hours.
   b. Until the gag reflex returns.
   c. Until the possibility of perforation has been ruled out.
   d. For 8 hours.
5. During dilatation with Eder-Puestow olives, the nurse is responsible for:
   a. Inserting the endoscope.
   b. Inserting the guidewire.
   c. Advancing the dilator.
   d. Keeping the guidewire stable.
6. One advantage of polyvinyl chloride dilators compared with the Eder-Puestow system is that:
   a. They are less likely to damage the patient's teeth.
   b. They are radiopaque.

   c. There is no risk of perforation.
   d. Fewer passes through the pharynx are needed.
7. The method used most often for dilatation of pyloric stenosis is:
   a. The Eder-Puestow system.
   b. A pneumatic balloon.
   c. A hydrostatic balloon.
   d. A rubber bougie.
8. A hydrostatic dilating balloon is filled with dilute contrast medium because:
   a. Full-strength contrast medium could crystallize, thereby damaging the balloon.
   b. Full-strength contrast medium may cause an allergic response.
   c. It helps stimulate peristalsis, thus aiding passage of the balloon through the upper GI tract.
   d. It exerts more pressure than water or saline.
9. The primary use of hydrostatic balloons in the biliary tract may be to:
   a. Permanently treat biliary strictures.
   b. Dilate the duct before long-term stent placement.
   c. Treat sphincter of Oddi dysfunction.
   d. Remove retained common bile duct stones.
10. In pneumatic dilatation, the balloon remains inflated:
    a. For up to 1 minute.
    b. For up to 10 minutes.
    c. Until the patient experiences chest pain.
    d. Until the preset pressure is obtained.

## BIBLIOGRAPHY

Bongiovanni, G, ed. *Essentials of Clinical Gastroenterology.* 2nd ed. New York: McGraw-Hill, 1988.

Cotton, P, and Williams, C. *Practical Gastrointestinal Endoscopy.* 3rd ed. Boston: Blackwell Scientific Publications, Inc., 1990.

Graham, D. "Dilatation for the Management of Benign and Malignant Strictures of the Esophagus." In *Therapeutic Gastrointestinal Endoscopy,* Silvis, S, ed. 1-30. New YorK; Igaku-Shoin, 1985.

Hardick, M, and Beck, M, eds. *Manual of Gastrointestinal Procedures.* 2nd ed. Rochester, N.Y.: Society of Gastroenterology Nurses and Associates, 1989.

Ravenscroft, M, and Swan, C. *Gastrointestinal Endoscopy and Related Procedures: A Handbook for Nurses and Assistants.* Baltimore: Williams & Wilkins, 1984.

Sivak, M, Jr., and Petrini, J, eds. *Gastrointestinal Endoscopy: Old Problems, New Techniques.* Gastroenterology Series, Volume 4. New York: Praeger, 1986.

Sleisenger, M, and Fordtran, J, eds. *Gastrointestinal Disease: Pathophysiology, Diagnosis, Management.* 4th ed. Philadelphia: W.B. Saunders, 1989.

Waye, J, Geenen, J, Fleischer, D, and Venu, R. *Techniques in Therapeutic Endoscopy.* Philadelphia: W.B. Saunders, 1987.

Webb, W, and Graham, D. "Modern Approach to Esophageal Dilatation." In *SGA Journal Reprints,* Trivits, S, ed. 55-58. Rochester, N.Y.: Society of Gastrointestinal Assistants, 1988.

# Chapter 30

# HEMOSTASIS AND TUMOR ABLATION

This chapter will acquaint the gastroenterology nurse with endoscopic and other techniques that are used to stop gastrointestinal bleeding.* Indications, contraindications, techniques, and potential complications of monopolar and bipolar electrocoagulation, heater probes, laser photocoagulation, esophageal-gastric balloon tamponade, injection sclerotherapy, and variceal ligation are all described in detail. Nursing considerations for managing these patients are outlined as they relate to the role of the gastroenterology nurse.

## Learning objectives

After reviewing the content of this chapter, the gastroenterology nurse should be able to:
1. Discuss the general principles and the role of the gastroenterology nurse in thermal coagulation procedures and methods, including monopolar and bipolar electrocautery, heater probes, and laser photocoagulation.
2. Discuss indications, contraindications, and techniques for esophageal-gastric tamponade.
3. Explain the use of injection sclerotherapy, variceal ligation, and chemical injection therapy in the treatment of esophageal and gastric varices.

## BASIC PRINCIPLES

In planning endoscopic therapy for gastrointestinal bleeding, it is important first to confirm the location of the hemorrhage (upper or lower GI tract). Most of the causes of upper GI bleeding and some of the causes of lower GI bleeding are amenable to endoscopic therapy.

---

* All techniques in this chapter, except bipolar ablation of obstructing gastrointestinal tumors and endoscopic variceal ligation, are also discussed in the SGNA *Manual of Gastrointestinal Procedures*. 2nd ed. Rochester, N.Y.: Society of Gastroenterology Nurses and Associates, 1989.

Causes of upper GI bleeding include esophageal, gastric, and duodenal ulcers; erosive esophagitis, gastritis, and duodenitis; Mallory-Weiss tears; varices; tumors; and arteriovenous malformations (AVMs). Although approximately 70% to 80% of upper GI bleeding episodes are self-limited, the overall mortality rate for patients with upper GI bleeding remains at 6% to 10%. Factors that increase this risk include the severity of bleeding, significant coexisting medical illness, age above 60 years, need for surgery, and continued or recurrent bleeding. At the time of diagnostic endoscopy, the physician should be prepared to treat the bleeding site with injection therapy or with photocoagulation or electrocoagulation.

Several factors affect the timing of the endoscopic examination. The likelihood of finding the source of the bleeding is higher when the procedure is done within 24 hours of the bleed. Ongoing upper GI bleeding requires urgent endoscopy as soon as the patient is medically stable. For upper GI bleeding that is not thought to be active, endoscopy should be performed as soon as personnel and equipment become available. For active lower GI bleeding, colonoscopy should not be performed until the colon has been cleansed properly.

Causes of lower GI bleeding include hemorrhoids, diverticulosis, polyps, cancer, AVMs, and colitis. Of these, endoscopic management is most often used for bleeding cancers, AVMs, and polyps.

Premedication for endoscopic hemostasis is similar to that administered for diagnostic endoscopy. However, because patients with major blood loss may be hypotensive, the blood pressure-lowering effects of commonly used narcotics and sedatives must be considered. Antiperistaltic agents such as glucagon may be administered to diminish motility when searching for or treating nonbleeding angiodysplasia.

A number of endoscopic methods are available to control gastrointestinal hemorrhage, including monopolar and bipolar electrocautery, heater probes, and laser therapy. Variceal bleeding may be treated with intravenous vasopressin (Pitressin), injection sclerotherapy, injection of hypertonic or epinephrine solutions, esophageal variceal ligation, or esophageal-gastric tamponade.

## ELECTROCAUTERY

Electrosurgery can be used to produce cutting and/or **coagulation** (**fulguration** and **desiccation**) effects. When both **cutting** and **coagulating current** are applied, the resulting energy is referred to as a "blended" current.

**Electrocoagulation (electrocautery)** occurs when current flows through resistant tissue, thereby coagulating protein and producing hemostasis. It is used to treat active bleeding from a visible vessel, visible vessels without bleeding, or blood oozing from a clot in the base of an ulcer. It is also used in conjunction with the excision of polyps, large mucosal biopsies, and endoscopic retrograde sphincterotomy. Polypectomy and sphincterotomy are discussed in detail in Chapter 32.

In addition, electrocoagulation is used for treatment of hereditary hemorrhagic telangiectasias (Osler-Weber-Rendu syndrome) of the GI tract and for acquired vascular abnormalities of the stomach, duodenum, or cecal area (angiodysplasia). For AVMs in the stomach and duodenum, electrocoagulation is accomplished by placing an electrode on the peripheral border of the malformation, applying moderate pressure, and moving circumferentially until a complete circle has been made. If the center of an AVM is electrocoagulated before its periphery has been treated, torrential bleeding may occur.

Electrocautery is contraindicated in patients with torrential bleeding, esophageal varices, or coagulopathy, and in uncooperative patients. It can be performed safely with the majority of newer model pacemakers, but a case-by-case determination must be made before the procedure.

**Electrosurgical units (ESUs)** are all different, even those that are provided by the same manufacturer. It is important to thoroughly understand the tissue effects caused by the use of each individual unit.

All electrosurgical equipment should be inspected regularly for frayed or cracked cords, loose connections, or deterioration in the power cord and plug. A working backup for the ESU should be readily available. Unit functioning should be checked before each use.

Before attempting electrocoagulation in the upper GI tract, the stomach must be free of blood, and the patient's condition must be stabilized. An oral bite block

should be placed, and IV sedation should be achieved as necessary. Diagnostic esophagogastroduodenoscopy (EGD), using a therapeutic scope if available, should be performed to determine the cause of the bleeding.

Before electrocoagulation of the colon or rectum, it is important that the colon be well prepped to eliminate the risk of exploding the hydrogen and methane gases that are normally present in the stool. It is also important to remember that the colon is thinner than the upper GI tract and thus the risk of perforation is greater, particularly if the lumen is overdistended.

Both before and during electrosurgical procedures, it is the nurse's responsibility to perform the following activities:
- Inspect all equipment to make sure it works properly
- Position the grounding pad on the patient (for monopolar electrocoagulation only)
- Turn on the power when the physician is ready to use the ESU and turn it off immediately after use.
- Check the placement of the foot pedal
- Verbally confirm the physician's orders for mode of operation (coagulation, cutting, or blended current) and settings
- Reassure and encourage the patient, keeping him or her as still as possible

After the procedure is completed, it is important to check for skin damage or burns near and under the grounding pad (in the monopolar modality); monitor the patient's vital signs and document results; monitor the patient for abdominal pain and/or distention; and document power settings.

Potential complications of electrocautery include thermal injury, hemorrhage, perforation, transmural burns, and explosion.

Following are two ways of applying electrocoagulation:
- In the monopolar modality, electrical current flows from a small, active electrode that is in contact with the target tissue, through the patient, and toward a grounding pad that is attached to the patient's skin. The site chosen should be muscular and well-vascularized and not over bony prominences or where circulation is likely to be impaired. The preferred site is the upper thigh. The high current density at the relatively small electrode site generates a significant amount of heat in the resistor (the target tissue), thereby causing coagulation. The current density at the grounding pad is lower because the amount of tissue in contact with the grounding plate is much larger.
- In the bipolar modality, the current flows between two small electrodes that are in contact with the tissue and are separated by a space of only a few

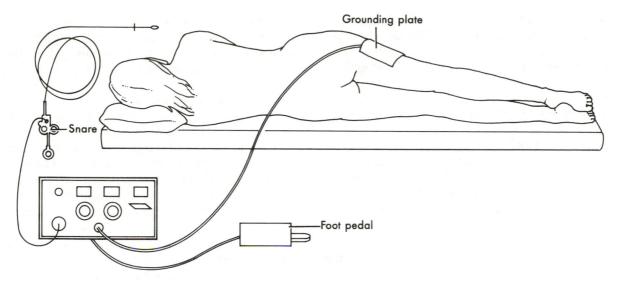

**Fig. 30-1.** Patient setup for electrocautery.

millimeters. The localized current pathway between the two electrodes results in tissue heating. The bipolar modality therefore does not require a grounding pad.

### Monopolar electrocoagulation

There are certain safety factors associated with the use of the grounding pad in **monopolar electrocoagulation**. Before the procedure the nurse should explain the purpose of the grounding pad to the patient. The patient should be instructed not to touch side rails, IV poles, or other metal objects during the procedure (Fig. 30-1).

A number of different types of grounding pads are available. Disposable pads with gel and adhesive edges are preferred because they conform to patient contours and do not have to be repositioned if the patient's position is changed. The nurse should apply the grounding pad according to the manufacturer's guidelines. The pad should have generous contact on healthy tissue, avoiding bony prominences and large scars that could decrease skin area contact. Excessive hair should be removed from the site of attachment.

Incorrect application of a grounding plate may result in "hot spots" where current density remains high because of limited skin contact. Spot burning can also occur. To avoid pacemaker malfunction and burns from internal metal prostheses, the grounding pad should be as far away as possible from any pacemaker, hip pin, or artificial joint, and as close as possible to the site of use.

With the use of high-frequency currents, current leakage can be a problem.

- Current may pass through the accessory, leak through the fiberoptic endoscope, and pass back to the endoscopist, causing burns to the operator.

- Current may pass through the accessory, leak through the scope, and pass to the patient at an internal point in which the patient is in contact with the scope, and then continue to the grounding pad, presenting the potential for a burn at a scope–patient contact point.
- Current may also pass through the accessory, through the tissue at the site of electrosurgery, and through the patient's body to a part that is in contact with a grounded piece of metal (e.g., table edges, Mayo stands, or IV poles).

It is important to remember that any personnel in contact with equipment or the patient during use of the generator can become part of the electrical circuit.

To avoid these problems, the gastroenterology nurse should take the following steps:

- Securely attach the grounding pad to the patient.
- Wear rubber gloves to decrease conduction and contact with the scope.
- Use a protective rubber covering on the eyepiece of the scope.
- Avoid touching the patient during activation of the ESU.
- Place metal objects far enough away from the x-ray table or exam table to prevent accidental patient contact.
- Prevent patient contact with metal railings or litter edges.

### Bipolar electrocoagulation

A bipolar electrode is a specialized, hemostatic probe that is inserted through an endoscope channel to control gastrointestinal hemorrhage and bleeding. The **bipolar** probe does not require a grounding pad because the current travels back through the bipolar electrode. Because there are two electrodes, coagulation takes place only between the two points. One point delivers the current and the other closes the circuit returning to the generator. Electrical energy is converted into thermal energy on contact with the tissue, thereby producing a predictable depth of injury.

The tip of the bipolar probe consists of an array of longitudinal or circumferential microelectrodes. The probes are 7 and 10 Fr in size; the 10-Fr probe can only be used with a large-channel scope. Through a hole in the center of the tip, a powerful water jet can be delivered intermittently or constantly to irrigate the bleeding lesion and to increase the precision of targeting. Coagulation is possible with the top and sides of the probe tip.

**Bipolar electrocoagulation** has certain advantages over the monopolar modality. Depth of tissue penetration is limited, thus reducing the risk of perforation and avoiding full-thickness burns. There is a rapidly decreasing energy and heating effect at short distance from the electrodes. Two additional features of the bipolar probe are its ability to tamponade the vessel before delivering thermal energy and the fact that the thermal energy can be delivered from the sides of the probes. Studies have shown that although bipolar electrocoagulation is technically more difficult to use, it produces less mucosal injury and is equally effective as monopolar electrocoagulation.

The bipolar probe also has certain advantages over laser photocoagulation.

- No special installation is necessary.
- The set can be used at bedside.
- There is no gas evacuation.
- No special endoscopic adaptation is necessary, although a bichannel scope or one with a large instrument channel is preferred.
- The bipolar probe is relatively inexpensive.
- It is technically easier to use and does not require special credentialing.

Use of the bipolar probe is indicated for actively bleeding lesions in the upper or lower GI tract, to destroy neoplastic cells and relieve symptoms of obstruction, and to destroy hemorrhoidal tissue.

Use of a bipolar probe is contraindicated in combative, uncooperative patients; in cases of massive hemorrhage, which require immediate surgery; where visualization of the bleeding site is inadequate; and where free peritoneal air is observed on x-ray films.

As in any endoscopic procedure that involves sedation, the nurse should establish an IV line as ordered. To set up the bipolar unit, the water bottle should be filled with sterile water and connected to the port on the machine. The probe and foot pedal should be connected to the unit, and the probe should be primed with water. The bipolar probe should be tested by placing several drops of normal saline on a glass slide, putting the tip in the saline, and depressing the bipolar pedal. If the probe is working properly, the saline will heat up and bubble. After testing, the unit should be turned off. The probe should be lubricated with silicone to help it pass smoothly through the endoscope.

For application of a bipolar probe, the electrode is placed within 2 to 3 mm of the vessel and firm pressure is applied. The probe is activated in 1- to 2-second bursts until circumferential coagulation has occurred. During the procedure the nurse's responsibilities are to maintain the water level in the water bottle, set the energy levels and water pressure designated by the physician, wipe secretions from the probe with gauze as it is withdrawn from the endoscope, and clean the probe tip as needed during the procedure. The patient should be monitored for abdominal distention caused by the instillation of large amounts of air and water.

After the procedure is completed, the nurse should again monitor the patient's vital signs, observing the patient for bleeding, vomiting, abdominal pain, and distention. The bipolar cautery unit should be cleaned and disassembled, and water should be flushed from the unit. The water bottle should be emptied and sterilized in accordance with institutional policy. Probes should be maintained and processed according to the manufacturer's directions.

Potential complications of bipolar electrocoagulation include perforation, delayed hemorrhage, and deep ulcerations.

### Bipolar ablation of obstructing gastrointestinal tumors

For palliative ablation of obstructing esophageal or rectal tumors, a specialized bipolar probe may be used to ablate the strictured area. The local delivery of heat to the site of the cancer may destroy neoplastic cells and relieve symptoms.

The standard bipolar tumor probe kit has five probes of different diameters. Each probe has four sections; a distal flexible, slinkylike tip that is 6 cm in length; an electrically activated bipolar probe that is similar to the Eder-Puestow olives in shape and size; a flexible shaft that is 60 cm in length and has markings at centimeter intervals; and the electrical connection, which attaches by a cord to a 50-watt bipolar electrocoagulating generator.

Preliminary screening tests are needed to confirm that the patient is a good candidate for the procedure. The tumor should be symmetrical, and there should be no contraindications to therapy. Preliminary testing should include the following:

- A screening endoscopy to determine the location, size, and shape of the tumor
- A contrast radiographic study of the esophagus to define the length, location, and shape of the tumor and to exclude the presence of a tracheoesophageal fistula
- An imaging study to determine the extent of the disease, the thickness and symmetry of the esophageal wall at the tumor site, and tumor's proximity to critical structures

Before the procedure the patient may be premedicated with both an IV analgesic and a sedative. An anticholinergic medication may also be used if the tumor is in the proximal esophagus.

A small-caliber endoscope is passed into the stomach, and a guidewire is inserted to the junction of the body and the antrum. Although fluoroscopic guidance is not absolutely necessary, it adds an extra measure of safety. The guidewire is then left in place while the endoscope is withdrawn. If the endoscope cannot advance beyond the proximal margin of the tumor, polyvinyl dilators are passed over the guidewire to dilate the tumor until the probe can pass beyond the distal margin of the tumor. It is important not to "overdilate" the tumor, however, because good contact between the probe and the tumor is necessary.

Thermal treatments are begun distally and proceed stepwise in a cephalad direction. Once the tumor probe reaches the proximal margin of the tumor and the last burn is delivered, the probe and guidewire are removed, and the treated area is evaluated endoscopically. If the burn has been delivered perfectly, a circumferential white burn should be seen. When the burn is incomplete, or if the probe pulls tissue with it as it advances, some areas will appear white and others will be friable and hemorrhagic.

After the procedure the tumor probe should be cleaned and processed according to the manufacturer's instructions. The patient should be NPO for at least 4 hours, and vital signs should be monitored for evidence of perforation or bleeding. If there is any concern about these complications, a chest x-ray examination may be done. If there are no complications, clear liquids may be given after 4 hours. In some institutions, patients remain NPO until the following morning, after a barium swallow is complete.

Some dysphagia is to be expected in the first 24 hours following the procedure. It is not uncommon for the patient to have a low-grade fever, mild leukocytosis, and chest pain. A second endoscopy is carried out 48 hours after the first to determine whether or not a second treatment is necessary. Once luminal patency has been achieved, monthly follow-up is conducted.

## HEATER PROBES

The **heater probe** is very similar in application to the bipolar probe. It consists of a hollow aluminum cylinder with an inner heat coil and an outer coating of Teflon. The aluminum has high thermal conductivity, which provides for a precise and uniform distribution of heat to tissue from its end or sides. A coaxial channel is provided to wash away blood and debris. Heater probes are available with diameters of 3.2 or 2.4 mm; the 3.2-mm size must be used with a large channel endoscope.

Positive features of the heater probe are its portability, absence of electrical hazard, coaxial channel for application of a water jet, capability for controlling and presetting the rate of pulses, effectiveness, low cost, and capability for use at angles other than directly vertical. Like the bipolar probe, the heater probe also permits direct tamponade of bleeding sites. Moreover, because of its Teflon coating, the tip does not require frequent wiping. In addition to controlling gastrointestinal bleeding, heater probes have been used successfully to treat patients with hemorrhoids.

Steps in the application of the heater probe unit and bipolar unit are very similar. One difference is that the heater probe is tested by submerging the tip in water and depressing the Coag pedal on the unit. If the unit is malfunctioning in any way, an alarm will sound and a fault light will be activated.

The heater probe is applied directly to a vessel with firm pressure. Several brief applications of thermal energy may be required to produce hemostasis. The probe must be allowed to cool before it is withdrawn through the scope; if it is still hot, it can melt the channel lining.

## LASER THERAPY

The word *laser* is an acronym for light amplification by stimulated emission of radiation. Because laser light is coherent and collimated it can be intensely focused, which allows it to be precisely aimed. To date, only argon and neodymium:yttrium-aluminum-garnet (**Nd:YAG**) lasers have been widely used in endoscopy. Carbon dioxide lasers are not adaptable to the current generation of flexible endoscopes.

In endoscopic applications, laser light energy is transmitted through a flexible quartz waveguide, which is usually protected by a plastic catheter passed through a flexible endoscope. Between the fiber and the catheter is free space, through which coaxial air, carbon dioxide, or helium flows, thus keeping the fiber and the surface of the treatment site clear of blood and other debris. Because this coaxial gas can lead to problems with overdistention, a two-channel endoscope is preferred so the gas can be exhausted through the suction channel.

More than 95% of the lasers used for gastrointestinal work are Nd:YAG lasers. The depth of penetration of the **argon** laser is less than that of the Nd:YAG lasers (approximately 1 mm, compared with 4 mm). Unlike the Nd:YAG laser, the argon laser is absorbed by hemoglobin and therefore will not penetrate clots. The argon laser beam is visible; the Nd:YAG beam is not visible and thus requires an additional xenon or helium–neon aiming beam. The Nd:YAG laser also carries the greater risk of potential damage to the eye of the examiner, observer, or patient.

Flexible endoscopes may be damaged if laser energy is reflected from the target surface to the tip of the endoscope. This can be avoided by the following preventive measures:

- Using endoscopes that are designed for laser therapy and are manufactured with stainless-steel or white porcelain reflective tips, rather than black tips
- Making sure that the laser fiber is well outside the endoscope channel and clearly visualized before activating the laser
- Not working too closely to the target surface during extensive coagulation

The effect of the laser on tissue is determined by the temperature generated at the treatment site. Generally speaking, protein coagulates at 60° C (photocoagulation), and tissue vaporizes at 100° C (photovaporization).

- **Photocoagulation** creates a white, blanched appearance with edema. The coagulative effect of lasers allows them to be used to achieve hemostasis for acute gastrointestinal bleeding and to treat gastrointestinal lesions that are not actively bleeding (e.g., angiodysplasia or ulcers with visible vessels).
- **Photovaporization** may cause a divot, charring of tissue, and smoke. The photovaporization effect of lasers allows them to destroy neoplastic tissue and to cut through normal tissue to achieve therapeutic goals.

Conventional laser therapy differs from heater probe and electrocoagulation treatment in that it is a noncontact method. The laser waveguide does not come into contact with the tissue. Newly developed sapphire endoprobes, however, permit the laser to be used as a contact device. These tips, which attach to the tip of the standard laser waveguide, serve as lenses to concentrate the energy at the tip of the waveguide, so much lower wattages are required.

Laser treatment may be used for hemorrhagic conditions of the GI tract, such as Mallory-Weiss tears, bleeding peptic ulcers, angiodysplasia, or Osler-Weber-Rendu syndrome. Patients with stigmata of recent hemorrhage, including active bleeding, a visible vessel, or a fresh clot, are ideal candidates for laser photocoagulation. In addition, laser photovaporization has been used for neoplastic disease, benign esophageal webs and anastomotic strictures, intrahepatic and extrahepatic biliary obstruction, and gallstones. In the colorectal area, the laser may be used for benign pedunculated polyps or sessile lesions, tumor vaporization, and photocoagulation of hemorrhoids.

Endoscopic laser therapy is contraindicated in uncooperative patients or in patients with coagulopathy, extremely large vessels in the field, or inaccessible lesions.

Before laser therapy the power emission from the laser probe must be checked. Patients usually receive IV sedation and are placed in the left lateral decubitus position. Everyone in the room, including the patient, should wear safety glasses or goggles. Endoscopists may use goggles or may rely on the protective ocular lens cover once the laser is inserted. Laser masks should be worn to protect personnel against smoke and possible aerosolization of tissue particles. The water cooling system should be in operation. The power emission from the laser probe should be checked. "Laser in use" warning signs should be placed at all doors. A smoke evacuator may also be beneficial.

During the procedure it is the responsibility of the gastroenterology nurse or assistant to maintain the laser on standby mode when it is not in the firing position, to set power and duration as ordered by the physician, and to clean the tip of the fiber frequently with hydrogen peroxide and a soft-bristled brush. Removal of the fiber from the biopsy channel allows an excellent opportunity to remove excess smoke and debris. The nurse also assists the physician with use of biopsy forceps for possible debridement of the treatment site. The patient should be monitored during the procedure for abdominal distention and possible vasovagal reaction. Pain level should be observed so additional IV sedation can be administered as necessary.

After the procedure is completed, the entire exterior of the fiber, including the brass tip, is wiped with a gauze pad saturated with hydrogen peroxide. The interior is cleaned by lavaging with hydrogen peroxide in a syringe without a needle, while a constant flow of carbon dioxide is maintained. The flow of carbon dioxide prevents the peroxide from traveling more than a few centimeters up the fiber. The peroxide can be removed by depressing the foot pedal, with the laser lamps off, to produce a burst of carbon dioxide gas. Fibers should be reprocessed according to the manufacturer's instructions.

The patient is kept NPO, except for ingestion of ice chips, for 4 hours after the procedure or until the physician's orders permit intake of clear liquids. Vital signs should be checked hourly at first and then routinely. Swallowing is often worse immediately after laser therapy of the esophagus because of edema. If there is odynophagia, antacids may relieve symptoms. If ordered by the physician, a nasogastric tube may be inserted to relieve abdominal distention. Narcotic analgesics may be necessary to relieve chest pain. Chest x-ray films and/or abdominal films may be ordered to exclude the possibility of perforation. It is not uncommon for patients to experience a low-grade fever and mild leukocytosis 12 to 36 hours after laser therapy.

To obtain adequate patency of a tumor site with laser therapy, several treatments may be required. After the final treatment, a water-soluble x-ray contrast swallow may be obtained to rule out perforation and to document the effects of therapy. The first follow-up endoscopy is usually carried out in 3 to 4 weeks.

Potential complications of endoscopic laser treatments include hemorrhage, tissue slough, perforation, gaseous abdominal distention, ulceration, delayed healing, and fistula formation. If perforation and/or bleeding are suspected, they should be treated as described in Chapter 33. Complications from endoscopic laser therapy increase with the amount of energy delivered and the length of the procedure. Minor increases in bleeding during laser therapy are relatively common, but laser-induced massive gastrointestinal bleeding is also possible and may require emergency surgical intervention.

### Laser treatment of gastrointestinal bleeding

Before laser photocoagulation of upper GI bleeding, a large-bore tube is used for thorough lavage of the stomach. Vasopressin (Pitressin) should be available for IV use if uncontrollable bleeding occurs, and a snare or grasper should be available for transecting and removing large adherent clots. A syringe irrigator may be used to remove smaller clots. A blood pump is necessary to allow rapid blood infusion if needed.

For the treatment of bleeding ulcers, the laser fiber is held 1 to 2 cm from the target, and pulses of high power and short duration are used for coagulation. If a vessel is visible, the beam is aimed circumferentially around it. When visible edema develops, the vessel itself is treated.

### Laser therapy for vascular abnormalities

Endoscopic obliteration and clinical benefit have been reported in patients with angiodysplasia after use of both the argon and the Nd:YAG laser. When the laser beam strikes a large, abnormal vessel, it may initially cause a dormant lesion to bleed, but further laser therapy can bring this hemorrhage under control. Although angiodysplastic lesions may be seen in both the stomach and intestines, gastric and proximal duodenal lesions are responsible for the majority of upper GI bleeding.

Angiodysplasia of the colon, particularly the cecum, has also been treated with argon and Nd:YAG laser therapy. Results are best when it has been established that the colonic lesion has bled and the lesion is not just an incidental finding. Risk of perforation is greater in the right colon because it is thinner than other areas of the GI tract.

In patients with Osler-Weber-Rendu syndrome, laser therapy may reduce treatment time when many lesions are present. Laser treatment has also been shown to significantly reduce the rebleeding rate and transfusion requirements.

### Laser coagulation of hemorrhoids

Nd:YAG laser photocoagulation and obliteration is a viable alternative to surgical removal of internal and external hemorrhoids. This technique delivers extensive heat therapy directly to the hemorrhoidal structures. It attempts to both fix the mucosa and remove some or all of the internal hemorrhoidal tissue. Compared with a surgical approach, laser therapy requires only local, rather than general, anesthesia; there is less trauma; and laser therapy causes less pain.

The infrared photocoagulator is another recent innovation for the treatment of hemorrhoids. This device is *not* a laser; it focuses infrared radiation on the tissue via a specially made polymer tip. The source is a low-voltage tungsten-halogen lamp. The light source is directed at the base of the hemorrhoid and is used to produce a visible eschar. It is generally painless for patients receiving treatment on an outpatient basis and is expected to have minimal long-term sequelae or serious complications.

### Laser treatment of gastrointestinal tumors

Endoscopic laser treatment is also indicated for palliative or curative treatment of benign or malignant tumors of the esophagus, stomach, duodenum, ampulla, colon, or rectum. When palliative treatment is undertaken, the goal is usually to relieve obstruction or to reduce blood loss; attempts to relieve pain have generally not been successful. Blood loss may be reduced by coagulating tumor bleeding sites or by destroying the tumor vasculature. Palliation of bleeding and/or obstruction with laser photocoagulation appears to be a true alternative to bypass surgery. In some cases, intended curative treatment has been achieved.

The use of laser therapy may be indicated in the following situations and types of malignant and premalignant lesions:
- Benign polyps and large villous adenomas that are sessile, at least 5 mm in transverse diameter, and not amenable to electrosurgical snaring
- Periodic removal of polyps to prevent development of rectal cancer in patients with Gardner's syndrome or familial polyposis who have had subtotal colectomies with ileorectal anastomoses

- Palliative treatment of malignancies in which there is widespread disease and no chance for surgical cure
- To reestablish luminal patency and relieve dysphagia in patients with incurable esophageal cancer
- To relieve gastric outlet obstruction, control chronic bleeding, or reduce tumor bulk in patients with gastric cancer
- To relieve obstruction, control bleeding, or reduce tumor bulk in patients with colorectal cancer who are not surgical candidates or who decline surgery

To determine whether or not a patient with gastrointestinal cancer is a candidate for laser therapy, the following three preliminary examinations are required:

- A barium swallow to define the location and extent of the tumor
- Diagnostic endoscopy to view the gross appearance of the tumor, and to obtain biopsies and cytology
- A computed tomography (CT) or nuclear magnetic resonance (NMR) scan to define the extent of the disease

If there is any possibility of a cure for gastrointestinal cancer, and there are no medical contraindications, exploratory surgery should be performed. In patients whose functional status is so poor that even if the lumen were opened it would not greatly improve the quality of life, laser therapy should not be considered.

It is preferred that laser treatment begin at the distal margin of the tumor. When laser therapy is begun distally, the resultant edema will not impede treatment because the scope will be pulled cephalad. If treatment is begun at the proximal margin, edema may prevent advancement of the scope in a caudad direction, and more laser sessions may be required to treat the entire lesion.

If a two-channel endoscope cannot be advanced to the distal margin of the tumor, the esophagus may be dilated with progressively larger polyvinyl tapered dilators passed over a guidewire. Dilatation is usually sufficient to allow for treatment to begin at the distal tumor margin. If not even the smallest endoscope will pass beyond the obstruction, the endoscopist may begin treatment at the proximal tumor margin.

To begin laser therapy, the quartz waveguide that carries the laser beam is passed out of the biopsy channel of the scope. The beam is aimed at the portion of the neoplastic tumor closest to the lumen, and treatment progresses in increasingly larger concentric circles toward, but not to, the wall of the target organ. Usually the tumor is destroyed by vaporization. Some endoscopists prefer to accomplish tumor destruction by coagulation because, although this is a slower process, less smoke is generated. At the end of treatment, the tissue is often edematous and charred black secondary to thermal damage. Major blood loss is not usually a problem.

It is uncommon for any patient with esophageal tumors to require more than three laser sessions. Patients are usually treated every other day until maximal luminal opening is achieved. The 48-hour period between treatments allows for maximal tissue necrosis and is well tolerated by most patients. In subsequent sessions, surveillance endoscopy is used to observe the effects of the last treatment. If necessary, necrotic tissue can be pushed distally into the stomach, and dilatation may be conducted.

Patients with rectal tumors are generally more amenable to outpatient treatment than patients with esophageal cancer, who are often more debilitated. When the colonic lumen is almost completely obliterated by the tumor, a temporary opening may be provided by dilatation with a through-the-scope balloon dilator. For rectal cancers, a rigid proctoscope and hand-held laser fiber may be used. If the lesion has advanced to the anal verge, treatment with the Nd:YAG laser is painful and a saddle block may be required. If a rectal lesion is circumferential, treating only 270 degrees of the lesion can reduce the risk of rectal stenosis.

## INJECTION THERAPY

Endoscopic injection therapy was first used to stop variceal bleeding in 1939. After being supplanted temporarily by portacaval shunt techniques, it was reintroduced in 1974 and has become increasingly popular since then. This therapy method involves the injection of a chemical agent through a needle injector into or around a bleeding site to stop bleeding through variceal thrombosis or local edema.

Injection therapy is contraindicated in uncooperative patients or in patients with severe coagulopathy. The procedure is performed under direct endoscopic visualization, most often by using a flexible upper endoscope. A double-channel endoscope is helpful to permit suction when the patient is actively bleeding.

The injectors used in injection therapy are disposable. The greatest flexibility is obtained with a simple tubular system made of synthetic material, into one end of which the needle is fixed. A second outer sheath is added, into which the needle may be withdrawn when not in use.

In addition to the choice of agent, the volume, rate of injection, and placement of injections are all important in determining the overall effect.

Before the procedure it is important to verify the patency of a large-bore IV line, to verify blood type and cross-match, and to obtain the results of laboratory testing. The patient should be instructed to remain still and to refrain from coughing. IV sedation should be administered to maximize patient cooperation and minimize patient movement. Because some of the agents

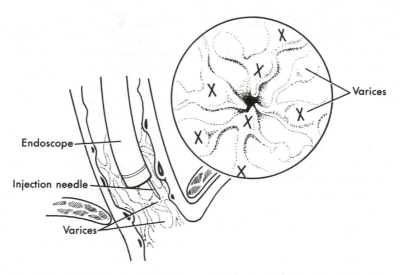

**Fig. 30-2.** Variceal sclerosing. Insert shows accepted sites for sclerosing.

used in this procedure can cause corneal ulcerations, the patient's eyes should be covered by a small towel during the procedure, and all personnel should wear protective eyewear, gloves, and masks.

A 5- or 10-ml syringe containing the chemical agent should be attached to the proximal end of the needle injector. The injector should be flushed with the agent to rid it of air and to check for patency and leaks. The needle injector should be checked to ensure that the needle properly protrudes from and retracts into the sheath.

A complete endoscopic examination of the esophagus, stomach, and duodenum is performed to locate the bleeding site or varices. The injector is passed through the biopsy port of the endoscope. (A gauze sponge held around the injector-syringe connection will prevent leakage.) With the patient in the left lateral position, the endoscope is positioned at the bleeding site. Air is insufflated to distend the esophageal lumen, thus enhancing visualization. The needle is advanced. Once the needle tip is visualized, it should be maneuvered into position, and the needle should be thrust directly into the desired site by rapidly advancing the injector and plunging the needle into the wall up to its junction with the sheath.

As soon as entry has been achieved, the nurse rapidly injects 0.5 to 3 ml of the chemical agent at the physician's direction, using slow, steady pressure. The nurse should verbally state the amount of injection in increments of 0.5 ml, and should say "stop" as soon as the injection has been completed.

Throughout the procedure the patient should be monitored for abdominal distention, and the number and amount of injections should be documented. Following the last injection, the needle should be removed from the accessory channel and discarded in an appro-

priate sharps container. The stomach should be suctioned to decompress the gastric distention caused by continuous insufflation of air.

**Nonvariceal injection therapy**

Nonvariceal gastrointestinal bleeding, such as with Mallory Weiss tears, angiodysplasias, ulcers, and post-polypectomy bleeds, has been treated with a hypertonic saline-epinephrine solution or dehydrated alcohol. Injection of hypertonic saline-epinephrine is a relatively simple maneuver and has satisfactory hemostatic efficacy in the endoscopic treatment of nonvariceal gastrointestinal bleeding.

The most common sclerosing agent used for hemostatic control of bleeding ulcers is dehydrated (98%) ethanol (Alcohol). Alcohol works by dehydrating and fixating the exposed blood vessel and surrounding tissue. The resulting local vasoconstriction, vascular wall degeneration, and endothelial destruction lead to thrombosis.

**Variceal sclerotherapy**

Injection **sclerotherapy** involves the injection of a sclerosing (hardening) agent into a blood vessel (Fig. 30-2). It is indicated for the following:
- Temporary control of acute bleeding from esophageal varices pending shunt placement or in patients who are poor surgical risks
- Eradication of esophageal varices to prevent rebleeding
- Treatment of small hemorrhoids with bleeding
- Temporary control of acute hemorrhage from gastric varices

Gastric varices do not respond as well to sclerotherapy as those in the esophagus. Needle puncture of a gastric varix may be associated with prolonged bleeding from the injection site that is difficult to tamponade.

Injection sclerotherapy is rarely used as a prophylactic measure for patients who have never bled from varices. In children who are awaiting liver transplantation, however, Grade III or IV varices are injected prophylactically.

The physician chooses the sclerosing agent. Ideally, it should induce rapid thrombosis followed by intimal damage to the vein and ending in obliteration with minimal damage to the underlying esophageal musculature. It should be innocuous when it reaches the extraesophageal vascular system and other organs. The sclerosing agents used most commonly in the United States for control of variceal bleeding are morrhuate sodium (Scleromate), sodium tetradecyl sulfate (Sotradecol), and ethanolamine oleate (Ethamolin). Sodium tetradecyl sulfate may be less ulcerogenic than morrhuate sodium, and ethanolamine oleate may be the least ulcerogenic of the three. Allergic reactions have been reported with all three of these agents. If skin comes into contact with the sclerosant, it should be rinsed immediately with water.

Sclerotherapy is difficult if there is active hemorrhage, because blood must be cleared from the field to make precise injections. It is usually started 4 to 6 hours after relative hemodynamic stability has been achieved by transfusion, IV vasopressin, and/or **balloon tamponade**. The currently accepted practice is to control acute bleeding by IV vasopressin (Pitressin). This procedure usually relieves acute bleeding in 50% to 75% of cases and allows the patient to be stabilized.

As soon as the sclerosant is injected, the needle is withdrawn and rapidly reinserted into another site. The needle is fully withdrawn into the sheath after each injection. If undue pressure is needed to inject, it usually means that the needle is against the wall or that the varix has been injected previously. Forcing sclerosant into the wall of the esophagus will probably result in a superficial, esophageal ulcer.

The number and pattern of injections is determined by the endoscopist. Injections may be given intravariceally or paravariceally or using a combination of both methods. Because it can be difficult to determine the exact location of the needle, the actual effect may be a combination of both intravariceal and paravariceal injections. Paravariceal (submucosal) injection can be recognized if the site blanches after injection; intravariceal injection results in ballooning of the blood vessel with a characteristic dark blue color within a few minutes of the injection.

In patients with active hemorrhage, when the bleeding point can be identified, the first injection should be made immediately above the bleeding point in the same column, and then to the right and left. As the flow subsides, an injection may be made distally to the bleeding point. Even if injection therapy is unsuccessful in stopping active bleeding, it is important to make an injection below the varix.

After each injection, there is frequently some back-bleeding. Oozing is permissible and stops in 1 to 2 minutes. If a stream of blood arises from a puncture site, the puncture pattern for active hemorrhage should be followed.

After the procedure an extended period of observation follows, in which the patient should be monitored for signs of gastrointestinal blood loss and esophageal perforation. A patent IV line should be maintained until discharge. The patient may need additional pain medication, as ordered. After the procedure the physician may order laboratory work and antacids or sucralfate (Carafate) slurry.

Transient side effects of injection sclerotherapy include mild to severe chest pain, dysphagia, and fever. Chest pain usually subsides within 24 hours. Severe pain that lasts more than 24 hours may be indicative of perforation. Esophageal ulceration should also probably be considered a side effect of sclerotherapy because up to 78% of these patients have some degree of ulceration. Another frequent complication is esophageal stricture. Many of these patients suffer chronic dysphagia, which responds well to esophageal dilatation with polyvinyl tapered dilators. A low-grade fever can be observed in about 28% of patients and also usually subsides in 24 hours.

More serious potential complications of injection sclerotherapy include hemorrhage, aspiration, ulceration and/or necrosis of the esophagus, mediastinitis, stricture formation, esophageal perforation, pleural effusion, sepsis, or portal vein thrombosis. Perforation is manifested by persistent chest pain, dysphagia, fever, and pleural effusion. Septicemia is rare, but prophylaxis is probably warranted for patients with clinically significant heart disease, prosthetic heart valves, or other internal prostheses. Pleural effusion seems to be related to the amount of sclerosant used and the amount of chest pain the patient experiences; it usually resolves without therapy.

Complete eradication of varices may require several endoscopic sessions, or may occur early in the patient's course, with an average of five sessions for complete eradication of varices. Varices recur in 10% of these patients, even once they are varix-free. Annual checkups are recommended.

## ENDOSCOPIC VARICEAL LIGATION (EVL)

A newer method for the treatment of bleeding varices is **endoscopic variceal ligation (EVL),** a technique that has also been used successfully for the eradication of hemorrhoids. With EVL, rubber bands or O-rings are applied around the varices. The tensile strength created by the bands is sufficient to eradicate the varices.

Because the patient must be reintubated for each band, an overtube is used to facilitate multiple intubations. The overtube is backloaded onto the endoscope sheath, and the esophageal and gastric anatomy is viewed endoscopically to confirm that EVL is required.

With one manufacturer's ligator, the outer cylinder of a friction-fit adaptor is carefully attached to the distal tip of the endoscope. A trip wire is inserted down the biopsy channel of the scope. The inner cylinder of the adaptor, with a latex O-ring attached, is attached to the trip wire and then to the outer cylinder.

With the overtube properly positioned, and the need for EVL confirmed, the preloaded ligator and endoscope are introduced. The varix is aspirated into the inner cylinder, and the trip wire is pulled to release the O-ring. Suction is released, and the endoscope is withdrawn. At the physician's discretion, serial ligations may be performed after removing the spent inner cylinder and reloading a new one.

One disadvantage of this technique is that when the trip wire is passed through the endoscope's biopsy channel, the use of endoscopic suction is limited. This is particularly a problem if the patient is actively bleeding. Compared to injection sclerotherapy, however, EVL seems to result in less ulcer and stricture formation.

## ESOPHAGEAL-GASTRIC TAMPONADE

Esophageal-gastric tamponade involves the insertion of specialized tubes to provide pressure on bleeding areas of the esophagus or esophagogastric junction. It is indicated in patients with acute upper GI bleeding from esophageal varices or tears at the esophagogastric junction. Because of the variety of potential complications and because it is more difficult to use than vasopressin (Pitressin), it is generally performed in patients with variceal bleeding after the administration of vasopressin, sclerotherapy, or EVL has failed. It is used rarely for Mallory-Weiss tears that are unresponsive to medical therapy.

Esophageal-gastric tamponade is contraindicated for patients with cardiopulmonary failure, recent surgical trauma to the esophagogastric junction, or when variceal bleeding has stopped. It should not be attempted when the source of upper GI bleeding cannot be identified. It is also contraindicated in patients who are surgical candidates and in whom prior tamponade has failed.

Before the procedure it is important to establish and confirm a patent oral airway, monitor vital signs, and establish one or two large-bore IV lines for fluid and blood replacement. Because patients with acute upper GI bleeding may become extremely agitated, it is important to explain the benefits of the procedure, assure the patient of constant nursing care and monitoring, and explain that some pressure will be felt when the tube balloons are inflated.

Following are the three different types of tubes that may be used for this procedure:

- The **Sengstaken-Blakemore tube** is a three-lumen tube with esophageal and gastric balloons. It provides a gastric aspiration port to allow drainage from below the gastric balloon. Esophageal aspiration is accomplished by a secondary tube, such as a Levin or Salem sump tube, that is inserted orally or nasally to rest above the esophageal balloon. A manometer is used to insufflate the balloons and to measure pressure.

- The **Linton tube** is a three-lumen tube that uses a gastric balloon but no esophageal balloon and provides ports for both esophageal and gastric aspiration. Elimination of the esophageal balloon reduces the risk of esophageal necrosis. A manometer is used to measure pressures from the gastric inflation port.

- The **Minnesota tube** is a rubber, radiopaque, 18-French, four-lumen, double-balloon tube. The four lumens are used for gastric lavage and aspiration, esophageal aspiration, esophageal tamponade, and gastric tamponade. Medications may be instilled through the gastric lavage port. Lavage and gastric and esophageal suction may be performed while the balloon is inflated.

Before insertion, all balloons should be inflated and examined for defects. They should be checked for air leaks by submerging in water. The patient should be placed in a semi-Fowler's or left lateral position. If a Sengstaken-Blakemore tube is used, a nasogastric tube should be attached above the esophageal balloon to provide esophageal suction. Intermittent suction should be attached to the nasogastric tube.

The lubricated balloon tube should be inserted through the patient's mouth or nose, and the position of the tube should be confirmed by x-ray examination. Gastric contents should be aspirated, and the gastric balloon should be inflated in increments of 100 cc of air until the balloon is full (250 to 500 cc for a Sengstaken-Blakemore tube; 450 to 500 cc for a Minnesota tube; and 700 to 800 cc for a Linton tube). If the patient complains of sudden substernal pain or if insufflation of air is not audible over the epigastric area, inflation should be stopped immediately.

Once the gastric balloon is inflated, the tube should be pulled back gently until resistance is felt against the gastroesophageal junction. The balloon inlet should be clamped, and the tube should be secured with 1 to 2 pounds of traction. Traction may be initiated by the use of a nasal sponge guard, an over-the-bed traction set-up with 1 pound of weight, and a football helmet or catcher's mask. External traction may cause ulceration of the nasal mucosa and should not be used for prolonged periods.

Suction should be connected to the gastric and esophageal lumens, and drainage from each port should be observed.

If bleeding continues after the gastric balloon is inflated, the esophageal balloon should be attached to a manometer and inflated with air to 25 to 45 mm Hg. The esophageal balloon inlet should be clamped, and the nasogastric tube should be changed to constant suction. If bleeding is clearly from esophageal varices above the gastroesophageal junction, the esophageal balloon may be inflated simultaneously with the gastric balloon. If bleeding continues during esophageal tamponade, it may be from a gastric varix.

The procedure for insertion of a Linton tube is the same as for a Sengstaken-Blakemore tube, except there is no esophageal balloon, and the esophageal suction lumen obviates the need for a secondary nasogastric tube. The Minnesota tube also has an esophageal suction lumen.

Regardless of the type of tube used, scissors should be taped to the head of the bed so they are within easy reach in case transection and emergency removal of the tube becomes necessary.

While the tube is in place it is important to check the traction on the tube regularly, monitor vital signs, irrigate the gastric tube as ordered and assess fluid return, recheck and adjust the esophageal balloon pressure every 2 hours, provide good oral care, and keep the patient NPO.

After 24 hours, if bleeding is controlled, the esophageal balloon should be deflated. The nurse should check for rebleeding per the physician's orders. The gastric balloon should be deflated if no bleeding recurs over the next 6 to 12 hours. Frequent oral care should be provided, and frequent coughing and deep breathing should be encouraged.

Potential complications of esophageal-gastric tamponade include aspiration, rupture of the esophagus from pressure secondary to a misplaced gastric balloon, tissue necrosis from excessive pressure and/or prolonged inflation time, and airway obstruction secondary to dislodgement of the esophageal tube.

## NURSING CONSIDERATIONS

Nursing considerations for patients with gastrointestinal bleeding require special attention. Gastrointestinal bleeding is usually the result of another, less obvious problem.

A thorough nursing history is of paramount importance. It is necessary to obtain as much information as possible about the patient's current health problems. In addition, a family health history can help to determine whether there is any family history of alcohol abuse or other problems that can cause gastrointestinal bleeding. The patient's past and current work environments should be assessed to determine if exposure to chemicals or inhalants of any type might be a causative factor.

A physical assessment including weight, skin quality, and muscle tone provides data specific to the general appearance of the patient. Any discoloration of the skin should be documented.

Once a total physical assessment is completed and documented, the gastroenterology nurse can formulate the nursing diagnosis. Nursing diagnoses that may apply to patients with gastrointestinal bleeding include the following:

- Anxiety, related to uncertainty of prognosis, multiple diagnostic procedures, and treatment regimen
- Ineffective breathing pattern, related to decreased lung expansion, decreased energy, and fatigue
- Potential for injury: bleeding, related to altered clotting mechanisms
- Chronic low self-esteem, related to unknown etiology
- Knowledge deficit with respect to treatment regimen

The gastroenterology nurse must work with the patient and family members to identify outcomes that will be realistic for the patient. The overall goal is to prevent further damage and to improve the patient's overall physical and mental condition. Examples of desired outcomes for patients with gastrointestinal bleeding might include the following:

- Patient is free of injuries and bleeding
- Skin integrity is good
- Patient has normal respiratory function
- Family demonstrates support for patient
- Patient is free of infection

Patient care must be planned specifically for the individual patient. For patients with bleeding problems, it is important to implement nursing care that assists in controlling hemorrhage. Patient comfort is maintained by assessing the need for pain medication. Fluid and electrolyte status is constantly assessed. The patient and family members and/or significant others must be taught appropriate self-care techniques. Potential problems and solutions are reviewed. The patient should be made aware of helpful community resources.

**CASE SITUATION**

Mr. Ben Harrison, age 54, was offered an executive physical when he was promoted. As a routine part of his physical, a stool test was done to check for blood, and a flexible sigmoidoscopy was performed. The stool was positive for occult blood and a small polyp was found at 30 cm from the anus on sigmoidoscopy. Mr. Harrison's internist knows that findings of stool positive for occult blood and a polyp in the sigmoid may indicate a synchronous lesion higher in the large bowel. For this reason, he refers Mr. Harrison to the gastroenterology department for a colonoscopy.

### Points to think about

1. Mr. Harrison exhibits the following signs and symptoms:
   - Increased heart and respiratory rates
   - Increased systolic blood pressure
   - Profuse palmar sweating
   - Increased muscular tension
   - Urinary frequency and urgency
   - Anger concerning need for various diagnostic tests
   
   To what nursing diagnosis do these data seem most applicable?
2. What interventions might the gastroenterology nurse use before and during the colonoscopy to reduce Mr. Harrison's anxiety?
3. The procedure has started, and the doctor has passed the first small polyp at 30 cm. The patient is tolerating the procedure very well. As the doctor advances to the ascending colon, he finds a larger, more vascular appearing polyp. He moves on to the cecum, which is normal, and comes back to the ascending colon to remove the polyp. What are the responsibilities of the nurse operating the ESU?
4. The body uses its own mechanisms to achieve hemostasis. Three of these mechanisms are local reactions, which would be a response to cell disruption, as in a cut. What are they?
5. By what mechanism does electrosurgery help to provide hemostasis?
6. The heat produced by a monopolar electrode is dependent on four factors. What are they?
7. When using an electrocautery device during a procedure, what should the nurse chart on the record specific to electrocautery?
8. Colonoscopy with polypectomy is a safe outpatient procedure. Barring any complication, Mr. Harrison will go home when he has recovered from sedation. What instructions will the nurse give him?

### Suggested responses

1. The most applicable nursing diagnosis is anxiety related to threat to bodily health and lack of control over events.
2. Appropriate anxiety-reducing interventions the nurse may take might include:
   - Providing a relaxing, reassuring, professional atmosphere
   - Discussing with Mr. Harrison the types of feelings he may experience during the exam, such as slight crampy abdominal pain caused by air insufflation or stretching of the bowel by moving the colonoscope
   - Telling the patient that she will be there throughout the procedure to take care of his needs
   - Speaking softly to the patient during the procedure and rubbing his back gently
3. The nurse responsible for the ESU should:
   - Set up and check the unit before the procedure and establish that it is working correctly
   - Place the grounding pad on the patient (because the nurse is using a monopolar unit); disconnect the heart monitor, because it can be an alternate pathway for current (this is debatable, but better to be safe than sorry); and move the patient's hands and legs away from the side rails
   - Be sure that the unit is plugged in, that all connections are secure, and that all personnel are wearing gloves
   - Hand the snare to the physician to feed through the scope, and open and close the snare per the physician's instructions
   - Once the polyp is removed, turn off the machine while removing the snare
4. The body's own mechanisms for achieving hemostasis include:
   - Vessel spasm. Vessels contract in an effort to diminish blood loss; spasm lasts from a few seconds to 30 minutes, so suspected bleeding vessels must be watched.
   - Platelet aggregation. Circulating platelets have an affinity for the moist, irregular endothelium that is exposed in a broken vessel and will adhere there, thus forming a platelet plug.
   - Clot formation. Within seconds or minutes after damage, platelet aggregates and altered blood structure release activator substances; this triggers formation of fibrin threads, thus forming a network in which plasma and red blood cells can coalesce into a clot.
5. Electrosurgery helps provide hemostasis by the following mechanism:
   - Kinetic energy relayed to the cells from the ESU excites the ions in the cells, and they collide with other cellular particles, thereby creating heat in the cell. The effect on tissue is thermal, not electrical.
6. The heat produced by a monopolar electrode depends on the following factors:
   - The power setting.
   - Tissue resistance. The heat in the tissue increases in relation to the resistance of the tissue. Tissue with a lot of water content has low resistance. Dry tissue has higher resistance. When heat dries out the tis-

sue, it may take a higher setting to continue cutting.

- Current density. Heat varies according to current density. When the snare loop is closed, it increases the current density and raises the temperature to the adjacent tissue. In the monopolar modality, the current density diminishes as it spreads out to the larger surface area of the dispersive electrode (grounding pad). If the surface area is large enough, the return electrode disperses the current and the patient does not feel the heat. If the large electrode were to come loose at the edges and have only a small contact with skin, the current density going to that small spot could be great enough to cause a burn.
- Time. The longer the physician depresses the foot pedal, the greater the heating depth will be.

7. When using an electrocautery device, the following should be documented:
- The equipment and accessories used, including brand name and whether it was monopolar or bipolar
- A description of the lesion and any tissue that was recovered and sent to pathology
- Machine settings and number of applications
- How the lesion looked after heat application; any bleeding that is present
- How the patient tolerated the procedure; any complications

8. Instructions the nurse should give Mr. Harrison when he goes home include:
- Not to drink alcohol, drive a car, or operate machinery until the next day
- Any dietary or medication restrictions the physician has ordered. For instance, the use of aspirin may be restricted after polypectomy because it interferes with blood clotting.
- That some bloating is normal because of the air instilled during the procedure and that it will subside as air is expelled
- To call the physician if any rectal bleeding occurs, or if there is severe abdominal pain or temperature elevation

---

### REVIEW TERMS

**argon, balloon tamponade, bipolar probe, bipolar electrocoagulation, coagulating current, coagulation, cutting current, desiccation, electrocautery, electrocoagulation, electrosurgical unit (ESU), endoscopic variceal ligation (EVL), fulguration, heater probe, laser, Linton tube, Minnesota tube, monopolar electrocoagulation, Nd:YAG, photocoagulation, photovaporization, sclerotherapy, Sengstaken-Blakemore tube, tamponade**

---

### REVIEW QUESTIONS

1. Thermal coagulation of bleeding vessels is achieved in gastroenterology patients by using:
   a. Monopolar electrocautery.
   b. Bipolar electrocautery.
   c. Lasers.
   d. All of the above.

2. Leakage of current in monopolar electrocoagulation can cause burns to the:
   a. Endoscopist.
   b. Patient.
   c. Nurse/associate.
   d. All of the above.

3. One advantage of bipolar over monopolar electrocoagulation is:
   a. Depth of penetration is greater.
   b. No grounding pad is needed.
   c. The unit is portable.
   d. It is easier to use.

4. Potential complications of bipolar electrocoagulation include:
   a. Perforation.
   b. Spot burning of the patient's skin.
   c. Sepsis.
   d. Eye damage.

5. The type of laser used most often in endoscopic applications is:
   a. Carbon dioxide.
   b. Nd:YAG.
   c. Argon.
   d. KTP/532.

6. Laser fibers used in endoscopic applications are cleaned with:
   a. Alcohol.
   b. Glutaraldehyde.
   c. Hydrogen peroxide.
   d. Sterile water.

7. The specialized three-lumen tube with esophageal and gastric balloons that is used for esophageal-gastric tamponade is called a:
   a. Sengstaken-Blakemore tube.
   b. Linton tube.
   c. Minnesota tube.
   d. Salem sump tube.

8. In esophageal-gastric tamponade, the esophageal balloon should be inflated to what pressure?
   a. 2.5 to 4.5 mm Hg.
   b. 25 to 45 mm Hg.
   c. 125 to 145 mm Hg.
   d. 1 psi.

9. The first line of treatment in patients with actively bleeding esophageal varices is usually:
   a. Intravenous vasopressin (Pitressin).
   b. Balloon tamponade.

c. Injection sclerotherapy.

d. Electrocoagulation.

10. Severe chest pain that persists for more than 24 hours in patients who have undergone sclerotherapy for esophageal varices is most likely a result of:

a. Myocardial infarction.

b. Residual effects of the sclerosing agent.

c. Aspiration pneumonia.

d. Perforation.

## BIBLIOGRAPHY

Chen, P, Wu, C, and Liaw, Y. "Hemostatic Effect of Endoscopic Local Injection with Hypertonic Saline-Epinephrine Solution and Pure Ethanol for Digestive Tract Bleeding." *Gastrointestinal Endoscopy* 32(October 1986): 319-23.

Dennison, A, Whiston, R, Rooney, S, and Morris, D. "The Management of Hemorrhoids." *American Journal of Gastroenterology* 84(May 1989): 475-81.

Fleischer, D. "BICAP Tumor Probe Therapy for Esophageal Cancer: A Practical Guide." Reprinted from *Endoscopy Review*. 5(March-April 1988): 2-13.

Fleischer, D. "The Therapeutic Use of Lasers in GI Disease." In *SGA Journal Reprints*, ed. Trivits, S, 191-201. Rochester, N.Y.: Society of Gastrointestinal Assistants, 1988.

Gruber, M, and Camara, D. "Injection Sclerotherapy: Seven Years' Experience." In *SGA Journal Reprints*, ed. Trivits, S, 127-29. Rochester, N.Y.: Society of Gastrointestinal Assistants, 1988.

Hardick, M, and Beck, M, eds. *Manual of Gastrointestinal Procedures*. 2nd ed. Rochester, N.Y.: Society of Gastroenterology Nurses and Associates, 1989.

Kidwell, J. "The Nurse's Role in the Laser Unit." *SGA Journal* 12(Winter 1989): 196.

Kirby, D. "Management of Esophageal Varices: A Review of Treatment Options and the Role of the Gastroenterology Nurse and Associate." *Gastroenterology Nursing* 12(Summer 1989): 10-14.

McFarland, P, and McFarlane, J. "Self-Perception — Self-Concept Pattern, Anxiety." In *Nursing Diagnosis and Intervention*, 597-612. St. Louis: Mosby–Year Book, 1990.

Schapiro, M. "The Gastroenterologist and the Treatment of Hemorrhoids: Is It About Time?" *American Journal of Gastroenterology* 84(May 1989): 493-95.

Sheck, P. "GI Assistant's Role in Laser Therapy." In *SGA Journal Reprints*, ed. Trivits, S, 203-05. Rochester, N.Y.: Society of Gastrointestinal Assistants, 1988.

Shields, N. "The Role of the G.I.A. in Electrosurgery." In *SGA Journal Reprints*, ed. Trivits, S, 185-89. Rochester, N.Y.: Society of Gastrointestinal Assistants, 1988.

Short, N. "Gastrointestinal Intubations: Nursing Considerations." *Gastroenterology Nursing* 12(Summer 1989): 43-49.

Silvis, S, ed. *Therapeutic Gastrointestinal Endoscopy*. New York: Igaku-Shoin, 1985.

Sivak, M, Jr., and Petrini, J, eds. *Gastrointestinal Endoscopy: Old Problems, New Techniques*. Gastroenterology Series, Volume 4. New York: Praeger, 1986.

Sleisenger, M+, and Fordtran, J, eds. *Gastrointestinal Disease: Pathophysiology, Diagnosis, Management*. 4th ed. Philadelphia: W.B. Saunders, 1989.

Swartz, M, Carey, K, and Danzi, J. "Laser Therapy of the Gastric Lesions of the Osler-Weber-Rendu Syndrome." *SGA Journal* 12(Winter 1989): 143-44.

Waye, J, Geenen, J, Fleischer, D, and Venu, R. *Techniques in Therapeutic Endoscopy*. Philadelphia: W.B. Saunders, 1987.

Zinberg, S, Stern, D, Furman, D, and Wittles, J. "A Personal Experience in Comparing Three Nonoperative Techniques for Treating Internal Hemorrhoids." *American Journal of Gastroenterology* 84(May 1989): 488-92.

# Chapter 31

# INTUBATION AND DRAINAGE

This chapter will acquaint the gastroenterology nurse with indications, contraindications, and techniques for gastrointestinal intubation and drainage. A variety of intubation and drainage procedures are covered, including nasogastric intubation, gastric lavage, insertion of nasobiliary catheters, biliary stent placement, intestinal intubation, colon decompression, and abdominal paracentesis.*

Intubation for esophageal-gastric tamponade is discussed in Chapter 30. The use of feeding tubes and percutaneous endoscopic gastrostomy/jejunostomy (PEG/PEJ) devices for long-term enteral nutrition are discussed in Chapter 23.

## Learning objectives

After reviewing the content of this chapter, the gastro-enterology nurse should be able to:

1. Discuss techniques for the insertion of nasogastric and nasoenteric tubes.
2. Explain indications and techniques for the insertion of esophageal prostheses.
3. Describe the use of nasobiliary catheters and biliary stents.
4. Discuss procedures for gastric lavage, colonic decompression, and abdominal paracentesis.

## NASOGASTRIC TUBE INSERTION

Nasogastric intubation is indicated for the following:
- Treatment of gastric distention or gastric outlet obstruction
- Assessment and treatment of upper GI bleeding

- Gastric tube feeding
- Certain gastric/esophageal tests
- Gastric lavage
- Aspiration of gastric secretions
- Administration of medications and feedings
- Prevention of vomiting by decompressing the stomach after major surgery
- Emptying the upper GI tract before emergency surgery

Insertion of a **nasogastric tube** must be performed cautiously in pregnant patients, and in patients with an aortic aneurysm, recent myocardial infarction, gastric hemorrhage, or esophageal varices. It is contraindicated in patients with nasopharyngeal or esophageal obstruction, severe maxillofacial trauma, or severe uncontrolled coagulopathy.

The nasogastric tubes used for normal adults are usually 14 or 16 French (Fr) and 22 to 26 inches (55 to 66 cm) long. The length of tubing needed to reach the stomach should be determined by placing the end of the tube at the tip of the patient's nose and extending it to the earlobe and down to the xiphoid process.

The most commonly used nasogastric tubes are the Levin and the Salem sump tubes.
- The Levin tube has only one lumen. If a vacuum forms, causing the tube to adhere to the stomach lining, the gastric mucosa may be damaged. Intermittent low suction is recommended for the Levin tube.
- The Salem sump tube has a primary suction-drainage lumen and a smaller vent lumen. Continuous air flow through the vent lumen prevents a vacuum from forming. When a Salem sump tube is used with suction, the larger lumen is connected to

---

* All techniques in this chapter, except intestinal intubation, are also discussed in the SGNA *Manual of Gastrointestinal Procedures*. 2nd ed. Rochester, N.Y.: Society of Gastroenterology Nurses and Associates, 1989.

the suction equipment. Intermittent high suction or continuous low suction may be used with the Salem sump tube.

Before insertion of a nasogastric tube, the patient should be questioned regarding any history of nasal surgery, fractures, or a deviated septum and to verify the length of the patient's NPO status.

To facilitate insertion, a limp rubber tube may be placed on ice for about 3 minutes, or a stiff plastic tube may be softened by immersion in warm water. The tube should be inserted in the nostril with the greatest airflow while the patient is in a high Fowler's or left lateral decubitus position. Before insertion the nostrils should be examined for any obvious obstruction. To determine which nostril has the greatest airflow, the nurse should perform the following activities:

- Question the patient about any previous nasal surgery, trauma, or a deviated septum.
- Inspect the nostrils with a penlight for any obvious obstruction.
- Occlude one nostril at a time while the patient breathes through the nose.

A topical anesthetic should be applied if ordered. Dentures should be removed so they will not be dislocated if the patient gags. While wearing disposable gloves, the nurse should lubricate the nasogastric tube with a water-soluble lubricant. With the patient's head tilted slightly back, the tube should be inserted into the nostril and rotated gently toward the center. When the tube is in the back of the patient's throat, the chin should be tipped toward the chest to close the trachea and open the esophagus. If the patient's condition or test permits, the patient may sip water through a bendable straw while the tube is guided gently down the esophagus and into the antrum. The tube should then be taped to the nose and correct placement confirmed by:

- Asking the patient to talk. If the patient cannot talk, the tube may be coiled in the throat or may have passed through the vocal cords.
- Using a tongue depressor and penlight to confirm that the tube is not curled in the mouth or throat, especially in unconscious patients.
- Injecting air through the tube and using a stethoscope to auscultate a "whooshing" sound just below the xiphoid process. If the patient belches, the tube may be in the esophagus.
- Attempting to aspirate the stomach contents.
- Performing an x-ray examination or fluoroscopy.

If the patient coughs frequently or experiences dyspnea during insertion, the tube should be removed immediately because it may be in the trachea or coiled in the pharynx.

Once proper placement is confirmed, the tube should be clamped or attached to intermittent suction or gravity drainage as ordered by the physician.

In some patients, such as those with a deviated septum, the tube can be placed orally. In such cases, the distal tip of the tube should be placed on the back of the patient's tongue. The patient should be asked to tip the chin toward the chest and swallow, keeping the upper and lower teeth slightly apart. If the patient is unconscious or cannot swallow for any reason, the tube should be advanced between respirations. It may be helpful to stroke the patient's neck to facilitate passage down the esophagus. Again, the tube should be inserted gently with each swallow.

After insertion the tube should be taped to the nose with adhesive tape. A pin or tape will support the weight of the tube on the patient's clothing. Adequate tubing should be used to allow the patient free movement and turning.

Patency of the tube should be confirmed periodically by irrigating with normal saline. The frequency of irrigation and the amount of solution should be specified by the physician. Fluid inserted during irrigation should be removed and measured.

The nares should be cleansed, and the tube should be retaped as necessary. Mouth care should be provided once a shift or as necessary. Depending on the patient's condition, lemon-glycerin swabs may be used to clean the teeth, or the patient may brush them. The lips should be coated with petroleum jelly to prevent dryness. The patient may be allowed to chew gum, suck on sour balls, or use throat lozenges to promote comfort.

Bowel sounds should be assessed regularly to check gastrointestinal function. The color, consistency, and odor of gastric drainage should be observed. Normal gastric secretions are colorless or yellow-green from bile and have a mucoid consistency. Gastric drainage that has the color of coffee grounds may be an indication of bleeding and should be reported immediately. Nausea, vomiting, a feeling of fullness, epigastric discomfort, or distention may be indications that the tube is not patent. Patients should also be observed for fluid and electrolyte imbalances.

If medications are to be instilled through the tube, it is important to irrigate the tube before and after instillation. Suction should be omitted for 30 to 45 minutes after instillation to permit absorption of the medication.

Before removing a nasogastric tube, it should be flushed with a small amount of air to clear the tube of stomach contents that would cause irritation during removal. The tube should be untaped from the patient's nose, and the patient should be instructed not to breathe to ensure closure of the epiglottis. The tube should be withdrawn gently and steadily until the distal end reaches the nasopharynx, when it can be pulled quickly. If possible, the tube should be quickly covered and removed. The patient should be assisted with mouth care, and tape residue should be cleaned from the nose with adhesive remover. If signs of gastrointestinal dysfunction recur, reinsertion of the tube may be necessary.

Potential complications of nasogastric tube insertion include respiratory distress caused by incorrect tube placement, pulmonary aspiration, epistaxis (nosebleed), necrosis of the nasal mucous membrane caused by incorrect taping of the tube, skin erosion at the nostril, sinusitis, esophagitis, esophagotracheal fistula, gastric ulceration, pulmonary and oral infection, and esophageal or gastric hemorrhage or perforation. An additional complication of nasogastric intubation is otitis media caused by eustachian tube irritation. The use of suction can cause electrolyte imbalance and dehydration.

## ESOPHAGEAL PROSTHESES

To provide a patent lumen for purposes of nourishment and oral secretions in patients with terminal, obstructive esophageal cancer, a prosthesis may be inserted endoscopically through the obstruction.

A variety of esophageal prostheses are available, most of which are made of latex or silicone rubber, polyvinyl chloride, or other plastics. Most have outside diameters of 14 to 16 mm. Some of the available models include the Celestin tube, the Keymed prosthesis, the Proctor-Livingstone tube, and "home-made" Tygon prostheses. The home-made types have the advantage of individualized length, thickness, rigidity, and position of extra shoulders for better anchoring.

Insertion of an esophageal prosthesis is indicated in patients with circumferential stenosis resulting from malignant carcinoma of the lower two thirds of the esophagus when dilatation, radiation, or laser therapy has failed to provide satisfactory relief from dysphagia. The procedure may also be indicated in patients with esophageal-pulmonary fistulae or extrinsic compression of the esophagus.

Use of an endoprosthesis is contraindicated in the following situations:

- In patients with any medical condition that takes priority over the prosthesis
- For cancers that are less than 2 cm below the upper esophageal sphincter, because of the constant awareness of a foreign body.
- If tumor invasion compresses the trachea and/or bronchus
- In patients who have had recent chemotherapy
- When the stricture cannot be dilated adequately
- In uncooperative or unmotivated patients
- In patients with a life expectancy of less than 6 weeks (relative)

Before insertion of an esophageal prosthesis, it is important to verify that the patient has been NPO for at least 8 hours. The nurse should assess the patient for any indication of cardiopulmonary compromise, establish a patent IV line, administer antibiotics as ordered, and remove dentures. The patient should be informed that he or she will feel the prosthesis in the chest for a few hours following the procedure.

The patient should be placed in the left lateral position. The throat should be anesthetized as ordered. During the procedure the gastroenterology nurse's responsibilities are to provide emotional support to the patient; maintain the oral airway and manage oral secretions; assist the physician; monitor vital signs; observe the color, warmth, and dryness of the patient's skin; and monitor the patient's level of consciousness, pain tolerance, and respiratory status.

The esophageal lumen should be dilated with mercury-filled, or preferably polyvinyl, dilators of 15 to 16 mm in diameter. One or more dilatations are usually performed in addition to the one carried out on the day of stent placement.

The proximal and distal margins of the tumor are identified by using a small-caliber endoscope. It is important to measure the length of the tumor and the distance of each landmark from the incisors for choosing the appropriate stent. Because most stents have a proximal flange that is 3 to 4 cm in length, it is also important to measure the location of the upper esophageal sphincter (UES) and its distance from the proximal tumor margin. The shaft of the stent should be 3 cm longer than the tumor, and the proximal flange will add another 3 cm. For example, a 7-cm tumor requires the use of a 13-cm stent. If there is a tracheoesophageal fistula that is not within the narrowed tumor segment, it should be determined whether or not the stent flange will cover it.

Once an appropriate size stent is determined, stent placement method should be chosen. There are several methods of placing esophageal stents. One of these methods is described below:

1. A silk thread is passed through a puncture site in the upper part of the flange to aid in stent removal in the event of a problem.
2. The thread is passed through the inside of a pusher tube that exits through its proximal end.
3. The inside of the stent and pusher tube are lubricated with silicone. The pusher tube is marked with an indelible pen so key points will be recognized during the passage of the stent and pusher.
4. For insertion, an introducing device is passed over the guidewire into the stomach.
5. The stent and pusher tube are positioned over the introducing device, advanced through the phar-

ynx, and seated in place. If placement is satisfactory, the introducing device and guidewire are removed.

Next, the pusher tube is gently twisted before removal to minimize the chance of pulling the stent proximally with it.

After the stent is positioned, a small-caliber endoscope is passed to confirm proper placement and to make certain that the lumen of the stent is easily traversed.

Chest radiography is used to confirm the position of the stent and to rule out perforation. After the effects of IV sedation have worn off, a barium swallow may be performed to confirm that contrast flows freely and no perforation exists.

The patient should be monitored for changes in vital signs, symptoms of compromised respirations, respiratory depression, aspiration, bleeding, or perforation. The patient should be NPO except for ice chips for 12 hours, after which clear liquids can be started. To be certain that no coughing occurs to dislodge the stent, a codeine preparation is administered as ordered. After 24 to 36 hours the diet may be advanced. When the prosthesis extends into the stomach, the patient is treated with antacids and antireflux measures to prevent reflux esophagitis.

After discharge the patient ingests a regular to soft diet, provided dentition is adequate. The patient must chew food well and drink liquids often during the meal.

Potential early complications of inserting an esophageal prosthesis include perforation, displacement, pressure necrosis, bleeding, airway obstruction, retrosternal pain, and respiratory depression secondary to medication or displacement of the prosthesis. Later complications may include food bolus obstruction, an obstruction secondary to tumor overgrowth, or esophagitis secondary to reflux if the prosthesis extends across the gastroesophageal junction.

Some of these complications may require removal of the prosthesis, which can be done endoscopically with grasping forceps, a polypectomy snare, or in other ways. Removal of the prosthesis rarely creates a major problem, except when a dislodged tube has to be removed from a tumorous stomach.

## GASTRIC LAVAGE

Gastric **lavage** involves insertion of a gastric tube through the nose or mouth for the purpose of washing toxic substances, blood, or secretions from the stomach. It is indicated in patients with acute gastrointestinal bleeding; when preparing the stomach for endoscopy after barium or food ingestion; and for evacuating the stomach after ingestion of toxic substances. In patients

with acute gastrointestinal bleeding, lavage gives a good indication of the rapidity of bleeding, cleanses the stomach for possible later endoscopy and, in patients with cirrhosis, removes blood to lessen the likelihood of hepatic encephalopathy. A smaller-diameter nasogastric tube is used to localize the bleeding, and a large-bore orogastric tube is placed for instillation of aliquots of fluid.

Gastric lavage is contraindicated in patients with possible esophageal or gastric perforation, known esophageal obstruction, or maxillofacial trauma. It is also contraindicated after ingestion of corrosive substances, such as lye and some cleaning compounds, because the nasogastric tube may perforate the esophagus.

The setup required for gastric lavage includes a container of irrigation solution to which is attached a piece of tubing ending in a Y-connector. One side of the Y-connector is attached to the patient's nasogastric or orogastric tube, and the other side is attached to another piece of tubing that is connected to a calibrated collection container.

A number of gastric tubes are available.

* The Levacuator, which is the basic orogastric "stomach pump" tube, is a sterile, single-use, double-lumen, polyvinyl tube that is 48 inches long and available in sizes of 18, 22, 28, 32, and 36 Fr. The Levacuator is indicated in situations where intermittent gastric lavage and evacuation are required. The larger lumen is used for evacuation of gastric contents, and the smaller is used for instillation of an irrigant. It is especially suitable for emergency removal of toxic agents, overdose of oral medications, or ingestion of hazardous substances. Activated charcoal slurries may be administered through the large suction lumen. In situations where there is a high risk of aspiration, such as loss of consciousness, seizures, or delirium, a cuffed endotracheal tube should be inserted before insertion of the Levacuator.
* The Ewald tube is a reusable, single-lumen, rubber tube with several openings at the distal end. It is usually passed orally, but can be inserted nasally. Single-lumen tubes allow rapid lavage and evacuation of large volumes of fluid, but continuous irrigation is not possible because the same lumen must be used for both instillation and evacuation of fluid. During an emergency the Ewald tube may be used to aspirate large amounts of gastric contents quickly.
* The Edlich tube is a single-lumen tube with four openings near the closed distal tip. A funnel or syringe may be connected at the proximal end. Like the Ewald tube, it is used to aspirate large amounts of gastric contents quickly.

Before inserting a gastric tube for lavage it is important to obtain baseline vital signs, ensure an adequate airway, and establish a large-bore IV line for volume replacement as ordered. Patients should be informed that the tube may cause some gagging, but they will be able to breathe. The importance of remaining on the left side should be emphasized.

The patient should be placed in the left lateral position. If a nasogastric tube is being used, the patient may be in Fowler's position. The nasogastric intubation procedure just described should be used for inserting a nasogastric tube. If the tube is inserted orally, the well-lubricated tube should be guided into the back of the mouth while the patient is encouraged to suck on the tube and swallow. To check tube placement, 20 to 40 cc of air (5 cc in children) should be injected, and the epigastric area should be auscultated with a stethoscope. Before instilling any irrigation solution, the stomach contents should be aspirated to ensure correct placement.

If the patient begins to cough or experiences dyspnea and nothing is aspirated from the tube, the tube may be in the trachea. The tube should be removed immediately and another insertion attempted. It is important to provide frequent patient reassurance and support during the procedure.

The irrigating solution container is hung from the highest level of an IV pole. The inflow tube is unclamped and 250 ml of irrigation are instilled gradually to evaluate the patient's tolerance and prevent vomiting. (Iced saline lavage is no longer recommended because it has a tendency to lower the patient's core temperature.) After instillation, continuous negative pressure should be applied with a syringe or by removing the clamp on the outflow tube, thereby allowing the fluid to flow via gravity into a collection container that is lower than the patient's head. The procedure should be repeated, increasing the amount of irrigating solution to 500 ml, until the return is clear or of acceptable clarity. In patients with upper GI bleeding, lavage should be continued until bleeding stops or until it becomes evident that other measures will be necessary. If the amount instilled is significantly greater than the amount recovered, the tube should be repositioned.

The patient should never be left alone during gastric lavage. He or she should be observed continuously for changes in level of consciousness, and vital signs should be monitored frequently. Throughout lavage, frequent suctioning of the oral cavity may be needed to prevent aspiration. When lavaging the stomach after ingestion of poisons or drugs, all return fluid should be saved for possible laboratory analysis.

When the return is of acceptable clarity, the tube should be withdrawn slowly, and aspiration of any fluid in the stomach or esophagus should be continued. The patient should exhale slowly as the tube is withdrawn.

Potential complications of gastric lavage include aspiration of gastric contents, which is most likely to occur in groggy patients; perforation; electrolyte imbalance from prolonged lavage; and hemorrhage. Bradyarrhythmias may also occur. If the gastric tube becomes clogged, unrelieved gastric distention may occur, thus leading to potentially fatal shock.

## NASOBILIARY CATHETERS

A **nasobiliary catheter (NBC)** is a long, thin, polyethylene tube that is placed endoscopically over a guidewire into the common bile duct or the pancreatic duct. The proximal end of the tube is brought out through the patient's nostril and connected to a bile drainage bag. The tip of the NBC that is placed in the duct has several side holes to facilitate adequate bile flow. Older models had a pigtail curl at the end, while the newer types have a straight tip with an alpha loop in the duodenum to prevent dislodgement.

Placement of an NBC is indicated for the following:

- Decompression of an obstructed bile duct in acute suppurative cholangitis.
- Temporary or short-term decompression of the common bile duct, similar to that which follows unsuccessful stone extraction after endoscopic sphincterotomy.
- Prevention of stone impaction after endoscopic sphincterotomy.
- Infusion of contrast medium for repeat cholangiography.
- Instillation of various therapeutic solutions, including monooctanoin (Moctanin, used for gallstone dissolution), antibiotics (for acute bacterial cholangitis), corticosteroids (for sclerosing cholangitis), or saline (to flush sludge or small stones after endoscopic sphincterotomy).
- Preoperative biliary decompression to decrease jaundice (thereby decreasing perioperative complications) in patients undergoing elective biliary tract surgery.
- Temporary biliary decompression in patients who are septic or who have severe coagulopathy. Once infection has been controlled or coagulopathy corrected, sphincterotomy can be performed, and a large stent can be inserted for long-term therapy.
- Access for intraluminal irradiation therapy, using iridium.
- Aspiration of bile for chemical and bacteriologic studies (e.g., to identify causative agents in bacterial cholangitis or to determine the lithogenicity of bile in patients with cholestasis).
- Facilitating the healing process in traumatic or surgical biliary fistulae.

Nasobiliary catheter placement is contraindicated in patients with coagulopathy, sepsis, active pancreatitis or other infection, recent food ingestion, or any other contraindication to esophagogastroduodenoscopy (EGD). Some physicians will insert an NBC in the presence of the first three contraindications, if leaving the patient untreated would cause further harm.

Endoscopic retrograde cholangiopancreatography (ERCP) is performed with a side-viewing endoscope to define the level and extent of obstruction. An endoscopic sphincterotomy is usually performed before NBC placement, except in patients with fulminant cholangitis or severe coagulopathy. The diseased duct is cannulated, and a guidewire with a flexible tip is inserted through the cannula. The cannula is withdrawn under fluoroscopic guidance while the nurse continues to feed the guidewire.

The portion of the guidewire that protrudes from the duodenoscope is lubricated with silicone spray. A 5- or 7-Fr nasobiliary catheter is then advanced over the guidewire until the desired position is reached above the obstruction in the bile duct. The guidewire is slowly withdrawn, the endoscope is removed, and the position of the NBC is adjusted, with one end of the NBC left protruding from the patient's mouth and the other end in the obstructed duct. A small loop in the duodenum helps to prevent displacement of the catheter. Loops or extra length are removed under fluoroscopic control.

The NBC must be rerouted through the patient's nose to allow normal ingestion of foods and liquids while the NBC is in place. A specially designed 25- to 30-cm, 14-Fr nasopharyngeal tube or a nasogastric tube is advanced through the nose, grasped with a pair of forceps in the posterior oropharynx, and pulled out through the patient's mouth. The tip of the NBC is threaded inside the oral end of the nasopharyngeal tube and advanced until it exits through the nasal end of the larger tube. The tube in the oropharynx is held firmly by the endoscopist or assistant to maintain its position during withdrawal through the nose, thereby preventing dislodgement of the drainage tube from the bile duct. The nasopharyngeal tube is then withdrawn slowly through the nostril until the tip of the NBC emerges from the nose. The nasopharyngeal tube is discarded. The excess portion of the NBC at the nose is transected and a luer lock valve is attached, thus creating an adapter for an appropriate biliary tract drainage system. The end of the NBC is taped to the cheek and connected to a drainage bag.

An NBC can remain in place indefinitely and will provide continuous access to the biliary tree. Two to four hours after the procedure, the patient may be permitted a soft diet.

Following insertion of the NBC, it is important to monitor and record the patient's vital signs; observe the patient for abdominal pain or distention; administer antibiotics as ordered; tape the NBC to the patient's cheek, avoiding sharp angles and kinks; and place adapters and a drainage bag on the catheter and secure the apparatus to the patient's gown, allowing enough tubing to prevent traction when the patient turns his or her head. The patient may experience some minor throat discomfort and green or yellow fluid may appear in the tube. Some movement of the tube is to be expected during eating and drinking.

In addition to the complications that are associated with ERCP, endoscopic sphincterotomy, or insertion of biliary stents, potential complications of inserting an NBC include blockage of the catheter, nasal irritation, and/or sore throat. Minor complications can be managed by proper care of the nostril and use of throat lozenges and mild analgesics. To prevent mucus from plugging the side holes of the NBC, it may be helpful to irrigate the NBC with 10 ml sterile saline every 3 to 4 hours. To straighten out a kink, a guidewire may be passed through the entire NBC under fluoroscopic control, followed by irrigation. If this fails, the NBC must be replaced.

## BILIARY STENTS

To provide permanent palliative biliary drainage, a thin, hollow Teflon or polyethylene tube can be placed endoscopically during ERCP (Fig. 31-1). The objective of a biliary stent or endoprosthesis is to create between two normal anatomic sites a bridge that bypasses the diseased or obstructed portion of the duct. **Stents** are most often placed in the common bile duct but may also be placed in the pancreatic duct.

Two basic types of stents are currently in use; the pigtail stent and the barbed stent. The length of the stent between the barbs may be 5 to 15 cm (2 to 6 inches), and the outside circumference ranges from 5 to 12 Fr. The larger the diameter of the stent, the better the drainage,

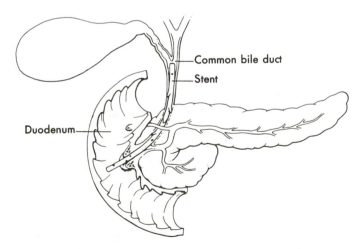

**Fig. 31-1.** Straight stent placement in common bile duct, draining to duodenum.

but the scope channel size must accommodate the diameter of the stent. Each stent is provided with a number of side holes to facilitate drainage.

- In the 5- or 7-Fr **pigtail stent,** one or both ends of the tube is coiled. This coiled shape disappears when the stent is pulled taut, but quickly returns when allowed to relax. Pigtail stents can be introduced through a lateral-viewing endoscope with an instrument channel of 2.8 mm. These stents provide inadequate drainage in many cases and are used primarily to facilitate drainage when unremovable intraductal stones are present.
- Straight **barbed,** or Amsterdam, **stents** have projections, or "barbs," at each end that result from a diagonal cut of the stent wall. They range in size from 7 to 12 Fr and can be inserted by using lateral-viewing endoscopes with instruments channels of 3.7 and 4.2 mm. Barbed stents are used primarily for strictures of the common and/or pancreatic duct. Barbed stents have been shown to decrease morbidity, maintain their position with infrequent dislodgement, provide maximal flow, and decrease the risk for occlusion by sludge, stones, or tumor.
- The newest barbed stents are curved to conform to curves or bends in the duct. Prepackaged stent sets contain all of the essential accessory items, including a guidewire, push catheter, and stent.

Regardless of the type of stent used, one end of the tube is seated above the ductal obstruction, and the other end protrudes into the duodenum. The configuration of the stent itself serves to secure it. The purpose of the stent is to allow free drainage or transhepatic **decompression.**

Placement of a biliary stent is indicated for the following:

- Relief of obstructive jaundice in patients with benign or malignant strictures of the bile duct
- Palliative treatment of inoperable or metastatic pancreatic or periampullary neoplasms
- Preoperative decompression to decrease complications associated with high bilirubin levels
- Prevention of stone impaction in the ampulla in patients who are at high risk for surgery and have had unsuccessful endoscopic sphincterotomy and stone extraction
- Maintaining biliary decompression in cases of sclerosing cholangitis with stricture of the extrahepatic bile ducts
- Protecting the area into which a biliary fistula drains

Compared with the traditional methods of relieving bile duct obstruction, insertion of a biliary stent is associated with fewer major complications, a decreased incidence of procedure-related mortality, and a reduced number of hospital days.

The use of biliary stents is contraindicated in patients with coagulopathy, sepsis, active pancreatitis or other infection, recent food ingestion, and with any other contraindication to EGD.

Before the procedure it is important to determine whether the patient has had biliary surgery in the past. Electronic monitoring should include an ECG. At least two gastroenterology nurses will assist with the procedure; one monitors the patient and one assists the endoscopist.

ERCP is performed first, to define the level and extent of the obstruction. A 5-mm sphincterotomy may be performed to allow easier passage of the stent (especially larger stents) and/or to facilitate drainage.

When placing a 5- or 7-Fr stent, a cannula is passed through a side-viewing duodenoscope with a 2.8-mm instrument channel and into the diseased duct. A 480-cm guidewire is passed through the cannula. The cannula is removed over the guidewire, which remains in place. The portion of the guidewire that protrudes from the duodenoscope is wiped to remove residual dye. Silicone may be applied to facilitate passage of the stent.

The stent is advanced over the guidewire, followed by a pusher tube that is the same diameter as the stent but of a different color. Once the stent has bypassed the obstructed area, the pusher tube and the guidewire are removed. These maneuvers are all performed under fluoroscopic guidance. At this point, the distal end of the stent anchors itself in the duct, the midportion of the stent traverses the obstruction, and the proximal end lies free in the duodenum. Once the continuity of the duct is reestablished, the patient's condition should improve.

When placing a stent that is 10, 11.5, or 12 Fr, a guide catheter is used. A guide catheter is a long, polyethylene tube with a tapered tip. Most guide catheters measure 350 cm in length and 6 to 8 Fr. Guide catheters with increasing diameters are available to progressively dilate strictures to pass larger stents.

The guide catheter is passed over the guidewire through the channel of a 4.2-mm channel duodenoscope. The endoscopist guides the catheter through the stricture. A stent of predetermined size is passed over the guide catheter, followed by a pusher tube of the same size. The pusher tube should slide freely over the guide catheter but not over the stent. The stent is advanced over the guide catheter, into the common bile duct, and through the stricture. The properly positioned stent should protrude 1 cm into the duodenum. The gastroenterology nurse must assist the endoscopist with coordinated movements and constant tension on the guidewire and guide catheter. After proper placement is determined, the pusher tube, guide catheter, and the guidewire are removed. Bile mixed with contrast medium should immediately escape through the stent.

Because endoscopic placement of biliary stents can be a lengthy process, it is important to use as little fluoroscopy as possible during the procedure.

During and after the procedure, the nurse should monitor and record the patient's vital signs, observe the patient for abdominal pain or distention, and administer antibiotics as ordered. Serial blood studies are usually performed after placement of large stents to follow the patient's progress and to monitor the effectiveness of decompression. The serum bilirubin level usually declines progressively until it is nearly normal.

The patient may be observed in the hospital for 48 to 72 hours, followed by outpatient observation. After about 6 hours, a soft diet may be permitted. IV antibiotics should be continued for 24 to 48 hours. Some physicians recommend changing stents every 3 to 6 months to avoid plugging or breakage of stent material. Because the proximal portion of the stent protrudes into the duodenum, it can be withdrawn endoscopically by using a snare, and can be replaced fairly easily.

Potential early complications of stent placement include bleeding from the sphincterotomy or the tumor, cholangitis, pancreatitis, trauma to the biliary tract or duodenum, and obstruction of the pancreatic duct. Failure to place a stent properly is most commonly caused by either tumors involving the papilla of Vater, in which case the bile duct orifice cannot be identified, or hepatic neoplasms that cause a tight stricture of the intrahepatic ducts.

Recurrent jaundice is the most common delayed complication of biliary stent placement and is usually caused by clogging of the stent. Rarely, it may be a result of tumor growth along the prosthesis or metastatic spread of a malignant tumor to the liver. If occlusion of the prosthesis by cell detritus and viscous bile causes recurrent cholestasis and cholangitis, the endoprosthesis can be extracted with the aid of a polypectomy snare and replaced by a new prosthesis during the same session. Migration of the stent or erosion of the duodenal wall by the stent with ulcer formation or duodenal perforation are also potential delayed complications.

## INTESTINAL (NASOENTERIC) INTUBATION

Nasoenteric tubes are longer than nasogastric tubes and typically have a balloon or rubber bag at one end that is filled with air, mercury, or water to stimulate peristalsis and facilitate passage through the pylorus into the intestinal tract. The type and size of the tube depends on its purpose, on the size of the patient's nostrils, and on the estimated length of time the tube will be in place. There are four types of tubes used for intestinal intubation.

- The Miller-Abbott tube is used to aspirate intestinal contents and in patients with bowel obstruction. It is a 10-foot, rubber, double-lumen tube with a metal Y-shaped connector at the proximal end. The two lumens are for suction and for instillation of mercury or water into the balloon at the distal end. It is available in sizes of 12, 14, 16, or 18 Fr. The tube is passed nasally and advanced into the stomach. After it has been passed through the pylorus, it is filled with mercury or water, which is removed before extubation. The tube should be irrigated with 30 ml saline every 6 to 8 hours to prevent blockage. Its position should be assessed radiographically.
- The Cantor tube is also used for bowel obstruction and to allow aspiration of intestinal contents. It is a 10-foot, single-lumen, rubber tube with a balloon on the distal tip for injecting mercury. It is available in sizes of 12 and 16 Fr. Mercury must be instilled into the bag before insertion of this nasointestinal tube, using a needle no larger than 21 gauge. Patients with active peristalsis require 5 ml of mercury, whereas patients with ileus or absent bowel sounds may require 7 to 9 ml. The position of the Cantor tube must be confirmed radiographically.
- The Kaslow tube is a single-lumen tube with a balloon of natural latex. Because latex is more permeable to various gases than neoprene rubber, the Kaslow balloon is more prone to overdilatation and resultant complications than the Cantor or Miller-Abbott tubes.
- The Harris tube is a 6-foot, single-lumen tube with a balloon for the injection of mercury. It is used for bowel obstruction and also allows lavage of the intestinal tract, usually with a Y-tube attached.

**Nasoenteric intubation** is used for the following reasons:
- To aspirate intestinal contents for examination
- To treat intestinal obstruction by providing intestinal decompression, relieving dilatation proximal to the obstruction, decreasing and diverting intestinal secretions and gas formation, and providing intestinal stenting
- To prepare the intestinal tract for surgery by removing intestinal contents
- To prevent postoperative nausea, vomiting, and abdominal distention
- To provide enteral alimentation postoperatively until edema at the operative site has subsided or until peristalsis returns

For nasoenteric intubation, the patient should be in the semi-Fowler's position. A local anesthetic may be applied to the nostril or back of the throat to dull sensations and the gag reflex. To determine the length of tube required to reach the pylorus, the physician may place the distal end of the tube at the tip of the patient's nose, extend the tube to the earlobe and down the xiphoid process, and then mark the tube at this point. A water-soluble lubricant is applied to the first few centimeters of the tube.

While the patient pants or breathes through the mouth, the physician inserts the balloon into the nostril that has the greatest airflow. When the tube reaches the nasopharynx, the patient should lower the chin to the chest, swallow, and sip water through a straw. To confirm passage of the tube into the stomach, stomach contents are aspirated with a syringe, or air may be injected through the tube while auscultating the patient's stomach with a stethoscope.

Only water-soluble lubricants and sprays should be used for lubrication of nasointestinal tubes. These tubes depend primarily on normal peristalsis to carry them distally. If passage from the stomach is delayed or impossible, a gastroscope may be used to directly grasp the tip of the tube and advance it into the duodenum. This maneuver can be accomplished by tying a loop of silk suture around the tip of the tube and grasping it with forceps passed through the biopsy channel of an endoscope. The forceps may then direct the tube into the duodenum or more distal small bowel. The endoscope must be removed with care to avoid inadvertent removal of the adjacent tube. The same method may be used to pass small-bore nasogastric tubes into the duodenum in children or to guide a tube through a gastroenterostomy or Billroth II anastomosis to deliver distal alimentation or for selective decompression.

Distal movement of the tube can be facilitated by changing the patient's position. Usually the patient lies on the right side until the tube passes through the pylorus, then on the back in the Fowler's position for 30 minutes as the tube passes through the first and second portions of the duodenum, and then on the left side for 2 hours. Throughout the procedure the tube may be advanced manually, 2 to 3 inches each hour. To confirm passage into the duodenum, the pH of an aspirated sample can be tested with litmus paper. The pH of intestinal fluid should be less than 7. Once the tube has passed the pylorus, movement may also be aided by ambulation.

After the tube has been inserted the necessary distance, its position is confirmed radiographically. Then the tube is taped to the patient's nostril, and suction is applied as ordered. If a two-lumen Miller-Abbott tube is used, the lumen to the mercury balloon should be labeled "do not touch," and the other lumen should be labeled "suction."

While the tube is in place, tube patency must be checked frequently. Suction should be checked at least every 2 hours. The patient should be observed for signs or symptoms of fluid and electrolyte imbalance, and for signs or symptoms of pneumonia, which may occur because of the patient's inability to cough effectively with the tube in place. Accurate intake and output records must be kept, and frequent mouth and nostril care should be given, including mouth care every 4 hours, and application of petrolatum to the opening of the nostrils. The amount, color, consistency, and odor of the drainage should be noted.

Once the tube is in the intestines, if the patient is not nauseated or vomiting, a light diet of clear and cream soups, custards, gelatins, milk, and fruit juices may be allowed. The tube should be clamped for about an hour after the patient eats to allow nutrients to be absorbed.

The amount of mercury instilled should be documented in the nursing notes. Ingested mercury is not toxic. If it escapes into the GI tract, it should be permitted to pass normally. Because mercury is a biohazardous material, however, it must be collected after the tube is removed from the patient and disposed of according to hospital guidelines. Tubes containing mercury cannot be incinerated, because mercury produces a toxic vapor when burned, but should be disposed of by a licensed hazardous-waste disposal company.

To remove a nasoenteric tube, it should be disconnected from suction and clamped. Miller-Abbott tubes should be deflated before withdrawal, while a Cantor or Harris tube should be withdrawn with the mercury still in the balloon. While in the intestines, the tube should be removed only 6 to 8 inches at a time, followed by a 10-minute rest period. After the tube reaches the stomach, it may be withdrawn gently but steadily. At times, the intestinal tube may be allowed to pass entirely through the bowel and to the rectum.

After removal of the tube, the patient is usually given food gradually, progressing from fluids to a regular diet. Initial feedings are small and frequent, and the amount of liquid given at any one time is limited.

Potential complications of intestinal intubation include otitis media resulting from eustachian tube irritation, although this is rare with small-bore tubes; intussusception; knotting of the tube; pressure necrosis with perforation; and rupture of esophageal varices. Indwelling nasoenteric decompression tubes may cause reflux esophagitis, inflammation of the nose or mouth, and ulceration of the nose and larynx.

## COLON DECOMPRESSION

Colon decompression involves placement of a tube in the rectum or colon to relieve colonic distention. It is indicated in patients with colonic pseudoobstruction (nontoxic megacolon or Ogilvie's syndrome); postoperative ileus; or colon distention secondary to flexible sigmoidoscopy or colonoscopy. Ogilvie's syndrome occurs in elderly patients who have a preexisting disease that necessitates bed rest. Without decompression, cecal perforation may result. Insertion of a rectal tube may be ordered every 2 to 3 hours in these patients.

Colon decompression is contraindicated in patients with recent rectal surgery, organic colon obstruction, recent surgical anastomosis, recent myocardial infarction, or diseases of the rectal mucosa.

Colon decompression can be accomplished by using a 22- to 32-Fr rectal tube of soft rubber or plastic, a small-lumen decompression tube, a large-lumen decompression tube, or an over-the-guidewire decompression tube. Tubes can be purchased in kits from different manufacturers.

- If a rectal tube is to be used, the patient is placed in Sims' position and draped appropriately. The tube is lubricated with a water-soluble lubricant. The patient breathes slowly and deeply, and then bears down as for a bowel movement to relax the anal sphincter and facilitate insertion. The tube is inserted into the rectum and then advanced 15 cm. The proximal end of the tube should be taped to the lower buttock, and the end of the tube should be covered with a waterproof absorbent pad or connected to a drainage bag. Rectal tubes should be left in place for a maximum of 30 minutes. If no gas has been expelled, the procedure may be repeated in 2 to 3 hours.
  NOTE: Rectal tubes may also be used to minimize excoriation and skin breakdown in incontinent patients who have watery diarrhea, or in incontinent patients who have significant lower GI bleeding.
- A small-lumen decompression tube can be passed through the biopsy channel of a colonoscope to the cecum. The colonoscope is removed while continuing to advance the tube through the channel. Tube placement is confirmed fluoroscopically and the proximal end is secured to the buttock and attached to a drainage bag.
- If a large-lumen decompression tube is to be used, biopsy forceps are passed through the channel of the colonoscope, and a suture is tied around the distal end of the decompression tube. The suture is grasped with the biopsy forceps, and the colonoscope and tube are passed side-by-side. Once the desired area is reached the tube is released, and the forceps are withdrawn from the colonoscope. The colonoscope is then withdrawn with care to avoid dislodging the tube, and confirmation is made of its placement fluoroscopically. The proximal end of the tube is secured to the buttock and attached to a drainage bag.
- If an over-the-guidewire decompression tube is to be used, the colonoscope is inserted, and a 480-cm guidewire is passed through the channel. The colonoscope is removed while advancement of the guidewire is continued. The position of the guidewire is confirmed, the decompression tube is advanced over the guidewire, and placement is

confirmed fluoroscopically. The guidewire is removed, and the proximal end of the tube is secured to the buttock and attached to a drainage bag.

Massive colonic distention may also be relieved by colonoscopic suction.

After placement of a rectal or decompression tube, it is important to assure the patency of the tube and to assess the patient for relief of symptoms. The color, consistency, and amount of drainage and the character of the patient's abdomen should be noted. The patient should be told to expect drainage from the tube. The physician may order a rectal tube to be removed once the abdomen is flat and soft or if the tube is ineffective after 30 minutes.

Potential complications of decompression include perforation and clogging of the tube with stool.

## ABDOMINAL PARACENTESIS

Abdominal **paracentesis** involves withdrawal of fluid from the peritoneal space for diagnostic and therapeutic purposes, using a large-bore needle or a trocar and cannula inserted in the abdominal wall. It may be performed at bedside or in a treatment room.

Paracentesis is indicated for the following:

- Evaluation of ascites
- Determination of a perforated viscus following blunt trauma or symptoms of acute abdomen
- Relief of dyspnea or abdominal pain secondary to tense ascites

It is contraindicated in uncooperative patients and for patients with the following:

- Severe coagulopathy
- Thrombocytopenia
- Intestinal obstruction
- Abdominal wall infection
- Previous multiple abdominal surgeries
- Portal hypertension with abdominal collateral circulation

Paracentesis may be performed in patients with coagulopathy if small-gauge needles in the vascular midline are used. It must be performed cautiously in pregnant patients and in patients with unstable vital signs.

Before paracentesis, it is important to have the patient void to reduce the risk of accidental injury to the bladder when the needle or trocar and cannula are inserted. Baseline vital signs, weight, and abdominal girth at the umbilical level should be recorded.

Depending on the physician's preference, the patient may be positioned in Fowler's position, the knee-hand position, or sitting on the side of the bed with the feet supported. The preferred position is usually sitting, with the feet and back firmly supported. In this position, gravity causes fluid to accumulate in the lower abdominal cavity, and the pressure created by the

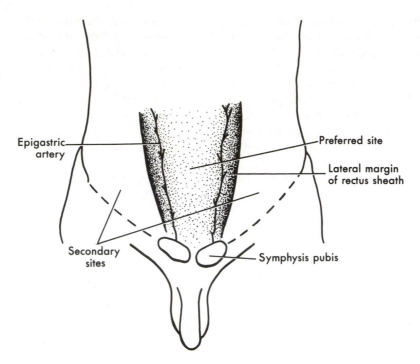

**Fig. 31-2.** Sites for paracentesis.

abdominal organs facilitates fluid flow. The patient should be draped with a sheet exposing the abdomen. He or she should be cautioned to remain as still as possible to avoid injury from the needle or trocar and cannula.

During the procedure the gastroenterology nurse should disinfect the skin, assist the physician in establishing and maintaining a sterile field, and draw up the local anesthetic. Specimen containers should be ready to receive fluid. The first 10 ml of fluid should be collected separately, followed by 50 ml aliquots. Pulse and respiratory status should be monitored throughout the procedure.

With sterile technique and under local anesthesia, the needle or catheter is introduced in the midline between the umbilicus and pubis (Fig. 31-2). The risk of hemorrhage is reduced by entering through the avascular linea alba, but the catheter may be introduced laterally if necessary. The rectus muscles, upper abdomen, collateral venous channels, and areas of surgical scars should be avoided.

Only a small amount of fluid is needed for diagnosis. If larger volumes are to be withdrawn, a larger gauge needle or catheter/needle assembly should be used. The physician may make a small incision with the scalpel before inserting the needle or trocar and cannula, usually 1 to 2 inches below the umbilicus.

After paracentesis is completed, an elasticized, adhesive dressing should be applied to the site. The patient should be helped to a comfortable position and vital signs should be monitored and documented every 15 minutes. The patient should be observed closely for vertigo, faintness, diaphoresis, pallor, heightened anxiety, tachycardia, dyspnea, and hypotension. The physician should be notified if the patient's pulse rate increases and systolic blood pressure decreases, respiratory status changes, temperature is elevated, there is leakage of peritoneal fluid from the site, or if scrotal edema develops.

The color, amount, viscosity, and odor of any drainage should be noted. Specimens should be labeled and sent to the laboratory with the appropriate requisition slip. The patient's weight and abdominal girth should be compared with baseline figures.

Complications are rare in abdominal paracentesis, but may include hemorrhage, perforation of the abdominal organs by the needle or the trocar and cannula, peritonitis, hepatic coma from decreased systemic circulation, reduced tissue perfusion, and wound infection. Aspiration of more than 1,500 ml of peritoneal fluid may induce hypovolemic shock because of the sudden shift of fluid from the circulatory system to replace aspirated fluid.

If the patient shows signs of hypovolemic shock, the drainage rate should be slowed by reducing the vertical distance between the needle or trocar and cannula and the collection container. If necessary, the drainage may be stopped altogether. Colloid replacement with albumin is recommended with large-volume paracentesis.

Mr. Jason Ruggles comes to his internist complaining of vague abdominal pain that is causing him some distress. He is willing to undergo whatever tests are necessary to find out what the problem is.

### Points to think about

1. Mr. Ruggles presents with abdominal pain. What might his internist do first?
2. If the internist refers Mr. Ruggles to a gastroenterologist, what type of diagnostic test might the gastroenterologist do?
3. If the gastroenterologist believes that Mr. Ruggles has inflammation caused by overproduction of gastric acid, what tests could he do to confirm his suspicions?
4. If Mr. Ruggles is not treated properly, what consequences can he expect?
5. If Mr. Ruggles must go through a lengthy series of tests and therapeutic procedures, he may become disheartened and discouraged. Periodically, the nurse must reevaluate and, if necessary, intervene in Mr. Ruggles' struggle to cope during this stressful time. What are some behaviors that might indicate that intervention is needed?

### Suggested responses

1. The internist sends Mr. Ruggles for an upper GI radiographic series, which outlines his esophagus, stomach, and duodenum. Although the films reviewed by the radiologist are normal, the internist knows that this normal x-ray examination does not necessarily mean there is nothing wrong with Mr. Ruggles, so he refers the patient to a gastroenterologist.
2. The gastroenterologist conducts a full history and physical examination and decides that an EGD is in order. The EGD is done, uneventfully, and the diagnosis is moderate duodenitis, gastritis, and esophagitis.
3. To confirm his suspicion that Mr. Ruggles is producing too much gastric acid, the gastroenterologist might order the following:
   - A gastric analysis, which measures the amount of acid produced. The nurse must know how to place a nasogastric tube appropriately for best drainage of the stomach (along the greater curvature with the tip in the antrum) and must collect specimens of gastric juice before and after stimulation with pentagastrin. Some gastroenterology nurses and associates also know how to titrate and calculate the acid content of these specimens; others have these measurements done by the chemistry lab.
   - An intraesophageal acid drip test (Bernstein test),

which determines if the esophagitis is symptomatic. This also requires a nasogastric intubation with precise placement of the tube in the esophagus.
   - An intragastric instillation of acid, which can determine if acid is causing the abdominal pain. This test also requires placement of a nasogastric tube.
   - Serial blood tests, conducted over an hour after the administration of a pancreatic stimulant (secretin), which can determine if the excess acid production is caused by a tumor in the pancreas (Zollinger-Ellison syndrome).
   - An esophageal motility study, which will show whether the esophagus contracts properly to clear acid from the esophagus.
   - 24-Hour pH monitoring, which will document the number of reflux episodes that occur. The motility study and the pH monitoring require two more nasogastric intubations.
4. If Mr. Ruggles is not treated properly, the following events could occur:
   - Mr. Ruggles could develop scarring and strictures from reflux of acid in the esophagus; this could require dilatation of the esophagus, perhaps on an ongoing basis.
   - Overacidity in the stomach can lead to peptic ulcerations, particularly in the prepyloric and pyloric channel area. This can lead to scarring and deformity or stenosis of the pyloric channel, causing gastric outlet obstruction, which would need to be dilated. Because dilatation of the pylorus is not usually as effective as dilatation of the esophagus, this may lead to gastric surgery to correct the problem.
   - If medications do not control Mr. Ruggles' acid production, he may progress from inflammation to ulcerations with bleeding and attendant complications. This may require surgical intervention to control acid production (vagotomy and pyloroplasty, vagotomy and antrectomy, highly selective vagotomy).
5. These are all difficult tests for the patient, and require that the nurse be patient, caring, and establish a supportive, trusting relationship with the patient. Nasogastric intubation can be uncomfortable, but a skilled person can make the procedure much more tolerable. Following are some signs that may indicate Mr. Ruggles is not effectively coping with the stress involved:
   - Nonperformance of activities of daily living
   - Purposelessness
   - Self-absorption
   - Inflexibility
   - Hopelessness
   - Unconcern and detachment from usual social supports

- Nonproductive lifestyle
- Excessive use of denial

Indifference to social supports and demoralization are two negative manifestations of coping with the stress caused by illness. The nursing diagnosis "ineffective individual coping" is defined as impairment of adaptive behaviors and problem-solving abilities of a person in meeting life's demands and roles. Coping is a continual process and numerous factors influence it, so the assessment of a person's coping mechanisms becomes an ongoing nursing responsibility.

## REVIEW TERMS

**barbed stents, decompression, lavage, nasobiliary catheter (NBC), nasoenteric intubation, nasogastric tube, paracentesis, pigtail stent, stents**

## REVIEW QUESTIONS

1. If the patient belches after air is injected into a nasogastric tube, what is the most likely cause?
   a. The tube is curled in the patient's mouth or throat.
   b. The tube is in the patient's esophagus.
   c. Stomach contents are blocking the tube.
   d. The tube is blocking the patient's airway.

2. After insertion of an esophageal prosthesis, the patient should be able to feel the presence of the prosthesis:
   a. For a few hours.
   b. For a few days.
   c. Indefinitely.
   d. The patient should not be aware of the presence of the prosthesis.

3. The main advantage of using a Levacuator orogastric tube for gastric lavage is that:
   a. It permits continuous instillation of an irrigant.
   b. It permits rapid aspiration of large amounts of gastric contents.
   c. It can be inserted nasally if necessary.
   d. It is easier to insert.

4. After the patient's tolerance of gastric lavage has been established, what volume of irrigation solution is used for each subsequent instillation?
   a. 50 ml.
   b. 250 ml.
   c. 500 ml.
   d. 1,000 ml.

5. Monooctanoin (Moctanin) is sometimes instilled through a nasobiliary catheter. Why?
   a. To treat bacterial cholangitis.
   b. To flush out small stones after endoscopic sphincterotomy.
   c. For gallstone dissolution.
   d. To treat sclerosing cholangitis.

6. For biliary decompression, a polyethylene tube (inserted via a duodenoscope) exits and drains to the outside through the patient's:
   a. Mouth.
   b. Nose.
   c. Abdominal wall.
   d. Gastrostomy tube.

7. The most common delayed complication of biliary stent placement is:
   a. Recurrent jaundice.
   b. Duodenal perforation.
   c. Hemorrhage.
   d. Pancreatitis.

8. The mercury that is instilled into the balloon at the tip of a nasoenteric tube should be:
   a. Left in the balloon and disposed of with other nonhazardous waste.
   b. Removed from the balloon and emptied into the sewer system.
   c. Handled as biohazardous waste.
   d. Incinerated.

9. An ineffective rectal tube should be left in place:
   a. Until decompression is achieved.
   b. For a maximum of 3 minutes.
   c. For a maximum of 30 minutes.
   d. For 2 to 3 hours.

10. Before abdominal paracentesis, it is important for the patient to void. Why?
    a. To keep the patient comfortable during the procedure.
    b. To reduce intraabdominal pressure.
    c. To give a more accurate measure of abdominal girth.
    d. To avoid injury to the bladder when the needle is inserted.

## BIBLIOGRAPHY

Bernard, M, and Forlaw, L. "Complications and Their Prevention." In *Clinical Nutrition: Enteral and Tube Feeding,* Volume 1. eds. Rombeau, J, and Caldwell, M. Philadelphia: W.B. Saunders, 1984.

Given, B, and Simmons, S. *Gastroenterology in Clinical Nursing.* 4th ed. St. Louis: Mosby–Year Book, 1984.

Hamilton, H, editorial director. *Procedures.* Nurse's Reference Library. Springhouse, Pa.: Intermed Communications, 1983.

Hardick, M, and Beck, M, eds. *Manual of Gastrointestinal Procedures.* 2nd ed. Rochester, N.Y.: Society of Gastroenterology Nurses and Associates, 1989.

McFarland, G, and McFarlane, E. *Nursing Diagnosis and Intervention.* St. Louis: Mosby–Year Book, 1989.

Miller, L. "Endoscopic Stent Placement; A Nursing Perspective." In *SGA Journal Reprints,* ed. Trivits, S, 95-99. Rochester, N.Y.: Society of Gastrointestinal Assistants, 1988.

Ravenscroft, M, and Swan, C. *Gastrointestinal Endoscopy and Related Procedures: A Handbook for Nurses and Assistants.* Baltimore: Williams & Wilkins, 1984.

Short, N. "Gastrointestinal Intubations: Nursing Considerations." *Gastroenterology Nursing* 12(Summer 1989): 43-49.

Silvis, S, ed. *Therapeutic Gastrointestinal Endoscopy.* New York: Igaku-Shoin, 1985.

Sivak, M, Jr., and Petrini, J, eds. *Gastrointestinal Endoscopy: Old Problems, New Techniques.* Gastroenterology Series Volume 4. New York: Praeger, 1986.

Sleisenger, M, and Fordtran, J. *Gastrointestinal Disease: Pathophysiology, Diagnosis, Management.* 4th ed. Philadelphia: W.B. Saunders, 1989.

Waye, J, Geenen, J, Fleischer, D, and Venu, R. *Techniques in Therapeutic Endoscopy.* Philadelphia: W.B. Saunders, 1987.

# Chapter 32

# EXCISION AND EXTRACTION

This chapter will acquaint the gastroenterology nurse with endoscopic procedures that are used for the removal of foreign bodies, polyps, and retained common bile duct stones from the GI tract. The use of lithotripsy for the disruption of gallstones is also discussed.*

## Learning objectives

After reviewing the content of this chapter, the gastroenterology nurse should be able to:

1. Describe techniques used for removal of foreign bodies and bezoars from the GI tract.
2. Explain the indications, contraindications, procedures, and potential complications of endoscopic polypectomy.
3. Describe the indications, contraindications, procedures, and risks of endoscopic sphincterotomy.
4. Discuss the investigational use of biliary lithotripsy for the disruption of gallstones, and the use of pulsed-dye laser lithotripsy.

## FOREIGN BODY REMOVAL

Endoscopic techniques may be used for extraction of foreign bodies from the esophagus, stomach, duodenum, or colon. Foreign bodies may be deliberately or accidentally swallowed or may be introduced into the lower GI tract from the rectum. Most foreign objects lodge at areas of anatomic or physiologic narrowing, such as the cricopharyngeal or the lower esophageal sphincter. (LES). If a foreign body passes the esophagus, it will usually pass through the remainder of the GI tract

* All techniques in this chapter, except bezoar removal and lithotripsy, are also discussed in the SGNA *Manual of Gastrointestinal Procedures.* 2nd ed. Rochester, N.Y.: Society of Gastroenterology Nurses and Associates, 1989.

without incident. Other sites of potential hang-up are the pylorus, the duodenal C-loop, the ligament of Treitz, the ileocecal valve, and the anus.

The most frequent victims of foreign body ingestion are young children who are between the ages of 6 months and 4 years, persons with dentures, and inebriated or mentally impaired individuals. Children most often ingest coins, toys, crayons, and ballpoint pen caps. Adults present with bones and meat impacted in the esophagus. Prisoners and psychiatric patients may ingest a variety of objects. In the lower GI tract, foreign objects are found predominantly in males who are between the ages 24 and 65 years, and who are either homosexuals or the victims of criminal assault. Foreign bodies may also be iatrogenic in origin, such as dental instruments, parts of nebulizers, tubes, prosthetic devices, or biopsy instruments, including small-bowel biopsy capsules that have been lost in the GI tract.

Of the foreign bodies that enter the GI tract, 80% to 90% pass through without incident, often within 48 hours; 10% to 20% need to be removed endoscopically, and 1% require surgery. Most foreign-body obstructions involve the esophagus, especially above a benign or malignant stricture, web, or ring.

Foreign bodies in the stomach cause few, if any, symptoms. Conservative management is in order for most foreign objects that have reached the stomach. Endoscopic or surgical removal of foreign bodies should not be attempted unless a week has passed without progress. Exceptions to this rule are objects containing lead or mercury or objects with sharp points, because of the risk of bleeding, obstruction, or perforation. Most ingested objects that have passed into the stomach will pass uneventfully through the pylorus and the rest of the

GI tract. In children, pennies, nickels, and dimes will pass, but quarters usually will not.

Objects that have passed beyond the second portion of the duodenum cannot be retrieved endoscopically. Their progress may be followed radiologically, with surgical exploration as a last resort.

Swallowed objects that hang up in the cecum or sigmoid colon may be retrieved with a colonoscope. Biopsy forceps, pronged polyp-retrieval forceps, and special foreign-body forceps may be useful in removing foreign bodies from the colon, but the polypectomy snare is the most versatile instrument.

Objects that have been inserted into the rectum and the sigmoid colon may be retrieved by using a flexible or rigid sigmoidoscope. In the case of large objects, the patient may require general anesthesia for cooperation and for relaxation of the anal sphincter. No cathartics or enemas should be given. Objects lying below the peritoneal reflection of the rectum can usually be grasped and removed by using a rigid anoscope or proctoscope. Early surgical consultation is advised for high colorectal foreign bodies.

Endoscopic or surgical removal of foreign bodies is indicated for the following:
- Most foreign bodies lodged in the esophagus, with the possible exception of round objects or food boluses in the distal esophagus, which may pass spontaneously
- Sharp or pointed objects that could result in obstruction or perforation, such as pins, toothpicks, and bones, even if they have entered the stomach
- Long, narrow objects, such as wires (more than 6 cm in length for children and more than 13 cm in adults), that may not be able to negotiate the fixed duodenal angles
- Gastric foreign bodies greater than 2 cm in diameter, or any gastric foreign bodies that do not pass after a 2-week observation period
- Toxic foreign bodies, such as alkaline button batteries
- Duodenal foreign bodies that do not pass within 6 days of ingestion

Foreign body removal is contraindicated when the risk associated with removing the object is greater than the risk posed by the object itself. It is also contraindicated in uncooperative patients or in patients with a known or suspected perforated viscus.

Patients with foreign bodies may present with pain, sepsis, mediastinitis, peritonitis, hemorrhage, abscess, or an abdominal mass. It is important to obtain a history and description of the foreign body, including its location, length of time lodged, type and location of pain, previous x-ray examinations, any history of dysphagia, previous foreign body removal, or other pertinent history information or symptoms.

The physician should confirm the location of the foreign body with X-ray films of the neck, chest, and abdomen. Serial films may be helpful to monitor the progression of the object. It is also important to establish the time of last food or fluid ingestion. Barium swallows should be avoided if there is any evidence that the object is located at or just below the cricopharyngeus, but a thin suspension of barium may be given in small sips to help locate radiolucent foreign bodies in the lower esophagus.

A wide assortment of endoscopic snares and retrieval devices are available, including the following:
- Laryngoscopes and curved forceps such as Kelly clamps for removal of objects that are lodged in the hypopharynx or are accidentally dropped into the hypopharynx during extraction.
- Rat-tooth, alligator, or shark-tooth forceps to grasp and secure flat, metallic objects or objects that may be difficult to remove
- Tripod-type forceps to remove food boluses
- W-shaped forceps or polypectomy snares to remove coins
- Polypectomy snares to remove long, narrow objects, such as opened paper clips, stiff pieces of wire, or injector razor blades
- Pelican-type forceps, which are available in graduated sizes, for breaking up and removing food obstructions
- Stainless steel wire basket-type forceps for a variety of round objects, such as marbles or stones, or for meat boluses that can be removed in one piece
- Snares, grasping forceps, and baskets for removal of gastric foreign bodies
- Rubber-tip forceps for grasping needles and nails
- Magnetic extraction devices for removal of metallic objects (although caution is advised when withdrawing the object through the cricopharyngeus)
- Standard biopsy forceps for objects with a small central opening, through which closed biopsy forceps will pass but opened forceps will not

It is important to confirm that the retrieval device will fit the channel size of the endoscope. It may also be helpful to obtain a similar object and practice grabbing it with various forceps, snares, and baskets to simulate the endoscopic situation and to determine which instrument is best suited in a particular case.

Use of a foreign body hood or **overtube** is optional. Endoscopic overtubes are polyvinyl sleeves that are used to facilitate various upper endoscopic procedures, including extraction of foreign bodies. The overtube protects the esophageal mucosa and the airway as the object is pulled out with the endoscope. An overtube should be used when sharp or pointed foreign bodies must be removed or when the endoscope must be passed several times, as for piecemeal removal of a soft bolus of meat. Overtubes cannot be used in the duodenum.

If an overtube is needed, one with an inner diameter approximately 2 mm larger than the outside diameter of the endoscope should be chosen. After it has been lubricated both inside and outside, it is slipped over the endoscope insertion tube. The patient is intubated in the usual manner with the overtube covering the endoscope as it is passed into the patient's esophagus. A mouthguard or bite block prevents the overtube from slipping into the patient's mouth.

In situations where a large or dangerous foreign body cannot be pulled far enough into the overtube, it is safer to use a latex hood. The hood is placed on the distal tip of the scope and folded back toward the controls for insertion. When the endoscope is withdrawn into the esophagus, the hood catches on the LES and is forced distally, thereby covering the object.

For removal of foreign bodies from the upper GI tract, the patient is placed in the left lateral position and antibiotic prophylaxis is administered if ordered. To reduce anxiety and promote cooperation, the patient may be premedicated. Administration of atropine may be helpful in patients with esophageal obstruction and excessive salivation. Infants, children, or uncooperative patients may require general anesthesia with endotracheal intubation.

During the procedure the nurse should monitor the patient's vital signs; the color, warmth, and dryness of the skin; and the level of consciousness and pain tolerance. It is also important to observe the patient for symptoms of perforation. Oral secretions should be suctioned. The airway must be protected and maintained and steps should be taken to prevent aspiration.

Extraction of a foreign body from the esophagus requires good visibility, a firm grasp of the object, and removal without force. Pointed objects should be withdrawn with the point trailing. If the object is pointed on both ends, the proximal sharp end must be completely covered by the grasping forceps. If the object has a single pointed end that is directed cephalad, it can be carried into the stomach and turned so the pointed end trails before it is removed. Objects with sharp edges should be extracted with the aid of an overtube or hood.

Great care must be taken to avoid dropping the foreign body into the laryngopharynx on withdrawal. The object should be grasped quickly from the patient's mouth to prevent it from falling into the trachea. Institutional policies should be followed for disposal of the retrieved foreign body.

After the object has been removed, it is important to monitor the patient's vital signs and to observe for bleeding, vomiting, abdominal or chest pain, continued abdominal distention, subcutaneous emphysema, or aspiration. After it is determined that the object has been removed without complications, the patient should be reevaluated to rule out any underlying disease that may have caused the obstruction, especially in the esophagus.

Although rare, potential complications of endoscopic foreign body removal include perforation, impaction of the foreign object, hemorrhage, localized inflammation or pressure necrosis, and aspiration of the object.

For patients with food impacted above an esophageal stricture, hydrostatic balloon dilatation of the stricture is an alternative method of treatment, providing the food bolus does not totally occlude the lumen. Once the stricture is dilated, the bolus can be pushed into the stomach. Medications such as glucagon should be available to promote relaxation of the esophagus, thereby facilitating passage of the foreign object into the stomach.

It is important to act quickly if a patient has swallowed a small, button-type battery. The alkaline substance from the battery acts rapidly on the mucosa, causing direct corrosive action, burns, and pressure necrosis. Direct corrosive activity frequently leads to perforation. Potentially catastrophic complications, such as esophagotracheal or esophago-aortic fistula, can ensue.

Occasionally, packets of cocaine are swallowed, often encased in condoms, in an attempt at concealment. The ingestion of 1 to 3 g of powdered cocaine can be fatal. Because rupture of even one packet carries the risk of death, the use of ipecac, lavage, enema, or cathartics should be avoided. Surgical removal is the treatment of choice in such cases.

## BEZOAR REMOVAL

Bezoars are concretions of food or foreign matter that have undergone digestive change(s) in the GI tract. They include trichobezoars, which consist of matted hair, and phytobezoars, which consist of plant material. Symptoms associated with the presence of a bezoar range from a feeling of fullness in the upper quadrants to epigastric pain and periodic attacks of nausea and vomiting. Gastric outlet and intestinal obstruction are common complications.

The best way to diagnose and differentiate between bezoars is by gastroscopy. The standard treatment methods for phytobezoars include the following:

- Physical disruption methods, including manual attempts at external disruption, a liquid diet, suction and lavage, and endoscopic internal fragmentation by using biopsy forceps and polypectomy snares.
- Chemical attack with papain, acetylcysteine, or cellulase.
- Gastrotomy, if medical treatment fails.

Trichobezoars cannot be dissolved in vivo. Treatment of these large intragastric masses is always surgical.

## POLYPECTOMY

Gastrointestinal **polyps** are lesions that may project from the mucosal surface into any part of the gastrointestinal lumen. Some polyps are **pedunculated;** that is, they are attached to the mucosa by a stemlike pedicle or stalk, and some are **sessile;** that is, they are attached to the mucosa by a broad base. Because of their protrusion into the lumen and the stresses of the fecal stream to which colonic polyps are subject, polyps occasionally bleed or cause abdominal pain or obstruction. However, symptomatic polyps are uncommon. The greatest concern is with their potential to become malignant.

Most polyps are removed by wire snares or with hot biopsy forceps, which are opened and closed by a gastroenterology nurse or associate. Commercial **polypectomy snares** come in various sizes and shapes.

Polyps are usually transected by use of a high-frequency current, which is produced by a generator attached to the sheathed snare. The current is applied for brief pulses until the polyp is transected. Electrical currents that have a pure cutting effect are never used in colonoscopic polypectomy. Electrocoagulation current alone may be used if the polyp is attached by a thin pedicle, but a blend of cutting and coagulation current is usually applied to thick-based polyps.

It is important to remember that different electrosurgical units (ESUs) may not provide the same current output as other types of units. In addition, the characteristics of the snare used may alter the power setting on a given ESU. For example, a thin wire cuts through tissue more quickly than a thick wire. The operator must be familiar with the units that are available, and guidelines must be developed for each unit.

To guard against electrical hazards, a ground system must be established. The electrocautery equipment, including the connections and ground plate, should be checked before each use. The snare should be checked to ensure that it is in working order and is conducting current. One way of testing the circuitry is to set the ESU at half power and then check for sparking between the side of the snare loop and the patient plate. ESU cutting and coagulation controls should be set in accordance with the physician's instructions.

### Colonic polyps

Colonoscopic **polypectomy** is indicated for all polyps with a diameter of 1 cm or larger. Smaller polyps can usually be handled with hot biopsy forceps, particularly if the polyp is sessile.

Contraindications to colonic polypectomy include the following:
- Use of aspirin, nonsteroidal antiinflammatory drugs (NSAIDs), or anticoagulants
- Coagulopathy
- Polyps that appear malignant and are probably invasive
- Inadequate bowel preparation
- Uncooperative patients

Coagulation screening should always be done before polypectomy. Blood count, blood typing, cross-match and appropriate blood chemistry studies may be needed, in addition to a history and physical examination. The patient should be told how to obtain the results of pathologic studies. Compliance with instructions for thorough bowel preparation is critical and must be confirmed.

The patient should be placed in the left lateral recumbent position, and a disposable gelled grounding pad should be applied to the patient, usually on the upper thigh or lower trunk, whichever is the largest tissue mass. All leads on the ESU should be checked for secure attachment. Cords and attachments should be inspected for fraying and wear. Cut and coagulation dials should be set according to the endoscopist's instructions, and verbal orders should be repeated back to the operator.

A colonoscope should be advanced as it would be for diagnostic colonoscopy. If diagnostic colonoscopy to the cecum has not been performed previously, it should be carried out before polypectomy. At a minimum, the scope should be advanced 20 to 25 cm beyond the polyp to remove fecal fluid.

When the polyp is in view, its shape, size, and the length of its stalk must be evaluated. Based on these factors, the appropriate technique for polypectomy can be determined.

- Small, sessile polyps less than 8 mm in diameter may be completely removed, recovered for biopsy examination, and ablated with hot biopsy forceps. The polyp is grasped between the jaws of the insulated forceps and lifted away from the intestinal wall by manipulating the angulation controls. This maneuver pulls the mucosa away from the submucosa and muscularis propria so the application of current causes only slight heating of the deeper tissues. With the grasped polyp pointed toward the lumen, coagulation current is applied, destroying the polyp. When the whitish area encircling the polyp base is 1 to 2 mm wide, the current is discontinued, and the polyp is pulled off its base.
- Sessile polyps less than 1 cm in diameter can be removed in one piece by using the snare-cautery technique if their bases are not wide, and if a reasonable "pseudo-stalk" can be created at the base.
- For most pedunculated polyps, a polypectomy snare is advanced so a wire loop is created, and the polyp is "lassoed" with the snare wire. The tip of the catheter is advanced to the base of the polyp, and

the loop is gently tightened. The polyp is tented slightly into the center of the lumen to be certain that no adjacent normal mucosa is caught in the loop. If the polyp has a long stalk, it is best to leave at least 1 cm of the stalk. Polyps with short stalks are ensnared as close to their necks as possible. Pedunculated polyps are usually transected within 2 to 4 seconds; mucosal blanching is noted adjacent to the snare wire during transection. Following closure of the snare, the polyp will fall into the lumen and the coagulated stalk will be visible.

- For pedunculated polyps with large or lobulated heads, segmental resection of the head may be necessary before complete polypectomy can be done.
- Broad-based pedunculated polyps may be bunched to acceptable resection size to permit single transection, or they may be managed by segmental resection.
- Large sessile polyps more than 2 cm in diameter are also removed in a piecemeal fashion, beginning with two oblique cuts made at right angles to each other across one quarter to one third of the polyp. The remaining base of the polyp may be transected during the initial polypectomy or 4 to 8 weeks later, after the area of mucosal ulceration has healed.
- If a polyp is awkwardly located for snaring, it may be helpful to bypass it and advance the colonoscope through the rest of the colon. As the instrument is removed, the colon is straightened, thereby providing a better view of the polyp for removal. The patient may also be repositioned to improve the orientation of the polyp.
- Snaring and retrieving multiple polyps requires passing the colonoscope several times, which can be facilitated through the use of an overtube.
- Ideally, the scope is first advanced to the cecum, and the polyps are removed as the scope is withdrawn.

When the physician is ready to use the ESU, the nurse should turn on the power and turn it off immediately after use. The nurse must also open and close the snare or biopsy forceps at the request of the physician. It is important to close the snare slowly while maintaining continual communication with the physician. The use of a lecture scope or video monitor is absolutely necessary.

After polypectomy is complete, the next important step involves retrieval of the polyp. The polyp may be retrieved by taking the following measures:

- Removing it in the cup of the forceps, if hot biopsy forceps were used for polypectomy.
- Placing the tip of the colonoscope flush against the head of the polyp and applying suction.
- Resnaring the cut polyp and withdrawing it by use of the colonoscope. If the resnared polyp is kept 3

to 5 cm from the instrument tip, the colon can be visualized during withdrawal.
- Entrapment of the polyp with a basket or by a three-pronged polyp retriever.
- Suction aspiration of the polyp through the suction line and into a pulmonary sputum/mucus trap or one of the newer filtered polyp retrieval traps

To locate a lost polyp, a bolus of water may be squirted through the biopsy channel to identify the path of gravity in the colon and thus determine the probable location of the resected polyp.

It may not be possible to pull large polyps through the anus with the colonoscope, but if the patient bears down, the polyp can be expelled. Sometimes, the polyp must be removed from the rectum by passing a rigid sigmoidoscope and grasping it with forceps.

Once the polyp has been retrieved, the colonoscope may be reinserted to inspect the polypectomy site and to determine that there is no serious complication at the polypectomy site.

A thorough histologic examination of the entire polyp is essential to determine whether there is a possibility of malignant change. The specimen should be prepared and labeled in accordance with institutional policy. The polyp itself should be fixed in formalin solution and examined by serial section to determine the presence of epithelial atypia or frank cancer within the polyp or invading the stalk. A fine, 25-gauge needle may be inserted into the base of the polyp stalk to assist the pathologist in orientation of the specimen. A final determination must be made by the pathologist.

The most common types of polyps encountered in the distal portion of the colorectum are hyperplastic or metaplastic polyps. Hyperplastic polyps are characterized by an abnormal multiplication or increase in the number of normal cells in a tissue, whereas metaplasia refers to a change in the adult cells in a tissue to an abnormal form. Hamartomatous polyps, including juvenile polyps and Peutz-Jeghers polyps, are those in which the cells of a circumscribed area grow faster than those of surrounding areas. There is no evidence that routine follow-up examination is necessary for patients with hyperplastic, inflammatory, or hamartomatous polyps. Carcinoma in situ does not recur or metastasize and requires no treatment other than polyp removal. Patients with sessile polyps that harbor invasive carcinoma and patients with pedunculated polyps with invasive carcinoma and no clear margin of resection should undergo surgery if feasible.

After the polypectomy procedure is completed, it is important to observe the patient for abdominal pain or distention. The nurse should monitor vital signs and instruct the patient regarding dietary and medication restrictions. For instance, aspirin, NSAIDs, or other medications that alter the clotting mechanism should be avoided for a period of time after the procedure to minimize the risk of delayed hemorrhage.

Polyps in the rectum and lower sigmoid colon can be resected more safely than those in the cecum and right side of the colon, where the wall is thinner. There are a number of potential complications of colonoscopic polypectomy.

- Bleeding is the most common complication and may occur immediately or as much as 21 days after polypectomy.
- Adverse reactions to sedation include hypotension, respiratory depression, bradycardia, nausea, vomiting, and sweating.
- Vasovagal attack usually occurs when colonoscopy causes serious discomfort or pain or from excessive abdominal distention. Clinical manifestations include hypotension, bradycardia, and cold, clammy skin. Depending on the extent of the adverse response, intervention may include oxygen, atropine, or termination of the procedure.
- Transmural burns are manifested by abdominal pain, leukocytosis, and fever without evidence of free air or diffuse peritoneal signs. If any portion of the polyp head is permitted to come in contact with the intestinal wall, heat may be transferred through this point of contact, causing a burn of the wall adjacent to the polyp. To avoid this, the polyp may be jiggled to and fro, to move a small point of contact to various areas on the wall. Pedunculated polyps may be manipulated with the tip of the catheter or with suction, or the patient's position may be changed to provide better access and to bring the head of the polyp away from the bowel wall. If no perforation is present, the patient should be observed and treated with antibiotics if ordered, and solid food should be withheld. The syndrome usually resolves in 24 to 48 hours.
- Perforation can occur if a portion of the wall of the colon is ensnared, if too much current is applied, or if there is substantial disruption of tissue by mechanical force during colonoscopy. Exploratory laparotomy with closure is the procedure of choice for the management of free perforation. Transmural burns and/or perforation from excessive coagulation is a more serious and more common complication with sessile polyps, compared to pedunculated polyps.
- The risk of explosion of flammable gases, such as hydrogen and methane, can be minimized by a good bowel preparation and by avoiding electrocautery in the presence of stool.
- Current leakage from the ESU can cause thermal injury to the endoscopist, the patient, or the nurse.

Hemorrhage is a potential occurrence during any polypectomy, but is most likely to occur when the polyp is large, in a difficult position, and/or has a thick stalk. Once the snare has been tightened around the polyp or its stalk, it should not be released or loosened, because if the tissue has been partially excised with the wire and it cannot be removed, bleeding may occur and vision may be impaired. Malfunctioning electrocoagulation equipment may also be a cause of postpolypectomy bleeding. If bleeding is suspected, IV fluids should be maintained throughout the night. A large-bore needle should be used in case the patient needs blood.

If there is active pumping of blood from the stalk of a pedunculated polyp following polypectomy, the stalk may be regrasped with the snare, which should be tightened until the bleeding is stopped, and then coagulation current should be reapplied at successive intervals until hemostasis is achieved. If bleeding occurs following transection of a sessile polyp, a catheter can be inserted through the instrument and an infusion of dilute epinephrine given. A bipolar probe or heater probe or injection therapy may also be used to stop the bleeding.

During this emergency situation, it is best to have at least two nurses in attendance to control the situation. One nurse or associate should prepare equipment for coagulation, while another nurse attends to the patient and checks vital signs at frequent intervals. An IV line should be established as soon as possible because intravenous fluids will act to restore volume, transport oxygen, and remove waste products. The patient should be prepared for a blood transfusion. Intake and output records should be established immediately. Blood loss should be assessed through the amount seen in the suction canister and rectal discharge. If not done before the procedure, laboratory work should be ordered, including hematocrit, hemoglobin, and coagulation studies. Blood should be typed and cross-matched. Oxygen should be administered via nasal cannula. The patient should be calmly reassured and should lie flat to encourage blood flow to the brain and other vital organs. The patient should be kept warm. Most of the time, bleeding can be controlled without surgery, but a surgeon should be notified in case surgery is needed. The patient should be prepared for admission to the hospital for observation.

**Peutz-Jeghers syndrome**

If the gastrointestinal hamartomatous polyps typical of Peutz-Jeghers syndrome are fairly well localized to a short segment of intestine, segmental resection may be all that is required. Usually, however, polyposis is extensive and the patient requires multiple enterotomies throughout his or her life. The physician should target the larger polyps, which are most likely to be responsible for symptoms.

### Gastric polyps

Gastric polyps are uncommon; most are solitary, small, hyperplastic polyps that may be either sessile or pedunculated. The majority are discovered in radiographic or endoscopic examinations in patients complaining of nausea, abdominal pain, and other gastrointestinal symptoms, although it is unlikely that the polyps are responsible for these symptoms.

It is important to note that the gastric mucosa is more vascular than that of the colon, and slower closure of the snare handle is necessary during electrocautery to ensure hemostasis.

To enhance retrieval of resected polyps after polypectomy in the antrum and duodenum, IV glucagon may be given just before resection to inhibit peristalsis. Once located, the polyp should be grasped with a wire snare to provide additional traction as the polyp and instrument pass back through the cricopharyngeus. A foreign-body hood can be helpful during polyp removal to keep the polyp from falling into the trachea.

Gastroscopic polypectomy is indicated for most gastric polyps, but surgical excision is indicated for the following:

- Sessile or broad-based polyps, in which no definitive diagnosis can be made by endoscopic biopsy examination
- Intramural polypoid lesions, such as leiomyomas
- Any polypoid lesion that is believed to be responsible for symptoms and cannot be removed by endoscopic polypectomy

Following removal of the gastric polyp, the denuded mucosa creates an iatrogenic ulcer. An antiulcer regimen with H2 antagonists for 1 to 2 weeks following gastric polypectomy has been recommended.

Patients with adenomatous gastric polyps should undergo repeat endoscopic surveillance every 1 to 2 years. Patients with hyperplastic gastric polyps do not require surveillance.

## SPHINCTEROTOMY

Endoscopic retrograde sphincterotomy, also known as papillotomy, is an electrosurgical incision of the papilla of Vater and the fibers of the sphincter of Oddi during endoscopic retrograde cholangiopancreatography (ERCP). The terms *sphincterotomy* and *papillotomy* are often used interchangeably. The term papillotomy may be used by some to indicate only a mucosal cut rather than a submucosal cut, but this is difficult to determine endoscopically.

The objective of sphincterotomy is to sever the sphincter fibers and any soft tissue that impedes the passage of bile and/or common duct stones. It is the procedure of choice for management of recurrent common bile duct (CBD) stones after cholecystectomy. In fact, retained or recurrent CBD stones account for 83% of the sphincterotomies performed.

In addition to postcholecystectomy choledocholithiasis, indications for endoscopic sphincterotomy include the following:

- Choledocholithiasis in patients with an intact gallbladder who are poor surgical risks or before laparoscopic cholecystectomy.
- Papillary stenosis in patients with prolonged symptoms and severe disability who have been unresponsive to symptomatic treatment. Sphincterotomy in these patients serves to enlarge the papillary opening and decrease ductal pressure.
- Obstruction of the CBD by ampullary tumors or distal CBD lesions. In this case, sphincterotomy is done to relieve ductal obstruction caused by tumor growth and to reduce the resultant jaundice. It may be performed in preparation for more extensive surgery or as palliation.
- Gallstone pancreatitis.
- Acute suppurative (purulent) cholangitis.
- Sphincter of Oddi dysfunction.
- Choledochocele.
- Sump syndrome, a rare clinical entity involving the accumulation of gallstones or food debris in the defunctionalized segment of the distal CBD in patients who have had a side-to-side choledochoduodenostomy.
- In preparation for stent placement, Gruntzig balloon dilatation, or nasobiliary catheterization.

Contraindications for sphincterotomy include:

- An uncooperative patient. (The patient must be able to lie still, follow directions for posturing for radiographs, and follow other directions as needed.)
- Significant coagulopathy.
- Recent myocardial infarction or severe pulmonary disease.
- Allergy to the contrast medium.
- The presence of an extremely large stone (greater than 20 or 25 mm in diameter), unless a lithotripter is available or stent placement is planned instead of surgery.
- Inability to properly position the **sphincterotome (papillotome).**

Periampullary diverticula do not necessarily constitute a contraindication to sphincterotomy, but patients with this condition are at additional risk.

In preparation for the procedure, a side-viewing duodenoscope with a nonmetal head should be checked for movement of the tip, good visibility, functioning of the forceps elevator, suction, and water channels. If the forceps elevator sticks, the tip of the scope should be soaked in tepid water until freed. Once it moves freely, silicone should be applied to maintain its motion. Also, silicone applied to the biopsy port just before the procedure ensures easy passage of the cannula.

The cannulating catheters used for dye injection should be filled with radiopaque contrast material and cleared of air bubbles. Sphincterotomes should be flexed to confirm full range of motion and smoothness of function. The sphincterotome should also be filled with the contrast medium. Balloon catheters should be filled with contrast material, cleared of air bubbles, and tested for balloon inflation.

Although ERCP can be safely performed on an outpatient basis, patients are usually hospitalized postsphincterotomy, because of the additional risks involved. Patients should be NPO for 6 to 12 hours before the procedure. Dentures or bridges should be removed, and a bite block should be used to protect the teeth and the scope. A topical anesthetic should be used to numb the throat. Prophylactic antibiotics usually are not necessary unless the patient has an underlying valvular heart disease, sepsis, biliary tract obstruction, or a pancreatic pseudocyst. It is recommended that two nurses assist during sphincterotomy to help ensure patient safety.

In patients with underlying coagulation abnormalities, necessary precautions should be taken, such as vitamin K injections, administration of fresh frozen plasma, or specific coagulation factors. Patients with abnormal coagulation studies should also be treated during the healing phase for 7 to 10 days following the procedure.

An IV line should be started in the patient's right hand or forearm and kept open with normal saline. The patient is then placed in the left lateral position to the far right side of the table, thereby making it relatively easy to roll the patient into the prone position once the scope is passed into the duodenum. The patient's left arm may be placed behind him/her to further facilitate prone positioning.

In preparation for sphincterotomy, the nurse applies the grounding pad and set up the ESU as described in the section on polypectomy. The cutting currents used in sphincterotomy are composed of continuous sinusoidal waves or bursts that are active most of the time. These cutting currents produce intense heat at the point of contact, thus vaporizing and exploding cells.

The medications used will vary with the physician. Before intubation and during the procedure, the patient is sedated. Glucagon may be given to reduce duodenal motility before cannulation and sphincterotomy. Atropine may be needed to control the pulse rate if vagal response occurs. Pediatric patients may require general anesthesia. Opiates are generally avoided when sphincter of Oddi manometric studies are anticipated because these agents may cause sphincter spasms, which alter the sphincter pressure and make cannulation difficult.

Narcotic and sedative antagonists should be on hand for reversal of drug effects. Emergency equipment should be available and functioning in the event of respiratory or cardiac arrest.

During the procedure the nurse should help the patient lie as still as possible, give emotional support, and monitor the patient's blood pressure; respirations; pulse; skin color, warmth, and dryness; oral secretions; and position. Pillows may be needed to support the patient in the required position.

Once the ampulla of Vater is sighted, glucagon is administered and a high-quality cholangiogram is obtained. The appropriate sphincterotome is selected, inserted into the scope, and introduced into the CBD. The sphincterotome should be advanced only a short distance before contrast material is injected to confirm placement in the CBD.

Fluoroscopy demonstrates proper placement of the sphincterotome within the bile duct. The physician then directs the nurse to flex the sphincterotome slowly, and the cannula is withdrawn from the duct far enough so that approximately one half to two thirds of the wire is visible in the duodenum, outside the papillary orifice. The wire is oriented in a 12 o'clock position in relation to the papilla so the wire is held against the roof of the papilla during cutting.

Before starting the electrocautery incision, voice checks should be made between the endoscopist and the gastroenterology nurse concerning the following:

- Application of the grounding pad on the patient and its connection. (On most units an alarm warns personnel of these problems.)
- Attachment of the sphincterotome handle to the ESU
- Presetting of the ESU with the desired blended current setting
- Correct positioning of the foot pedal
- Control of duodenal motility using glucagon
- Degree of wire flexion required on the sphincterotome
- Switching on the power just before cutting

Cutting is usually done with a partially flexed sphincterotome, with very short bursts of current (less than 1 second) to carry the incision through the sphincter 1 to 2 mm at a time.

The length of the sphincterotomy should be tailored to the size of the common duct stones. The apparent length of the intraduodenal segment of the CBD and the length of the narrow portion of the duct until the point where the duct becomes dilated are of great importance. The sphincterotomy must be extended to the dilated portion of the duct, but it must also remain within the intraduodenal segment of the duct. The usual length of

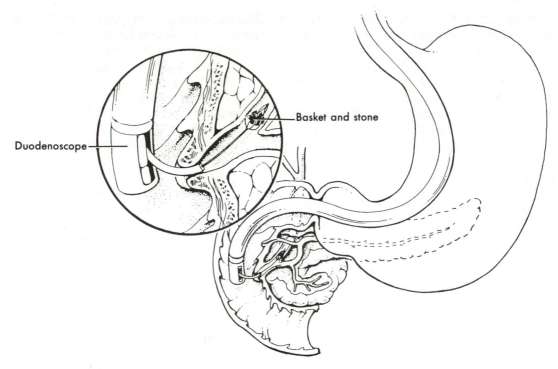

**Fig. 32-1**. Stone retrieval while basket is in common bile duct.

the incision is 10 to 12 mm. As the current is being applied, the endoscopist may order changes in the flexion of the sphincterotome. The entire procedure should be done under direct visual guidance.

The completion of a sphincterotomy is usually signaled by a gush of bile that contains some blood, thus indicating that the sphincter fibers have been severed and usually that the sphincterotomy is adequate. After sphincterotomy is completed, the operator determines the size of the opening and patency to the bile duct by using a flexed sphincterotome or an inflated balloon catheter.

The ESU should be turned off as soon as the sphincterotomy is complete. If stones are present and do not pass spontaneously, a retrieval device should be passed into the duct to retrieve the stones. Alternative retrieval devices include occlusion balloons (the preferred method), baskets, or mechanical lithotripters:

- Stones up to 12 mm in diameter can be extracted by using a balloon catheter. Balloons are passed up beyond the stone and then inflated to pull the stone down and drag it through the sphincterotomy incision. Balloons may also be used for determining the size of the incision, for determining the presence of and removing gravel, and for performing cholangiography after sphincterotomy or chole- dochoduodenostomy. Considerable traction is often required for pulling a stone through a sphincter- otomy incision.

- A basket can trap stones up to 15 mm in size (Fig. 32-1). Baskets are more difficult to intro- duce into the CBD than is a balloon or sphinc- terotome. Occasionally, the operator has diffi- culty entrapping stones in a basket, and there have been reports of impaction of baskets with en- trapped stones in the distal portion of the CBD. Some patients have required surgical intervention for removal of impacted baskets with entrapped stones.

- A modified sphincterotome, similar to a polypec- tomy snare, can be used to hook the stone in a wire loop and extract it.

- A mechanical lithotripter functions on the same principle as the basket, capturing the stone and then applying pressure against the trapped stone, caus- ing fragmentation. The device is composed of a basket with high tensile strength wires with a Teflon sheath that can be removed and replaced by a coil spring sheath to allow application of traction on the stone. Mechanical cutting through the stone is accomplished by using wires for mechanical cutting and a coil spring sheath for firm traction on the stone.

- Electric spark pulsing lithotripsy, which has been useful for removing stones from the urinary tract, is being studied to determine its effectiveness in the removal of gallstones.

Gallstones have also been destroyed with lasers, but this method is not widely used at this time. Occasionally, large stones that cause ductal obstruction and cannot be removed endoscopically may be bypassed with a biliary stent.

If stones cannot be removed immediately after sphincterotomy, it is usually advisable to allow them to remain until the edema and reaction to the sphincterotomy have subsided. A nasobiliary catheter may be placed as a prophylactic measure to avoid obstruction. The patient is reexamined in 5 to 14 days to determine whether the stones have passed. During this second examination, the operator may again consider extending the sphincterotomy and attempting extraction of the stones.

If these methods are unsuccessful, cholesterol stones may be dissolved by using monooctanoin (Moctanin) infusion through a nasobiliary catheter. This method dissolves the stones in approximately 50% of cases or may soften large calculi so they can be extracted a few days later as "mud." Infusions of monooctanoin take 6 to 14 days, must be done on an inpatient basis, and frequently cause epigastric distress and/or diarrhea.

If all attempts to remove stones fail, a stent can be inserted to facilitate biliary drainage and to keep the stone from impacting and causing biliary obstruction.

In patients with Billroth II gastrectomies, endoscopic access to the papilla and its subsequent cannulation and sphincterotomy can be difficult. Specially designed sphincterotomes are needed in this case.

Following endoscopic sphincterotomy, antibiotics should be administered according to the physician's order. The patient should be monitored for 1 hour for pulse, respiration, and blood pressure, attending to any abdominal discomfort, nausea, or vomiting. Clear fluids are usually given on the same evening and the patient is discharged on the following day if there are no adverse reactions and at least one full meal has been tolerated.

The mortality rate for endoscopic sphincterotomy is considerably lower than for surgical removal of retained common duct stones. Reported complications include the following:

- Bleeding, which is the most common complication and is responsible for half of the deaths. Bleeding can usually be managed by observation and/or transfusion.
- Pancreatitis, which usually can be adequately treated with antibiotics and conservative follow-up
- Free retroduodenal perforation
- Cholangitis, which can be prevented by placing a stent in the bile duct or by adding a nasobiliary catheter

- Entrapment of baskets, which can be eliminated by using balloons to extract stones or by ensuring that the sphincterotomy is adequate to allow the passage of a basket with a trapped stone

If the papilla becomes edematous as a result of excessive probing or electrocoagulation, the retroduodenal artery may be displaced. Accidental severing of the artery caused by anatomical aberration may occur.

## EXTRACORPOREAL SHOCK WAVE LITHOTRIPSY

For selected patients, extracorporeal shock wave lithotripsy (ESWL) is a noninvasive alternative to cholecystectomy. ESWL involves the use of shock waves generated in a specially designed table to fragment larger stones into smaller particles, most of which can then be passed spontaneously. The Food and Drug Administration (FDA) is presently conducting a research study into the safety and effectiveness of this procedure in the treatment of gallstones.

Patients who are candidates for ESWL must be screened according to criteria approved by the FDA. Approximately 25% of patients with gallbladder stones and most common duct stones that are referred for ESWL can be accepted as suitable candidates. ESWL is usually done on an outpatient basis under local anesthesia and conscious sedation. Patients can return to their normal activities the following day.

**Lithotripsy** is generally applied in combination with dissolution therapy. Success of stone fragmentation is dependent on the size, composition, and number of stones. Stone clearance depends on the ability of the gallbladder to contract and expel the stone fragments. ESWL has been most successful with solitary stones that are less than 2 cm in size.

There have been no serious complications from ESWL, and no significant damage to surrounding organs has been reported. If large stone fragments remain following ESWL, common bile duct obstruction is a potential complication. Endoscopic sphincterotomy may be required in these patients. Compared with patients treated with cholecystectomy, patients who are treated with ESWL generally appear to have less pain, a shorter recovery period, and less chance of infection.

## PULSED-DYE LASER LITHOTRIPSY

Stones in the gallbladder and common bile duct can also be destroyed with a pulsed-dye laser beam. With this new technology a quartz fiber is pushed up against the stone, and the laser fires. The beam creates a high-energy shock wave (a photo-acoustic effect) at the point of contact, and the stone is fragmented. The only contraindication for treatment of gallstones with this method is cirrhosis of the liver.

A number of successful options have been developed for reaching the stones with the laser fiber.

- Lasertripsy can be used during ERCP to treat ductal stones, either by threading the laser catheter through a smaller, flexible "baby" scope that is passed through the duodenoscope or by introducing a flexible radiopaque laser catheter through the duodenoscope.
- In a percutaneous approach to fragmentation of ductal stones, the procedural cannula that leads the laser fiber to the stones can be inserted through either the tract formed by a T-tube left in place after cholecystectomy or the skin under fluoroscopic guidance.
- Stones in the gallbladder can be fragmented by catheterizing the gallbladder through its free wall (cholecystolithotomy), and 2 weeks later replacing this drainage catheter with a procedural catheter, through which an endoscope and a laser fiber are inserted.

Compared to ESWL, lasertripsy is less time consuming; eliminates the need for long-term dissolution therapy; and can be used for patients with a greater number of stones.

---

### CASE SITUATION

Mr. Thomas Freeman is a 69-year-old man with a history of insulin-dependent diabetes. During his last visit to his internist, he complained of abdominal discomfort with early satiety and a general feeling of fullness in his stomach. The internist ordered an upper GI series. The x-ray film showed a gastric mass in the antrum, so the internist referred Mr. Freeman to a gastroenterologist, who will perform an esophagogastroduodenoscopy (EGD).

### Points to think about

1. The gastroenterology nurse has done her assessment of Mr. Freeman before his EGD. Based on her knowledge of his symptoms and history, the most likely causes of the patient's symptoms are either a tumor or a bezoar. What equipment will the nurse set up for the procedure?
2. The nurse knows that this is a potentially time consuming and resource intensive procedure. What can she do to plan ahead?
3. The EGD confirms that Mr. Freeman has a phytobezoar. The gastroenterologist breaks up the bezoar, allows it to pass, and withdraws the scope. What might happen next?
4. Why would the gastroenterologist schedule Mr. Freeman for a repeat endoscopy?

5. What patient education would be helpful for Mr. Freeman?

### Suggested responses

1. In setting up for Mr. Freeman's EGD, the gastroenterology nurse should consider the following:
   - The UGI series shows a mass in the antrum. This could be a malignant lesion, so the nurse will set up to collect specimens for biopsy and cytology.
   - Because Mr. Freeman is a diabetic, he may have decreased gastric motility caused by diabetic autonomic neuropathy and gastroparesis. This condition can allow food to remain in the stomach and collect into a phytobezoar. The nurse will set up equipment to be used to break up this concretion and allow it to pass through the stomach (e.g., rat-tooth forceps, snare, grasper).
   - Some bezoars form because pyloric strictures prevent passage of food into the duodenum. It is possible that the nurse will need balloons to dilate the pyloric sphincter.
2. To plan for a potentially time consuming and resource intensive procedure, the nurse should complete the following steps:
   - Place the procedure at the end of the schedule, rather than in the busiest part, to avoid feeling rushed. Allow at least an hour.
   - Have all equipment readily available and checked with regard to proper working order.
   - The procedure is much easier if the patient is comfortable and cooperative. The nurse should assess medication needs appropriately throughout the procedure and give additional doses as needed. The nurse should also monitor vital signs carefully and vigilantly, maintain the airway, and suction secretions.
3. After the bezoar has been broken up, and the endoscope has been removed, the nurse might expect the following:
   - If the endoscopist has been able to ascertain that the pyloric sphincter is not stenosed, the particles should pass through. If not, the pyloric sphincter may need to be dilated.
   - The physician may place Mr. Freeman on a full liquid diet for several days to help passage.
   - Metoclopramide (Reglan) may be ordered to increase peristalsis.
   - A repeat endoscopy may be ordered.
4. A repeat endoscopy might be ordered for the following reasons:
   - It is often difficult to properly visualize the mucosa because of the bezoar, and it may be difficult to get past it to view the antrum and pylorus.
   - Pyloric stenosis may require further evaluation and dilatation.

- Gastric carcinomas may be found distal to the bezoar, thereby causing obstruction. These should be examined by biopsy.
- Ulcerations may have been missed because of the presence of the bezoar.
- It is a good idea to check to be sure that the material has passed successfully through the pyloric sphincter.

5. Patient education considerations for Mr. Freeman could include the following:
   - Poor dentition is often a problem in phytobezoars. The nurse might question Mr. Freeman about teeth and gum problems. He may have ill-fitting dentures or teeth in poor repair. The nurse might suggest a trip to the dentist.
   - Poor eating habits may contribute to the formation of bezoars. Question Mr. Freeman about his diet and caution him to chew his food very well before swallowing. Consultation with a dietician may be in order.

---

REVIEW TERMS

---

**lithotripsy, overtube, papillotome, papillotomy, pedunculated polyp, polypectomy, polypectomy snares, sessile polyp, sphincterotome, sphincterotomy**

---

REVIEW QUESTIONS

---

1. Objects that are accidentally dropped into the hypopharynx during extraction should be removed using:
   a. A polypectomy snare.
   b. A wire basket.
   c. A laryngoscope and curved forceps.
   d. Biopsy forceps.
2. A polyvinyl overtube is useful for endoscopic removal of:
   a. Foreign bodies from the duodenum.
   b. Pointed objects.
   c. Extremely large objects.
   d. Small, round objects.
3. Individuals who have swallowed packets of cocaine in an attempt at concealment should be treated:
   a. Endoscopically.
   b. Surgically.
   c. With observation only, permitting the packets to pass unimpeded.
   d. With syrup of ipecac.
4. Polyps that are attached by a thin pedicle are usually transected by use of:
   a. Cutting current alone.
   b. Coagulation current alone.
   c. Blended current.
   d. Hot biopsy forceps.

5. Endoscopic polypectomy is contraindicated in patients with:
   a. Gastric polyps.
   b. Hyperplastic polyps.
   c. Sessile polyps more than 2 cm in diameter.
   d. Coagulopathy.
6. The grounding pad used for electrocautery is placed:
   a. On the table.
   b. On the patient's upper thigh or lower trunk.
   c. On the side rails.
   d. On the patient's upper arm.
7. For endoscopic retrograde sphincterotomy, the electrosurgical unit is turned on:
   a. Only when the endoscopist indicates that he or she is ready to begin cutting.
   b. As soon as the grounding pad is securely attached.
   c. Once the patient is in position.
   d. As soon as fluoroscopy demonstrates proper placement of the sphincterotome within the bile duct.
8. The preferred method of retrieving stones that do not pass spontaneously after endoscopic retrograde sphincterotomy is:
   a. A mechanical lithotripter.
   b. A retrieval basket.
   c. A balloon catheter.
   d. Nasobiliary drainage.
9. Extracorporeal biliary lithotripsy disrupts gallstones using what mechanism?
   a. Ultrasonography.
   b. Chemical agents.
   c. Shock waves.
   d. Endoscopic removal.
10. Compared to ESWL, lasertripsy has the following advantages:
    a. It is faster.
    b. It does not require dissolution therapy.
    c. It can be used in patients with a greater number of stones.
    d. All of the above.

BIBLIOGRAPHY

Brumm, J, and Crim, B. "Biliary Lithotripsy: A Smashing Solution." *Today's OR Nurse* 12(April 1990): 4-8.

Chobanian, S. "Gastrointestinal Foreign Bodies." In *Manual of Clinical Problems in Gastroenterology,* eds. Chobanian, S, and Van Ness, M, 94-96. Boston: Little, Brown & Co., 1988.

Cotton, P, and Williams, C. *Practical Gastrointestinal Endoscopy.* 3rd ed. Oxford: Blackwell Scientific Publications, Inc., 1990.

Eastwood, G, and Avunduk, C. *Manual of Gastroenterology: Diagnosis and Therapy.* Boston: Little, Brown & Co., 1988.

Hardick, M. "Foreign Body Removal in the Gastrointestinal Tract." In *Journal Reprints II,* ed. Trivits, S, 95-102. Rochester, N.Y.: Society of Gastroenterology Nurses and Associates, 1990.

Holland, P, and Hussain, I. "Biliary Lithotripsy: Nonsurgical Treatment of Gallstones." In *Journal Reprints II,* ed. Trivits, S, 135-39. Rochester, N.Y.: Society of Gastroenterology Nurses and Associates, 1990.

LaFleur, S. "Will Candela's LaserTripter Replace Conventional Gallbladder Surgery?" *Laser Medicine & Surgery News and Advances.* December 1989: 14-17.

Nord, H. "Diagnosis and Management of UGI Foreign Bodies." In *Gastrointestinal Endoscopy: Old Problems, New Techniques,* eds. Sivak, M, Jr., and Petrini, J, 13-17. Gastroenterology Series, Volume 4. New York: Praeger, 1986.

Ringrose, J, and Tyllia, P. "ERCP and Sphincterotomy: Responsibilities of the GI Assistant." In *SGA Journal Reprints,* ed. Trivits, S, 87-94. Rochester, N.Y.: Society of Gastrointestinal Assistants, 1988.

Shields, N. "Endoscopic Retrograde Sphincterotomy: Special Challenge for the GIA." *Journal Reprints II,* ed. Trivits, S, 115-19. Rochester, N.Y.: Society of Gastroenterology Nurses and Associates, 1990.

Shields, N, and Dreyer, M. "Endoscopic Sphincterotomy: The Role of the Gastrointestinal Assistant." *SGA Journal Reprints,* ed. Trivits, S, 89-94. Rochester, N.Y.: Society of Gastrointestinal Assistants, 1988.

Silverman, A, and Roy, C. *Pediatric Clinical Gastroenterology.* 3rd ed. St. Louis: Mosby–Year Book, 1983.

Silvis, S, ed. *Therapeutic Gastrointestinal Endoscopy.* New York: Igaku-Shoin, 1985.

Sleisenger, M, and Fordtran, J, eds. *Gastrointestinal Disease: Pathophysiology, Diagnosis, Management.* 4th ed. Philadelphia: W.B. Saunders, 1989.

Sugawa, C, and Schuman, B. *Primer of Gastrointestinal Fiberoptic Endoscopy.* Boston: Little, Brown & Co., 1981.

Waye, J, Atchison, M, Talbott, M, and Lewis, B. "Suction Retrieval of the Small Colon Polyp." *SGA Journal* 10(Spring 1988): 199-201.

Waye, J, Geenen, J, Fleischer, D, and Venu, R, eds. *Techniques in Therapeutic Endoscopy.* Philadelphia: W.B. Saunders, 1987.

# Chapter 33

# COMPLICATIONS AND EMERGENCIES

This chapter will acquaint the gastroenterology nurse with some of the complications and emergency situations that can occur in gastroenterology settings and will describe appropriate interventions for each situation. The topics covered include endoscopic and spontaneous perforations, hemorrhage, shock, adverse drug reactions, cardiac arrest, respiratory depression, vasovagal reactions, and aspiration.

**Learning objectives**

After reviewing the content of this chapter, the gastroenterology nurse should be able to:
1. Discuss the causes and risk factors for eight of the most important emergency situations and complications that are encountered in the gastroenterology lab.
2. Recognize the symptoms of these complications.
3. Explain the steps that must be taken to avoid or treat complications and emergencies associated with endoscopic procedures.

## PERFORATION OF THE UPPER GI TRACT

After cardiopulmonary complications, the second most common complication associated with endoscopic examination of the upper GI tract is **perforation.** Predisposing factors include anastomoses, strictures, and weakening of the wall from diverticula, inflammation, ischemia, neoplasms, or caustic ingestion.

Therapeutic endoscopy carries a greater risk of perforation than diagnostic procedures. Upper GI perforation may occur in the esophagus, stomach, or duodenum, but it frequently affects the cervical esophagus, the thoracic esophagus, or neoplastic stricture sites. Esophageal perforations most often result from trauma with an instrument, mainly after dilatation of a stricture or after pneumatic dilatation for achalasia. Gastric or duodenal perforation may be a complication of peptic ulcers.

The type of pain and other signs and symptoms are determined by the site of the perforation.
- If perforation has occurred in the cervical esophagus, the patient will have dysphagia, crepitus or stiffness of the neck, and neck and throat pain that is aggravated by swallowing or moving the cervical spine. The patient may also experience fever, tenderness in the affected area, or neck swelling.
- Perforation of the thoracic esophagus typically results in substernal or epigastric pain that increases with respirations and movement of the trunk. Shortness of breath, cyanosis, pleural effusion, and back pain may also be present.
- Perforation at the distal area of the esophagus, near the diaphragm, may lead to shoulder pain, dyspnea, severe back and abdominal pain, tachycardia, cyanosis, diaphoresis, and hypotension.
- Boerhaave's syndrome is a spontaneous (nontraumatic) rupture of the esophagus that is commonly associated with dyspnea after a vomiting episode. It may cause severe chest and/or abdominal pain. The patient appears acutely ill, and has hypotension, fever, subcutaneous emphysema, unilateral absence of breath sounds, or evidence of pleural effusion.
- Gastric perforation causes severe back and abdominal pain, tachycardia, cyanosis, diaphoresis, and hypotension with a drop in temperature, followed by a high fever. Patients may also experience prolonged distention of the abdomen following gastroscopy or disappearance of liver dullness on percussion.
- After duodenal perforation, vital signs may remain

341

stable initially. The patient then experiences sudden local or general abdominal pain. Although a brief period of improvement follows, peritonitis develops. The patient's abdomen becomes rigid, and he or she has a high fever, hypotension, tachycardia, and severe pain that inhibits abdominal movement and the ability to breath deeply. Both gastric and duodenal perforation can produce indications of leaking gastric or duodenal contents, such as acute upper abdominal pain and subsequent signs of guarding, rebound tenderness, or absent bowel sounds.

Esophageal perforation is often diagnosed using plain radiographs, with the neck hyperextended to remove the clavicular shadow from the esophageal inlet. The results of plain radiographic films of the neck are positive in virtually all patients, with cervical esophageal perforations showing air in the prevertebral space. Chest x-ray films may show mediastinal air, subcutaneous air, pneumothorax, pleural effusion, or mediastinal widening. An esophagogram with water-soluble contrast agents may help localize the perforation, but is only positive in 50% of patients with cervical perforations and in 75% to 85% of patients with thoracoabdominal perforations. If the water-soluble material does not reveal a perforation, a barium swallow may be ordered.

Close observation and symptomatic treatment are important if perforation is suspected. Surgical advice should be sought immediately, even though perforations that are recognized early may be treated conservatively with nasogastric or pharyngeal suction, IV feeding, and broad-spectrum antibiotics. Conservative management is contraindicated if a major leak is apparent on contrast radiology, or if perforation occurs through an ulcer or tumor.

If necessary, cervical perforations may be sutured, and the patient may be treated with IV antibiotics. Surgery is more often recommended for intrathoracic perforations, which have a poorer prognosis. Contained thoracic perforations may be treated conservatively. If an intrathoracic perforation is not contained, urgent thoracotomy with chest and mediastinal drainage and esophageal suturing is indicated.

Gastric perforations are far less common than esophageal perforations and are usually related to biopsies of ulcerated lesions or to impaction of the endoscope in a hiatal hernia sac. Small perforations into the lesser sac of the peritoneal cavity can be managed conservatively. Anterior free gastric perforations with peritoneal signs and abdominal free air shown on x-ray film require surgical management.

## PERFORATION OF THE LOWER GI TRACT

Underlying conditions that increase the risk of colonic perforation include diverticular disease, adhesions from pelvic surgery, pelvic carcinoma, colonic carcinoma, inflammatory bowel disease, colonic strictures, and radiation colitis. Lower GI perforations occur most often from mechanical trauma related to manipulation of the colonoscope itself, but pneumatic perforation may result from overdistention with insufflated air.

The risk of perforation with polypectomy is almost twice as high as with diagnostic colonoscopy. It may be related to electrical injury to the bowel from excessive coagulation of the base of the polyp before cutting the polyp, or it may be the result of injury to the bowel wall opposite the base of the polyp, if there is contact with the body of the polyp at that site. Perforation can also result from improper placement of polypectomy snare loops with resultant entrapment of normal mucosa and bowel wall. Perforations secondary to polypectomy may occasionally be delayed and have been reported to occur up to 2 weeks after the procedure.

Signs of lower GI perforation include sudden, severe abdominal pain that becomes generalized, possibly accompanied by signs of peritonitis, abdominal distention, pneumoperitoneum, increased tympany, loss of hepatic dullness, malaise, fever, a change in vital signs, and bloody or mucopurulent rectal drainage. A hole in the colon may be seen by the examiner, or omentum may be visualized. On occasion, a colonic perforation is diagnosed radiographically, using plain abdominal radiographs in the supine position.

Most free colonoscopic perforations need to be treated promptly with surgical exploration. Patients with retroperitoneal perforations, which are usually pneumatic perforations, should receive symptomatic treatment and close observation. Surgical intervention is indicated only if signs progress.

## GASTROINTESTINAL BLEEDING

Gastrointestinal **hemorrhage** may be associated with an underlying disease state or trauma or may arise as a rare complication of diagnostic endoscopy (Fig. 33-1). Therapeutic endoscopic procedures, including sclerotherapy, polypectomy, laser therapy, and dilatation are more likely to cause bleeding. Hemorrhage is the most common complication of polypectomy. Inexperience or lack of expertise on the part of the electrosurgical unit (ESU) operator and/or malfunction can contribute to the risk of polypectomy-related hemorrhage.

Other precipitating factors include traumatization of recently bleeding esophageal varices, esophagitis or gastritis, mucosal tears in patients with strictures, cardio-esophageal (Mallory-Weiss) tears, and a biopsy performed on a recently bleeding lesion or at the base of ulcers where larger vessels may be exposed. Less-common causes include Boerhaave's syndrome and Osler-Weber-Rendu disease. Common causes of lower

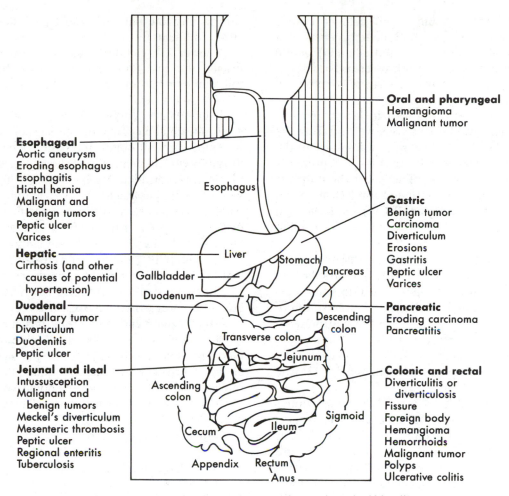

**Esophageal**
Aortic aneurysm
Eroding esophagus
Esophagitis
Hiatal hernia
Malignant and
benign tumors
Peptic ulcer
Varices

**Hepatic**
Cirrhosis (and other
causes of potential
hypertension)

**Duodenal**
Ampullary tumor
Diverticulum
Duodenitis
Peptic ulcer

**Jejunal and ileal**
Intussusception
Malignant and
benign tumors
Meckel's diverticulum
Mesenteric thrombosis
Peptic ulcer
Regional enteritis
Tuberculosis

**Oral and pharyngeal**
Hemangioma
Malignant tumor

**Gastric**
Benign tumor
Carcinoma
Diverticulum
Erosions
Gastritis
Peptic ulcer
Varices

**Pancreatic**
Eroding carcinoma
Pancreatitis

**Colonic and rectal**
Diverticulitis or
diverticulosis
Fissure
Foreign body
Hemangioma
Hemorrhoids
Malignant tumor
Polyps
Ulcerative colitis

Esophagus
Liver
Stomach
Pancreas
Gallbladder
Duodenum
Descending colon
Transverse colon
Jejunum
Ascending colon
Sigmoid
Cecum
Ileum
Appendix
Rectum
Anus

**Fig. 33-1.** Common sites and causes of gastrointestinal bleeding.

GI bleeding include diverticulosis, inflammatory bowel disease, colonic angiodysplasia, and hemorrhoids. Less-common causes include intussusception, rectal trauma, and anal disorders.

Upper GI bleeding is indicated by hematemesis, hypotension, and tachycardia, or melena (liquid, tarry, foul-smelling black stools). Lower GI bleeding is associated with increased pulse rate, decreased blood pressure, weakness, pallor, bright red rectal bleeding (hematochezia), maroon or black stools, and possibly abdominal pain and distention. Bleeding as a complication of polypectomy is most often intracolonic, resulting in obvious hematochezia.

To minimize the risk of bleeding and hemorrhage, laboratory tests are often performed before certain procedures, including biopsy and polypectomy, to confirm that coagulation is adequate. Coagulation parameters and platelet counts should be checked, and biopsies should be avoided when there are significant abnormalities.

The initial management of acute gastrointestinal bleeding involves taking a thorough history, including any history of hematemesis or hematochezia, pain and abdominal tenderness, or severe retching. Any concomitant heart, lung, renal, liver, or central nervous system (CNS) disease should be considered. Vital signs should be monitored, including postural signs. A physical examination should be performed, including a rectal examination.

Intervention in cases of upper GI bleeding should focus on maintaining the airway, providing oxygenation, establishing a large-bore IV catheter, maintaining adequate fluid volume, stabilizing the patient's condition, stopping the bleeding, and beginning appropriate therapy to prevent further bleeding. Invasive procedures may be indicated to make a prompt diagnosis. In general, a disproportionate share of the mortality is in patients who continue bleeding or experience recurrent bleeding after admission to the hospital and, in particular, in patients who are bleeding from esophageal and/or gastric varices.

A large-bore peripheral catheter and if necessary, a central venous line should be inserted. Blood should be withdrawn for initial laboratory studies. Crystalloids (such as normal saline or Ringer's lactate solution, which maintain intravascular volume) and colloids (whole blood, packed red blood cells, and blood products such as fresh-frozen plasma, platelets, and albumin) should be administered as ordered by the physician. The patient should be assessed frequently for signs and symptoms of electrolyte disturbances.

Nasogastric aspiration and gastric lavage may be required, using an Ewald tube to remove clots from the stomach, if necessary. If the return fluid from the nasogastric tube is clear initially, or if it clears promptly with lavage, the tube can be removed; if the return is bloody, lavage should be continued until clear. Nasal oxygen and an electrocardiogram (ECG) may be needed in patients with hypovolemia to assess and combat ischemic effects.

Depending on the cause and site of gastrointestinal bleeding, the physician may treat it with gastric lavage, drug therapy, balloon tamponade, injection sclerotherapy, thermal coagulation methods, or surgery. Endoscopic techniques for the management of gastrointestinal bleeding are discussed in detail in Chapter 30, including thermal coagulation methods, injection sclerotherapy, and esophagogastric tamponade. Gastric lavage is discussed in Chapter 31.

In patients with acute upper GI bleeding, upper endoscopy may reveal stigmata of recent hemorrhage, such as a visible vessel, fresh blood clot, black eschar, or active bleeding. If no signs of recent hemorrhage are visible, medical treatment may be sufficient. In patients with continuing bleeding or stigmata of recent hemorrhage, therapeutic endoscopy or surgery may be indicated, in addition to further diagnostic tests.

The following steps should be taken to determine the source of lower GI bleeding:

1. Perform anoscopy, sigmoidoscopy, and nasogastric aspiration.
2. If no obvious bleeding site is found and the patient continues to bleed, perform esophagogastroduodenoscopy (EGD) to exclude an upper GI lesion.
3. Perform technetium-99 tagged red blood cell scan, which can detect bleeding rates as low as 0.1 ml/min.
4. Perform a fluid purge and colonoscopy if bleeding slows sufficiently.
5. If bleeding remains brisk, perform mesenteric arteriography.
6. If extravasation of contrast is seen, infuse vasopressin (Pitressin) or consider embolization therapy; if bleeding persists despite vasopressin or embolization, perform surgery before blood losses become too great.
7. If no extravasation is noted, but significant bleeding persists, consider exploratory laparotomy.

In patients with postpolypectomy hemorrhage, management involves stabilizing the patient; monitoring blood pressure, urine output, and central venous pressure in unstable patients; and transfusion (in 25% to 50% of patients).

If lower GI bleeding ceases spontaneously, as is usually the case, colonoscopy should be performed, followed by a barium enema and possibly an EGD and small bowel series.

If emergency endoscopy is indicated to control gastrointestinal bleeding, the nurse should verify signed informed consent; obtain the patient's medical history, including current medications and allergies and a history of the present bleeding episode; remove dentures; monitor vital signs at least every 15 minutes; monitor the patient's cardiac status using a heart monitor; monitor oxygen saturation with a pulse oximeter; establish large-bore IV line(s); obtain blood samples for complete blood count (CBC) and type and cross-match as ordered; and start oxygen via nasal cannula as ordered. Staff should be prepared to perform gastric lavage using a large-bore orogastric or nasogastric tube.

After an emergency endoscopy, it is important for the nurse to monitor vital signs and observe the patient for bleeding, vomiting, or change in vital signs, pain, and abdominal distention. The type, amount, and times of replacement of IV fluids given should be documented.

Complications of gastrointestinal bleeding may include the following:

- Anemia from blood loss
- Hypovolemic shock from severe volume depletion
- Exsanguination from rapid massive intravascular blood loss
- Myocardial or cerebral infarction from acute hemoglobin depletion
- Disseminated intravascular coagulation from shock and clotting factor loss
- Peritonitis and sepsis from bowel rupture
- Aspiration from massive upper GI bleeding

## SHOCK

**Shock** is a condition of acute peripheral circulatory failure caused by derangement of circulatory control or loss of circulating fluid. It may be endocrine, neurogenic, bacterial, cardiogenic, or hypovolemic in origin, but is always characterized by decreased tissue perfusion and increased peripheral vasoconstriction. The two most common forms of shock in gastroenterology patients are hypovolemic shock and bacterial (septic) shock.

### Hypovolemic shock

In hypovolemic shock, the loss of circulating volume may result from loss of blood or plasma, intestinal obstruction, nephrotic syndrome, dehydration, or trauma. In patients undergoing paracentesis, hypovolemic shock may result from the rapid shift of fluid from the circulatory system to the peritoneum as the body attempts to replace the aspirated fluid.

**Hypovolemia** causes the body to respond to the perceived volume loss by decreasing urinary output and constricting the caliber of peripheral blood vessels. At the same time, blood flow to the cerebral and cardiovascular systems increases, thereby resulting in mental confusion and ECG changes.

Glycogen breakdown increases, insulin is suppressed, and hyperglycemia occurs. If cerebral blood flow is decreased and a subsequent loss of consciousness takes place, the central regulating centers may shut down.

Signs of shock include altered mental status; restlessness; increased anxiety; pale, cool, clammy skin; decreased capillary refill time, which is noted by pressing the fingernail; collapse of peripheral neck veins; and tachycardia. In the early stages, hypertension may occur. Hypotension is an advanced sign. The patient may also show diaphoresis, goose bumps, muscle weakness, decreased urinary output, hyperventilation, abdominal distention, and electrolyte imbalance.

Treatment should focus on restoring tissue perfusion and reducing peripheral vasoconstriction. The patient should be positioned in a way that facilitates the blood supply to the brain and promotes venous return from the rest of the body. To promote respiration, the patient should lie flat with the legs elevated 20 degrees at the hips or with the head elevated slightly. To decrease oxygen use, activity should be minimized.

Intravenous fluids should be administered to maintain the patency of the vascular system, to restore volume and an oxygen transport system, and to remove wastes. Depending on the patient's hematocrit, the fluid given may be blood, plasma, plasma expanders, or a balanced salt solution (Ringer's).

Vasoactive agents or steroids may be given. Steroids decrease peripheral resistance, increase tissue perfusion, increase venous return, and have a positive effect on the heart muscle. Metabolic acidosis is generally corrected by the administration of fluids. It may be necessary to use endotracheal intubation or a volume respirator to deliver oxygen.

Internal or external bleeding should be stopped. Methods of controlling external bleeding are direct pressure, ligation, cautery, or application of topical medication. Central venous pressure readings may be ordered to monitor the course and effectiveness of treatment.

### Septic shock

Septic or bacterial shock is produced by direct invasion of the bloodstream by an organism or, most commonly, by the accumulation of toxins in the blood. Septic shock may be associated with peritonitis, infections such as cholecystitis or pancreatitis, bowel surgery or trauma, reduction of volvulus, or hemorrhage.

Symptoms of septic shock vary from "warm shock," in which the skin is dry, pink, and warm, and urinary output is good, to "cold shock," in which catecholamine is released.

Treatment for septic shock focuses on removing the cause and starting massive antibiotic therapy.

### ADVERSE DRUG REACTIONS

In the gastroenterology lab, most morbidity and mortality from adverse drug reactions is associated with excitation or depression of the CNS, respiratory depression, cardiac arrhythmias, or loss of vascular tone. Individually or in combination, these reactions may result in aspiration of gastric contents, respiratory failure, and cardiovascular collapse. Table 33-1 lists a number of drugs commonly used in the gastroenterology lab and their potential adverse effects.

Whenever a drug is administered it is important to be aware of potential side effects, toxic reactions, and allergic responses.

- A side effect is any drug effect that is not intended. Some side effects are transient and subside as the patient develops a tolerance to the drug. In some patients, adjusting the drug dosage may control undesirable side effects, but in others, side effects contraindicate the use of a drug altogether.
- Toxic reactions can be acute, resulting from excessive doses, or chronic, resulting from progressive accumulation of the drug in the body. Toxic reactions can also result from impaired metabolism or excretion that can cause elevated blood levels.
- Drug allergy or hypersensitivity results from an antigen-antibody immune reaction in susceptible patients. Skin lesions (urticaria) and respiratory distress are the most common symptoms of drug allergies, but cardiovascular dysfunction and potentially fatal **anaphylaxis** may also be seen. Topical anesthetics used in upper endoscopy can cause rare anaphylactic reactions. (The need for pharyngeal anesthesia during endoscopy with small-caliber endoscopes is debatable, and many operators no longer use pharyngeal anesthetics.) It is vitally important to check for drug allergies before administering medications.

Antispasmodic and antisecretory agents, such as atropine, scopolamine, and glucagon, all have side effects. These agents have been associated with reports of ileus, urinary retention, arrhythmias (bradycardia, tachycardia, and atrioventricular block), vomiting, and hyperglycemia. Atropine or scopolamine can increase intraocular pressure in patients with narrow-angle glaucoma. Glucagon is used most often during endoscopic retrograde cholangiopancreatography (ERCP). Vomiting may be avoided by slow administration of small doses.

**Table 33-1.** Adverse effects of drugs used in the gastroenterology lab

| Agent | Adverse effects |
| --- | --- |
| diazepam (Valium) | Laryngospasm, respiratory depression, phlebitis |
| atropine | Tachycardia, hypertension |
| glucagon | Hypotension, vomiting |
| meperidine (Demerol) | Respiratory depression, hypotension, bradycardia tachycardia |
| benzocaine (Cetacaine), lidocaine (Xylocaine), benzonatate (Tessalon) | Laryngospasm, interference with gag reflex |
| physostigmine (Antilirium) | Bradycardia, hypersalivation leading to respiratory difficulties, convulsions |
| naloxone (Narcan) | Hypotension, hypertension, ventricular tachycardia and fibrillation, and pulmonary edema; excessive postoperative doses may result in excitement; drug withdrawal in patients who are using narcotics |
| cimetidine (Tagamet) | Potentiates diazepam |
| pentagastrin (Peptavlon) | Hypotension |
| betazole (Histalog) | Palpitations, hypotension, shock |
| butorphanol (Stadol) | Sedation, nausea, clamminess, overdosage producing respiratory depression and variable cardiovascular and CNS effects |
| midazolam (Versed) | Respiratory depression, fluctuation in vital signs |

Adapted from Adams, J: Emergencies in the GI Lab: The GIA Role. Presented at the 14th annual meeting of SGNA, 1986.

Sedatives can cause excessive depression of the CNS, particularly in elderly patients and in those with hypoalbuminemia. Physostigmine (Antilirium) may reverse central depression. Diazepam (Valium) may also cause superficial phlebitis at the injection site in 3.5% to 17% of patients. To avoid this common side effect, diazepam should be injected into a large vein, and the vein should be flushed with straight or heparinized saline.

Narcotic analgesics such as meperidine (Demerol) are used to achieve analgesia, sedation, and euphoria. Side effects of meperidine include nausea and vomiting, respiratory depression, hypotension, and spasm of intestinal smooth muscle. Allergic reactions, usually urticaria or rashes, are uncommon. Respiratory depression usually persists for 2 to 4 hours, but may last longer in patients with hypothyroidism, head trauma, or chronic pulmonary disease. Hypotension results from peripheral vasodilatation. It is usually treated by administering IV fluids and by placing the patient in Trendelenburg's position. The narcotic effects of meperidine can be reversed in 1 or 2 minutes with IV naloxone (Narcan). Naloxone's duration of action is dependent on the dose and route of administration. Intramuscular (IM) administration produces a more prolonged effect than IV administration. In one study, the serum half-life of parenteral naloxone in adults ranged from 30 to 81 minutes. In a neonatal study, the mean plasma half-life was $3.1 \pm 0.5$ hours.

Whenever analgesia is started, the patient's breathing pattern should be monitored by both the endoscopist and the nurse. The pulse, usually the temporal or carotid, should also be taken. Once endoscopy has begun, it is the nurse's responsibility to monitor the patient's vital functions.

To avoid adverse medication effects, it is important to administer medications cautiously. Titration should be performed slowly to the level of sedation required. The patient should be observed for signs of laryngospasm, bradycardia, excessive diaphoresis, hypotension, respiratory depression, or apnea. Resuscitation equipment and reversal agents should always be readily available. The staff should be alert to the danger of drug withdrawal when narcotic antagonists are given to drug users or patients who are being treated with narcotics.

Every endoscopy unit should have readily available a cart with equipment for cardiopulmonary resuscitation, including airway, ambu bag, oxygen supply tubing, suction, laryngoscope, IV infusion setup, drugs, and a defibrillator. This cart should be checked daily or in accordance with institutional policy and should be restocked if drugs are outdated. A supply of oxygen must be available whenever resuscitation is attempted.

Early diagnosis and treatment of anaphylactic reactions are necessary to avert death, which can occur within 15 minutes. There must be constant attention to an adequate airway and perfusion. Epinephrine and an antihistamine are usually used for treatment.

## CARDIAC ARREST

The most common complication of upper endoscopy, aside from miscellaneous medication reactions, is cardiopulmonary in nature. There is a mild to moderate amount of cardiovascular stress associated with upper GI endoscopy. Minor ECG changes during the procedure are common and can occur in up to 38% of patients. These are primarily sinus arrhythmias, S-T segment changes, and premature ventricular contractions. Some of the changes are related to anxiety and premedication rather than to the procedure itself. Patients with known heart disease should be monitored by ECG during upper GI endoscopy.

Some of the major causes of **cardiac arrest** in the gastroenterology unit are too-rapid administration or overdosage of medications, obstruction of the respiratory tract, and preexisting conditions, such as acute anxiety states, anemia, cardiac disease, dehydration, pulmonary edema, and shock.

Signs of impending cardiac arrest include the following:
- Signs of respiratory obstruction (cyanosis, gasping respiration, increased rate and shallowness of respiration)
- Pulse irregularities and rate changes
- Muscle twitching
- Cold and clammy skin

Initial signs of collapse of cardiopulmonary function are absent pulse and/or respiration and lifeless appearance. If these conditions are present, cardiopulmonary resuscitation (CPR) must begin immediately. In any situation, the most important principles of CPR include establishment of a patent airway, provision of ventilation, and restoration of cardiac pumping action.

When a patient experiences cardiac arrest, the nurse must act quickly. Brain damage or death can result if circulation is not restored within 3 to 6 minutes after cardiac and respiratory arrest. First, the resuscitation team or another source of assistance should be alerted. The patient should be placed on a flat, firm surface, and CPR should be initiated. The patient should be attached to an electrocardiograph or a defibrillator, and defibrillation should be performed by a qualified person. An IV line should be started by using a large-bore catheter, the oxygen apparatus should be set up, and oxygen should be administered. Tracheal suction apparatus and catheters should be prepared, and the patient should be suctioned as needed. The nurse may assist with intubation as needed. Events immediately preceding the crisis should be documented, and the necessary data should be provided to the resuscitation team. Vital signs should be monitored. The necessary equipment should be provided.

Any excess equipment and personnel should be removed from the area. Family members and visitors should be escorted to a waiting area and provided with emotional support. Other patients should be screened from activities. The attending physician should be notified if he or she is not in attendance.

If the resuscitation effort is successful, the patient should be transferred to a monitored area, and the physician should speak with the family. If unsuccessful, the physician should notify the family and provide emotional support. The physician may request a consent for autopsy. If the family agrees, consent forms need to be completed and documented. Resuscitation equipment should be checked and restocked. The established protocol for a death in the gastroenterology unit should be followed.

## RESPIRATORY DEPRESSION

In patients receiving anesthesia, sedatives, or narcotics, **respiratory depression** can occur, potentially leading to cardiovascular collapse. Symptoms of respiratory depression include a decrease in respiratory rate and/or tidal volume, Cheyne-Stokes respiration (rhythmic waxing and waning of respirations), periods of apnea, and cyanosis. These symptoms may be accompanied by extreme somnolence, skeletal muscle flaccidity, cold, clammy skin, and sometimes bradycardia and hypotension.

Narcotic drugs that are used to sedate the patient, most notably meperidine (Demerol), have been known to cause respiratory depression. When using medications that have been associated with respiratory depression, the gastroenterology nurse should be prepared to assist with intubation of the patient and to control respirations if necessary. Respiratory depression may be reversed with naloxone (Narcan) and/or flumazenil (Mazicon). With benzodiazepines, it is important to titrate the dosage carefully, using the smallest dose necessary to provide adequate sedation. Particular care should be used with elderly patients and in patients with underlying pulmonary disease.

If the patient stops breathing, the physician should be notified at once. The most important factors are the establishment and maintenance of the patient's airway. These goals are accomplished by placing the patient in a supine position and tilting the head back, taking care to avoid hyperextension and subsequent closing of the airway. An oropharyngeal airway should be inserted quickly.

An appropriate IV dose of naloxone (Narcan) and/or flumazenil (Mazican) should be administered simultaneously with efforts at respiratory resuscitation. The pulse should be checked. An ambu bag should be used. If the carotid pulse cannot be palpated, external cardiocompression should be begun. Usually, once the naloxone takes effect, the patient begins to awaken and breathe independently.

## VASOVAGAL SYNCOPE

**Vasovagal syncope** is the most frequent cause of transient loss of consciousness (fainting). The patient experiences nausea, profuse sweating, pallor, weakness, and possibly hypotension and bradycardia. Vasovagal syncope may be caused by sudden emotional stress or a sudden painful experience, such as when colonoscopy stretches the mesentery to such an extent that serious discomfort or pain results.

To treat a vasovagal reaction, the patient should be positioned with the head at a level with or lower than the rest of the body. Consciousness usually returns quickly once the patient is recumbent. Saline may be given intravenously. Sometimes a small dose of atropine is given. To help prevent a vasovagal attack from occurring, atropine or narcotic analgesics may be given before colonoscopy.

## POSTURAL HYPOTENSION

Postural hypotension may occur when the patient suddenly assumes an upright position. There is a fall in systolic and diastolic blood pressure, sometimes accompanied by weakness, dizziness, or syncope. Postural hypotension is commonly associated with prolonged bedrest, older people who are inactive and have peripheral venous insufficiency, and loss of intravascular volume from severe gastrointestinal hemorrhage.

## ASPIRATION

**Aspiration** occurs when liquids or solids mistakenly enter the pulmonary system. The incidence of aspiration is only 0.08%, but the mortality rate of this complication may reach 10%. Patients can aspirate saliva, gastric secretions, or blood.

Topical pharyngeal anesthesia, sedation, and supine positioning may all be contributing factors in aspiration and its sequelae. A full stomach, active bleeding, and retained gastric secretions caused by obstructive lesions are all risk factors. The elderly and any other patients who have depressed cough and gag reflexes are also at risk. Because of the increased length of the procedure, the amount of sedation involved, and the need to reposition the patient, ERCP involves a greater risk of aspiration than many other endoscopic procedures.

Aspiration is also a problem in patients who are receiving enteral nutrition. It may be minimized by placing the tube well beyond the pylorus into the duodenum, by controlling gastric volumes, and by elevating the patient's head and shoulders.

During upper endoscopy, the nurse suctions the patient if necessary to avoid aspiration. The risk of aspiration is also reduced by performing the procedure with the patient on the left side, with the head tilted to the side to allow secretions to run out. Immediately after the procedure, the patient is encouraged to cough.

All nursing measures that are taken to prevent aspiration should be documented.

## CONVULSIONS

Convulsions may be associated with hypovolemia, hypotension, sedation, hyperventilation, hypoglycemia, or alcoholic withdrawal. When convulsions occur, it is important to prevent self-injury, maintain an adequate airway, administer oxygen by face mask (if cyanosis is present), and treat the causative condition.

## ANXIETY

Signs of an anxiety state may include the following:
- Feelings of panic or impending danger, tenseness, and restlessness
- Hyperactivity, tremor, perspiration, dry mouth, wringing of hands, tachycardia, and possibly hyperventilation
- Marked agitation or a full panic state
- Fear of death or disaster

Nurses and other staff members should calmly approach anxious patients, and should give patients reassurance and explanations about what to expect. Direct physical contact may be useful, such as holding the patient by the hand or arm.

---

**CASE SITUATION**

It is midnight on a Friday night. The gastroenterology nurse on call awakens upon hearing her beeper go off. She checks the number and calls the hospital. The Intensive Care Unit (ICU) informs the nurse that they have just admitted a John Doe who is vomiting bright red blood. Dr. Hamilton, the gastroenterologist on call, is on his way in and has requested that the nurse on call meet him as soon as possible in the ICU. She rushes to get dressed. While driving to the hospital, she goes over what she will need to do.

*Points to think about*

1. Because this is a new patient, the gastroenterology nurse has no history on which to rely and must think of all possible causes of upper GI bleeding that she may be able to treat endoscopically. What will she take to the bedside?
2. Because this patient is a John Doe, he is either too disoriented to provide his name or is unconscious and has no identification. If the patient is conscious, some quick questions might help the nurse assess possible problems. What would she ask?
3. Dr. Hamilton arrives, and together he and the nurse plan the course of action. He decides the nasogastric aspirate is clear enough to proceed and the nurse

prepares the patient for endoscopy. During the procedure the patient will be at risk for the serious complication of aspiration. How should the nurse address this issue?

4. Assessing the amount of blood lost is important when judging the amount of fluid needed to reverse volume depletion. What can the nurse learn from lab data about this?

5. What should the nurse know about how each body system responds to massive gastrointestinal bleeding?

6. John Doe's inability to provide his name and address leads the nurse to the nursing diagnosis "altered thought processes caused either by loss of consciousness or disorientation to time, place, and person." (Data have not been provided to determine whether this patient is unconscious or disoriented.) What are the seven areas of cognitive assessment in which a nurse ordinarily endeavors to obtain data for this diagnosis?

*Suggested responses*

1. The gastroenterology nurse might take the following equipment to the bedside:
   - At least two injector needles, with the sclerosant that Dr. Hamilton prefers, and banding equipment, if the physician uses that technique. The vomiting of bright red blood may indicate variceal bleeding.
   - Gastric lavage equipment (Ewald tube and large irrigating syringes). Large amounts of blood in the stomach make it difficult to visualize bleeding sites, and it is often difficult to get supply items from central service in the middle of the night.
   - The electrocautery device that the gastroenterology department uses (bipolar probe, heater probe, or cautery unit) and an extra probe. The laser can be used for gastrointestinal bleeding, but it usually cannot be transported to the ICU because of its specific electrical and plumbing needs. Late at night is not an optimal time to do emergency endoscopy in the gastroenterology unit because there are usually not enough personnel present to handle any complications that occur.
   - The usual sedatives and emergency drugs. The ICU may stock most things, but it is better to plan ahead as the pharmacy may not be open.
   - Cover gowns, protective eyewear, masks, and enough gloves for the gastroenterology nurse, the physician, and the ICU nurse, who may have to help you.
   - The largest channel gastroscope available or a double channel gastroscope. The nurse should ensure that equipment is checked and working properly before going to bedside.

2. If the nurse was able to ask John Doe some questions, she might ask the following:

   - Whether he has had a bleeding episode such as this before, or has been previously diagnosed or treated for ulcer disease. Recurrent ulcerations are common; however, in 40% of patients, the new bleeding will stem from a different lesion.
   - If he is allergic to any medication, and what medications he has been taking at home. Many patients forget about over-the-counter medications, and the nurse should specifically ask about aspirin, cold remedies, or ibuprofen (Advil, Nuprin, Motrin). Also, she should ask about specific anticoagulants, which may prolong bleeding time.
   - If he had vomiting of gastric contents before the onset of vomiting of blood. Forceful vomiting can cause a tear in the lower esophagus or gastric cardia, which can bleed profusely (Mallory-Weiss tear).
   - If he consumes much alcohol. Sometimes it helps to ask about specific quantities; that is, "Do you drink beer? If so, one or two six-packs a day?" "Do you drink vodka, whiskey or rum? If so, one or two pints a day?" If a family member is present, he or she may give more accurate information than the patient. Excessive alcohol consumption can cause gastritis or ulcers that bleed excessively. Alcoholic liver damage may be evident on physical examination (ascites, spider angiomata, enlarged liver, or gynecomastia). If liver damage is probable, you may suspect esophageal varices as a cause of bleeding. Clotting mechanisms would also be affected.
   - What the state of his general health is, with particular attention to cardiac, respiratory, or renal problems. Patients with concomitant health problems are at higher risk for complications.

3. To address the issue of the possibility of aspiration during endoscopy, the gastroenterology nurse can take the following precautions:
   - Recognize that all patients undergoing upper endoscopy are at risk of aspirating saliva, gastric secretions, and blood. Patients most at risk are those who have recently eaten a meal, those who have active upper GI bleeding, those with recent stroke, and those with pyloric obstruction and gastric retention.
   - Use a topical throat anesthetic sparingly, if at all. Local pharyngeal anesthesia interferes with swallowing and gag reflex and alters coordination of the pharynx and upper esophageal sphincter.
   - Minimize the use of sedative medications in patients at high risk for aspiration. IV conscious sedation causes depression of the respiratory system and CNS and can also suppress the laryngeal closure reflex for 5 to 10 minutes.
   - Keep the patient in the left lateral position until sedation wears off. Have adequate, working oral

suction available with Yankauer suction tips. Monitor the patient carefully throughout the procedure and during recovery, with special attention to color, blood pressure, secretions, and sensorium.

4. Loss of 10% to 25% of blood volume is considered a moderate bleed; over 25% is considered a massive bleed. The normal adult has a circulating blood volume of 75 ml/kg body weight. A man who weighs 154 lb (70 kg) will have about 5,250 ml of circulating blood volume; 20% of that is about 1 L. Therefore, if he loses a single liter, he will experience a moderate bleed, with a corresponding drop in blood pressure, rapid pulse, labored breathing, loss of sensorium, anxiety, or a feeling of impending doom.

The following physical and laboratory data can help assess the amount of blood loss:

- Blood pressure. Lying and standing blood pressures can help determine extent of shock and hypotension. If, on standing, the blood pressure falls 30 mm/Hg or more from baseline or the apical pulse rate increases 20 to 30 beats per minute, there is significant postural hypotension. If the patient is "shocky" in the recumbent position, he may already have lost more than 50% of his circulating volume.

- Hemoglobin and hematocrit. Hemoglobin and hematocrit levels are always done and may give an indication of the duration of hemorrhage, rather than provide information about the amount of acute blood loss. The patient can exsanguinate with a normal hemoglobin and hematocrit. It can take from 12 to 36 hours for hemoglobin and hematocrit values to drop in acute bleeding.

- Blood urea nitrogen (BUN). A BUN level above 40 mg (in patients without previous renal disease) indicates a significant bleed. Blood in the gut is partially digested and proteins are absorbed, which elevate BUN, and volume depletion produces a prerenal azotemia with consequent elevation of BUN.

- Coagulation studies. Coagulation studies are important because clotting factors will be used up quickly, and patients with underlying liver disease will have difficulty keeping up with the demand.

- Arterial blood gases (ABGs). ABGs should be drawn to check for lactic acidemia, which can occur as a result of severe tissue hypoxia because there is less blood carrying less oxygen to cells. Hypoperfusion causes potential complications to each body system as a result of hemorrhage.

5. The different body systems respond to massive gastrointestinal bleeding in the following ways:

- Cardiovascular system. The heart's workload increases during periods of hypovolemia and reduced tissue oxygenation. A diseased heart may not be able to provide the increased output needed to maintain adequate tissue perfusion. The heart itself needs a lot of blood and oxygen and can suffer from myocardial ischemia during gastrointestinal bleeding.

- Respiratory system. Hemorrhage can worsen preexisting pulmonary disease. Ventilation and perfusion may be impaired by white blood cells clumping in the lung's tiny blood vessels, and ARDS (adult respiratory distress syndrome) may result. This may occur 12 to 28 hours after hemorrhage; the ABGs should be watched.

- Hematologic system. Coagulation problems frequently occur following hemorrhage because the clotting factors are used more rapidly than they are produced.

- Renal system. Prolonged low renal blood flow causing hypoxia leads to renal failure. Acute tubular necrosis can occur when large myoglobin molecules in the bloodstream (released from other cells being destroyed) become lodged in tiny tubules. Watch for decreased urine output. The serum creatinine is a more reliable indication of kidney function than the BUN.

- Metabolic system. When the compensatory hormone regulation fails to maintain fluid and electrolyte concentrations, metabolic derangement can follow, including decreased serum pH (acidosis), decreased potassium (hypokalemia), increased sodium (hypernatremia), and serum hyperosmolality, which causes movement of fluid into the vascular space from the extravascular space to maintain circulating volume. This must be corrected.

6. The seven areas of cognitive assessment are as follows:
- Level of consciousness
- Orientation
- Memory
- Judgment/intellectual functioning
- Thought flow
- Thought content
- Perception

---

**REVIEW TERMS**

**anaphylaxis, aspiration, cardiac arrest, hemorrhage, hypovolemia, perforation, respiratory depression, shock, vasovagal syncope**

---

**REVIEW QUESTIONS**

1. Substernal or epigastric pain that increases with respirations and movement of the trunk is associated with perforation of what portion of the GI tract?
   a. Cervical esophagus.
   b. Thoracic esophagus.

c. Distal esophagus, near the diaphragm.
d. Stomach.

2. Conservative management of upper GI perforations may include:
   a. Suction.
   b. IV nutrition.
   c. Administration of antibiotics.
   d. All of the above.

3. Hematochezia is a symptom of:
   a. Bleeding esophageal varices.
   b. Bleeding ulcers.
   c. Gastritis.
   d. Lower GI bleeding.

4. In a patient with upper GI bleeding, if the return fluid from gastric lavage promptly becomes clear, the next step is to:
   a. Continue lavage.
   b. Remove the nasogastric tube.
   c. Use an Ewald tube to remove clots from the stomach.
   d. Begin balloon tamponade.

5. In patients suffering from hypovolemic shock, circulation to the heart and the brain initially:
   a. Increases.
   b. Decreases.
   c. Remains the same.
   d. Stops.

6. An important side effect of topical pharyngeal anesthesia is:
   a. Vomiting.
   b. Increased intraocular pressure.
   c. Allergic reactions.
   d. Superficial phlebitis.

7. When a patient experiences cardiac arrest, what is the first action the gastroenterology nurse should take?
   a. Call for help.
   b. Initiate CPR.
   c. Attach the patient to a monitoring device.
   d. Remove family members and visitors from the room.

8. What drug is used to reverse narcotic-induced respiratory depression?
   a. Physostigmine (Antilirium).
   b. Naloxone (Narcan).
   c. Meperidine (Demerol).
   d. Epinephrine.

9. To treat a vasovagal attack, it is important to:
   a. Offer fluids.
   b. Begin CPR.
   c. Position the patient with the head at the level of or below the rest of the body.
   d. Keep the patient warm.

10. To avoid aspiration during upper endoscopy, the nurse usually:
    a. Maintains the patient in the supine position.
    b. Encourages the patient to breathe deeply.
    c. Provides suction as necessary.
    d. Intubates the patient.

**BIBLIOGRAPHY**

Adams, J. "Emergencies in the Gastrointestinal Diagnostic Laboratory." *SGA Journal* 8(Fall 1985): 14-16.

Adams, J. "Emergencies in the GI Lab: The G.I.A. Role." Presented at the 14th Annual Meeting of the Society of Gastrointestinal Assistants, May 1986.

Barnhart, E, publisher. *Physicians' Desk Reference.* Oradell, N.J.: Medical Economics, 1990.

Eastwood, G, and Avunduk, C. *Manual of Gastroenterology: Diagnosis and Therapy.* Boston: Little, Brown & Co., 1988.

Gitnick, G, and Hollander, D, eds. *Principles and Practice of Gastroenterology and Hepatology.* New York: Elsevier, 1988.

Given, B, and Simmons, S. *Gastroenterology in Clinical Nursing.* 4th ed. St. Louis: Mosby–Year Book, 1984.

Goldberg, K, ed. *Gastrointestinal Problems.* Nurse Review Series. Springhouse, Pa.: Springhouse Corporation, 1986.

Hamilton, H, editorial director. *Procedures.* Nurse's Reference Library. Springhouse, Pa.: Intermed Communications, 1983.

Hardick, M, and Beck, M, eds. *Manual of Gastrointestinal Procedures.* 2nd ed. Rochester, N.Y.: Society of Gastroenterology Nurses and Associates, 1989.

Lobitz, J, and Katon, R. "Complications of Gastrointestinal Endoscopic Procedures: Incidence, Recognition and Management." In *Handbook of Gastrointestinal Emergencies,* ed. Gitnick, G, 325-97. Garden City, N.J.: Medical Examination Publishing, 1982.

McFarland, P, and McFarlane, J. "Cognitive and Perceptual Pattern, Altered Thought Processes." In *Nursing Diagnosis and Intervention,* 557-72. St. Louis: Mosby–Year Book, 1990.

Polizzi, A. "GI Unit Emergency—Postpolypectomy Bleeding." *SGA Journal* 10(Summer 1987): 16-17.

Silvis, S, ed. *Therapeutic Gastrointestinal Endoscopy.* New York: Igaku-Shoin, 1985.

Sivak, M. *Gastroenterologic Endoscopy.* Philadelphia: W.B. Saunders, 1987.

Sleisenger, M, and Fordtran, J, eds. *Gastrointestinal Disease: Pathophysiology, Diagnosis, Management.* 4th ed. Philadelphia: W.B. Saunders, 1989.

Surowiec, F. "Respiratory Arrest in the Endoscopy Suite." In *SGA Journal Reprints,* ed. Trivits, S, 213-15. Rochester, N.Y.: Society of Gastrointestinal Assistants, 1988.

# PREPARATION FOR CERTIFICATION

# Chapter 34

# STUDY SKILLS AND TEST TAKING

This chapter will provide gastroenterology nurses and associates with the information needed to prepare systematically for their certification examinations and to perform successfully on the day of the examination. Given in this chapter are suggestions on developing good study habits and formulating a study plan. Different types of learning activities are suggested, including tips on taking practice tests. A day-of-test checklist is offered, relaxation exercises are outlined, and basic strategies are described for approaching a multiple-choice examination. The information provided should help the gastroenterology nurse or associate achieve an optimal score on the certification examination.

**Learning objectives**

After reviewing the content of this chapter, the gastroenterology nurse should be able to:
1. Develop productive study habits and routines.
2. List the content areas that will be covered on the examination, identify gaps in existing knowledge or experience, and obtain the appropriate resource materials.
3. Set realistic goals for preparing for the examination.
4. Select several different types of learning activities that will help build the necessary knowledge base, including the use of practice tests.
5. Generate a day-of-test checklist to ensure adequate preparation for taking the examination.
6. Use relaxation exercises to reduce test anxiety and optimize performance on the day of the examination.
7. Apply test-taking strategies that will enhance performance on multiple-choice tests.

The certification examination is given in two disciplines; one for the gastroenterology registered nurse (CGRN) and one for licensed practical or vocational nurses (CGNs), technologists or technicians (CGTs), and other associates (CGAs). The examinations are developed, administered, and evaluated by the **Certifying Board of Gastroenterology Nurses and Associates, Inc.,** which is a volunteer, nonprofit organization of certified gastroenterology clinicians and physicians. The Certifying Board is also responsible for formulating and adopting requirements for eligibility for admission to the examination, certification of candidates who successfully complete the exam, and certification renewal.

Following are the objectives of **certification:**
- To provide recognition to individuals who meet the requirements for certification.
- To encourage continued professional growth.
- To establish a standard requisite knowledge base for gastroenterology nurses and associates, thereby enhancing the quality of care given to patients.
- To promote a high standard of competency among gastroenterology nurses and associates.

Completion of the certifying exam provides successful candidates with an opportunity to evaluate their professional abilities both for self-satisfaction and for peer recognition. It does not permit certified gastroenterology professionals to expand their scope of practice beyond the patient-care activities sanctioned by their state nurse practice acts, educational licensure, or the policies and procedures in the workplace.

Certification in gastroenterology is open to nurses and other healthcare professionals who are engaged in gastroenterology and gastrointestinal endoscopy. Candidates must have been employed in a clinical, educational, supervisory, administrative, or research capacity in institutional or private-practice settings for a minimum of 2 years full-time or its part-time equivalent of 4,000 hours within the past 5 years. Candidates should contact the headquarters of the Society of Gastronenterology Nurses and Associates (SGNA) regarding specific information about the examination.

## PREPARING FOR THE EXAMINATION

Every year a large number of registered nurses, licensed practical nurses, technologists, technicians, and associates take examinations for certification in their discipline. Once the decision has been made to take the certification examination in gastroenterology and the appropriate application forms and fees have been forwarded to the testing office, the next step is to prepare for the examination.

Certification in gastroenterology requires study and experience. Anyone considering certification must have at least 2 years of clinical experience in the field. There is no substitute for this hands-on experience.

Some amount of studying is also advisable. Gastroenterology is a diverse field, with many experts and many sources of information. For most people, it is best to start the review process several months before the examination. Only a few rare individuals can benefit from cramming in the final hours. Trying to learn large amounts of information in a short period of time only produces anxiety in most people. This study technique is not recommended. Instead, an organized, systematic review of the material over a period of several months is advised.

### Developing good study habits

Study habits vary from individual to individual; what works for one person may not work for another. For any individuals who have not studied in several years, it is a good idea to try to recall the study methods that worked well in the past.

The study process may require retraining one's attention span. To assess current concentration abilities and study habits, the following methods are suggested:

- Study alone in different settings (e.g., at home or in a library)
- Study with another person who is preparing for the examination
- Study with a group of peers who are also preparing for the examination

Individuals should try to determine the optimal study environment; that is, whether studying is easiest in a quiet, secluded setting or in a setting with music or other people close by. In addition, it is important to make sure reference materials are available in the preferred study setting, including current textbooks and journals. The development of good study habits will help meet learning goals and shorten study time. Considerations in regard to the development of good study habits include the following:

- Deciding before sitting down whether or not studying will occur
- Deciding the content to study and how long to spend on it
- Providing the necessary information
- Allowing for sufficient breaks, incorporating active pursuits that totally relax the mind from study content, such as jogging, bicycling, or gardening; knowing when breaks are needed and looking forward to them
- Planning study time so that reviewing information already learned takes place right before sleep
- Realizing that simply reading or memorizing is *not* studying
- Outlining the material and underlining major points to facilitate retention, being careful not to waste time by rewriting the content while outlining
- Putting facts into meaningful associations with gastroenterology nursing, continually asking what implications the material has
- Stopping when the limit for retention has been reached; failure to stop studying when the limit has been reached reinforces negative study habits
- Planning the next study time before putting away the books

Other important considerations are the place of study, the frequency and type of distractions that might be encountered, and the ability to deal with distractions. To facilitate studying, it may be helpful to conduct studying endeavors in the same room, at the same desk or table, and in a comfortable chair that is not conducive to relaxation and sleep. One special location that represents the location of study will facilitate getting started. If, on the other hand, distractions become frequent at the study location, it may be a good idea to change locations and start over.

The choice of study locations must be augmented with a knowledge of how to study. Many people complain of distractions while studying and inappropriately blame their poor study habits. Distractions are things that divert one's attention. They can be either external or internal. Following are some of the common **distractors** that contribute to poor concentration, fatigue, and the inability to study:

- Music or television
- Answering the telephone
- Voices of children, family, or friends
- Uncomfortable furniture or surroundings
- Hunger or thirst

All of these external and internal distractions need to be eliminated or tuned out for learning to take place. It may be helpful to study behind closed doors, turn on the telephone answering machine, and ask friends and family members to refrain from distracting. It is a good idea to choose a well-lit area with a comfortable (but not too comfortable) chair, and to eat lightly before studying is begun.

If studying in the presence of distractions, relatively simple material should be studied first. Once simple material is mastered under these circumstances, more complex material can be studied. Soon, the ability to block external stimuli, prevent internal distractions, and study under a variety of adverse circumstances will also be mastered.

## What to study

The subject matter of the 200 multiple-choice test items is derived from the role-delineation statements for gastroenterology nurses and associates. Appendix 1 lists these competency statements in full for each group. Basically, the certification tests for gastroenterology nurses and associates will cover the following:
- Professional and practice issues (10%)
- Anatomy, physiology, and pathology of the gastrointestinal system (15%)
- Patient care (15% for associates; 20% for RNs)
- Pharmacology and IV therapy (15% for associates; 20% for RNs)
- Gastrointestinal diagnostic and therapeutic instrumentation (30% for associates; 20% for RNs)
- Emergency situations (10%)
- Research (5%)

To determine the amount of preparation needed, it is important for each individual to assess his or her present knowledge base in these areas. For someone who has been in practice for several years, he or she undoubtedly has extensive knowledge and clinical skills. If experience has been concentrated in certain areas, an individual may need to broaden his or her knowledge base by using the following steps:
- Assess knowledge in each area of gastroenterology nursing by reviewing a current textbook. The individual should list those areas in which he or she feels confident in the knowledge base; areas in which he or she has some knowledge, but infrequent clinical practice; and areas in which his or her knowledge and clinical skills are limited.
- Assess knowledge of issues and trends in health care that impact gastroenterology nursing by reading professional journals and talking to peers.
- Review the role delineation statements presented in Appendix 1 to assess level of skill in various patient-care areas.

It is important to remember that knowledge is the basis for responding to the test questions, and test candidates will be required to draw on their individual knowledge base to evaluate practice situations that reflect various patient-care concerns. The natural way to obtain this knowledge is to study and review all of the areas in which it has been determined that there is a need to strengthen skills.

## Resources

In addition to reviewing the content of this **core curriculum,** there are a number of other ways to prepare for the certification exam.

A critical look at one's own job is a good method of preparation. The individual should list every step involved in daily activities and then ask, "*Why* do I do this?" "*What* do I need to know to do this right?" "*How* is this supposed to be done?" The individual who can correctly answer "why," "what," and "how" for each action that is a part of his or her daily practice has made an excellent beginning in preparing for the examination.

In addition to evaluating one's own scope of practice, it is important to broaden horizons to include unfamiliar techniques and disease entities. No one professional is familiar with every disorder and every procedure in the complex, varied field of gastroenterology.

Important educational resources include the following:
- The regulations of the official agencies that govern the practice of endoscopy and patient care, including the Joint Commission on Accreditation of Healthcare Organizations (JCAHO) and the Centers for Disease Control (CDC)
- The SGNA *Standards for Practice,* which are excellent guidelines for safe, ethical, and optimal care of the gastroenterology patient
- Hospital or institutional policies that affect aspects of gastroenterology practice
- Textbooks that pertain to the scope of practice of a gastroenterology professional, including a basic anatomy and physiology text
- Journal articles related to gastroenterology practice, especially SGNA's journal *Gastroenterology Nursing.* It is a good idea to read about unfamiliar techniques, diseases, or drugs, and articles on patient assessment, interviewing techniques, patient education, patient care planning, and research.
- The SGNA *Manual of Gastrointestinal Procedures,* second edition
- The SGNA monograph series, which provides in-depth information on documentation, infection control, quality assurance, conscious sedation, and other topics
- SGNA's two compilations of journal reprints
- The American Hospital Association's patient bill of rights
- Educational courses provided by SGNA
- Study groups

No one book or journal is used to write the examination questions, but the references used by individuals to write the test items are current, well-known, and widely available textbooks and journals.

## Setting goals

In arranging a study routine, it is important to begin to study several months before the exam. It is not advisable to cram! It is a good idea to schedule regular study sessions that match personal study habits. It is also important to be realistic in scheduling study sessions and in making a firm personal commitment to stay on schedule. Realistic goals for study time and amount of material to cover should be set. For example, it may work for some individuals to study emergency procedures on one evening and to review the principles of disinfection and sterilization for 2 hours on the next evening. Setting unrealistic goals can only result in frustration, and possibly failure in the future. There is more self-satisfaction in setting and reaching realistic goals.

It may be helpful to write a study guide that includes identified learning needs. Such a study guide should clearly delineate the areas of knowledge that need to be covered and then specific steps that will be taken to acquire this knowledge, including the use of study materials, in-service programs, and resource persons. It might include the following considerations:

- Knowledge needed
- Ways to obtain knowledge
- Where to obtain it
- Specific goals and objectives
- Sources available for obtaining knowledge
- An evaluation of progress

Careful attention to the development of detailed study guides has proven to be a very effective test preparation method.

## Learning activities

For those individuals who would like to further develop and refine study skills, it may be helpful to use some or all of the following learning activities:

- Update knowledge in familiar areas by reviewing current textbooks and journals.
- Concentrate on the areas in which knowledge is needed; arrange for study sessions and/or clinical practice with a gastroenterology colleague, if possible.
- Use flash cards to assist in memorization of factual information.
- To review information that is more theoretical or abstract, form study groups in which each member takes responsibility for preparing multiple-choice questions in a particular content area. These questions can be shared among study group members and can form the basis for a practice test.
- Use cassette tape recordings of sample questions and their responses. The tape can be listened to at leisure, not necessarily only during study time. For example, it might help to listen to the tape in the car on the way to work or on the way home. Several tapes could be created, in which questions and answers are categorized by content area.
- Practice deep muscle relaxation by simultaneously tensing and relaxing entire muscle groups. The following exercises will be helpful in this area:
  1. Curl both fists, tighten biceps and forearms. Relax.
  2. Wrinkle the forehead. Press the head as far back as possible. Roll the head clockwise in a circle. Reverse. Wrinkle up the facial muscles: frown and squint and purse the lips. Hunch the shoulders. Relax.
  3. Arch the back as far as possible. Take in a deep breath and hold it. Relax. Take another deep breath and press out the stomach. Hold the breath. Relax.
  4. Pull the feet and toes back.
  5. Tighten the leg muscles. Hold and then relax. Curl the toes, tighten the calves, thighs, and buttocks. Hold and relax.
- Use the following breathing exercise to improve concentration:
  1. Sit erect, feet together, hands at each side with palms up, touching the sides of the body.
  2. Take a slow, even, deep breath through the nose and visualize a warm, golden yellow energy being drawn in through the top of the head, then going through the rest of the body right down to the toes. Think of the yellow energy as knowledge.
  3. While slowly breathing out, visualize cool blue energy being drawn up through the soles of the feet and going out through the top of the head. Think of this as negative energy that robs you of your concentration.
  4. Continue breathing in and out and visualizing the flow of yellow and blue energy for 5 to 10 minutes until a state of mental energy is reached.
- Attend continuing education programs that are focused on identified learning needs.
- Talk to other nurses who have taken the exam. They can suggest areas for study and provide helpful hints.

## Practice tests

To become more familiar with the kinds of questions to be encountered on the examination, it is advisable to take as many practice tests as possible by using simulated test conditions. It is helpful to use a quiet room, an answer sheet similar to the one that will actually be used, sample test questions, and the allotted time limit for test completion. Rehearse the situation and imagine successful results. Identify aspects of the testing situation that may be troublesome (e.g., answering questions under a time limit) and work toward eliminating negative behaviors and attitudes.

Another suggestion is to review performance on the study questions at the end of each of the preceding chapters of this core curriculum. Focus test preparation review on those content areas in which scores were lowest. (It is important to recognize that these review questions are only samples; they are not psychometrically sound, nor has their reliability been established.)

When studying for the exam by using sample questions, learn from each wrong answer. Examine each response and determine the reason for missing the correct answer. Try using the following format for analyzing wrong answers:

- Type 1. Did not read the question carefully; missed details; or missed key words.
- Type 2. Assumed additional data not in question; "read into" the situation or case study.
- Type 3. Identified priorities incorrectly, confused major and minor points, or placed events in the wrong order of importance.
- Type 4. Did not know concepts or facts needed to answer the question, resulting from an information deficit or lack of a sufficient data base.

If it is discovered that there are many Type 1 errors, it is advisable to slow down, examine the questions more carefully, and double-check answers.

Type 2 errors indicate that more is being read into the situation than is warranted. This is a common type of error among nurses. In this instance, it is advisable to select an answer slowly and carefully.

Type 3 errors are frustrating. It is upsetting to realize that the wrong priorities are being selected. It is a good idea to ask oneself, "Which of these steps must be done before the others are completed?"

Type 4 errors will help identify those content areas in which further study is needed.

## TEST TAKING

On the day of the test, it is important to relax. Challenges are always anxiety-provoking. Although a small amount of anxiety is productive, too much anxiety will interfere with the ability to think carefully and rationally. It is counterproductive to cram the night before. The best thing to do is to get a good night's sleep and eat a normal breakfast. During the test, it is important to relax, read each question carefully, and use one's best judgment.

### Day-of-test-checklist

The following is a checklist of points to be considered during the 24-hour period immediately before the examination.

1. Use stress reduction methods, such as relaxation, deep breathing, or visualization.
2. Get adequate rest and sleep.
3. Avoid stimulants and tranquilizers.
4. Avoid eating a large meal or drinking an excessive amount of liquid on the morning of the test. A heavy meal may cause feelings of lethargy, and frequent trips to the restroom may disrupt concentration during the test.
5. Arrive early at the testing center. It is impossible to anticipate traffic or weather conditions that may hinder travel, so plan on reporting to the test center well before the scheduled starting time. All candidates should report to the test center 30 minutes before the scheduled starting time. Individuals who arrive after the reading of the examination instructions have begun will not be admitted to the test center. Arriving early will allow time to park the car, find the testing location, and calm oneself before the start of the exam.
6. Dress comfortably and appropriately.
7. Bring the following materials to the testing center:
   - The admission card, which will contain the test date and address, including the location of the testing room
   - Several well-sharpened #2 pencils and a good eraser
   - Two forms of identification, at least one of which contains a picture
   - A watch
   - A nonprogrammable silent calculator that does not require an electrical outlet
     NOTE: No reference materials or visitors are permitted in the examination room.
8. Before the test date, review directions and instructions in detail. Candidates have been denied entrance after the test has begun or have even shown up on the wrong day because instructions were not read carefully.

### Relaxation

Most adults find paper-and-pencil tests anxiety-producing. The words *test, quiz,* and *examination* immediately call forth unpleasant memories for most of us. This frame of mind ultimately diminishes test performance.

It is an unfortunate fact of human physiology that when a person becomes distressed, the higher thinking processes, such as memory, logical thinking, reasoning, idea production, and decision making, tend to suffer. The nervous activation of the brain, combined with the increased flow of stress hormones, tends to cause whole portions of the brain to shut down mental activities. This means that complex mental tasks, such as answering exam questions, may be much more difficult for the individual than normal problem-solving situations.

Try the following breathing exercise immediately before beginning the examination:
1. Sit up straight.
2. Breathe out deeply, letting the air rush out of the lungs.
3. Do not think about inhaling; let the air come in naturally.
4. Repeat four to six times.

It may also be helpful to repeat the following affirmations before beginning the examination:
- "There is nothing to worry about. I'm going to be all right."
- "I know I can answer each and every one of these questions."
- "I'll jump right in and be all right. It's easier once I get started."

Once the exam has begun, repeat the following:
- "Take it step by step; don't rush."
- "I can do this. I'm doing it now. I can only do my best."
- "Relax! Breathe deeply. There's an end to it."

Knowing how feelings can affect thinking is important. Recognizing that any intense feelings, such as anger or the anxiety and frustration of taking a test, may alter critical thinking ability is often the first step to successful exam taking.

### During the test

Once the examination period has begun, it is important to give the test supervisor undivided attention. He or she will read instructions that describe the correct method for completing the answer sheet, and will be giving other information pertinent to the testing situation. If any aspects of the instructions are not understood, it is advisable to ask for clarification before the testing period begins. Test supervisors and proctors are instructed to answer only questions about testing procedures. They cannot respond to inquiries regarding test content.

The examination will be composed of 200 multiple-choice questions developed by the Certifying Board. Each test item consists of a **stem** (a question or incomplete statement) and four multiple-choice answers. Each item must be a clear and concise statement with bibliographic verification. New procedures and/or medications must be in general practice a minimum of 2 years before they can be addressed by test items on the examination.

The four responses listed for the multiple-choice questions always consist of one correct or best response and three incorrect responses. The correct or best response is called the "key" to the item. Candidates are credited with one point for each "keyed" or correct response that they select and no points for each "nonkeyed" response. A candidate's total score on the test is determined by the number of questions which are answered correctly. There is no penalty for guessing. It is not to the candidate's advantage to leave questions unanswered.

When considering an individual test item, remember the following general guidelines:
- There is only one correct answer for each question.
- Each question has a stem and four possible answers: one correct response and three others that are referred to as distractors. Each distractor is designed to seem reasonable if the correct answer is not known. If the correct response is known, distractors should appear less correct. Eliminate unlikely, implausible distractors first. If the correct answer is not known, it is a good idea to reason carefully and make an educated guess. There is no penalty for a wrong answer on this examination.
- If a question seems unfair, one should not get angry; anger will only detract from thinking abilities.
- It is advisable to refrain from panicking if a correct answer is not known. Try to examine the answers carefully and make a selection among the alternatives.
- Choose the answer that matches the question in scope: a general question should have a general answer, while a specific question should have a response that is specific.
- Select the answer that addresses the question, not one that is merely correct in itself.

The following steps should be included in overall test-taking strategy:
- Read each stem carefully, paying particular attention to words and phrases such as *major, most likely, primary, except, most appropriate,* and *not.* Such words often provide strong clues in relation to the correctness or incorrectness of a particular response.
- After reading the stem, try to answer the question or complete the statement mentally before reading the printed responses. Covering the responses to each item in the test booklet with the answer sheet may help to answer the item before reading the responses.
- After deciding on an answer to the question, uncover the printed responses and carefully read each of the four multiple-choice items before recording the selection on the answer sheet. Even if you think the first or second choice is the correct one, the third or fourth response may be a better answer to the question. Select the response that is closest in meaning to the answer. Record this response in the appropriate place on the answer sheet.
- Some items may be difficult to answer, or it may be that the responses listed don't correspond to the

test taker's own answers to such items. If this is the case and there is still uncertainty, leave this question's answer space blank and proceed to the next question.

- Another suggestion is to begin by answering the questions that you are sure about. After answering all of these questions, answer the questions that were troublesome the first time around. This strategy will help avoid spending too much time on any one question.
- To keep track of items left unanswered, circle the numbers of those questions in the test booklet so they can be easily identified. When skipping a particular question, be sure to skip the corresponding space on the answer sheet.
- Once finished with all of the questions that were easy to answer, go back to the troublesome ones. Reread these questions and try to eliminate the responses that may be incorrect. Place an "X" next to these incorrect responses in the test booklet.
- After identifying all of the responses that may be incorrect for a question, choose the best answer from among the remaining responses. Record the selection in the appropriate space on the answer sheet, and then proceed to the next item that was initially left unanswered. Repeat this process until every item on the test has been answered.

    NOTE: It is to the test taker's advantage to answer all items on the exam. The consequence of selecting an incorrect response or of not responding to an item is the same: no points are given for the item. Therefore, if unsure of an answer, it is better to select the best response to the item, rather than to leave the question unanswered.
- Monitor progress throughout the testing period. Consider the number of items in relation to the total amount of time provided for the examination. Work through the test at an even pace; do not fall behind by spending too much time on a difficult item. Remember, each item on the exam carries the same point value.
- If time remains after completing the exam, it is advisable to go back and check the work. Make sure all responses have been recorded on the answer sheet; all items on the test have been answered; only one response to each item has been indicated; all responses that have been changed have been completely erased. Make sure there are no stray pencil marks on the answer sheet.

Approximately 8 weeks after the examination, candidates will be notified of their scores. Initial certification will be valid for 5 years. Certification renewal will be by examination or continuing education credits from an approved provider.

REVIEW TERMS

**certification, Certifying Board of Gastroenterology Nurses and Associates, Inc., core curriculum, distractors, stem**

SAMPLE QUESTIONS

The following questions are actual sample test items from previous certification examinations. Although these specific questions will not appear on future examinations, they may be considered representative examples of the types of items that will be encountered.

1. In which of the following countries did endoscopy originate?
   a. United States.
   b. England.
   c. Germany.
   d. Japan.
2. Reports that document untoward incidents or procedural complications are necessary in order to:
   a. Identify trends that require changes in practice.
   b. Monitor physician competence.
   c. Identify morbidity outcome.
   d. Provide the basis for legal documentation.
3. The following statements about the role of saliva in digestion are correct *except:*
   a. It produces amylase.
   b. It lubricates food.
   c. It promotes hydrolysis of starch.
   d. It stimulates the taste buds.
4. In ulcerative colitis, the *most frequent* site of free perforation is the:
   a. Transverse colon.
   b. Sigmoid colon.
   c. Right colon.
   d. Cecum.
5. During endoscopy, the *primary* responsibility of the RN/associate is to:
   a. Assist the physician.
   b. Handle biopsy specimens.
   c. Monitor the patient's condition.
   d. Check equipment function.
6. Long-term treatment of the patient with esophageal varices should focus on:
   a. Mandatory attendance at Al-Anon meetings by the patient's family.
   b. Life-style changes, emphasizing total abstinence from alcohol.
   c. Elimination of all activities that could encourage alcohol consumption.
   d. Mandatory weekly attendance at Alcoholics Anonymous (AA) meetings.
7. The type of jaundice that is the result of a common bile duct stone is:

a. Hemolytic.
b. Pancreatic.
c. Obstructive.
d. Hepatocellular.

8. Which of the following emergency drugs reverses the actions of narcotics?
   a. Lidocaine hydrochloride (Xylocaine).
   b. Isoproterenol hydrochloride (Isuprel).
   c. Norepinephrine bitartrate (Levophed bitartrate).
   d. Naloxone hydrochloride (Narcan).

9. The risk of infection from endogenous organisms and from organisms contaminating the equipment is *greatest* during:
   a. Liver biopsy.
   b. Colonoscopy.
   c. Gastroscopy without biopsy.
   d. Esophageal bougienage.

10. The primary accessory in endoscopic extraction of a sharp foreign body is:
    a. Administer general anesthesia.
    b. The use of an overtube.
    c. The use of alligator-type forceps.
    d. The use of basket-type forceps.

11. For a patient who has active upper GI bleeding, the RN/associate's priority is to:
    a. Maintain an airway.
    b. Establish a peripheral IV line.
    c. Monitor vital signs.
    d. Remove blood from the stomach.

12. A 59-year-old male is admitted to the emergency room complaining of weakness, shortness of breath, and perspiration, and is vomiting blood clots. He is admitted to the intermediate-care unit for treatment of massive bleeding. The next step will be:
    a. Treating hypovolemia.
    b. Providing exercise.
    c. Monitoring arrhythmias.
    d. Restriction of fluids.

13. In starting a drug study, the following would be the *last* step to take:
    a. Review the literature.
    b. Purchase materials.
    c. Write a protocol.
    c. Obtain funds if necessary.

14. In research, the point on a distribution above and below which 50% of the cases fall is called the:
    a. Range.
    b. Median.
    c. Mode.
    d. Mean.

## BIBLIOGRAPHY

Certifying Board of Gastroenterology Nurses and Associates. *Role Delineation for Gastroenterology Associates.* NY, NY:CBGNA, 1990.

Certifying Board of Gastroenterology Nurses and Associates. *Role Delineation for Gastroenterology RNs.* NY, NY: CBGNA, 1990.

Certifying Council for Gastroenterology Clinicians. *Certification Examination for Gastroenterology Nurses and Associates: Handbook for Candidates.* New York: Professional Examination Service, 1990.

Connelly, N. "Certification: A Study Primer Covering the Basics." *Gastroenterology Nursing* 12(Fall 1989): 141-46.

Gruber, M. "Certification: How Do I Prepare? What Do I Study?" In *SGA Journal Reprints,* ed. Trivits, S, 5-6. Rochester, N.Y.: Society of Gastrointestinal Assistants, 1988.

Gruber, M. "Certifying Council for Gastroenterology Clinicians, Inc.: Questions and Answers." *SGA Journal* 10(Summer 1987): 48.

Kneedler, J, ed. *CNOR Study Guide.* Denver: National Certification Board: Perioperative Nursing, 1990.

# Answers to Review Questions

**Chapter 1**
1. C
2. A
3. B
4. A
5. D
6. B
7. B
8. C
9. A
10. A

**Chapter 2**
1. B
2. C
3. A
4. B
5. D
6. B
7. C
8. B
9. C
10. D

**Chapter 3**
1. B
2. B
3. B
4. A
5. D
6. A
7. C
8. B
9. B
10. C

**Chapter 4**
1. A
2. B
3. D
4. D
5. B
6. C
7. B
8. A
9. D
10. D

**Chapter 5**
1. D
2. C
3. C
4. D
5. C
6. A
7. B
8. B
9. D
10. B

**Chapter 6**
1. C
2. D
3. D
4. A
5. D
6. B
7. A
8. B
9. B
10. A

**Chapter 7**
1. A
2. B
3. B
4. D
5. C
6. C
7. B
8. B
9. A
10. C

**Chapter 8**
1. A
2. D
3. D
4. B
5. D
6. C
7. A
8. C
9. C
10. C

**Chapter 9**
1. C
2. B
3. C
4. D
5. A
6. C
7. B
8. C
9. B
10. A

**Chapter 10**
1. D
2. B
3. B
4. A
5. C
6. B
7. A
8. C
9. D
10. A

**Chapter 11**
1. A
2. D
3. D
4. A
5. D
6. C
7. C
8. C
9. A
10. C

**Chapter 12**
1. A
2. C
3. D
4. D
5. C
6. B
7. D
8. A
9. D
10. B

**Chapter 13**
1. A
2. D
3. C
4. C
5. A
6. B
7. B
8. D
9. C
10. A

**Chapter 14**
1. B
2. C
3. D
4. A
5. A
6. C
7. D
8. C
9. A
10. C

**Chapter 15**
1. A
2. C
3. B
4. C
5. B
6. A
7. A
8. D
9. C
10. C

**Chapter 16**
1. C
2. B
3. C
4. C
5. D
6. B
7. A
8. B
9. D
10. C

**Chapter 17**
1. B
2. A
3. D
4. B
5. D
6. B
7. C
8. C
9. B
10. D

**Chapter 18**
1. B
2. B
3. C
4. D
5. C
6. B
7. A
8. C
9. C
10. A

## Chapter 20

1. B
2. C
3. A
4. D
5. D
6. A
7. A
8. B
9. C
10. D

## Chapter 21

1. B
2. A
3. C
4. C
5. A
6. B
7. A
8. A
9. B
10. A

## Chapter 22

1. C
2. B
3. A
4. B
5. B
6. A
7. C
8. A
9. B
10. B

## Chapter 23

1. B
2. D
3. A
4. A
5. A
6. B
7. D
8. C
9. D
10. B

## Chapter 24

1. C
2. B
3. D
4. C
5. A
6. B
7. D
8. B
9. A
10. C

## Chapter 25

1. B
2. B
3. C
4. D
5. A
6. C
7. A
8. B
9. D
10. C

## Chapter 26

1. D
2. B
3. C
4. C
5. A
6. A
7. D
8. B
9. C
10. A

## Chapter 27

1. B
2. C
3. A
4. C
5. D
6. D
7. B
8. A
9. A
10. C

## Chapter 28

1. D
2. A
3. C
4. A
5. C
6. D
7. C
8. A
9. B
10. C

## Chapter 29

1. B
2. C
3. A
4. B
5. D
6. A
7. C
8. A
9. B
10. A

**Chapter 30**
1. D
2. D
3. B
4. A
5. B
6. C
7. A
8. B
9. A
10. D

**Chapter 31**
1. B
2. A
3. A
4. C
5. C
6. B
7. A
8. C
9. C
10. D

**Chapter 32**
1. C
2. B
3. B
4. B
5. D
6. B
7. A

8. C
9. C
10. D

**Chapter 33**
1. B
2. D
3. D
4. B
5. A
6. C
7. A
8. B
9. C
10. C

**Chapter 34**
1. C
2. A
3. A
4. B
5. C
6. B
7. C
8. D
9. B
10. B
11. A
12. A
13. B
14. B

# *Appendix*

The Certifying Board of Gastroenterology Nurses and Associates in conjunction with Professional Examination Service (PES) and members-at-large of the Society of Gastroenterology Nurses and Associates have developed the following role delineations for gastroenterology nurses and associates. The purpose of these statements is to define expected behaviors of the gastroenterology nurse and associate and to form the basis for the certification examinations. The general areas of knowledge required of the nurse and associate are similar, but the depth of knowledge tested is proportional to the level of expertise required for the performance of each role.

## ROLE DELINEATION FOR GASTROENTEROLOGY REGISTERED NURSES
### MARCH 1990
### Subject I. Professional and practice issues (10%)

**Master Competency 01**
The GRN will be knowledgeable about professional and practice issues related to the field of gastroenterology.

**Competency 0101**
The GRN will be knowledgeable about the history of gastroenterology/GI endoscopy.

**Competency 0102**
The GRN will be knowledgeable about principles of basic management pertinent to operating the GI unit, e.g., scheduling, record keeping, etc.

**Competency 0103**
The GRN will be knowledgeable about the standards of practice as set forth by SGNA, JCAHO, CDC, etc.

**Competency 0104**
The GRN will be knowledgeable about ethical, professional and legal standards inherent in patient care and professional conduct, e.g., patient Bill of Rights, advocate's role, those actions considered to be patient abuse, etc.

**Competency 0105**
The GRN will be knowledgeable about the quality assurance process.

### Subject II. Anatomy, physiology and pathology of the GI system (15%)
**Master Competency 02**
The GRN will distinguish between normal and abnormal GI anatomy, physiology, pathology, histology and microbiology, as well as those alterations which may be imposed by congenital anomaly and/or surgical intervention.

**Competency 0201**
The GRN will distinguish normal and abnormal structure and function of the esophagus or distortions thereof which may be naturally imposed through congenital anomaly or artificially imposed through surgical intervention.

    Knowledge required:
    k-1 Anatomy
        A. Gross structure
        B. Histology
    k-2 Physiology
        A. Motility
    k-3 Pathophysiology and microbiology
        A. Disease/disorder mechanism
        B. Signs and symptoms
        C. Related diagnostic examination
        D. Therapeutic interventions and their effects
        E. Effects of other normal or abnormal organ systems on the esophagus
    k-4 Alterations of structure imposed
        A. Congenital anomaly
        B. Surgical intervention
        C. Trauma
        D. Developmental defects

**Competency 0202**
The GRN will distinguish normal and abnormal structure and function of the stomach or distortions thereof which may be naturally imposed through congenital anomaly or artificially imposed through surgical intervention.

    Knowledge required:
    k-1 Anatomy
        A. Gross structure

B. Histology
k-2 Physiology
  A. Motility
  B. Secretion
  C. Absorption
k-3 Pathophysiology and microbiology
  A. Disease/disorder microbiology
  B. Signs and symptoms
  C. Related diagnostic examination
  D. Therapeutic interventions and their effects
  E. Effects of other normal or abnormal organ systems on the stomach
k-4 Alterations of structure imposed
  A. Congenital anomaly
  B. Surgical intervention
  C. Trauma
  D. Developmental defects

## Competency 0203

The GRN will distinguish normal and abnormal structure and function of the small bowel or distortions thereof which may be naturally imposed through congenital anomaly or artificially imposed through surgical intervention.

Knowledge required:
k-1 Anatomy
  A. Gross structure
  B. Histology
k-2 Physiology
  A. Motility
  B. Secretion
  C. Absorption
k-3 Pathophysiology and microbiology
  A. Disease disorder mechanism
  B. Signs and symptoms
  C. Related diagnostic examination
  D. Therapeutic interventions and their effects
  E. Effects of other normal or abnormal organ systems on the small bowel
k-4 Alterations of structure imposed
  A. Congenital anomaly
  B. Surgical intervention
  C. Trauma
  D. Developmental defects

## Competency 0204

The GRN will distinguish normal and abnormal structure and function of the large bowel or distortions thereof which may be naturally imposed through congenital anomaly or artificially imposed through surgical intervention.

Knowledge required:
k-1 Anatomy
  A. Gross structure
  B. Histology
k-2 Physiology

  A. Motility
  B. Secretion
  C. Absorption
k-3 Pathophysiology and microbiology
  A. Disease/disorder mechanism
  B. Signs and symptoms
  C. Related diagnostic examination
  D. Therapeutic interventions and their effects
  E. Effects of other normal and abnormal organ systems on the large bowel
k-4 Alterations of structure imposed
  A. Congenital anomaly
  B. Surgical intervention
  C. Trauma
  D. Developmental defects

## Competency 0205

The GRN will distinguish normal and abnormal structure and function of the gallbladder and extrahepatic biliary system or distortions thereof which may be naturally imposed through congenital anomaly or artificially imposed through surgical intervention.

Knowledge required:
k-1 Anatomy
  A. Gross structure
  B. Histology
k-2 Physiology
  A. Motility
  B. Secretion
k-3 Pathophysiology
  A. Disease/disorder mechanism
  B. Signs and symptoms
  C. Related diagnostic examination
  D. Therapeutic interventions and their effects
  E. Effects of other normal or abnormal organ systems on the gallbladder and extrahepatic biliary system
k-4 Alterations of structure imposed
  A. Congenital anomaly
  B. Surgical intervention
  C. Trauma
  D. Developmental anomalies

## Competency 0206

The GRN will distinguish normal and abnormal structure and function of the pancreas or distortions thereof which may be naturally imposed through congenital anomaly or artificially imposed through surgical intervention.

Knowledge required:
k-1 Anatomy
  A. Gross structure
  B. Histology
k-2 Physiology
  A. Secretion

1. Endocrine
2. Exocrine

k-3 Pathophysiology
  A. Disease/disorder mechanism
  B. Signs and symptoms
  C. Related diagnostic examination
  D. Therapeutic interventions and their effects
  E. Effects of other normal and abnormal organ systems on the pancreas

k-4 Alterations of structure imposed
  A. Congenital anomaly
  B. Surgical intervention
  C. Trauma
  D. Developmental defects

## Competency 0207

The GRN will distinguish normal and abnormal structure and function of the liver or distortions thereof which may be naturally imposed through congenital anomaly or artificially imposed through surgical intervention.

  Knowledge required:

k-1 Anatomy
  A. Gross structure
  B. Histology

k-2 Physiology
  A. Metabolism
  B. Secretion
  C. Absorption

k-3 Pathophysiology and microbiology
  A. Disease/disorder mechanism
  B. Signs and symptoms
  C. Related diagnostic examination
  D. Therapeutic interventions and their effects
  E. Effects of other normal or abnormal organ systems on the liver

k-4 Alterations of structure imposed
  A. Congenital anomaly
  B. Surgical intervention
  C. Trauma
  D. Developmental defects

## Subject III. Patient care (20%)

## Master Competency 03

The GRN will formulate a plan of care that will include assessments, prioritizations and interventions which are implemented and documented.

## Competency 0301

The GRN will perform an objective and subjective assessment.

  Knowledge required:

k-1 Health history
  A. General health
  B. Medical/surgical history
  C. Medication history
  D. Present medical complaints
  E. Allergies

  F. Preparation compliance

k-2 Physical exam
  A. Observation, e.g., skin color, temperature, vital signs, general behavior
  B. Auscultation, e.g., of heart, lungs, abdomen
  C. Palpation

## Competency 0302

The GRN will utilize the nursing process to develop and implement a plan of care.

  Knowledge required:

k-1 Nursing diagnosis
k-2 Pre-, intra-, postprocedure care
k-3 Potential problems
k-4 Therapeutic interventions
k-5 Expected outcomes
k-6 Evaluations
k-7 Patient and family teaching
k-8 Documentation

## Subject IV. Pharmacology and IV. therapy (20%)

## Master Competency 04

The GRN will have knowledge of pharmacology and I.V. therapy.

  Knowledge required:

k-1 Techniques and routes of administration
k-2 Indications and contraindications
k-3 Signs and symptoms of adverse reactions
k-4 Expected actions
k-5 Dosage calculations
k-6 Patient education
k-7 Documentation

## Competency 0401

The GRN will have knowledge of diagnostic, therapeutic and emergency medications.

  Knowledge required:

k-1 Techniques and routes of administration
k-2 Indications and contraindications
k-3 Signs and symptoms of adverse reactions
k-4 Expected actions
k-5 Dosage calculations
k-6 Patient education
k-7 Documentation

## Competency 0402

The GRN will have knowledge of IV medications used in the GI lab.

  Knowledge required:

k-1 Techniques and routes of administration
k-2 Indications and contraindications
k-3 Signs and symptoms of adverse reactions
k-4 Expected actions
k-5 Dosage calculations
k-6 Patient education
k-7 Documentation

**Competency 0403**

The GRN will have knowledge of transfusion of blood and blood products.

Knowledge required:

k-1 Techniques and routes of administration

k-2 Indications and contraindications

k-3 Signs and symptoms of adverse reactions

k-4 Expected actions

k-5 Patient education

k-6 Documentation

**Competency 0404**

The GRN will have knowledge of antibiotic prophylaxis

Knowledge required:

k-1 Techniques and routes of administration

k-2 Indications and contraindications

k-3 Signs and symptoms of adverse reactions

k-4 Expected actions

k-5 Dosage calculations

k-6 Patient education

k-7 Documentation

**Competency 0405**

The GRN will have knowledge of electrolyte, colloid and other I.V. solutions.

Knowledge required:

k-1 Techniques and routes of administration

k-2 Indications and contraindications

k-3 Signs and symptoms of adverse reactions

k-4 Expected actions

k-5 Dosage calculations

k-6 Patient education

k-7 Documentation

**Competency 0406**

The GRN will have knowledge of enteral and parenteral nutritional therapy.

Knowledge required:

k-1 Techniques and routes of administration

k-2 Indications and contraindications

k-3 Signs and symptoms of adverse reactions

k-4 Expected actions

k-5 Dosage calculations

k-6 Patient education

k-7 Documentation

k-8 Care of central lines

**Subject V. GI diagnostic and therapeutic instrumentation (20%)**

**Master Competency 05**

The GRN will have knowledge of GI diagnostic and therapeutic modalities.

**Competency 0501**

The GRN will assist with diagnostic and therapeutic endoscopic procedures.

Knowledge required:

k-1 Indications/contraindications

k-2 Potential complications

k-3 Patient care and teaching

k-4 Documentation

k-5 Capabilities and limitations of equipment

k-6 Cleaning/disinfection/sterilization and storage of equipment

k-7 Repair and maintenance of equipment

k-8 Required safety measures

k-9 Specimen collection and handling

**Competency 0502**

The GRN will perform or assist the physician with manometric procedures.

Knowledge required:

k-1 Indications/contraindications

k-2 Potential complications

k-3 Patient care and teaching

k-4 Documentation

k-5 Capabilities and limitations of equipment

k-6 Cleaning/disinfection/sterilization and storage of equipment

k-7 Repair and maintenance of equipment

k-8 Required safety measures

**Competency 0503**

The GRN will perform or assist the physician in the performance of nonendoscopic specimen collection and will administer patient care specific to procedure.

Knowledge required:

k-1 Indications/contraindications

k-2 Potential complications

k-3 Patient care and teaching

k-4 Documentation

k-5 Capabilities and limitations of equipment

k-6 Cleaning/disinfection/sterilization and storage of equipment

k-7 Repair and maintenance of equipment

k-8 Required safety measures

k-9 Specimen collection and handling

**Competency 0504**

The GRN will assist in the performance of esophageal dilatation.

Knowledge required:

k-1 Indications/contraindications

k-2 Potential complications

k-3 Patient care and teaching

k-4 Documentation

k-5 Capabilities and limitations of equipment

k-6 Cleaning/disinfection/sterilization and storage of equipment

k-7 Repair and maintenance of equipment

k-8 Required safety measures

**Competency 0505**

The GRN will perform or assist in the performance of secretory studies and GI tests.

Knowledge required:

k-1 Indications/contraindications

k-2 Potential complications

k-3 Patient care and teaching
k-4 Documentation
k-5 Capabilities and limitations of equipment
k-6 Cleaning/disinfection/sterilization and storage of equipment
k-7 Repair and maintenance of equipment
k-8 Required safety measures
k-9 Specimen collection and handling

## Competency 0506
The GRN will have knowledge of related GI diagnostic studies, e.g., contrast X-rays, nuclear scans, etc.

## Subject IV. Emergency situations (10%)

## Master Competency 06
The GRN will recognize life-threatening situations and respond appropriately.
    Knowledge required:
    k-1 Observation and monitoring of patients
    k-2 Emergency procedures
    k-3 Subjective and objective assessment
    k-4 Acute care interventions

## Competency 0601
The GRN will recognize signs and symptoms of vasovagal reaction and respond appropriately.

## Competency 0602
The GRN will recognize respiratory depression and will respond appropriately.

## Competency 0603
The GRN will recognize signs and symptoms of adverse drug reactions, including anaphylaxis, and will respond appropriately.

## Competency 0604
The GRN will recognize signs and symptoms of hemorrhage and respond appropriately.

## Competency 0605
The GRN will recognize signs and symptoms of aspiration and will respond appropriately.

## Competency 0606
The GRN will recognize signs and symptoms of procedural and spontaneous perforations and will respond appropriately.

## Competency 0607
The GRN will recognize signs and symptoms of shock and respond appropriately.

## Competency 0608
The GRN will recognize signs and symptoms of cardiopulmonary arrest and respond appropriately.

## Subject VII. Research (5%)

## Master Competency 07
The GRN will be knowledgeable about the basic research process.
    Knowledge required:

k-1 Basic terminology of research design, e.g., double-blind, random sampling, placebo effect, hypothesis, null hypothesis, dependent variable, independent variable, etc.
k-2 Elementary data analysis, e.g., measures of central tendency, dispersion, etc.

## ROLE DELINEATION FOR GASTROENTEROLOGY ASSOCIATES
## APRIL 1990
## Subject I. Professional and practice issues (10%)

## Master Competency 01
The GA will be knowledgeable about professional and practice issues related to the field of gastroenterology.

## Competency 0101
The GA will be knowledgeable about the history of gastroenterology/GI endoscopy.

## Competency 0102
The GA will be knowledgeable about principles of basic management pertinent to operating the GI unit, e.g., scheduling, record keeping.

## Competency 0103
The GA will be knowledgeable about the standards of practice as set forth by SGNA, JCAHO, CDC, etc.

## Competency 0104
The GA will be knowledgeable about ethical, professional, and legal standards inherent in patient care and professional conduct, e.g., patients' Bill of Rights, advocates' role, those actions considered to be patient abuse.

## Competency 0105
The GA will be knowledgeable about the quality assurance process.

## Subject II. Anatomy, physiology, and pathology of the GI system (15%)

## Master Competency 02
The GA will distinguish between normal and abnormal GI anatomy, physiology, pathology, histology, and microbiology, as well as those alterations which may be imposed by congenital anomaly and/or surgical intervention.

## Competency 0201
The GA will distinguish normal and abnormal structure and function of the esophagus or distortions thereof which may be naturally imposed through congenital anomaly or artificially imposed through surgical intervention.
    Knowledge required:
    k-1 Anatomy
        A. Gross structure
        B. Histology
    k-2 Physiology
        A. Motility

k-3 Pathophysiology and microbiology
  A. Disease/disorder mechanism
  B. Signs and symptoms
  C. Related diagnostic examination
  D. Therapeutic interventions and their effects
  E. Effects of other normal or abnormal organ systems on the esophagus
k-4 Alterations of structure imposed
  A. Congenital anomaly
  B. Surgical intervention
  C. Trauma
  D. Developmental defects

**Competency 0202**

The GA will distinguish normal and abnormal structure and function of the stomach or distortions thereof which may be naturally imposed through congenital anomaly or artificially imposed through surgical intervention.

  Knowledge required:
  k-1 Anatomy
    A. Gross structure
    B. Histology
  k-2 Physiology
    A. Motility
    B. Secretion
    C. Absorption
  k-3 Pathophysiology and microbiology
    A. Disease/disorder mechanism
    B. Signs and symptoms
    C. Related diagnostic examination
    D. Therapeutic interventions and their effects
    E. Effects of other normal or abnormal organ systems on the stomach
  k-4 Alterations of structure imposed
    A. Congenital anomaly
    B. Surgical intervention
    C. Trauma
    D. Developmental defects

**Competency 0203**

The GA will distinguish normal and abnormal structure and function of the small bowel or distortions thereof which may be naturally imposed through congenital anomaly or artificially imposed through surgical intervention.

  Knowledge required:
  k-1 Anatomy
    A. Gross structure
    B. Histology
  k-2 Physiology
    A. Motility
    B. Secretion
    C. Absorption
  k-3 Pathophysiology and microbiology
    A. Disease/disorder mechanism

B. Signs and symptoms
C. Related diagnostic examination
D. Therapeutic interventions and their effects
E. Effects of other normal or abnormal organ systems on the small bowel
k-4 Alterations of structure imposed
  A. Congenital anomaly
  B. Surgical intervention
  C. Trauma
  D. Developmental defects

**Competency 0204**

The GA will distinguish normal and abnormal structure and function of the large bowel or distortions thereof which may be naturally imposed through congenital anomaly or artificially imposed through surgical intervention.

  Knowledge required:
  k-1 Anatomy
    A. Gross structure
    B. Histology
  k-2 Physiology
    A. Motility
    B. Secretion
    C. Absorption
  k-3 Pathophysiology and microbiology
    A. Disease/disorder mechanism
    B. Signs and symptoms
    C. Related diagnostic examination
    D. Therapeutic interventions and their effects
    E. Effects of other normal and abnormal organ systems on the large bowel
  k-4 Alterations of structure imposed
    A. Congenital anomaly
    B. Surgical intervention
    C. Trauma
    D. Developmental defects

**Competency 0205**

The GA will distinguish normal and abnormal structure and function of the gallbladder and extrahepatic system or distortions thereof which may be naturally imposed through congenital anomaly or artificially imposed through surgical intervention.

  Knowledge required:
  k-1 Anatomy
    A. Gross structure
    B. Histology
  k-2 Physiology
    A. Motility
    B. Secretion
  k-3 Pathophysiology
    A. Disease/disorder mechanism
    B. Signs and symptoms
    C. Related diagnostic examination
    D. Therapeutic interventions and their effects

E. Effects of other normal or abnormal organ systems on the gallbladder and extrahepatic biliary system

k-4 Alterations of structure imposed
   A. Congenital anomaly
   B. Surgical intervention
   C. Trauma
   D. Developmental anomalies

## Competency 0206

The GA will distinguish normal and abnormal structure and function of the pancreas or distortions thereof which may be naturally imposed through congenital anomaly or artificially imposed through surgical intervention.

Knowledge required:
k-1 Anatomy
   A. Gross structure
   B. Histology
k-2 Physiology
   A. Secretion
      1. Endocrine
      2. Exocrine
k-3 Pathophysiology
   A. Disease/disorder mechanism
   B. Signs and symptoms
   C. Related diagnostic examination
   D. Therapeutic interventions and their effects
   E. Effects of other normal or abnormal organ systems on the pancreas
k-4 Alterations of structure imposed
   A. Congenital anomaly
   B. Surgical intervention
   C. Trauma
   D. Developmental defects

## Competency 0207

The GA will distinguish normal and abnormal structure and function of the liver or distortions thereof which may be naturally imposed through congenital anomaly or artificially imposed through surgical intervention.

Knowledge required:
k-1 Anatomy
   A. Gross structure
   B. Histology
k-2 Physiology
   A. Metabolism
   B. Secretion
   C. Absorption
k-3 Pathophysiology and microbiology
   A. Disease/disorder mechanism
   B. Signs and symptoms
   C. Related diagnostic examination
   D. Therapeutic interventions and their effects
   E. Effects of other normal or abnormal organ systems on the liver

k-4 Alterations of structure imposed
   A. Congenital anomaly
   B. Surgical intervention
   C. Trauma
   D. Develomental defects

## Subject III. Patient care (15%)

### Master Competency 03

The GA will implement a plan of care that includes assessment, observation, intervention and documentation.

## Competency 0301

The GA will perform an objective assessment.
   Knowledge required:
   k-1 Health history
      A. General health
      B. Medical/surgical history
      C. Medication history
      D. Present medical complaints
      E. Allergies
      F. Preparation compliance
   k-2 Observation, e.g., skin color, temperature, vital signs, general behavior

## Competency 0302

The GA will provide preprocedure, intraprocedure and postprocedure care.
   Knowledge required:
   k-1 Observation
   k-2 Monitoring
   k-3 Intervention
   k-4 Patient and family teaching
   k-5 Documentation

## Subject IV. Pharmacology and I.V. therapy (15%)

### Master Competency 04

The GA will have basic knowledge of pharmacology and I.V. therapy.
   Knowledge required:
   k-1 Routes of administration
   k-2 Indications and contraindications
   k-3 Signs and symptoms of adverse reactions
   k-4 Expected actions
   k-5 Patient education
   k-6 Documentation

## Competency 0401

The GA will have basic knowledge of diagnostic, therapeutic, and emergency medications.
   Knowledge required:
   k-1 Routes of administration
   k-2 Indications and contraindications
   k-3 Signs and symptoms of adverse reactions
   k-4 Expected actions
   k-5 Patient education
   k-6 Documentation

**Competency 0402**

The GA will have basic knowledge of I.V. medications and solutions used in the GI laboratory.

Knowledge required:
- k-1 Routes of administration
- k-2 Indications and contraindications
- k-3 Signs and symptoms of adverse reactions
- k-4 Expected actions
- k-5 Patient education
- k-6 Documentation

**Competency 0403**

The GA will recognize signs and symptoms of transfusion reactions and respond appropriately.

Knowledge required:
- k-1 Indications and contraindications
- k-2 Signs and symptoms of adverse reactions
- k-3 Expected actions
- k-4 Patient education
- k-5 Documentation

**Competency 0404**

The GA will have basic knowledge of indications for antibiotic prophylaxis.

Knowledge required:
- k-1 Routes of administration
- k-2 Indications and contraindications
- k-3 Signs and symptoms of adverse reactions
- k-4 Expected actions
- k-5 Patient education
- k-6 Documentation

**Subject V. GI diagnostic and therapeutic instrumentation (30%)**

**Master Competency 05**

The GA will have knowledge of GI diagnostic and therapeutic modalities.

**Competency 0501**

The GA will assist with diagnostic and therapeutic endoscopic procedures.

Knowledge required:
- k-1 Indications and contraindications
- k-2 Potential complications
- k-3 Patient care and teaching
- k-4 Documentation
- k-5 Capabilities and limitations of equipment
- k-6 Cleaning/disinfection/sterilization and storage of equipment
- k-7 Repair and maintenance of equipment
- k-8 Required safety measures
- k-9 Specimen collection and handling

**Competency 0502**

The GA will perform or assist the physician with manometric procedures.

Knowledge required:
- k-1 Indications/contraindications

- k-2 Potential complications
- k-3 Patient care and teaching
- k-4 Documentation
- k-5 Capabilities and limitations of equipment
- k-6 Cleaning/disinfection/sterilization and storage of equipment
- k-7 Repair and maintenance of equipment
- k-8 Required safety measures

**Competency 0503**

The GA will perform or assist the physician in the performance of nonendoscopic specimen collection and will administer patient care specific to the procedure.

Knowledge required:
- k-1 Indications/contraindications
- k-2 Potential complications
- k-3 Patient care and teaching
- k-4 Documentation
- k-5 Capabilities and limitations of equipment
- k-6 Cleaning/disinfection/sterilization and storage of equipment
- k-7 Repair and maintenance of equipment
- k-8 Required safety measures
- k-9 Specimen collection and handling

**Competency 0504**

The GA will assist in the performance of esophageal dilatation.

Knowledge required:
- k-1 Indications/contraindications
- k-2 Potential complications
- k-3 Patient care and teaching
- k-4 Documentation
- k-5 Capabilities and limitations of equipment
- k-6 Cleaning/disinfection/sterilization and storage of equipment
- k-7 Repair and maintenance of equipment
- k-8 Required safety measures

**Competency 0505**

The GA will perform—or assist in the performance of—secretory studies and GI tests.

Knowledge required:
- k-1 Indications/contraindications
- k-2 Potential complications
- k-3 Patient care and teaching
- k-4 Documentation
- k-5 Capabilities and limitations of equipment
- k-6 Cleaning/disinfection/sterilization and storage of equipment
- k-7 Repair and maintenance of equipment
- k-8 Required safety measures
- k-9 Specimen collection and handling

**Competency 0506**

The GA will have knowledge of related GI diagnostic studies, e.g., contrast X-rays, nuclear scans.

**Subject VI. Emergency situations (10%)**

**Master Competency 06**
The GA will recognize life-threatening situations and will respond appropriately.
　Knowledge required:
　k-1 Observation and monitoring of patients
　k-2 Emergency procedures

**Competency 0601**
The GA will recognize signs and symptoms of vasovagal reaction and will respond appropriately.

**Competency 0602**
The GA will recognize respiratory depression and will respond appropriately.

**Competency 0603**
The GA will recognize signs and symptoms of adverse drug reactions, including anaphylaxis, and will respond appropriately.

**Competency 0604**
The GA will recognize signs and symptoms of hemorrhage and will respond appropriately.

**Competency 0605**
The GA will recognize signs and symptoms of aspiration and will respond appropriately.

**Competency 0606**
The GA will recognize signs and symptoms of procedural and spontaneous perforation and will respond appropriately.

**Competency 0607**
The GA will recognize signs and symptoms of shock and will respond appropriately.

**Competency 0608**
The GA will recognize signs and symptoms of cardiopulmonary arrest and will respond appropriately.

**Subject VII. Research (5%)**

**Master Competency 07**
　Knowledge required:
　k-1 Basic terminology of research design: double-blind, random sampling, placebo effect, hypothesis, null hypothesis, population, sample, experimental group, control group, variable, dependent variable, independent variable, etc.
　k-2 Elementary data analysis: measures of central tendency, dispersion, etc.

# Glossary

*abetalipoproteinemia.* A hereditary syndrome characterized by a lack of beta-lipoproteins in the blood, acanthocytosis, hypocholesterolemia, progressive ataxic neuropathy, atypical retinitis pigmentosa, and malabsorption.

*achalasia.* A combined defect of absent peristalsis of the esophageal body and elevated lower esophageal sphincter pressure.

*achlorhydria.* Absence of free hydrochloric acid in the stomach. May be caused by gastric cancer, ulcer, pernicious anemia, adrenal insufficiency, or chronic gastritis.

*acinus.* A small saclike dilatation, especially a functional unit of the liver, which is supplied by terminal branches of the portal vein and the hepatic artery, and drained by a terminal branch of the bile duct.

*activated partial thromboplastin time.* A measure of the rapidity of blood clotting, which examines Factors I, II, V, VIII, IX, X, XI, and XII.

*actual health problem.* A health condition that is identified as presently causing some difficulty for the patient.

*adenomatous polyp.* A benign polypoid adenoma.

*advocacy.* The act of speaking or writing in support of another or in protection of another's rights.

*Alagille's syndrome.* See **Intrahepatic Biliary Dysplasia.**

*α1-antitrypsin deficiency.* Lack of a plasma protein that is produced in the liver.

*ambulatory pH monitoring.* A 24-hour test that records fluctuations in esophageal pH and correlates them with symptoms of esophageal reflux.

*amebiasis.* The state of being infected with **Entamoeba histolytica.**

*American dilator.* One of a series of radiopaque, tapered, polyvinyl dilators that are passed over a guidewire for the purpose of widening a gastrointestinal lumen.

*American Nurses' Association (ANA).* A professional society for nursing in the United States.

*amino acid.* A class of organic compounds containing an amino group and a carboxyl group. Amino acids form the chief structural components of proteins and several are essential in human nutrition.

*ampulla of Vater.* The dilatation formed by the junction of the common bile duct and the pancreatic duct proximal to their opening into the duodenum.

*anabolism.* Any constructive process by which simple substances are converted by living cells into more complex compounds, especially into living matter.

*anaphylaxis.* An unusual or exaggerated allergic reaction to a foreign protein or other substance.

*anemia.* A reduction below normal in the number of erythrocytes. See also **pernicious anemia.**

*anesthetic.* A drug or agent used to abolish the sensation of pain, particularly before surgery or other painful procedures.

*angiography.* The roentgenographic visualization of blood vessels following introduction of contrast material.

*annular pancreas.* A developmental anomaly in which the pancreas forms a ring entirely surrounding the duodenum.

*anorexia.* Lack or loss of appetite for food.

*anoscopy.* Examination of the anus and lower rectum using a specially designed speculum.

*antacid.* A substance that counteracts or neutralizes acidity, usually gastric acidity.

*antibiotic.* An agent that inhibits the growth of or kills microorganisms, used in the treatment of infectious diseases.

*anticholinergic.* An agent that blocks the parasympathetic nerves.

*antidiarrheal.* An agent that combats abnormally frequent and liquid fecal discharges.

*antiemetic.* An agent that prevents or alleviates nausea and vomiting.

*antiflatulent.* An agent that disperses or prevents the formation of air or gas pockets in the gastrointestinal tract.

*antifungal.* An agent that is destructive to fungi, suppresses their growth or reproduction, or is effective against fungal infections.

*antrum.* The constricted, elongated, lower portion of the stomach.

*anus.* The terminal orifice of the gastrointestinal tract.

*argon.* An inert gas that is used in lasers.

*arteriography.* Roentgenography of an artery after injection of a contrast medium.

*ascending colon.* The portion of the large intestine

between the cecum and the right colic (hepatic) flexure.

*ascites*. The effusion and accumulation of serous fluid in the abdominal cavity.

*aspiration*. (1) The act of inhaling, including the accidental inhalation of solids or liquids; (2) the removal of fluids or gases from a cavity by the application of suction. See also **fine-needle aspiration.**

*aspiration biopsy*. A biopsy in which the tissue is obtained by the application of suction through a needle attached to a syringe.

*assessment*. Continuous, systematic collection, validation, and communication of patient data for the purpose of planning, implementing, and evaluating nursing care directed toward the attainment of specific patient outcomes.

*atresia*. Congenital absence or closure of a normal body orifice or tubular organ.

*audit*. A review of documentation for the purpose of determining whether or not specific objectives were met (i.e., patient goals were achieved, nursing standards of care were met, or structural or environmental criteria were attained) during the period of time outlined in a goal or standard. See also **concurrent audit, nursing audit,** and **retrospective audit.**

*Auerbach's plexus*. The part of the enteric plexus that is within the muscularis. Also called the myenteric plexus.

*authority*. The legal or rightful power to command or act.

*balloon tamponade*. Esophageal-gastric tamponade, involving exertion of pressure against bleeding esophageal varices by inflation of esophageal and usually gastric balloons.

*barbed stent*. A stent with projections or "barbs" at each end that result from a diagonal cut in the stent wall and serve to hold the stent in place.

*barium enema*. A suspension of barium that is injected into the rectum and retained in the intestines during roentgenologic examination. Also called a contrast enema.

*barium sulfate*. A bulky, fine, white powder without odor or taste, and free from grittiness, which is used as a contrast medium in roentgenography of the digestive tract.

*barium swallow*. Ingestion of a thick barium solution for the purpose of radiographic examination of the esophagus.

*Barrett's esophagus*. Replacement of the normal squamous epithelium of the esophagus by columnar epithelium.

*Bernstein test*. Attempted simulation of noncardiac chest pain by instillation of hydrochloric acid through one of the ports of a manometry catheter or a nasogastric tube that is positioned in the esophagus.

*bezoar*. A concretion of foreign material that builds up in the stomach.

*bile*. An alkaline golden brown to greenish-yellow fluid that is secreted by the liver and poured into the small intestine via the bile ducts. Important constituents include conjugated bile salts, cholesterol, phospholipid, bilirubin diglucuronide, and electrolytes.

*biliary colic*. Paroxysms of pain and other severe symptoms resulting from the passage of gallstones along the bile duct.

*biopsy*. The removal and examination, usually microscopic, of tissue from the living body, performed to establish a precise diagnosis. See also **aspiration biopsy, percutaneous liver biopsy,** and **suction biopsy.**

*biopsy forceps*. An instrument that can be passed through the biopsy channel of an endoscope for the purpose of excising pieces of living tissue from a suspected pathologic site. See also **hot biopsy forceps.**

*bipolar electrocoagulation*. An electrocoagulation method in which the electrical current flows between two small electrodes on the tip of the probe, both of which are in contact with the target tissue.

*bipolar probe*. A specialized bipolar hemostatic probe that is inserted through the instrument channel of an endoscope.

*body*. The largest and most important part of the stomach, lying between the fundus and the antrum.

*borborygmi*. Rumbling noises caused by the propulsion of gas through the intestines.

*bougie*. A slender, flexible, cylindrical instrument for introduction into a tubular organ, usually for the purpose of calibrating or dilating a constricted area. See also **Hurst bougie** and **Maloney bougie.**

*bougienage*. The passage of a slender, flexible cylindrical instrument into a tubular organ to dilate a stricture.

*Brunner's gland*. A tubulo-alveolar gland in the submucosa of the duodenum, which opens into a crypt of Lieberkühn.

*candidiasis*. Infection with a fungus of the genus *Candida*.

*cannula*. A tube for insertion into a duct or cavity; sometimes passed over a guidewire.

*carbohydrate*. An aldehyde or ketone derivative of a polyhydric alcohol; the hydrogen and oxygen are usually in the proportion to form water. The most important carbohydrates are the starches, sugars, celluloses, and gums.

*cardia*. The portion of the stomach surrounding the esophagogastric junction, which contains cardiac glands but lacks parietal and chief cells.

*cardiac arrest*. Sudden cessation of cardiac function, with disappearance of arterial blood pressure, connoting either ventricular fibrillation or ventricular standstill.

*cardiac gland*. A gland located distal to the esophagogastric junction which secretes mucus and pepsinogens.

*cardiac sphincter*. See **lower esophageal sphincter.**

*carey capsule*. A specially designed capsule that is inserted into the small bowel over a guidewire for the purpose of obtaining a biopsy specimen.

*catabolism*. Any destructive process by which complex substances are converted by living cells into more simple compounds.

*cathartic*. An agent that causes evacuation of the bowels by increasing bulk (bulk cathartic), stimulating peristaltic action (stimulant cathartic), softening the feces and reducing friction between them and the intestinal wall (lubricant cathartic), or increasing fluidity of the intestinal contents by retention of water by osmotic forces and indirectly increasing motor activity (saline cathartic).

*catheter*. A tubular, flexible surgical instrument for withdrawing fluids from, or introducing fluids into, a cavity of the body. See also **nasobiliary catheter (NBC), solid-state catheter,** and **water-infusion catheter.**

*cecum*. The first part of the large intestine, forming a dilated pouch into which open the ileum, the colon, and the vermiform appendix.

*celestin dilator*. A stepped dilator that is passed over an endoscopically placed guidewire for the purpose of widening a gastrointestinal lumen.

*celiac sprue*. A malabsorption syndrome affecting both children and adults, precipitated by the ingestion of gluten-containing foods. Pathologically, the proximal intestinal mucosa loses its villous structure, surface epithelial cells exhibit degenerative changes, and their absorptive function is severely impaired.

*cell*. Any one of the minute protoplasmic masses that make up organized tissue, consisting of a nucleus surrounded by cytoplasm which contains the various organelles and is enclosed in the cell or plasma membrane. A cell is the fundamental structural and functional unit of living organisms. See also **chief cell, enterochromaffin cell, g-cell, goblet cell, Kupffer cell, oxyntic cell, paneth's cell, parietal cell, red blood cell, white blood cell,** and **zymogen cell.**

*Centers for Disease Control (CDC)*. The federal public health agency within the Public Health Service that investigates specific disease outbreaks and formulates general guidelines for disease control.

*central tendency*. The grouping or score that occurs with the greatest frequency, used in describing a mass of data.

*certification*. The process by which a nongovernmental agency or association grants recognition to an individual who has met certain qualifications that have been predetermined by that agency or association.

*Certifying Board of Gastroenterology Nurses and Associates, Inc*. A volunteer, nonprofit organization of gastrointestinal clinicians and physicians formed for the purpose of testing the knowledge, understanding, and skill of practitioners engaged in the field of gastroenterology and endoscopy.

*chief cell*. A cell located in the parietal glands of the stomach; chief cells secrete pepsinogens.

*cholangiogram*. A roentgenogram of the gallbladder and bile ducts, following intravenous injection of contrast medium. See also **percutaneous transhepatic cholangiogram.**

*cholangitis*. An inflammation of a bile duct. See also **primary sclerosing cholangitis.**

*cholecystitis*. Inflammation of the gallbladder.

*cholecystokinin*. A polypeptide hormone secreted by the mucosa of the upper small bowel, which stimulates contraction of the gallbladder (with release of bile) and secretion of pancreatic enzymes.

*choledocholithiasis*. The presence of gallstones in the common bile duct.

*cholelithiasis*. The presence or formation of gallstones.

*cholestasis*. Stoppage or suppression of the flow of bile, having either intrahepatic or extrahepatic causes.

*cholinergic*. Stimulated, activated or transmitted by choline (acetylcholine); a term applied to nerve fibers that liberate acetylcholine at a synapse when a nerve impulse passes; an agent that produces such effects.

*chyme*. A relatively homogeneous semiliquid combination of food and digestive juices found in the stomach and small bowel.

*cirrhosis*. A liver disease characterized pathologically by loss of the normal microscopic lobular architecture, with fibrosis and nodular regeneration.

*coagulating current*. An electric current that is applied for the purpose of coagulating tissue.

*coagulation*. The process of clot formation; in surgery, the disruption of tissue by physical means to form an amorphous residuum, as in electrocoagulation and photocoagulation.

*colitis*. Inflammation of the colon. See also **Crohn's colitis, ischemic colitis, pseudo-membranous colitis,** and **ulcerative colitis.**

*collaborative diagnosis*. Statements of actual or potential health problems which occur from complications of disease, diagnostic studies, or therapeutic procedures, for which the nurse identifies a need to work with other members of the healthcare team toward resolution. See also **medical diagnosis; nursing diagnosis.**

*colloid*. A state of matter made up of very small, insoluble, nondiffusible particles that remain in suspension in a dispersion medium. The particles in a colloid are larger than ordinary crystalloid molecules, but are not large enough to settle out under the influence of gravity. See also **crystalloid.**

*colon.* The part of the large intestine that extends from the cecum to the rectum. See also **ascending colon, descending colon, sigmoid colon,** and **transverse colon.**

*colonoscopy.* Endoscopic examination of the colon.

*common bile duct.* The duct formed by the union of the cystic duct and the hepatic duct.

*comparison group.* A group of subjects whose scores on a dependent variable are used as the basis for evaluating the scores of an experimental group or the group of primary interest. "Comparison group" is used rather than "control group" when the investigation does not use a true experimental design. See also **control group.**

*computed tomography.* The process of moving an x-ray source in one direction as the film is moved in the opposite direction, thus showing in detail a predetermined plane of tissue while blurring or eliminating detail in other planes. The emergent x-ray beam is measured by a scintillation counter and the electronic impulses are recorded on a magnetic disk, then processed by a minicomputer for reconstruction display of the body in cross-section on a cathode-ray tube. Also called a CT scan.

*concurrent audit.* An evaluation of nursing care and patient outcomes performed while the patient is receiving care. It is performed by using direct observation of nursing care, patient interview, and/or chart review.

*constipation.* Infrequent or difficult evacuation of feces; passage of unduly hard or dry fecal material.

*consultation.* A meeting of two or more professionals to exchange ideas concerning patient care or to seek advice, instruction, or information.

*contrast roentgenography.* Roentgenography performed after the administration of a contrast medium, often barium sulfate, which facilitates interpretation of the film by accentuating differences in the densities of different regions and structures.

*control group.* The subjects not receiving an experimental treatment or intervention, whose performance provides a baseline against which the effects of the treatment can be measured. See also **comparison group.**

*corticosteroid.* Any of the steroids elaborated by the adrenal cortex (excluding sex hormones of adrenal origin) in response to the release of corticotropin by the pituitary gland, or any of the synthetic equivalents of these steroids.

*counseling.* The act of rendering short-term, long-term, or motivational guidance to a patient/significant other, an act which may involve the patient in problem solving.

*criterion.* A measurable quality, attribute, behavior, or characteristic that specifies a skill, knowledge, or

health state that is met at the point a health goal is achieved.

*critical item.* An instrument or object that is introduced directly into the bloodstream or into other normally sterile areas of the body.

*Crohn's colitis.* Crohn's disease, confined to the colon.

*Crohn's disease.* A chronic granulomatous inflammatory disease involving any part of the GI tract, but commonly involving the terminal ileum, with scarring and thickening of the bowel wall. It frequently leads to intestinal obstruction and fistula and abscess formation and has a high rate of recurrence after treatment. Also known as regional enteritis.

*cryoprecipitate.* Any one of a group of serum proteins, including factors VIII, XIII, and fibrinogen, that settle out of solution at temperatures below 20° C.

*crypt of Lieberkühn.* A simple tubular gland in the mucous membrane of the intestine, opening between the bases of the villi and containing argentaffin cells.

*crystalloid.* A substance that, in solution, passes readily through animal membranes, lowers the freezing point of the solvent containing it, and is generally capable of being crystallized. See also **colloid.**

*culture.* The propagation of microorganisms or of living tissue cells in special media conducive to their growth.

*Curling's ulcer.* A stress ulcer that appears in patients with serious burn injuries.

*Cushing's ulcer.* A stress ulcer that appears in patients with intracranial trauma.

*cutting current.* An electrical current applied for the purpose of dissection or fulguration.

*cystic duct.* The passage connecting the neck of the gallbladder and the common bile duct.

*cystic fibrosis.* A hereditary disorder of infants, children, and young adults, in which there is widespread dysfunction of the exocrine glands. It is characterized by signs of chronic pulmonary disease caused by excess mucus production in the respiratory tract, pancreatic deficiency, abnormally high levels of electrolytes in the sweat, and occasionally by biliary cirrhosis.

*cytology.* The study of cells, their origins, structure, function, and pathology. See also **exfoliative cytology.**

*cytology brush.* A sheathed, disposable brush that can be passed through the biopsy channel of an endoscope for the purpose of obtaining specimens for microscopic examination.

*data.* The material or collection of facts upon which a discussion or an inference is based. See also **objective data** and **subjective data.**

*data base.* A foundation of subjective and objective patient information which enables the design and implementation of a comprehensive and effective plan of care.

*decompression*. The removal of pressure, as in the removal of excess gas from the intestinal tract.

*decontamination*. The removal of gross soils and the reduction of the number of microorganisms to the point where an item may be considered safe for handling.

*dependent intervention*. Nursing action performed under the supervision or direction of a physician.

*dependent variable*. . A concept capable of taking on different values whose value is affected by, or determined by, other variables.

*descending colon*. The portion of the colon between the splenic flexure and the sigmoid colon at the pelvic brim.

*desiccation*. The act of drying up, especially the treatment of a tumor or other disease by drying up the part by the application of laser or electrical energy.

*dextrose*. D-Glucose monohydrate. A monosaccharide that occurs as colorless crystals or as a white, crystalline or granular powder; used chiefly as a fluid and nutrient replenisher, usually administered by IV infusion. Also used as a diuretic and alone or in combination with other agents for other clinical purposes.

*diaphragmatic hiatus*. An opening in the diaphragm where the esophagus enters the abdominal cavity.

*diarrhea*. Abnormally frequent and liquid fecal discharges.

*diffuse esophageal spasm*. Repetitive, prolonged simultaneous contractions along the length of the esophagus, with intermittent normal peristalsis.

*dilator*. An instrument that is used to enlarge an orifice or canal by stretching. See also **American dilator, celestin dilator, Eder-Puestow dilator, Savary-Gilliard dilator, Bougie-Hurst dilator, and Maloney dilator.**

*disaccharide*. Any of a class of sugars that yield two monosaccharides on hydrolysis and have the general formula

$$C_n(H_2O)_{n-1}.$$

*disinfection*. A physical or chemical process that kills or destroys most pathogenic microorganisms, but rarely kills all spores.

*distractor*. One of the incorrect responses listed on a multiple-choice test question; distractors are designed to seem plausible if one does not know the answer to the question.

*diverticulitis*. Inflammation of a diverticulum, especially inflammation related to colonic diverticula, which may undergo perforation with abscess formation.

*diverticulosis*. The presence of diverticula, particularly colonic diverticula, in the absence of inflammation.

*diverticulum*. An outpouching of one or more layers of the wall of a tubular organ. See also **Meckel's diverticulum.**

*documentation*. The act of collecting, abstracting, and coding of patient data and therapeutic processes for the purposes of communicating patient care, supplying a supporting reference concerning the status or progress of a patient, and archiving evidence of care rendered.

*double-blind*. An experiment in which neither subjects nor investigators are aware of which subjects are in the experimental group and which subjects are in the control group.

*double-contrast roentgenography*. Mucosal relief roentgenography; involves injection and evacuation of a barium enema, followed by inflation of the intestine with air under light pressure. The light coating of barium on the walls of the inflated intestine in the roentgenogram clearly reveals even small abnormalities.

*duct*. A passage with well-defined walls, especially a tube for the passage of excretions or secretions. See also **common bile duct, cystic duct, duct of Santorini, duct of Wirsung,** and **hepatic duct.**

*duct of Santorini*. The minor pancreatic duct, draining a part of the head of the pancreas into the minor duodenal papilla.

*duct of Wirsung*. Pancreatic duct; the main excretory duct of the pancreas, which usually unites with the common bile duct before entering the duodenum at the major duodenal papilla (papilla of Vater).

*dumping syndrome*. A group of disabling symptoms associated with rapid gastric emptying that mimic the symptoms of hypoglycemia.

*duodenum*. The first, or proximal, portion of the small bowel, extending from the pylorus to the jejunum.

*dyspepsia*. Impairment of the power or function of digestion, usually applied to epigastric discomfort following meals.

*dysphagia*. A sensation of difficulty in swallowing.

*D5W*. Five percent dextrose in water; given as an intravenous solution

*Eder-Puestow dilator*. One of a graduated series of metal olives that is screwed onto a semiflexible metal wand and passed over a guidewire for the purpose of widening a gastrointestinal lumen.

*edrophonium chloride*. Tensilon; a cholinesterase inhibitor that is administered by IV bolus in a provocative test designed to reproduce noncardiac chest pain caused by esophageal dysmotility.

*electrocautery*. An instrument used to destroy tissue, using an electrical current.

*electrocoagulation*. Coagulation of tissue, using either a monopolar or a bipolar electrical current. See also **bipolar electrocoagulation** and **monopolar electrocoagulation.**

*electrolyte*. A substance that dissociates into ions when fused or in solution and thus becomes capable of conducting electricity.

*electrosurgical unit (ESU)*. An apparatus for cutting or coagulating tissue, using a high-frequency electrical current.

*endoscopic retrograde cholangiopancreatography (ERCP)*. An endoscopic technique for radiologic visualization of the biliary and/or pancreatic ducts.

*endoscopic variceal ligation (EVL)*. The endoscopic introduction of rubber bands or O-rings for the treatment of bleeding varices.

*endoscopy*. Visual inspection of any cavity of the body by means of an endoscope.

*enema*. A liquid injected into the rectum. See also **barium enema.**

*enteral nutrition*. Administration of a prescribed diet by means of a flexible tube inserted into the stomach or small bowel either transnasally, surgically, or endoscopically.

*enteric plexus*. A plexus of autonomic nerve fibers within the wall of the digestive tube, and made up of the submucosal, myenteric, and subserosal plexuses.

*enteritis*. Inflammation of the intestine, especially of the small bowel. See also **radiation enteritis** and **regional enteritis.**

*enterochromaffin cell*. A basal granular cell whose granules stain readily with silver and chromium salts and which is a site of synthesis and storage of serotonin; includes argentaffin cells and agyrophilic cells.

*enteroclysis*. The injection of a nutrient or a medicinal liquid into the bowel.

*enterocolitis*. Inflammation involving both the small bowel and the colon.

*Environmental Protection Agency (EPA)*. The federal agency that, among other things, approves products for disinfectant registration by review of labeling and supporting data submitted by the registrants.

*erythrocyte*. A red blood cell; one of the elements found in peripheral blood; normally, in humans, the mature form is a nonnucleated, yellowish, biconcave disk, adapted, by virtue of its configuration and its hemoglobin content, to transport oxygen.

*esophageal reflux*. Reflux of gastric or duodenal contents back into the esophagus.

*esophageal rings and webs*. Thin, circumferential mucosal shelves appearing in the esophagus. See also **schatzki ring.**

*esophagitis*. An inflammation of the esophageal mucosa.

*esophagogastroduodenoscopy (EGD)*. Endoscopic examination of the esophagus, stomach, and duodenum.

*esophagus*. The musculomembranous tubular portion of the GI tract that extends from the pharynx to the stomach.

*ethylene oxide*. A colorless, flammable gas used to sterilize instruments.

*evaluative statement*. A statement defining an actual outcome; for example, skills developed, knowledge obtained, or change in health status.

*exfoliative cytology*. Microscopic examination of cells desquamated from the body surface or a lesion as a means of detecting malignancy and microbiologic changes, to measure hormonal levels, etc. Cells may be obtained by such procedures as aspiration, washing, smears, and scraping, and the technique may be applied to vaginal secretions, sputum, urine, abdominal fluid, prostatic secretions, etc.

*experimental group*. The subjects receiving an experimental treatment or intervention.

*familial polyposis*. Multiple adenomatous polyps with high malignant potential lining the mucous membrane of the intestine, particularly the colon, beginning at about puberty.

*fatty acid*. Any monobasic aliphatic acid containing only carbon, hydrogen, and oxygen and made up of an alkyl radical attached to the carboxyl group. Saturated fatty acids have the general formula $C_nH_{2n}O_2$. There are also several series of unsaturated fatty acids having one or more double bonds, and a few cyclic acids.

*fiber optics*. The transmission of an image along flexible bundles of coated parallel fibers that propagate light by internal reflections.

*fine-needle aspiration*. Sampling of pancreatic tissue for the purpose of cytologic examination. Used in the diagnosis of pancreatic cancer.

*fistula*. An abnormal passage between two internal organs. See also **pancreatic fistula.**

*fluoroscopy*. Examination of deep structures by means of roentgen rays; uses a screen covered with crystals of calcium tungstate, on which are projected the shadows of x-ray beams passing through the body placed between the body and the source of irradiation.

*Food and Drug Administration (FDA)*. The federal regulatory agency responsible for controlling the safety and effectiveness of drugs, devices, and instrumentation.

*french unit*. A unit for denoting the size of catheters or other tubular instruments, each unit being roughly equivalent to 0.3 mm in diameter, (i.e., 18 French (Fr) indicates a diameter of 6 mm).

*frozen section*. A tissue biopsy obtained during endoscopy which is sent for immediate microscopic examination by a pathologist to determine the type of abnormal tissue present.

*fulguration*. Destruction of living tissue by electric sparks generated by a high-frequency current.

*fulminant hepatic failure*. Massive liver cell death that occurs within 2 months of the development of acute hepatitis.

*functional organization*. A form of organizational structure that is designed to allow specialists in given areas to give and enforce recommendations within a clearly defined scope.

*fundus*. The proximal portion of the stomach, which lies above and to the left of the lower esophageal sphincter.

*g-cell*. A cell type located in the pyloric glands of the stomach; G-cells secrete gastrin.

*gallbladder*. The pear-shaped reservoir for bile on the posteroinferior surface of the liver, between the right and the quadrate lobe; from its neck, the cystic duct projects to join the common bile duct.

*Gardner's syndrome*. Familial polyposis of the colon (with malignant potential), supernumerary teeth, fibrous dysplasia of the skull, osteomas, fibromas, and epithelial cysts.

*gastric ulcer*. Ulcer of the gastric mucosa.

*gastritis*. An inflammation of the gastric mucosa.

*gastroenterology associate*. A non-RN healthcare professional with varied educational background who is engaged in the field of gastroenterology.

*gastroenterology nurse*. A registered nurse who specializes in the field of gastroenterology.

*gastroesophageal sphincter*. See **lower esophageal sphincter.**

*giardiasis*. Infection with the flagellate protozoan *Giardia lamblia*, characterized by protracted, intermittent diarrhea with symptoms suggesting malabsorption, and by abdominal pain, distention, and flatulence; light infections are usually asymptomatic.

*gland*. An aggregation of cells, specialized to secrete or excrete materials not related to their ordinary metabolic needs. See also **Bruner's gland, cardiac gland,** and **pyloric gland.**

*glucose*. A monosaccharide, $C_6H_{12}O_6$, found in certain foodstuffs, especially fruits, and in the normal blood of all animals. It is the chief source energy for living organisms, its utilization being controlled by insulin.

*glutaraldehyde*. A high-level disinfectant that is effective against vegetative gram-positive, gram-negative, and acid-fast bacteria, some bacterial spores, some fungi, and viruses.

*glycerol*. A trihydric sugar alcohol that is the alcoholic component of the fats; it is soluble in water and alcohol and is an intermediate in the metabolism of fatty acids.

*glycogen*. A polysaccharide that is the chief carbohydrate storage material in animals. It is a long-chain polymer of glucose, formed in and largely stored in the liver and to a lesser extent in muscles, being depolymerized to glucose and liberated as needed.

*goal*. (1) A desired outcome that should reflect the mission statement of an organization. (2) A desired patient outcome, which must be realistic, usable, observable, and specific.

*goblet cell*. A unicellular mucous gland found in the epithelium of various mucous membranes, especially in the respiratory passages and the intestines. Droplets of mucigen collect in the upper part of the cell and distend it, while the basal end remains slender and the cell assumes the shape of a goblet.

*greater curvature*. The lower lateral border of the stomach.

*greater omentum*. A layer of visceral peritoneum that hangs from the greater curvature of the stomach over the anterior side of the abdominal viscera.

*grounding pad*. A dispersive electrode that is securely attached to the patient's skin and serves to complete the current flow from a monopolar electrosurgery probe, through the patient's body, and back to the generator. Also known as a grounding plate.

*halon*. Bromotrafluoromethane. A commercial product used in fire extinguishers that are safe for use in high break areas.

*haustrum*. Sacculation in the wall of the colon produced by adaptation of its length to that of the tenia coli, or by the arrangement of the circular muscle fibers. Plural: haustra.

*health problem*. A condition related to health which requires intervention if disease or illness is to be prevented or resolved and if coping and wellness are to be promoted. See also **actual health problem, possible health problem,** and **potential health problem.**

*heartburn*. A retrosternal sensation of warmth or burning that occurs in waves and tends to rise toward the neck. Also known as pyrosis.

*heater probe*. A hollow aluminum cylinder with an inner heat coil and an outer coating of Teflon which is applied directly to a bleeding vessel to produce hemostasis.

*helicobacter pylori*. A gram-negative curved or special rod that is microaerophilic. Formerly Campylobacterital pylori.

*hematochezia*. The passage of bloody stools.

*hematocrit*. The volume percentage of red blood cells in whole blood.

*Hemoccult*. The trademark for a modification of the guaiac test for occult blood, in which guaiac-impregnated filter paper is used; the test is positive if the specimen turns blue.

*hemochromatosis*. A disorder of iron metabolism characterized by excess deposition of iron in the tissues, especially in the liver and pancreas, and by bronze pigmentation of the skin, cirrhosis, diabetes mellitus, and associated bone and joint changes.

*hemoglobin*. The oxygen-carrying pigment of the red blood cells.

*hemolysis*. The liberation of hemoglobin from the red blood cells and its appearance in the plasma.

*hemorrhage*. Bleeding; the escape of blood from the blood vessels.

**hepatic duct**. The duct that is formed by the union of the right and left hepatic ducts, and in turn joins the cystic duct to form the common bile duct.

**hepatic encephalopathy**. A condition usually occurring secondary to advanced liver disease, but also seen in the course of any severe disease or in patients with porta-caval shunts. Marked by disturbances of consciousness which may progress to deep coma (hepatic coma), psychiatric changes, flapping tremor, and fetor hepaticus. Also called portal-systemic encephalopathy.

**hepatic flexure**. The right flexure of the colon; the bend in the large intestine at which the ascending colon becomes the transverse colon.

**hepatitis**. The inflammation of the liver.

**hepatocyte**. A parenchymal liver cell.

**hepatorenal syndrome**. A syndrome characterized by functional renal failure, oliguria, and low urinary sodium concentration, without pathological renal changes, associated with cirrhosis and ascites or with obstructive jaundice.

**hiatus hernia**. Occurs when a portion of the stomach protrudes through the diaphragmatic hiatus into the thoracic cavity.

**Hirschsprung's disease**. Megacolon due to congenital absence of myenteric ganglion cells in a distal segment of the colon. The resultant loss of motor function causes massive hypertrophic dilatation of the normal proximal colon; the aganglionic segment usually remains narrowed, but may dilate passively. The condition appears soon after birth, is more common in males, and causes extreme constipation, abdominal distention, sometimes vomiting, and when severe, growth retardation. Also known as congenital megacolon or aganglionic megacolon.

**histamine**. A decarboxylation product of histidine found in all body tissues. Cellular receptors of histamine include H1 receptors, which mediate the effects of histamine on smooth muscle and capillaries; and H2 receptors, which mediate the acceleration of heart rate and the promotion of gastric acid secretion.

**histamine-2 (H2) blocker**. An agent that blocks the cellular receptor site for histamine that is responsible for stimulating the heart rate and gastric secretion.

**histology**. The study of the minute structure, composition, and function of the tissues; also called microscopical anatomy.

**hot biopsy forceps**. A type of biopsy forceps that is insulated by a nonconducting sheath and attached to an electrocoagulation snare handle.

**Hurst bougie**. One of a series of blunt-tipped, mercury-filled tubes of graded diameter used for dilating esophageal strictures.

**hydrogen breath test**. A measure of the amount of hydrogen expelled in the breath after ingestion of a carbohydrate drink; used to detect carbohydrate malab-sorption, abnormal gastrointestinal transit time, or bacterial overgrowth in the small bowel.

**hydrostatic balloon**. A polyethylene balloon that can be inserted into the GI tract, and inflated with fluid to a specified pressure; used primarily for the dilatation of strictures.

**hypertonic**. A term denoting a solution which, when bathing body cells, causes a net flow of water across the semipermeable cell membrane out of the cell. Also denotes a solution having a greater tonicity than another solution, (e.g., the blood, to which it is being compared).

**hypoalbuminemia**. An abnormally low albumin content in the blood.

**hypoglycemia**. An abnormally low glucose content in the blood, which may lead to tremulousness, cold sweat, piloerection, hypothermia, and headache, accompanied by confusion, hallucinations, bizarre behavior, and ultimately, convulsions and coma.

**hypopharyngeal sphincter**. See **upper esophageal sphincter.**

**hypothesis**. A declarative conjectured statement posing a relationship between two or more variables; hypotheses lead to empirical studies that seek to confirm or disconfirm the relationships. See also **null hypothesis.**

**hypotonic**. A term denoting a solution which, when bathing body cells, causes a net flow of water across the semipermeable cell membrane into the cell; also denotes a solution having less tonicity than another solution; for example, the blood, to which it is being compared.

**hypovolemia**. Abnormally decreased volume of circulating fluid in the body.

**ileocecal valve**. A functional valve at the junction of the ileum and cecum, consisting of circular muscle of the terminal ileum.

**ileum**. The distal portion of the small intestine, extending from the jejunum to the cecum.

**independent intervention**. Nursing action initiated without direction or supervision of other healthcare professionals. Independent nursing intervention is instituted as the result of a nursing assessment.

**independent variable**. A concept capable of taking on different values whose value is unaffected by other variables in a given study.

**indicator**. A measurable variable that is used to measure the degree to which standards are met.

**infectious waste**. Waste capable of producing an infectious disease; includes human, animal, or biologic wastes and any items that may be contaminated with pathogens.

**infiltration**. The diffusion or accumulation in a tissue or cells of substances not normal to it or in amounts in excess of the normal.

**inflammatory bowel disease**. A general term for inflammatory diseases of the bowel of unknown etiology, including Crohn's disease and ulcerative colitis.

*informed consent*. An interaction between physician and patient in which a meaningful exchange of information concerning an impending healthcare ministration occurs. Consent is not valid without fulfillment of these four requirements: full disclosure, competent judgment and decision-making ability, comprehension of the procedure and its associated risks and aftereffects, and free will.

*insufflation*. The act of blowing a vapor, gas, or air into a body cavity.

*interdependent intervention*. Nursing action performed in concert with the efforts of other healthcare professionals.

*intervention*. All those activities the nurse identifies that directly relate to the nursing diagnosis and are directed towards improving the patient's problem. See also **dependent intervention, independent intervention, and interdependent intervention.**

*interview*. A meeting of patient and nurse to gather data concerning a patient's health status, health problems, risks, weaknesses, strengths, and need for nursing care.

*intestinal pseudoobstruction*. A condition characterized by constipation, colicky pain, and vomiting, but without evidence of organic obstruction.

*intrahepatic biliary dysplasia*. A rare autosomal dominant liver disease that incorporates a combination of anomalies in conjunction with chronic cholestasis.

*intussusception*. The prolapse of one part of the intestine into the lumen of an immediately adjoining part.

*ionizing radiation*. High-energy radiation which interacts with matter to produce ion pairs.

*irritable bowel syndrome*. A chronic noninflammatory disease characterized by excessive secretion of mucus and disordered colonic motility with consequent colic, constipation, and/or diarrhea with the passage of mucus. It is a common disorder with a psychophysiologic basis.

*ischemic colitis*. Acute vascular insufficiency of the colon usually involving the portion supplied by the inferior mesenteric artery. The classic radiologic sign is thumbprinting caused by localized elevation of the mucosa by submucosal hemorrhage or edema. Ulceration may follow.

*islet of Langerhans*. One of the irregular microscopic structures scattered throughout the pancreas and comprising the endocrine portion of the pancreas.

*isotonic*. A term denoting a solution in which body cells can be bathed without a net flow of water across the semipermeable cell membrane. Also denotes a solution having the same tonicity as another solution; for example, the blood, to which it is being compared.

*jaundice*. A syndrome characterized by hyperbilirubinemia and deposition of bile pigment in the skin, mucous membranes, and sclera with resulting yellow appearance of the patient.

*jejunum*. The portion of the small bowel that extends from the duodenum to the ileum.

*Joint Commission on the Accreditation of Healthcare Organizations (JCAHO)*. An independent credentialing agency that grants approval to healthcare facilities that voluntarily comply with the agency's standards for public and patient health and safety.

*kupffer cell*. A large, star-shaped or pyramidal cell with a large oval nucleus and a small prominent nucleolus. These intensely phagocytic cells line the walls of the sinusoids of the liver and form part of the reticuloendothelial system.

*lactase deficiency*. A deficiency in the brush-border enzyme lactase, which causes malabsorption of the disaccharide lactose; patients typically experience distention, flatulence, cramping, and diarrhea within minutes of ingesting milk or milk products.

*lamina propria*. The connective tissue coat of a mucous membrane.

*laparoscope*. A fiberoptic instrument that permits inspection of the peritoneal cavity.

*laparoscopy*. Examination of the interior of the abdomen using a laparoscope.

*laparotomy*. A surgical incision made through the abdomen.

*laser*. Light Amplification by Stimulated Emission of Radiation. A device that transforms light of various frequencies into an extremely intense, small, and nearly nondivergent beam of monochromatic radiation in the visible region with all the waves in phase. Capable of mobilizing immense heat and power when focused at close range, it is used as a tool in surgical procedures, in diagnosis, and in physiologic studies.

*lavage*. The irrigation or washing out of an organ, such as the stomach or bowel.

*laxative*. An agent that acts to promote evacuation of the bowel.

*lesser curvature*. The upper lateral border of the stomach.

*lesser omentum*. A layer of visceral peritoneum that attaches the lesser curvature of the stomach to the underside of the liver.

*leukocyte*. A white blood cell.

*liability*. Legal responsibility for one's acts (or failure to act), including the responsibility for financial restitution in the event of demonstrable damages resulting from negligent acts.

*ligament of Treitz*. Suspensory muscle of the duodenum; a flat band of smooth muscle originating from the diaphragm and continuous with the muscular coat of the duodenum at its junction with the jejunum.

*line organization*. A traditional form of organizational

structure, in which each position has authority over a lower one in the organization.

*Linton tube*. A three-lumen tube used for esophageal-gastric tamponade; it has a gastric balloon but no esophageal balloon, and ports for both gastric and esophageal aspiration.

*lipid*. A fat or fatlike substance that is easily stored in the body and serves as a source of fuel. They include the fatty acids, neutral fats, waxes, and steroids; compound lipids include glycolipids, lipoproteins, and phospholipids.

*lithotripsy*. The crushing of gallstones or bladder calculi, either by using a mechanical lithotripter or by focusing shock waves on the stone.

*lower esophageal sphincter (LES)*. A group of thickened circular muscles at the distal end of the esophagus, which regulate the entry of food into the stomach. Also known as the cardiac sphincter or gastroesophageal sphincter.

*malabsorption*. Impaired intestinal absorption of nutrients.

*maldigestion*. Impaired digestion.

*Mallory-Weiss tear*. A mucosal rent at the gastroesophageal junction that is associated with prolonged forceful vomiting.

*malnutrition*. Any disorder of nutrition, whether caused by unbalanced or insufficient diet or by defective assimilation or utilization of foods.

*Maloney bougie*. One of a series of mercury-filled bougies similar to the Hurst bougie but with a conical tip.

*malrotation*. Failure of normal rotation of an organ, as of the gut, during embryologic development.

*manometry*. Measurement of pressure or contraction, especially within the GI tract.

*matrix organization*. A type of organizational structure that looks at individual subsystems within a complex structure. These subsystems can be viewed anywhere on the continuum from totally dependent to totally autonomous.

*mean*. The index of central tendency usually referred to as the average; it is the sum of the values in a set, divided by the total number of elements in the set.

*Meckel's diverticulum*. An occasional sacculation or appendage of the ileum, derived from an unobliterated yolk stalk.

*median*. That point in a set of values above which and below which 50% of the values lie.

*medical diagnosis*. Classification of a patient's medical condition, based on interpretation of data related to pathology and etiology; usually implies a course of treatment.

*megacolon*. Abnormally large or dilated colon; the condition may be congenital or acquired, acute or chronic. See also **toxic megacolon.**

*Meissner's plexus*. The part of the enteric plexus that is situated in the submucosa. Also called the submucosal plexus.

*microorganism*. A minute living organism, usually microscopic, including bacteria, viruses, fungi, and protozoa.

*microvillus*. A minute cylindrical process on the free surface of a cell, especially in the intestinal epithelium.

*mineral*. A nonorganic, homogeneous solid substance, usually a constituent of the earth's crust.

*Minnesota tube*. A four-lumen tube used for esophageal-gastric tamponade; it has both gastric and esophageal balloons and ports for gastric and esophageal aspiration.

*mission statement*. A statement that describes the intent of a specific organization. The statement should include the unit's overall goals, objectives, services, and the intent of the quality to be delivered.

*mode*. The numerical value in a set of values that occurs most frequently.

*monoglyceride*. A compound consisting of one molecule of fatty acid esterified to glycerol.

*monopolar electrocoagulation*. An electrocoagulation method in which the electrical current flows between a small, active electrode that is in contact with the target tissue and a larger grounding pad that is attached to the patient's skin.

*monosaccharide*. A simple sugar; a carbohydrate that cannot be decomposed by hydrolysis. The monosaccharides are colorless crystalline substances, with a sweet taste, and which have the general formula $CH_2O$.

*narcotic*. An agent that depresses the central nervous system, reduces pain, and sometimes produces sleep.

*narcotic antagonist*. An agent that opposes the action of narcotics on the nervous system.

*nasobiliary catheter (NBC)*. A catheter that is inserted endoscopically into the common bile duct during ERCP, with the opposite end brought out through the patient's nostril. Its purpose is to provide drainage or to allow the instillation of therapeutic solutions.

*nasoenteric intubation*. Insertion of a tube that is passed through the nares, into the stomach, and then into the intestinal tract; used primarily to remove intestinal contents or to provide for tube feeding (enteral nutrition).

*nasogastric tube*. A soft rubber or plastic tube that is inserted through a nostril and into the stomach, for instilling liquid foods or other substances, or for withdrawing gastric contents.

*Nd:YAG (neodymium:yttrium/aluminum/garnet)*. A mineral crystal that is used as a laser medium to produce 1060-nm light.

*needle*. A sharp instrument used for suturing or puncturing. See also **verres needle.**

*nitrogen balance*. A state of the body in regard to ingestion and excretion of nitrogen. In negative nitrogen balance the amount of nitrogen excreted is greater than the quantity ingested; in positive nitrogen balance the amount excreted is smaller than the amount ingested.

*noncritical item*. An item that either does not ordinarily touch the patient or touches only intact skin. Washing with a detergent is often sufficient for these items.

*normal saline*. An isotonic solution of sodium chloride for temporarily maintaining living cells. Also known as physiologic saline.

*null hypothesis*. The hypothesis that states that there is no relationship between the variables under study. It is used primarily in connection with tests of statistical significance as the hypothesis to be rejected.

*nursing audit*. The method of evaluating care, the outcomes of care, or the process by which these outcomes are achieved by using a review of patient records.

*nursing care conference*. A collaborative meeting of nurses and possibly other health and allied health professionals for the purposes of planning and evaluating nursing management of a patient's health problem or set of problems. It represents a brainstorming effort to generate creative, comprehensive, or more aggressive approaches to care, usually for long-term patients with complicated problems whose previous management has failed to bring about desired outcomes.

*nursing diagnosis*. A statement of an actual or potential health problem that can be alleviated or prevented by independent nursing intervention.

*nursing examination*. A physical assessment focused on functional abilities, usually performed in head-to-toe format, during which objective data about a patient's health status is gathered; steps in the examination include inspection, auscultation, percussion, and palpation.

*nursing history*. An interview-style assessment that is performed to evaluate a patient's health status, health problems, risks, weaknesses, strengths, and need for nursing care.

*nursing order*. A prescription for the nursing care that is to be given to achieve patient health goals.

*nursing process*. A systematic approach to nursing care using problem-solving techniques. It encompasses assessment, diagnosis, outcome identification, planning, implementation, and evaluation.

*nutcracker esophagus*. Esophageal peristalsis with a contractile amplitude two to three times the normal volume.

*nutrition*. The processes involved in taking nutriments and assimilating and using them. See also **enteral nutrition, peripheral parenteral nutrition,** and **total parenteral nutrition.**

*objective*. An observable activity that is developed to help achieve the established goals of an organization.

*objective data*. Facts perceptible by the senses of one observer which can be verified by another person observing the same data.

*observation*. Systematic, deliberate use of the five senses to gather data.

*obstipation*. Intractable constipation.

*occult blood*. Blood present in such small quantities that it can be detected only by chemical tests of suspected material, or by microscopic or spectroscopic examination.

*Occupational Safety and Health Administration (OSHA)*. The federal regulatory agency responsible for enforcing safety and health regulations in the workplace.

*odynophagia*. Painful swallowing.

*oral*. Pertaining to the mouth; taken through or applied in the mouth.

*organizational structure*. A structure that determines the process by which a group of people distribute responsibilities, establish lines of communication, identify relationships, and establish accountability. See also **functional organization, line organization, matrix organization, project organization,** and **staff organization.**

*osmosis*. The passage of a solvent from a solution of lesser to one of greater solute concentration when the two solutions are separated by a membrane which selectively prevents the passage of solute molecules, but is permeable to the solvent.

*outcome*. The end product of nursing care; measurable changes in a patient's health or behavior.

*outcome identification*. Is an actual or potential health problem exhibited by an individual through the process of clinical reasoning and judgement functions that nurses by virtue of their education and experience are capable and licensed to treat independently.

*outcome standard*. A patient-focused standard that addresses changes in the patient's health status or the results of nursing care.

*overtube*. A polyvinyl sleeve that fits over an endoscope and serves to protect the esophageal mucosa and the airway during various upper GI procedures, including extraction of foreign bodies.

*oxyntic cell*. See parietal cell.

*pancreas*. A large, elongated gland situated transversely behind the stomach, between the spleen and the duodenum. See also **annular pancreas** and **pancreas divisum.**

*pancreas divisum*. A developmental anomaly in which the pancreas is present as two separate structures, each with its own duct.

*pancreatic enzyme insufficiency*. A deficiency in pancreatic exocrine function, leading to malabsorption of fats and other nutrients.

*pancreatic fistula*. An abnormal passage between the pancreas and another organ or, more often, between the pancreas and the exterior, often following pancreatic trauma, external drainage of a pseudocyst, or pancreatic surgery.

*pancreatitis*. Acute or chronic inflammation of the pancreas.

*paneth's cell*. A narrow, pyramidal, or columnar epithelial cell with a round or oval nucleus close to the base of the cell, occurring in the fundus of the crypts of Lieberkühn; Paneth's cells contain large secretory granules that may contain peptidase.

*papillotome*. A cutting instrument for incising the papilla of Vater.

*papillotomy*. Incision of a papilla.

*paracentesis*. Surgical puncture of a cavity for the aspiration of fluid, especially the abdominal cavity.

*paralytic ileus*. Obstruction of the intestines resulting from inhibition of bowel motility, which may be produced by numerous causes, most frequently by peritonitis.

*parenteral*. Administration of medications or nutrition by an injection route, such as subcutaneous, intramuscular, or intravenous.

*parietal cell*. A cell type located in the parietal glands of the stomach and secrete hydrochloric acid and intrinsic factor. Also known as oxyntic cells.

*pathology*. The structural or functional manifestations of disease.

*pedunculated polyp*. A polyp that is attached to the mucosa by a stemlike pedicle or stalk.

*peptic ulcer*. An ulceration of the mucous membrane of the esophagus, stomach, or duodenum, caused by the action of the acid gastric juice.

*percutaneous endoscopic gastrostomy (PEG)*. A technique for the endoscopic insertion of a gastrostomy feeding tube, for the purpose of providing enteral feeding.

*percutaneous endoscopic jejunostomy (PEJ)*. A technique for the endoscopic insertion of a feeding tube through a PEG tube and into the jejunum, for the purpose of providing enteral feeding.

*percutaneous liver biopsy*. Aspiration biopsy of the liver by using a needle that has been inserted through a small incision in the skin.

*percutaneous transhepatic cholangiogram*. A roentgenogram of the hepatic and biliary ductal systems following injection of contrast directly into an intrahepatic bile duct, using a needle that is introduced percutaneously into the liver, through the eighth or ninth intercostal space.

*perforation*. A hole made through a body part.

*peripheral parenteral nutrition (PPN)*. Intravenous administration of a prescribed diet by means of a catheter inserted into a peripheral vein.

*peristalsis*. A distally progressive band of circular muscle contraction that causes the gradual progression of digestive contents through the GI tract.

*peritoneoscopy*. Examination of the peritoneal cavity by an instrument (laparoscope) that is inserted through the abdominal wall.

*peritoneum*. The serous membrane that lines the abdominopelvic walls and holds the viscera in place.

*pernicious anemia*. A megaloblastic anemia occurring in children or more commonly in later life, characterized by histamine-fast achlorhydria; laboratory and clinical manifestations are based on malabsorption of vitamin B12 due to a failure of the gastric mucosa to secrete adequate and potent intrinsic factor.

*Peutz-Jeghers syndrome*. A hereditary syndrome characterized by gastrointestinal polyposis associated with excessive melanin pigmentation of the skin and mucous membranes; gastrointestinal bleeding and intussusception are common complications.

*Peyer's patch*. An oval elongated area of lymphoid tissue on the mucosa of the small intestine, composed of many lymphoid nodules closely packed together.

*philosophy*. Major beliefs held by an individual or the members of a group.

*phlebitis*. Inflammation of a vein.

*photocoagulation*. Condensation of protein material by the controlled use of an intense beam of light.

*physiograph*. Device that produces a graphic display of test results.

*pigtail stent*. A stent that is coiled at one or both ends. The coiled shape straightens out when the stent is pulled taut, but returns when it is allowed to relax.

*placebo effect*. An assumed psychologic response to administration of a treatment suggested by the process of taking a medicine; usually encountered in drug testing, these effects are discounted from the real effects of the drug under study.

*planning*. The development of patient goals based on nursing diagnoses for the purpose of preventing, reducing, or resolving health problems through nursing intervention.

*plasma*. The fluid portion of the blood, in which the particulate components are suspended.

*plasmolysis*. Contraction or shrinking of a cell caused by the loss of water by osmotic action.

*platelet*. A disk-shaped structure found in the blood of all mammals and chiefly known for its role in blood coagulation.

*plexus*. A general term for a network of lymphatic vessels, nerves, or veins. See also **Auerbach's plexus, enteric plexus,** and **Meissner's plexus.**

*pneumatic balloon*. A balloon that is inserted over a guidewire into the lower esophageal sphincter and then inflated to a preset pressure and left in place for a period of time; used in the treatment of patients with achalasia.

*pneumoperitoneum*. The presence of gas or air in the peritoneal cavity; it may occur spontaneously, as in a subphrenic abscess, or be deliberately introduced as an aid to radiologic examination and diagnosis.

*polyp*. A protruding growth from any mucous membrane; includes gastric polyps. See also **adenomatous polyp, pedunculated polyp,** and **sessile polyp.**

*polypectomy*. Surgical or endoscopic removal of a polyp.

*polypectomy snare*. A sheathed wire loop that can be passed through the instrument channel of an endoscope; it may be attached to an electrosurgical unit and used to apply coagulation current for removal of gastrointestinal polyps or it may be used to remove foreign bodies.

*polyposis*. The development of multiple polyps on a part. See also **familial polyposis.**

*population*. All of the members of a group in which a survey researcher is interested; the entire set of people, objects, etc., with characteristics in common.

*porphyria*. Any of a group of disturbances of porphyrin metabolism, characterized by marked increase in formation and excretion of porphyrins or their precursors.

*portal hypertension*. Abnormally increased blood pressure in the portal venous system, a frequent complication of cirrhosis of the liver.

*portal triad*. The grouping of the tributaries of the hepatic artery, hepatic vein, and bile duct at the angles of the lobules of the liver.

*position description*. A delineation of the responsibilities of an individual in an organization, including the title of the position, the department, the person to whom the individual is responsible, a job summary, job qualifications, and specific duties and functions.

*possible health problem*. A health condition that has a high probability of developing because of an existing condition or disease.

*potential health problem*. A health condition that does not presently exist, but because of the presence of identified risk factors, requires that the nurse take preventive measures.

*pressure transducer*. A transducer is a device that translates one form of energy to another; in the case of manometric pressure transducers, changes in pressure are translated into electrical signals.

*primary schlerosing cholangitis*. A rare and serious condition in which inflammation involves the entire biliary tract; often related to GI or biliary tract infection.

*priority setting*. The activity concerned with ranking nursing diagnoses in order of actual or potential threat to the patient's well-being.

*process standard*. A standard that focuses on the nature and sequence of activities carried out by nurses implementing the nursing process; describes an acceptable level of performance of nursing actions.

*proctoscopy*. Inspection of the rectum with a speculum or tubular instrument with appropriate illumination.

*proctosigmoidoscopy*. Examination of the rectum and sigmoid colon with an instrument designed for illuminating and viewing those areas.

*project organization*. An organizational structure that is designed to complete a specific task.

*prostaglandin*. A group of naturally occurring, chemically related, long-chain hydroxy fatty acids that stimulate contractility of smooth muscle and have the ability to lower blood pressure, regulate acid secretion of the stomach, regulate body temperature and platelet aggregation, and control inflammation and vascular permeability; they also affect the action of certain hormones. There are six types: A,B,C,D,E, and F, with the degree of saturation of the side chain of each being designated by subscripts 1, 2, and 3.

*protein*. Any of a group of complex organic compounds, which contain carbon, hydrogen, oxygen, nitrogen, and usually sulfur, the characteristic element being nitrogen. Proteins are of high molecular weight and consist essentially of combinations of $\alpha$-amino acids in peptide linkages.

*prothrombin*. Coagulation Factor II, a protein present in the plasma that is converted to thrombin. See also **prothrombin time.**

*prothrombin time*. A measure of the rapidity of blood clotting that examines coagulation factors I, II, V, VII, and X.

*pseudocyst*. An abnormal or dilated space resembling a cyst but not lined by epithelium as is a true cyst. A pancreatic pseudocyst is an encapsulated collection of pancreatic juice and cellular debris that has escaped from the pancreas, the wall being formed by inflammatory fibrosis of serosal surfaces of adjacent organs; pseudocysts most commonly occur in the lesser sac of the peritoneum.

*pseudomembranous colitis*. An acute inflammation of the bowel mucosa with the formation of pseudomembranous plaques overlying an area of superficial ulceration and the passage of the pseudomembranous material in the feces; may result from shock and ischemia or be associated with antibiotic therapy. Also called necrotizing enterocolitis.

*pyloric gland*. A gland located in the antrum or pylorus of the stomach, which contains mucous cells and G-cells.

*pyloric sphincter*. The thickened muscular sphincter that controls the passage of food from the stomach into the duodenum.

*pyloric stenosis*. Obstruction of the pyloric sphincter at the outlet of the stomach.

*pylorus*. The most distal portion of the stomach, lying between the antrum and the duodenum.

*pyrosis*. See **Heartburn.**

*qualitative*. Pertains to describing or analyzing qualities, attributes, or characteristics.

*quality*. In health care, the degree to which actions

taken or not taken maximize the probability of beneficial outcomes.

*quality assurance (QA)*. An ongoing process of review in which data collected over a period of time are used to compare actual practice against standards of practice to determine if the care actually rendered meets a level of quality deemed acceptable within a practice setting.

*quality improvement*. A method established to monitor and evaluate the appropriateness and effectiveness of patient care services.

*quantitative*. Pertaining to or measuring quantity.

*radiation enteritis*. Radiation injury to the intestines, usually occurring as a result of radiotherapy for pelvic, intraabdominal, or retroperitoneal malignancies.

*radiography*. The making of film records (radiographs) of internal structures of the body by passage of x-rays or gamma rays through the body to act on specially sensitized film. See also **roentgenography.**

*random sample*. Selection from the population (or a subpopulation) at large performed in such a way that each member of the population has an equal probability of being included in the sample.

*range*. The highest score (or value) minus the lowest score in a given set of values.

*rapid pull-through*. A technique whereby a manometry catheter is withdrawn steadily through the esophagus while the patient is not breathing or swallowing.

*rectosigmoidoscopy*. Endoscopic visualization of the lower portion of the sigmoid colon and the upper portion of the rectum.

*rectum*. The distal portion of the colon, beginning anterior to the third sacral vertebra as a continuation of the sigmoid and ending at the anal canal.

*red blood cell*. See **erythrocyte.**

*referral*. The process of sending a patient to another source for aid or to another professional for appropriate action; also, a patient received from another source.

*regional enteritis*. See **Crohn's disease.**

*regurgitation*. A backward flowing of undigested food.

*respiratory depression*. A decrease in the rapidity and depth of respirations.

*retrospective audit*. An evaluation of nursing care and patient outcomes performed after discharge of the patient. Postdischarge questionnaires, interviews (over the telephone or face-to-face), or chart review are retrospective auditing techniques.

*ringer's solution*. A sterile solution containing sodium chloride, potassium chloride, and calcium chloride in water for injection; used as a topical physiologic salt solution.

*roentgenography*. The making of a record (roentgenogram) of internal body structures by passing x-rays through the body to act on specially sensitized film. See also **contrast roentgenography** and **double-contrast roentgenography.**

*role delineation*. A statement of the behaviors that are expected of an individual in a certain position, as of a gastroenterology nurse or associate.

*ruga*. A wrinkled ridge in the interior wall of the stomach. Plural: rugae.

*sample*. The portion of a group or population that is targeted for a survey. See also **random sample.**

*sanitation*. A process capable of destroying or reducing the number of microbial contaminants to a relatively safe level, as judged by public health requirements.

*Savary-Gilliard dilator*. One of a series of semiflexible, tapered polyvinyl chloride bougies that are passed over a guidewire for the purpose of widening a gastrointestinal lumen.

*Schatzki's ring*. One of a series of thin, concentric membranes located at the esophagogastric junction.

*Schilling test*. A test for gastrointestinal absorption of vitamin B12, in which a measured amount of radioactive vitamin B12 is given orally and the percentage of radioactivity in the urine excreted over a 24-hour period is determined.

*Schindler, Gabriele*. The wife of pioneer gastroscopist Dr. Rudolph Schindler. She assisted her husband with gastroscopic procedures and is considered a role model for today's professional gastroenterology nurses and associates.

*scintigraphy*. The production of two-dimensional images of the distribution of radioactivity in tissues after the internal administration of radionuclide, with the images obtained by a scintillation camera.

*sclerotherapy*. The injection of sclerosing solutions in the treatment of hemorrhoids, varicose veins, or esophageal varices.

*scope of practice*. A statement of the dimensions of a professional practice which outlines the functions of individuals in that profession.

*secretin*. A strongly basic polypeptide hormone secreted by the mucosa of the duodenum and jejunum when acid chyme enters the intestine. Carried by the blood, it stimulates the secretion of a watery pancreatic juice high in salt content but low in enzymes. It has a lesser stimulatory effect on bile and intestinal secretion.

*sedative*. An agent that allays excitement.

*semicritical item*. An item or instrument (including endoscopes), that may come in contact with intact mucous membranes, but does not ordinarily penetrate body surfaces. Meticulous physical cleaning followed by high-level disinfection is required for these items.

*Sengstaken-Blakemore tube*. A three-lumen tube used for esophageal-gastric tamponade; it has both gastric and esophageal balloons and a port for gastric aspiration.

*serum*. The cell-free portion of the blood from which the fibrinogen has been separated in the process of clotting.

*sessile polyp*. A polyp that is attached to the mucosa by a broad base.

*shock*. (1) A condition of acute peripheral circulatory failure caused by derangement of circulatory control or loss of circulating fluid; marked by hypotension, coldness of the skin, usually tachycardia, and often anxiety. (2) An extreme stimulation of the nerves, muscles, etc., accompanying the passage of electrical current through the body.

*short bowel syndrome*. Any of the malabsorption syndromes resulting from massive resection of the small bowel, the degree and kind of malabsorption depending on the site and extent of the resection; characterized by diarrhea, steatorrhea, and malnutrition.

*sigmoid colon*. The S-shaped part of the colon, lying in the pelvis, extending from the pelvic brim to the third segment of the sacrum, and continuous above with the descending (iliac) colon and below with the rectum.

*sigmoidoscopy*. Inspection of the sigmoid colon through the use of an endoscope.

*sinusoid*. A form of terminal blood channel consisting of a large, irregular anastomosing vessel; found in the liver, suprarenals, heart, parathyroid, carotid gland, spleen, hemolymph glands, and pancreas.

*small bowel*. The proximal portion of the intestine.

*small bowel enteroscopy*. Visualization of the small bowel with a long, thin, extremely flexible endoscope.

*Society of Gastroenterology Nurses and Associates (SGNA)*. The professional society for registered nurses and other healthcare personnel involved in the practice of gastroenterology.

*solid-state catheter*. A long, flexible manometry catheter that contains a series of miniature pressure transducers that directly record gastrointestinal contractions.

*sphincter*. A ring-like band of muscle fibers that constricts a passage or closes a natural orifice. See also **cardiac sphincter, gastroesophageal sphincter, hypopharyngeal sphincter, lower esophageal sphincter, pyloric sphincter, sphincter of Oddi,** and **upper esophageal sphincter.**

*Sphincter of Oddi*. The sheath of muscle fibers surrounding bile and pancreatic ducts as they pass through the wall of the duodenum.

*sphincterotome*. An electrosurgical instrument for cutting through a sphincter, specifically the sphincter of Oddi.

*sphincterotomy*. Division of a sphincter, especially division of the sphincter of Oddi during ERCP.

*splenic flexure*. The left flexure of the colon; the bend at which the transverse colon becomes the descending colon.

*sprue*. A chronic form of malabsorption syndrome that occurs in both tropical and celiac forms. See also **celiac sprue** and **tropical sprue.**

*staff organization*. A type of organizational structure that requires staff to assist management, but allows them no authority.

*standard*. An acceptable, expected level of performance established by authority, custom, or consent. Standards in nursing define optimum levels of actual and expected performance. See also **outcome standard, process standard,** and **structural standard.**

*standard deviation*. An average size spread among values in a set around the average value in the set; how far away the numbers in a list are from their average.

*standard for practice*. An authoritative statement of the expected outcomes of professional practice, established through research and/or professional consensus.

*standard of care*. A measurable statement that defines the means to accomplish a practice outcome.

*station pull-through*. A technique whereby a manometry catheter is withdrawn through the esophagus in a step-wise fashion while the patient breathes slowly and evenly.

*steatorrhea*. Excessive amounts of fat in the feces, as in malabsorption syndromes.

*stem*. The first part of a multiple-choice question; it may consist of a question or an incomplete statement.

*stent*. A hollow tube or endoprosthesis that is inserted for the purpose of bypassing diseased or obstructed parts of a duct or tubular organ. See also **barbed stent.**

*sterilization*. The destruction of all microbial life, including spores.

*stoma*. An opening established in the abdominal wall by colostomy, ileostomy, etc.

*stress ulcer*. A form of acute gastritis that is related to a severe trauma, illness, or chronic ingestion of certain drugs.

*stricture*. A narrowing of a canal, duct, or other passage as a result of scarring or deposition of abnormal tissue.

*structural standard*. A standard concerned with the environment in which care is provided.

*subjective data*. Perceptions by an affected person that cannot be perceived or verified experimentally.

*suction biopsy*. A method of obtaining tissue specimens from the rectum or small bowel, by creating a vacuum in a specially designed capsule or tube.

*syncope*. A temporary suspension of consciousness caused by generalized cerebral ischemia; faint.

*syndrome*. A set of symptoms that occur together; the sum of signs of any morbid state; a symptom complex.

*tamponade*. Compression of a part. See also **balloon tamponade.**

*tenesmus*. Straining, especially ineffectual and painful straining at stool or in urination.

*tenia coli*. Three thickened flat bands, about one-sixth shorter than the colon, formed by the longitudinal fibers in the muscular tunic of the colon and extending from the root of the vermiform appendix to the rectum, where they spread out and form a continuous layer encircling the tube.

*tonicity*. The effective osmotic pressure equivalent.

*topical*. Pertaining to a particular surface.

*total parenteral nutrition (TPN)*. The intravenous administration of the total nutrient requirements of a patient with gastrointestinal dysfunction, accomplished via a central venous catheter, usually inserted in the superior vena cava.

*toxic megacolon*. Acute dilatation of the colon associated with amebic or ulcerative colitis; it may precede perforation of the colon.

*transverse colon*. The portion of the colon that runs transversely across the upper part of the abdomen, from the right to the left colic flexure.

*triglyceride*. A compound consisting of three molecules of fatty acid esterified to glycerol; it is a neutral fat synthesized from carbohydrates for storage in animal adipose cells. On enzymatic hydrolysis, it releases free fatty acids in the blood.

*trocar*. A sharp-pointed instrument contained in a cannula, used to puncture the wall of a body cavity; usually used for insertion of the cannula.

*tropical sprue*. A malabsorption syndrome occurring in the tropics and subtropics. Protein malnutrition is usually precipitated by the malabsorption, and anemia caused by folic acid insufficiency is particularly common.

*ulcer*. A local defect, or excavation, of the surface of an organ or tissue, which is produced by the sloughing of inflammatory necrotic tissue. See also **Curling's ulcer, Cushing's ulcer, gastric ulcer, peptic ulcer,** and **stress ulcer.**

*ulcerative colitis*. Chronic, recurrent ulceration in the colon, chiefly of the mucosa and submucosa, of unknown cause; manifested clinically by cramping, abdominal pain, rectal bleeding, and loose discharges of blood, pus, and mucus with scanty fecal particles.

*ultrasonography*. Mechanical radiant energy with a frequency greater than 20,000 hertz (cycles per second); ultrasonography is the visualization of deep structures of the body by recording the reflections (echoes) of ultrasonic waves directed into the tissues. Diagnostic ultrasonography uses a frequency range of 1 million to 10 million Hz, or 1 to 10 MHz.

*Universal Precautions*. A system of infection-control guidelines developed by the Centers for Disease Control that advise healthcare workers to take specific precautions that minimize exposure to blood and body fluids of all patients, regardless of their infective status.

*upper gastrointestinal (UGI) series*. A series of radiographs taken to visualize the esophagus, stomach, and sometimes the small bowel, following the ingestion of a barium solution.

*upper esophageal sphincter (UES)*. The sphincter located at the upper end of the esophagus. Also known as the hypopharyngeal sphincter.

*validation*. Verification; confirmation.

*Valsalva maneuver*. Forcible exhalation against a closed glottis, resulting in an increase in intrathoracic pressure.

*variability*. A concept concerned with how spread out or dispersed the data values are about the mean; the degree to which subjects in a sample vary from one another with respect to some critical attribute.

*variable*. A measured concept or construct; a characteristic or attribute of a person or object that takes on different values within the population under study. See also **dependent variable** and **independent variable.**

*varix*. An enlarged and tortuous vein or artery. Plural: varices.

*vasovagal reaction*. A transient vascular and neurogenic reaction marked by pallor, nausea, sweating, bradycardia, and rapid fall in arterial blood pressure which, when below a critical level, results in loss of consciousness and characteristic EEG changes. It is most often evoked by emotional stress associated with fear or pain.

*vermiform appendix*. A worm-like diverticulum of the cecum, ranging from 3 to 6 inches in length.

*verres needle*. A disposable or reusable needle that is used in laparoscopic procedures for the creation of pneumoperitoneum.

*videoendoscopy*. Visualization of gastrointestinal structures through an endoscope that has a distal sensing device in the tip, which electronically transmits an image to a video processor for display on a television monitor; the procedure is then performed by reference to the monitor.

*villus*. A small vascular process or protrusion, especially such a protrusion from the free surface of a membrane; the intestinal villi are the numerous thread-like projections that cover the surface of the mucosa of the small bowel and serve as the sites of absorption of fluids and nutrients.

*vitamin*. An organic substance that occurs in foods in small amounts and that is necessary in trace amounts for the normal metabolic functioning of the body.

*volvulus*. Intestinal obstruction caused by a knotting and twisting of the bowel.

*washing*. Collection of a specimen for culture or cytology by injecting and then aspirating 20 to 30 ml of nonbacteriostatic saline.

*water-infusion catheter*. A long, multilumen manometry catheter that is continuously perfused with water. Each lumen has a separate recording port that is attached to a separate external pressure transducer; when a port is occluded by gastrointestinal contractions, the resulting pressure change is recorded on a physiograph.

*webs.* See **esophageal rings and webs.**

*Whipple's disease.* A malabsorption syndrome characterized by diarrhea, steatorrhea, skin pigmentation, arthralgia and arthritis, lymphadenopathy, and central nervous system lesions.

*white blood cell.* See **leukocyte.**

*whole blood.* Blood from which none of the elements have been removed.

*Wilson's disease.* Hepatolenticular degeneration. A rare progressive disease, inherited as an autosomal recessive trait, and caused by a defect in the metabolism of copper; a pigmented ring at the outer margin of the cornea is pathognomonic.

*x-ray.* Electromagnetic vibrations of short wavelengths that are produced when high-velocity electrons impinge on various substances. X-rays are able to penetrate some substances much more readily than others and to affect a photographic plate, thus making them useful for taking roentgenograms of various parts of the body. They also cause certain substances to fluoresce, allowing fluoroscopic observation of the size, shape, and movements of various organs.

*Zollinger-Ellison syndrome.* A triad comprising intractable, sometimes fulminating and in many ways atypical peptic ulcers; extreme gastric hyperacidity; and gastrin-secreting, nonbeta islet cell tumors of the pancreas.

*zymogen cell.* See **chief cell.**

# Resources

## BOOKS AND MONOGRAPHS

American Medical Association, Department of Drugs, Division of Drugs and Toxicology. *Drug Evaluations Annual 1991.* Chicago: AMA, 1991.

American Nurses' Association. *Quality Assurance Workbook.* Kansas City, Mo.: ANA, 1976.

American Nurses' Association. *Standards of Clinical Nursing Practice.* Kansas City, Mo.: ANA, 1991.

Association of Operating Room Nurses. *AORN Standards and Recommended Practices for Perioperative Nursing.* Denver: AORN, 1991.

Barnhart, E, publisher. *Physicians' Desk Reference.* 44th ed. Oradell, N. J.: Medical Economics, 1990.

Beare, P, and Meyers, J. *Principles and Practice of Adult Health Nursing.* St. Louis: Mosby–Year Book, 1990.

Beck, M, ed. *Recommended Guidelines for Infection Control in Gastrointestinal Endoscopy Settings.* 2nd ed. SGNA Monograph Series. Rochester, N.Y.: Society of Gastroenterology Nurses and Associates, 1990.

Bernard, M, and Forlaw, L. "Complications and Their Prevention." In *Clinical Nutrition,* Volume 1: *Enteral and Tube Feeding,* eds. Rombeau, JL and Caldwell, MD. Philadelphia: W.B. Saunders, 1984.

Blake, R, and Mouton, J. *The Managerial Grid.* Houston: Gulf Publishing, 1964.

Blume, D. *Dosages and Solutions.* 3rd ed. Philadelphia: F.A. Davis, 1980.

Bodinsky, G. *Documentation: Charting to Standardize.* SGNA Monograph Series. Rochester, N.Y.: Society of Gastroenterology Nurses and Associates, 1989.

Bongiovanni, G, ed. *Essentials of Clinical Gastroenterology.* 2nd ed. New York: McGraw–Hill, 1988.

Brooks, F, ed. *Gastrointestinal Pathophysiology.* 2nd ed. New York: Oxford University Press, 1978.

Carpenito, L. *Nursing Diagnosis: Application to Clinical Practice.* 2nd ed. Philadelphia: J.B. Lippincott, 1987.

Castell, D, Richter, J, and Dalton, C, eds. *Esophageal Motility Testing.* New York: Elsevier, 1987.

Certifying Board of Gastroenterology Nurses and Associates. *Role Delineation for Gastroenterology Associates.* NY, NY: CBGNA, 1990.

Certifying Board of Gastroenterology Nurses and Associates. *Role Delineation for Gastroenterology RNs.* NY, NY:CBGNA, 1990.

Certifying Council for Gastroenterology Clinicians. *Certification Examination for Gastroenterology Nurses and Associates: Handbook for Candidates.* New York: Professional Examination Service, 1990.

Chobanian, S, and Van Ness, M, eds. *Manual of Clinical Problems in Gastroenterology.* Boston: Little, Brown & Co., 1988.

Chopra, S, and May, R, eds. *Pathophysiology of Gastrointestinal Diseases.* Boston: Little, Brown & Co., 1989.

Cleary, P, Faven, E, and Intenzo, D, eds. *Fundamentals of Nursing: The Art and Science of Nursing Care.* Philadelphia: J.B. Lippincott, 1989.

Coco, C. *Intravenous Therapy: A Handbook for Practice.* St. Louis: Mosby–Year Book, 1980.

Cotton, P, and Williams, C. *Practical Gastrointestinal Endoscopy.* 3rd ed. Oxford: Blackwell Scientific Publications, Inc., 1990.

Crocker, O, Charney, S, Chiu, L, and Sik, J. *Quality Circles: A Guide to Participation and Productivity.* New York: New American Library, 1984.

Crosby, P. *Quality is Free: The Art of Making Certain.* New York: New American Library, 1979.

Damsgard, C. *G.I.A. Certification Review Manual.* Rochester, N.Y.: Society of Gastrointestinal Assistants, 1985.

Eastwood, G, and Avunduk, C. *Manual of Gastroenterology: Diagnosis and Therapy.* Boston: Little, Brown & Co., 1988.

Emmert, P, and Barker, L. *Measurement of Communication Behavior.* New York: Longman Publishing, 1989.

Environmental Protection Agency. *EPA Guide for Infectious Waste Management.* EPA/530-SW-86-014, NTIS No. PB86-199130. Washington, D.C.: EPA, Office of Solid Waste, 1986.

Fielder, F. *A Theory of Leadership Effectiveness.* New York: McGraw–Hill, 1967.

Garfield, C. *Peak Performers.* New York: Avon Books, 1986.

Garner, J, and Favero, M. *Guideline for Handwashing and Hospital Environmental Control.* Atlanta: Centers for Disease Control, 1985.

"Gastrointestinal Disorders." In *Diseases.* Nurse's Reference Library Series. Springhouse, Pa.: Springhouse Corporation, 1986.

Gitnick, G, ed. *Handbook of Gastrointestinal Emergencies.* Garden City, N.J.: Medical Examination Publishing, 1982.

Gitnick, G, and Hollander, D, eds. *Principles and Practice of Gastroenterology and Hepatology.* New York: Elsevier, 1988.

Given, B, and Simmons. *Gastroenterology in Clinical Nursing.* 4th ed. St. Louis: Mosby–Year Book, 1984.

Goldberg, K, ed. *Gastrointestinal Problems.* Nurse Review Series. Springhouse, Pa.: Springhouse Corporation, 1986.

Gordon, M. *Nursing Diagnosis: Process and Application.* New York: McGraw-Hill, 1987.

Hamilton, H, editorial director. *Procedures.* Nurse's Reference Library. Springhouse, Pa.: Intermed Communications, 1983.

Hardick, M, and Beck, M, eds. *Manual of Gastrointestinal Procedures.* 2nd ed. Rochester, N.Y.: Society of Gastroenterology Nurses and Associates, Inc., 1989.

Hersey, P, and Blanchard, K. *Management of Organizational Behavior: Utilizing Human Resources.* Englewood Cliffs, N.J.: Prentice-Hall, 1982.

Hickman, C, and Silva, M. *Creating Excellence.* New York: New American Library, 1984.

Joint Commission on Accreditation of Healthcare Organizations. *Accreditation Manual for Hospitals, 1991.* Volume I. Standards. Oakbrook Terrace, Ill.: JCAHO, 1990.

Joint Commission on Accreditation of Healthcare Organizations. *Primer on Indicator Development and Application.* Oakbrook Terrace, Ill.: JCAHO, 1990.

Katsugai, T, ed. *Endoscopic Diagnosis in Gastroenterology.* New York: Igaku-Shoin, 1982.

Kim, M, McFarland, G, and McLane, A, eds. *Classification of Nursing Diagnosis: Proceedings from the Fifth National Conference.* St. Louis: Mosby–Year Book, 1984.

Kneedler, J, ed. *CNOR Study Guide.* Denver: National Certification Board: Perioperative Nursing, 1990.

Kneedler, J, and Dodge, G. *Perioperative Patient Care: The Nursing Perspective.* 2nd ed. Boston: Blackwell Scientific Publications, Inc., 1987.

Langfitt, D. *Critical Care: Certification Preparation and Review.* Bowie, Md.: Brady Communications, 1984.

Manuel, B. *The Nursing Process Series V: Evaluation.* Modular Independent Learning Systems for the Association of Operating Room Nurses. Denver: Association of Operating Room Nurses, 1979.

Marriner, A. *Guide to Nursing Management.* St. Louis: Mosby–Year Book, 1980.

Mayo, E. "Hawthorne and the Western Electric Company." In *The Social Problems of an Industrial Civilization,* 60-76. Boston: Routledge, 1949.

McFarland, G, and McFarlane, E. *Nursing Diagnoses and Intervention: Planning for Patient Care.* St. Louis: Mosby–Year Book, 1989.

Mikels, C, Calvette, B, and Dahl, C. *Quality Assurance for the Endoscopy Department.* 2nd ed. SGNA Monograph Series. Rochester, N.Y.: Society of Gastroenterology Nurses and Associates, 1990.

Misiewicz, J, Bartram, C, Cotton, P, Mee, A, Price, A, and Thompson, R. *Atlas of Clinical Gastroenterology.* London: Gower Medical Publishing, 1985.

North American Nursing Diagnosis Association. *Taxonomy I with Official Diagnostic Categories.* St. Louis: NANDA, 1989.

*Nursing90 Drug Handbook.* Nursing90 Books. Springhouse, Pa.: Springhouse Corporation, 1990.

Polit, B, and Hunger, B. "Essentials of Nursing Research." In *Methods and Applications.* Philadelphia: J.B. Lippincott, 1985.

Ravenscroft, M, and Swan, C. *Gastrointestinal Endoscopy and Related Procedures: A Handbook for Nurses and Assistants.* Baltimore: Williams & Wilkins, 1984.

Rayhorn, N, ed. *Manual of Gastrointestinal Procedures: Pediatric Supplement.* Rochester, N.Y.: Society of Gastroenterology Nurses and Associates, 1991.

Sachar, D, Waye, J, and Lewis, B, eds. *Gastroenterology for the House Officer.* Baltimore: Williams & Wilkins, 1989.

Sacher, R, ed. *Widmann's Clinical Interpretation of Laboratory Tests.* 10th ed. Philadelphia: F.A. Davis, 1991.

Seaman, C, and Verhoniak, P. *Research Methods for Undergraduate Students in Nursing.* Norwalk, Conn.: Appleton-Century-Crofts, 1982.

Silverman, A, and Roy, C, eds. *Pediatric Clinical Gastroenterology.* 3rd ed. St. Louis: Mosby–Year Book, 1983.

Silvis, S, ed. *Therapeutic Gastrointestinal Endoscopy.* New York: Igaku-Shoin, 1985.

Sivak, M. *Gastroenterologic Endoscopy.* Philadelphia: W.B. Saunders, 1987.

Sivak, M, Jr., and Petrini, J, eds. *Gastrointestinal Endoscopy: Old Problems, New Techniques.* Gastrointestinal Series, Volume 4. New York: Praeger, 1986.

Sleisenger, M, and Fordtran, J, eds. *Gastrointestinal Disease: Pathophysiology, Diagnosis, Management.* 4th ed. Philadelphia: W.B. Saunders, 1989.

Society of Gastroenterology Nurses and Associates. *Standards for Practice.* SGNA Monograph Series. Rochester, N.Y.: SGNA, 1991.

Society of Gastroenterology Nurses and Associates, Practice and Education Committees. *Nursing Care of the Patient Receiving Conscious Sedation in the Gastrointestinal Endoscopy Setting.* Rochester, N.Y.: Society of Gastroenterology Nurses and Associates, 1991.

Sugawa, C, and Schuman, B. *Primer of Gastrointestinal Fiberoptic Endoscopy.* Boston: Little, Brown & Co., 1981.

Sullivan, E, and Decker, P. *Effective Management in Nursing.* 2nd ed. Menlo Park, Calif.: Addison-Wesley, 1988.

Taylor, F. *Scientific Management.* New York: Harper & Row, 1947.

Thomson, E. "The Surgical Patient's Rights." In *A Commitment to Caring,* 139-45. Papers presented at the Second World Conference of Operating Room Nurses, Lausanne, Switzerland, August 12-15, 1980. Denver: Association of Operating Room Nurses, 1980.

Trivits, S, ed. *Journal Reprints II.* Rochester, N.Y.: Society of Gastroenterology Nurses and Associates, 1990.

Hardick, M, and Trivitts, S, eds. SGA *Journal Reprints.* Rochester, N.Y.: Society of Gastrointestinal Assistants, 1988.

Van Ness, M, and Gurney, M, eds. *Handbook of Gastrointestinal Drug Therapy.* Boston: Little, Brown & Co., 1989.

Waltz, C, and Bausell, R. *Nursing Research: Design, Statistics and Computer Analysis.* Philadelphia: F.A. Davis, 1981.

Watson, D. *Monitoring the Patient Receiving Local Anesthesia.* Denver: Association of Operating Room Nurses, 1990.

Waye, J, Geenen, J, Fleischer, D, and Venu, R. *Techniques in Therapeutic Endoscopy.* Philadelphia: W.B. Saunders, 1987.

## JOURNAL ARTICLES AND UNPUBLISHED PAPERS

Current volumes of *Gastroenterology Nursing* (formerly SGA *Journal*), published by the Society of Gastroenterology Nurses and Associates, provide an invaluable resource. Individual articles are cited in chapter reference lists but are not reproduced in this bibliography.

Adams, J. "Emergencies in the GI Lab: The G.I.A. Role." Presented at the 14th Annual Meeting of the Society of Gastrointestinal Assistants, May 1986.

"Advice for Users on Compliance with Devices Act." *OR Manager* 7(May 1991): 1, 14-15.

Beck, M. "Percutaneous Endoscopic Gastrostomy." *Nursing89* 19 (April 1989): 76-77.

Brider, P. "Who Killed the Nursing Care Plan?" *American Journal of Nursing* 91(1991): 35-39.

Brumm, J, and Crim, B. "Biliary Lithotripsy: A Smashing Solution." *Today's OR Nurse* 12 (April 1990): 4-8.

Chen, P, Wu, C, and Liaw, Y. "Hemostatic Effect of Endoscopic Local Injection with Hypertonic Saline-Epinephrine Solution and Pure Ethanol for Digestive Tract Bleeding." *Gastrointestinal Endoscopy* 32(October 1986): 319-23.

Crass, R, and Vanderveen, T. "IV Pumps & Controllers: New Technology Stimulates Increased Sophistication." *Journal of Healthcare Material Management* 6(January 1988): 52-61.

Davis, G, et al. "Treatment of Chronic Hepatitis C with Recombinant Interferon Alfa: A Multi-Center Randomized, Controlled Trial." *New England Journal of Medicine* 321(November 30, 1989): 1501-06.

Dennison, A, Whiston, R, Rooney, S, and Morris, D. "The Management of Hemorrhoids." *American Journal of Gastroenterology* 84(May 1989): 475-81.

Eddy, M. *Hepatitis A Through E.* Paper presented at the 17th National Meeting of the Society of Gastroenterology Nurses and Associates, San Antonio, Tex., 16 May 1990.

Edel, E, Johnson, P, and Tiller, S. "Perioperative Documentation: Incorporating Nursing Diagnoses into the Intraoperative Record." *AORN Journal* 50(1989): 596-600.

Flaherty, G, and Fitzpatrick, J. "Relaxation Techniques to Increase Comfort of Postoperative Patients." *Nursing Research* 27(1978): 352-55.

Fleischer, D. "BICAP Tumor Probe Therapy for Esophageal Cancer: A Practical Guide." *Endoscopy Review* 5(March-April 1988): 2-13.

Fralic, M, Kowalski, P, and Llewellyn, F. "The Staff Nurse as a Quality Monitor." *American Journal of Nursing* 91(1991): 40-42.

Gordon, M. "Nursing Diagnosis and the Diagnostic Process." *American Journal of Nursing* 76(1976): 1296.

Graham, G. "Decontamination: A Microbiologist's Perspective"

*Journal of Healthcare Material Management* 5(January-February 1988): 36-41.

Griffith, H, Thomas, N, and Griffith, L. "MDs Bill for These Routine Nursing Tasks." *American Journal of Nursing* 91(1991): 22-27.

Harris, F. "Sometimes Pediatric Home Care Doesn't Work." *American Journal of Nursing* 88(1988): 851-54.

Huey, F. "Working Smart." *American Journal of Nursing* 86(1988): 679-84.

Intravenous Nurses Society. "Intravenous Nursing Standards of Practice." *Journal of Intravenous Nursing* Supplement (1990): S1-S98.

Jakobsen, E. "Three New Ways to Deliver Care." *American Journal of Nursing* 90(1990): 24-26.

"Johns Hopkins Nurses Earn Salaries and Pursue Autonomy in New 'Professional Practice' Units." *American Journal of Nursing* 87(1987): 713-14, 730-34.

Kessler, D, Pape, S, and Sundwall, D. "The Federal Regulation of Medical Devices." *New England Journal of Medicine* 366(August 6, 1987): 317-57.

Kirsch, M, Blue, M, Desai, R, and Sivak, M, Jr. "Intralesional Steroid Injections for Peptic Esophageal Strictures." *Gastrointestinal Endoscopy* 37(1991): 180-82.

Kitz, D, Robinson, D, Schiavone, P, Walsh, P, and Conahan, T. "Discharging Outpatients." *AORN Journal* 48(1988): 87-91.

Kleinbeck, S. "Developing Nursing Diagnoses for a Perioperative Care Plan: A Classroom Research Project." *AORN Journal* 49(1989): 1613-25.

Kneedler, Julia. "A Standard: What Is It and How to Use It." *AORN Journal* 23(March 1976): 551-54.

Labar, C. "Filling in the Blanks on Prescription Writing." *American Journal of Nursing* 86(1986): 31-33.

LaFleur, S. "Will Candela's LaserTripter Replace Conventional Gallbladder Surgery?" *Laser Medicine & Surgery News and Advances* December 1989: 14-17.

MacKenzie P, and Beresford, L. "Planning and Documentation: Addressing Patient Needs in a Day Surgery Setting." *AORN Journal* 47(1988): 526-37.

Malen, A. "Perioperative Nursing Diagnoses: What, Why, and How." *AORN Journal* 44(1986): 829-39.

Marousky, R. "The Material Safety Data Sheet: A Guide to Chemical Safety in the OR." *Today's O. R. Nurse* 13(June 1991): 6-11.

McDonald, D. "Nurses on Ethical Teams—Expanding Their Decision-Making Role." *AORN Journal* 44(1986): 83-85.

Monroe, D. "Patient Teaching for X-Ray and Other Diagnostics." *RN* 53(1990): 52-56.

Ord, B. "Communication: Care Plan Sharing." *Nursing Times* 86(1990): 40-41.

Reeder, J. "Secure the Future: A Model for an International Nursing Ethic." Keynote address to the Sixth World Conference of Operating Room Nurses in Vienna, Austria. *AORN Journal* 50(1989): 1298-1307.

Reerink, E. "Defining Quality of Care: Mission Impossible?" *Quality Assurance in Health Care* 2(1990): 197-201.

Rothrock, J. "Perioperative Nursing Research, Part I: Preoperative Psychoeducational Intervention." *AORN Journal* 49(1989): 597-619.

Rowland, G, Marks, D, and Torres, W. "The New Gallstone Destroyers and Dissolvers." *American Journal of Nursing* 89(1989): 1473-76.

Rutala, W. "APIC Guidelines for Selection and Use of Disinfectants." *American Journal of Infection Control* 18(April 1990): 99-117.

Schapiro, M. "The Gastroenterologist and the Treatment of Hemorrhoids: Is It About Time?" *American Journal of Gastroenterology* 84(May 1989): 493-95.

Stachner, G, Kiss, A, and Wiesnagrotzki, S. "Oesophageal and Gastric Motility Disorders in Patients Categorized as Having Primary Anorexia Nervosa." *Gut* 27(1986): 1120-26.

Wheeler, B. "Crisis Intervention." *AORN Journal* 47(1988): 1242-48.

Wiggins, M, and Sesin, P. "Guidelines for Administering I.V. Drugs." *Nursing90* 20(April 1990): 145-52.

Williams, M, and Brett, S. "Discharge Surveys: A Quality Assurance Method for Ambulatory Surgery." *AORN Journal* 49(1989): 1371-80.

World Health Organization Working Group. "The Principles of Quality Assurance." *Quality Assurance in Health Care* 1(1989): 79-95.

Zinberg, S, Stern, D, Furman, D, and Wittles, J. "A Personal Experience in Comparing Three Nonoperative Techniques for Treating Internal Hemorrhoids." *American Journal of Gastroenterology* 84(May 1989): 488-92.

# Index

"t" Indicates material located in table.